Biomim

and

Biomimetic Materials and Design

Biointerfacial Strategies, Tissue Engineering,
and Targeted Drug Delivery

edited by

Angela K. Dillow

3M Corporation
St. Paul, Minnesota

Anthony M. Lowman

Drexel University
Philadelphia, Pennsylvania

MARCEL DEKKER, INC.   NEW YORK · BASEL

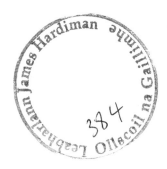

ISBN: 0-8247-0791-5

This book is printed on acid-free paper.

Headquarters
Marcel Dekker, Inc.
270 Madison Avenue, New York, NY 10016
tel: 212-696-9000; fax: 212-685-4540

Eastern Hemisphere Distribution
Marcel Dekker AG
Hutgasse 4, Postfach 812, CH-4001 Basel, Switzerland
tel: 41-61-260-6300; fax: 41-61-260-6333

World Wide Web
http://www.dekker.com

The publisher offers discounts on this book when ordered in bulk quantities. For more information, write to Special Sales/Professional Marketing at the headquarters address above.

Copyright © 2002 by Marcel Dekker, Inc. All rights reserved.
Neither this book nor any part may be reproduced or transmitted in any form or by any means, electronic, mechanical including photocopying, microfilming, and recording, or by any information storage and retrieval system, without permission in writing from the publisher.

Current printing (last digit):
10 9 8 7 6 5 4 3 2 1

PRINTED IN THE UNITED STATES OF AMERICA

Preface

Biomaterials science has evolved significantly since its birth little more than a quarter century ago. Biomaterials were originally designated to be any material that might provide structural and mechanical integrity in the body and when used in life-threatening situations. Polymers developed commercially for industrial applications were often utilized based on desirable physical properties including toughness and elasticity. Once biomaterials as a field emerged in the mid-1970s, new generations of biomaterials were designed with their medical use in mind. Biocompatibility—the ability to reside in the body without producing significant immune responses or toxicity issues—became the focus of the rational decision for materials to be used within the body. Biodegradable polymers also became (and still are) a focus of much research in the area of biomaterials science. Using biodegradable materials, the goal is to produce polymers with appropriate mechanical properties that degrade in a predictable manner in the body, leaving no toxic by-products.

We are currently in the embryonic stage of a new era of biomaterials research. Today we strive to produce biomaterials that interact with targets within the body or mimic tissue architecture. To design interactive biomaterials, or "biomimetic" materials, effectively, we look to nature to understand how cells interact with other cells, extracellular proteins, and tissue. "Biomimetic" is a term that has traditionally been applied to "hard" biomaterials, but biointerfacial scientists have adopted the terminology for "soft" biomaterials as well. Biomimetic strategies for rational design of functional, interactive biomaterials include biodegradable and "smart" materials used in targeted drug delivery applications and tissue engineering, as well as modification of biomaterials surfaces for implant or wound-healing applications.

Biomimetic materials are intended to elicit specific responses (adhesion, signaling, stimulation) in the body by incorporating peptides, nucleic acids, growth factors, cell surface receptors, or any active biomolecules as binding sites. True to the spirit of biomaterials science, engineers, materials scientists, chemists, molecular biologists, and medical professionals must work in close collaboration for successful design of effective biomimetic materials. First, the fundamental mechanisms of molecular biology must be understood. The transition from understanding a natural system to producing a synthetic biomimetic material involves a tremendous amount of research and understanding of how these fabricated materials function when compared to their natural analogs. We must understand how to incorporate the biomolecules into our biomaterial while maintaining a "natural" or recognizable binding site when placed in contact with the body. This work involves understanding how to control biomolecule activity by density, spatial arrangement, orientation, 3-dimensional configuration, presentation, and the chemical environment. Finally, this information must be combined with methods of synthesizing the biomaterial with these functional and appropriately located, oriented, and active molecules.

This book presents various strategies for successful design of biomimetic materials. Because so many areas must be researched and understood before the successful application of biomimetic materials, we have compiled the research and teachings of the leading drivers of this field of technology. The book is divided into three main parts, "Interfacial Strategies," "Tissue Engineering," and "Targeted Drug Delivery," representing three significant directions in the research. While each part contains contributions specific to a particular area, many of the chapters of this text are relevant not only to the three core areas described in this book, but also to the field of biomimetics as a whole.

In the first part of the book, "Interfacial Strategies," we examine structure–function relationships of biomimetic materials. In these chapters, experimental and theoretical strategies are explored for the rational design of new biomimetic materials. The work in this section focuses on the incorporation of active biomolecules into thin films and coatings, including self-assembled monolayers (SAMs) and Langmuir-Blodgett membranes, and evaluating their ability to elicit a particular response from a target cell or tissue. At the interface, we can closely examine how biomolecule chemistry, concentration, orientation, presentation, and density affect the activity of the biomimetic surface. This section places emphasis on the combination synthetic biomaterials with minimal peptide sequences that target specific cellular receptors to create novel "biomimetic" materials that may be used in tissue engineering and drug delivery applications.

The second part of the book focuses on biomimetic materials for use in tissue engineering. Specifically, this part includes a wide range of contributions that discuss current topics relevant to biomaterials scientists working in this area. The first focus of this section is the engineering of degradable and nondegradable polymeric scaffolds for tissue engineering. One emphasis of these contributions is strategies for continued development of synthetic and biological materials with improved properties in vivo. Included in these strategies is the use of hybrid materials consisting of synthetic and natural molecules that "signal" natural tissue in order to stimulate the desired response. A second emphasis of this part is a discussion of methods for application of biomaterials for neural tissue engineering.

The final part of the book focuses on methods for the synthesis and characterization of biomimetic materials for targeted drug delivery applications. A major emphasis is the design of "smart" biomaterials that have the ability to turn on or off depending on the physiological environment. Approaches for the design of such materials discussed here include micropatterning of biomaterials, as well as the synthesis of conjugates consisting of natural and synthetic materials. Other topics covered in this section include methods for improved drug delivery at the biomaterial/tissue interface and design of biological materials for site-specific delivery.

Angela K. Dillow
Anthony M. Lowman

Contents

Contributors

George A. Abrams, D.V.M. Department of Surgical Sciences, School of Veterinary Medicine, University of Wisconsin, Madison, Wisconsin

Thomas A. Barber, M.S. Department of Bioengineering, University of California–Berkeley, Berkeley, California

Annelise E. Barron, Ph.D. Department of Chemical Engineering, Northwestern University, Evanston, Illinois

Fiona Black, Ph.D. Illumina, Inc., San Diego, California

Paul Bornstein, M.D. Departments of Biochemistry and Medicine, University of Washington, Seattle, Washington

Benjamin A. Byers Woodruff School of Mechanical Engineering, Georgia Institute of Technology, Atlanta, Georgia

Mark E. Byrne, Ph.D. NSF Program on Therapeutic and Diagnostic Devices, Biomaterials and Drug Delivery Laboratories, Department of Biomedical Engineering, School of Chemical Engineering, Purdue University, West Lafayette, Indiana

Jean S. Campbell Department of Pathology, University of Washington, Seattle, Washington

Scott M. Cannizzaro, Ph.D. Department of Chemical Engineering, Massachusetts Institute of Technology, Cambridge, Massachusetts

Xudong Cao, Ph.D. Center for Engineering in Medicine, Harvard University, Boston, Massachusetts

Jeffrey D. Carbeck, Ph.D. Department of Chemical Engineering, Princeton University, Princeton, New Jersey

Elliot L. Chaikof, M.D., Ph.D. Department of Surgery, Emory University, Atlanta, Georgia

Charles Cheung Department of Bioengineering, University of Washington, Seattle, Washington

David M. Collard, Ph.D. School of Chemistry and Biochemistry, Georgia Institute of Technology, Atlanta, Georgia

Sarah M. Cutler Petit Institute for Bioengineering and Bioscience and GT/Emory School of Biomedical Engineering, Georgia Institute of Technology, Atlanta, Georgia

Angela K. Dillow, Ph.D. 3M Health Care, 3M Corporation, St. Paul, Minnesota

Zhongli Ding, Ph.D. Department of Bioengineering, University of Washington, Seattle, Washington

Thomas D. Dziubla Department of Chemical Engineering, Drexel University, Philadelphia, Pennsylvania

Keith M. Faucher, Ph.D. Department of Surgery, Emory University, Atlanta, Georgia

Nelson Fausto, M.D. Department of Pathology, University of Washington, Seattle, Washington

Gregg B. Fields Department of Chemistry and Biochemistry, Florida Atlantic University, Boca Raton, Florida

Nathan D. Gallant, M.E. Woodruff School of Mechanical Engineering, Georgia Institute of Technology, Atlanta, Georgia

Andrés J. García, Ph.D.   Woodruff School of Mechanical Engineering, Georgia Institute of Technology, Atlanta, Georgia

David W. Grainger, Ph.D.   Department of Chemistry, Colorado State University, Fort Collins, Colorado

Gregory M. Harbers, M.S.   Department of Bioengineering, University of California–Berkeley, Berkeley, California, and Department of Biomedical Engineering, Northwestern University, Evanston, Illinois

Kevin E. Healy, Ph.D.   Department of Bioengineering and Department of Materials Science and Engineering, University of California–Berkeley, Berkeley, California

David B. Henthorn   NSF Program on Therapeutic and Diagnostic Devices, Biomaterials and Drug Delivery Laboratories, Department of Biomedical Engineering, School of Chemical Engineering, Purdue University, West Lafayette, Indiana

Allan S. Hoffman, Sc.D.   Department of Bioengineering, University of Washington, Seattle, Washington

Yanbin Huang, Ph.D.   Biomaterials and Drug Delivery Laboratories, Department of Biomedical Engineering, School of Chemical Engineering, Purdue University, West Lafayette, Indiana

Jeffrey I. Joseph, D.O.   Department of Anesthesiology, Jefferson Medical College, Thomas Jefferson University, Philadelphia, Pennsylvania

Benjamin G. Keselowsky   W. H. Coulter Department of Biomedical Engineering, Georgia Institute of Technology, Atlanta, Georgia

Andrea L. Koenig, Ph.D.   Department of Chemistry, Colorado State University, Fort Collins, Colorado

Pamela K. Kreeger   Department of Chemical Engineering, Northwestern University, Evanston, Illinois

Themis R. Kyriakides, Ph.D.   Department of Biochemistry, University of Washington, Seattle, Washington

Chantal Lackey, Ph.D. Department of Bioengineering, University of Washington, Seattle, Washington

Robert Langer, Sc.D. Department of Chemical Engineering, Massachusetts Institute of Technology, Cambridge, Massachusetts

Anthony M. Lowman, Ph.D. Department of Chemical Engineering, Drexel University, Philadelphia, Pennsylvania

Kristyn S. Masters, Ph.D. Department of Chemical Engineering, Rice University, Houston, Texas

Howard W. T. Matthew, Ph.D. Department of Chemical Engineering and Materials Science, Wayne State University, Detroit, Michigan

Prabhas V. Moghe, Ph.D. Department of Chemical and Biochemical Engineering and Department of Biomedical Engineering, Rutgers University, Piscataway, New Jersey

Christopher J. Murphy, D.V.M., Ph.D. Department of Surgical Sciences, School of Veterinary Medicine, University of Wisconsin, Madison, Wisconsin

Niren Murthy, Ph.D. Department of Bioengineering, University of Washington, Seattle, Washington

Paul F. Nealey, Ph.D. Department of Chemical Engineering, University of Wisconsin, Madison, Wisconsin

Nicholas A. Peppas, Sc.D. NSF Program on Therapeutic and Diagnostic Devices, Biomaterials and Drug Delivery Laboratories, Department of Biomedical Engineering, School of Chemical Engineering, Purdue University, West Lafayette, Indiana

Sarah E. Ochsenhirt Department of Chemical Engineering and Materials Science, University of Minnesota, Minneapolis, Minnesota

Oliver W. Press, M.D., Ph.D. Department of Clinical Research, Fred Hutchinson Cancer Research Center, Seattle, Washington

Christine E. Schmidt, Ph.D. Department of Biomedical Engineering, University of Texas at Austin, Austin, Texas

James W. Schneider, Ph.D. Department of Chemical Engineering, Carnegie Mellon University, Pittsburgh, Pennsylvania

Jean E. Schwarzbauer, Ph.D. Department of Molecular Biology, Princeton University, Princeton, New Jersey

Lonnie D. Shea, Ph.D. Departments of Chemical Engineering and Biomedical Engineering, Northwestern University, Evanston, Illinois

Tsuyoshi Shimoboji, Ph.D. Department of Bioengineering, University of Washington, Seattle, Washington

Molly S. Shoichet, Ph.D. Departments of Chemical Engineering and Applied Chemistry, University of Toronto, Toronto, Ontario, Canada

Patrick S. Stayton, Ph.D. Department of Bioengineering, University of Washington, Seattle, Washington

Sean N. Stephansson Department of Chemical Engineering, Georgia Institute of Technology, Atlanta, Georgia

Ranee A. Stile Department of Biomedical Engineering, Northwestern University, Evanston, Illinois

Dale R. Sumner, Ph.D. Department of Anatomy, Rush Medical College, Chicago, Illinois

Xue-Long Sun, Ph.D. Department of Surgery, Emory University, Atlanta, Georgia

Ana I. Teixeira, B.S. Department of Chemical Engineering, University of Wisconsin, Madison, Wisconsin

Matthew Tirrell, Ph.D.* Department of Chemical Engineering and Materials Science, University of Minnesota, Minneapolis, Minnesota

---

* *Current affiliation*: Department of Chemical Engineering and Materials, University of California–Santa Barbara, Santa Barbara, California.

Jane S. Tjia, Ph.D. Department of Chemical and Biochemical Engineering, Rutgers University, Piscataway, New Jersey

Marc C. Torjman, Ph.D. Department of Anesthesiology, Jefferson Medical College, Thomas Jefferson University, Philadelphia, Pennsylvania

Jennifer L. West, Ph.D. Department of Bioengineering, Rice University, Houston, Texas

Jessica O. Winter, M.S. Department of Chemical Engineering, University of Texas at Austin, Austin, Texas

Cindy W. Wu Department of Chemical Engineering, Northwestern University, Evanston, Illinois

Biomimetic Materials
and Design

1

Use of Supported Thin Films of Peptide Amphiphiles as Model Systems of the Extracellular Matrix to Study the Effects of Structure–Function Phenomena on Cell Adhesion

Sarah E. Ochsenhirt and Matthew Tirrell*
University of Minnesota, Minneapolis, Minnesota

Gregg B. Fields
Florida Atlantic University, Boca Raton, Florida

Angela K. Dillow
3M Corporation, St. Paul, Minnesota

I. INTRODUCTION

The extracellular matrix (ECM) is an intricate network of multifunctional macromolecules that connect cells within a tissue and maintain the architecture of the body. Local cells secrete the polysaccharides and proteins that form the ECM. The temporal and spatial distributions of proteins in the ECM are critical for normal and pathological processes. The adhesion of cells to ECM proteins affects morphology, motility, gene expression, and survival of adherent cells (1–3). Interactions between ECM

---

*Current affiliation: University of California–Santa Barbara, Santa Barbara, California.

1

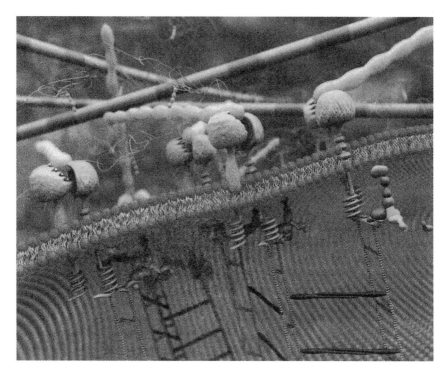

Figure 1   Integrin receptors connecting the extracellular matrix to the cellular cytoplasm.

proteins and integrin cell surface receptors also govern events such as adhesion, migration, proliferation, and metastasis.

Integrin receptors, a class of cell surface receptors, are transmembrane proteins with hydrophilic regions that extend into the ECM to provide binding sites to the ECM protein (Fig. 1). The "tail" of the integrin has a hydrophobic region that is buried in the cell's lipid bilayers and another hydrophilic region that extends into the cytoplasmic cellular domain. Binding between integrin receptors and ECM proteins (ligands) provides a means of signal transduction between the ECM and cytoplasm of the cell. The ability of the integrins to provide a mechanism for signal transduction, as well as structural integrity, makes this class of cell surface receptors critically important to our understanding of cell differentiation, growth, and regulation.

The adhesion of ECM ligands to integrin cell surface receptors is an important step in understanding the effects of a binding event on cellular behavior; accordingly, the ability to mimic ligand–receptor interactions is key to the rational development of biocompatible surfaces and therapeutic devices. The complexity of the microenvironment that modulates cell–matrix interactions makes development of a comprehensive, single-model system daunting; thus, a system capable of mimicking a specific variable(s) of this microenvironment is desirable. One approach is to immobilize peptides that mimic ECM proteins, rather than intact ECM proteins, onto an interface to render the surface bioactive. Immobilization of the ECM peptide to an interface may provide critical insight into the hierarchical control imbedded in the native extracellular protein or matrix. That control may reside in the primary amino acid sequence, secondary or tertiary orientation and conformation of the peptide, or synergistic contributions from noncontiguous domains of the ECM protein. Numerous functionalization techniques, such as surface grafting (4–13), self-assembled monolayers (14–18), and polymer–peptide hybrids (19–27), have effectively tethered single peptides to interfaces for the study of cell adhesion phenomena. While the strengths of each technique differ, each can provide unique insights about cell adhesion, signaling, and transformation events.

Assessment of subtle changes in peptide structure affecting cell signaling requires a model system that allows the control of peptide sequence, conformation, orientation, and presentation and provides the ability to systematically tether multiple ligands to an interface. The methods mentioned above meet some of these criteria but often lack the precise control of peptide orientation, density, and mobility. Our group has designed and synthesized amphiphiles with ECM-mimetic peptide headgroups that are incorporated into supported membranes using the Langmuir–Blodgett (LB) technique. The resulting bioactive membranes are ideal substrates for studying cell adhesion phenomena and for probing isolated ligand–receptor interactions. In this chapter, we demonstrate that the identity and structure as well as the controlled presentation of the ECM peptides can be modulated through lipidation (creation of "peptide amphiphiles"), multiple ECM ligands can be incorporated into the supported membrane at predetermined surface densities creating a precisely organized surface, and ligand accessibility can be controlled by molecularly engineering headgroups of membrane amphiphiles. We have created synthetic peptide amphiphiles that mimic the ECM proteins collagen and fibronectin. Characterization and interactions of these biomimetic surfaces with cells or isolated cell surface receptors will be discussed below.

II. CONSTRUCTION OF ECM-MIMETIC SURFACES

Many soluble amphiphilic molecules have been used as means to target drugs to cancer cells (28), to agglomerate circulating tumor cells (29) and prevent them from forming secondary tumors (30–32), and to deliver corrective genes to unhealthy nuclei (33); however, this discussion strictly focuses on deposited LB films of dialkyl-tailed peptide amphiphiles. Our peptide amphiphiles are made by chemically linking a hydrophilic peptide headgroup to a set of hydrocarbon tails, where the dialkyl tails are separated from the peptide by a spacer group, as shown in Fig. 2. In 1995 we reported the synthesis of peptide amphiphiles having synthetic dialkyl tails, using a highly efficient solid-phase approach (34). The dialkyl tails provide a mechanism for self-assembling of the peptide amphiphiles on hydrophobic surfaces or at the air–water interface.

The LB technique was used to create solid-supported biomimetic surfaces constructed from these peptide amphiphiles. Here the amphiphiles are spread in a monolayer onto the air–water interface of the Langmuir trough (Fig. 3). The monolayer is compressed until the molecules are assembled in a two-dimensional solid phase. The ability to vary this surface pressure (i.e., amphiphile density) gives a means of controlling the cell surface receptor's accessibility to the ligand (peptide headgroup) by changes in number, packing, and secondary conformation of the binding sequence. Once the monolayer is compressed to the desired density, a hydrophobic surface is passed vertically through the air–water interface in a downward stroke to transfer the amphiphiles onto the solid support (Fig. 3).

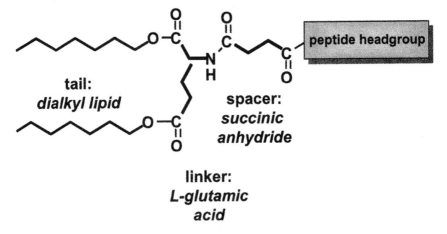

Figure 2 Chemical structure of peptide amphiphiles.

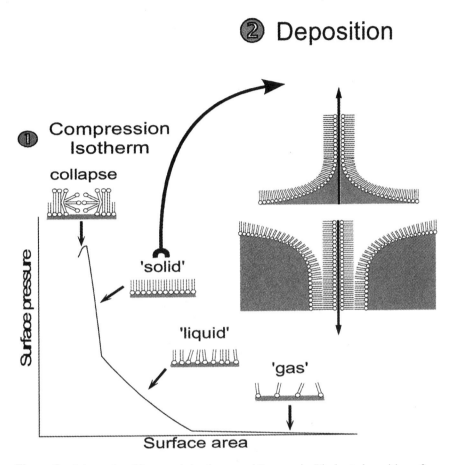

Figure 3 Schematic of Langmuir isotherm and Langmuir–Blodgett deposition of a bilayer on a solid substrate. In the first step, a monolayer of molecules is compressed to a two-dimensional solid on the air–water interface of a Langmuir trough. In the second step, a surface is passed vertically through the interface to transfer the monolayers onto a solid substrate.

III. COLLAGEN-MIMETIC PEPTIDE AMPHIPHILES

We first synthesized peptide amphiphiles composed of synthetic rather than phospholipid tails (34) in 1995. Using a solid-phase approach, novel dialkyl chain amphiphiles were coupled to a peptide derived from residues 1263– 1277 of type IV collagen. The peptide, having the sequence GVKGDKDNPDWPGAP and henceforth referred to as IV-H1, was discovered by Chelberg and coworkers (35). IV-H1 directly supports adhesion, spreading, and motility of highly metastatic K1735 M4 murine melanoma and other cell types in vitro (35). The triple helicity of the collagen domain was hypothesized to be essential to IV-H1's activity; thus, IV-H1 was an ideal candidate to study whether the conformation of a small peptide could be manipulated using our techniques and whether such structural changes would influence cellular adhesion. We used IV-H1 as a model template (Fig. 4) on which a library of adhesive collagen-like peptide amphiphiles was based.

A triple helix consists of three polypeptide chains staggered by one residue and supercoiled along a common axis in a right-handed manner (36,37). Because it is known that the Gly-X-Y motif geometrically enhances formation of the triple helix in native collagen (39), we modified the IV-H1 peptides by incorporating the helix initiator, $(GPP^*)_4$, at the N, C, or both termini of the IV-H1 peptide to determine the effect on the headgroup's ability to form triple helices. The corresponding $(GPP^*)_4$-IV-H1 hybrids were coupled to $1',3'$-didodecyl N-[O-(4-nitrophenyl)succinyl]-L-glutamate, designated as $(C_{12})_2GluC_2$-COOH, to yield IV-H1 peptide amphiphiles.

To investigate the ability of IV-H1 and peptide amphiphile head-groups to form triple helices with neighboring peptides, we employed circular dichroism (CD) to measure the ellipticity of our samples (38). The triple helix of native collagen has a positive ellipticity in the 215- to 245-nm range. While $(GPP^*)_4$ must flank both termini of the simple IV-H1 peptide to induce helix formation, lipidation of the unmodified IV-H1 peptides and the singly $(GPP^*)_4$-modified IV-H1 peptides enabled three amphiphiles to supercoil around one another to form a triple helix (38). Lipidating the IV-H1 sequence enhances triple helicity to such a degree that the $(C_{12})_2GluC_2$-$(GPP^*)_4$IV-H1 amphiphile approximates the native triple-helical sequence, $(GPP^*)_{10}$ (40), as demonstrated by the pronounced positive ellipticity in the 215- to 245-nm range that indicates polypro II helicity (Fig. 5a).

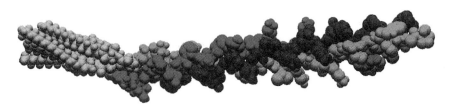

Figure 4 Computer-modeled structure of the IV-H1 peptide amphiphile. (Reproduced with permission from *JACS* 1996;118:12515–12520.)

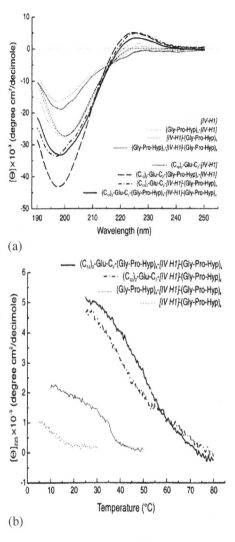

(a)

(b)

Figure 5 (a) Circular dichroism spectra of collagen-like peptides and peptide amphiphiles. Positive values of ellipticity in the λ range of 215–245 nm are attributed to an ordered, polypro II–like structure. The only peptide that shows appreciable ellipticity in this range is (GPP*)$_4$-[IV-H1]- (GPP*)$_4$; however, all peptide *amphiphiles* (except one) exhibit appreciable ellipticity in the range indicative of the formation of triple-helical structure. (b) Temperature dependence of positive molar ellipticity per amino acid residue in the wavelength range indicative of the formation of triple helices for peptides and peptide amphiphiles of IV-H1. (Reproduced with permission from *JACS* 1996;118:12515–12520.)

Heteronuclear single quantum coherence (HSQC) and inverse-detected ^{1}H-^{15}N NMR spectroscopy (41) also indicated that the peptide headgroup of the IV-H1 amphiphiles forms a continuous triple helix. The stability of the IV-H1 helix increases significantly when in the amphiphilic form, as evidenced by a 15–20° shift in the denaturation temperatures from the peptide to the peptide amphiphile (38) (Fig. 5b). Additional evidence that the amphiphilic form increases stability of the helix was provided by Fields and coworkers (42) who observed that the denaturation temperature of C_nGluC$_2$-(GPP*)$_4$IV-H1(GPP*)$_4$ amphiphiles increased by approximately 2.75 °C per tail methylene repeat.

The IV-H1 amphiphiles exhibit high degrees of triple helicity that resemble the native structure of type IV collagen; accordingly, it was of interest to determine whether LB films of IV-H1 amphiphiles would support cell adhesion, spreading, or migration similarly to native collagen. Once demonstrating that IV-H1 amphiphiles formed stable monolayers at the air–water interface using a Langmuir trough (34), a monolayer of closely packed amphiphiles was deposited on a solid support using the LB technique. Supported bioactive membranes composed of equimolar binary mixtures of $(C_{16})_2$GluC$_2$-(GPP*)$_4$IV-H1 and a PEGXXX lipid were deposited, where the molecular weight (XXX) of the PEG could be modulated to control the distance that the PEG molecules extend from the surface. PEG lipids were chosen as a diluent amphiphile because the PEG serves to minimize the occurrence of nonspecific adhesion and adsorption. A 50 mol % IV-H1 amphiphile and 50 mol % PEG120 amphiphile mixture supported M14#5 human melanoma cell adhesion and spreading (43). Similarly, mixtures of $(C_{16})_2$GluC$_2$-(GPP*)$_4$IV-H1 and $(C_{18})_2$GluC$_2$-COOCH$_3$ (44) support murine melanoma cell adhesion and spreading, with maximal cell response occurring at intermediate concentrations. In the absence of the active IV-H1 amphiphile [100% PEG-120 or $(C_{18})_2$GluC$_2$-COOCH$_3$ amphiphile], cell adhesion and spreading were eliminated. Together, these data demonstrate that IV-H1 peptide amphiphiles support specific cellular adhesion and provide model surfaces for studying targeted cell adhesion phenomena.

Cell adhesion to model surfaces depends on the accessibility of the ligand to the cell's receptor. The experiments above were taken one step further by varying the length of the PEG amphiphile headgroup (i.e., the number of repeat units of the ethylene glycol) that was to be mixed with the IV-H1 amphiphile. Recall that the molecular weight of the PEG determines its headgroup length or the distance that the PEG extends from the interface. Increasing the molecular weight (height) of the PEG headgroup allows masking (burying) of successive residues (amino acids) on the neighboring IV-H1 headgroup, as summarized in Table 1 and pictured in Fig. 6a. By covering up more and more of the amino acids in the IV-H1 peptide, the

Table 1 Summary of the Amphiphile Headgroup Lengths as Obtained from Neutron Reflectivity Data[a]

Amphiphile	Headgroup length (nm)
$(C_{16})_2$-Glu-C_2-(GPP*)$_4$-IV-H1	8.8
DSPE-PEG-120	1.6
DSPE-PEG-750	3.5
DSPE-PEG-2000	9.0
DSPE-PEG-5000	16.8

[a]The headgroup length of the peptide amphiphile refers to the Glu-C_2-(GPP*)$_4$-IV-H1 moiety. The headgroup length of the PEG lipids is the sum of the lengths of phosphate group, the ethanolamine group, and the PEG chain.

signal that tells the cells to bind should be diminished. This hypothesis was verified by cell adhesion assays. Neutron reflectivity measurements were used to determine the length of each amphiphile headgroup (Table 1) (45). From the cell adhesion assays, we found that when the length of the PEG headgroup is shorter than that of the IV-H1 headgroup (PEG-120 and PEG-750 < IV-H1), melanoma cells adhere and spread (Fig. 6b). When the lengths are approximately equal (PEG-2000 ≈ IV-H1), melanoma cells adhere but do not spread. Finally, when the length of the PEG is longer than IV-H1 (PEG-5000 > IV-H1), melanoma cells neither adhere nor spread. Length differences between amphiphile headgroups effectively modulate ligand accessibility and discriminate between cellular responses.

Griffith and coworkers demonstrated that clustering of RGD ligands significantly reduced the average ligand density required to support the migration of NR6 fibroblast cells (13). Because varying ligand organization at the nanoscale can regulate cell motility, LB films in which organization of the peptide headgroup (ligand) can be controlled may provide valuable insight into cell adhesion and migration phenomena. Our next set of experiments using the IV-H1 amphiphiles demonstrated that two-component membranes could be transformed from thermodynamically homogeneous to heterogeneous surfaces simply by changing the number of methylene groups in the tails of the respective peptide amphiphiles, as shown in Fig. 7 (45). The ability to control the phase behavior of the amphiphilic surface provides a means of controlling the "clustering" of ligands that may be required for desired cell signaling events. When the lipid tails were identical in number of hydrocarbon units and degree of saturation, the resulting two-component membrane was imaged as a homogeneous (single-phase) surface using atomic force microscopy in both contact and tapping modes. However, when the number of methylene

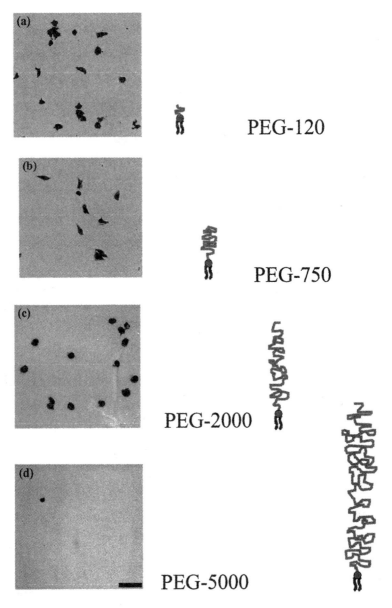

Figure 6 Relative heights of the PEGXXX amphiphiles obtained from neutron reflectivity measurements and images of M14#5 human melanoma cells after a 1-h adhesion assay on 50 mol % IV-H1 peptide amphiphile mixtures with (a) DSPE PEG-120, (b) DSPE PEG-750, (c) DSPE PEG-2000, and (d) DSPE PEG-5000 (From Ref. 43. Copyright © 2000 John Wiley & Sons, Inc.)

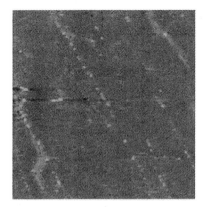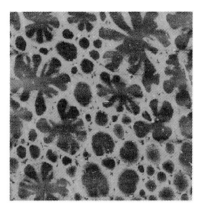

Figure 7 AFM image of 50 mol % $(C_{16})_2$-Glu-(GPP*)$_4$-IV-H1 amphiphile mixed with $(C_{16})_2$-Glu-C_2-COOCH$_3$ (left) or $(C_{18})_2$-Glu-C_2-COOCH$_3$. Changing the dialkyl tail length by two methylene groups changes the mixture from homogeneous (single phase) to heterogeneous (domain formation, phase separated) mixture.

units in one amphiphile was increased by two repeats, the membrane was imaged as heterogeneous (multiphase), having floral-shaped domains on a hexagonal lattice (45). Thus, utilizing the synthetic nature of peptide amphiphiles assembled into lipid bilayers may allow the biointerface to be tailored to a higher order than by covalently immobilizing the peptide to a surface. We believe that this methodology, where ligands are presented at an interface in a spatially and organizationally controlled manner and where ligand accessibility can be modulated, offers insights into many biomaterial–cell interface concerns; thus, a library of adhesive peptide amphiphiles was developed based on this original research using IV-H1 amphiphiles.

IV. FIBRONECTIN-MIMETIC PEPTIDE AMPHIPHILES

A. RGD Peptide Amphiphiles

The vision of mimicking an in vivo system using a mixture of peptide amphiphiles was realized with the synthesis of fibronectin-derived peptide amphiphiles in our laboratory. Several groups have attached alkyl tails to the classical adhesion motif, arginine-glycine-aspartic acid (RGD) (47). We (48) and others (49) have synthesized peptide amphiphiles based on the RGD template and characterized them using the Langmuir isotherms, while others (50,51) have synthesized RGD amphiphiles for incorporation into vesicles. Following our protocol (34), Chaikof and coworkers coupled dialkyl tails to the N terminus of GRGDSY, but used phosphatidylethanolamine to couple RGDY through the C terminus (52) and aggregated platelets using microstructures of phosphatidylethanolamine coupled to SFLLRN (49), an agonist toward the human thrombin receptor. However, no biological data were published on either of these RGD variants. Here we will discuss our research relating to biomimetic surfaces composed of RGD amphiphiles where bioactivity has been demonstrated and the effects of RGD orientation and presentation on cell signaling and integrin–receptor binding has been studied.

B. Cell Assays on RGD Peptide Amphiphiles

To investigate the effects of the orientation of linear RGD on cellular responses, we synthesized amino- and carboxy-coupled RGD amphiphiles (48), as shown in Fig. 8a. Because the RGD sequence is presented in a

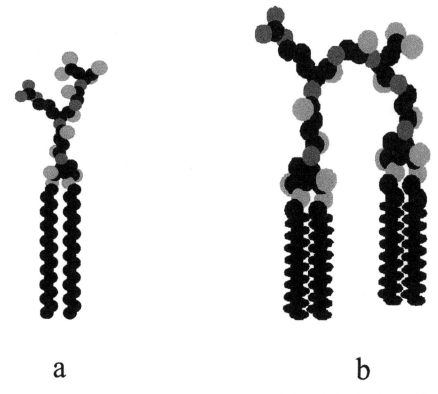

a   b

Figure 8 Schematic diagram of linear (a) and looped (b) RGD peptide amphiphiles.

conformationally constrained loop in fibronectin (47,53) and disintegrins (54), we coupled synthetic dialkyl tails to both termini of RGD using solution phase chemistries, as shown in Fig. 8b. Using the LB technique to deposit the RGD amphiphiles onto hydrophobic substrates, two conformations of the RGD peptide (linear and looped) and two orientations of the linear RGD (N and C grafted) were presented to cells. The surface density of looped RGD was adjusted by dilution using a looped RGE amphiphile, where an RGE amphiphile does not support cell adhesion (48). The N- and C-grafted linear RGD amphiphiles were diluted using a methylated amphiphile, $(C_{18})_2GluC_2\text{-}COOCH_3$.

We demonstrated that the supported monolayers of looped RGD support adhesion and spreading of M14#5 human melanoma cells and RHE-1A rat heart endothelial cells in a dose-dependent and specific manner (48). An equimolar mixture of looped RGD and looped RGE yielded the highest degree of cell spreading (Fig. 9a). Control surfaces of 100% looped RGE surfaces resulted in minimal cell adhesion and spreading (Fig. 9b). Inhibition assays using integrin-blocking antibodies identified $\alpha_3\beta_1$ as the primary receptor-mediating melanoma cell adhesion to the looped RGD construct. Cells did not spread on monolayers containing the amino-coupled RGD amphiphiles, whereas cells spread in a nonspecific manner on monolayers of the carboxy-coupled RGD amphiphiles. In both linear

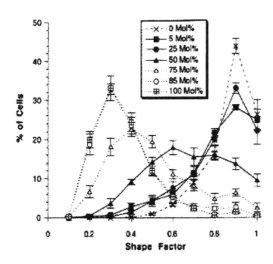

Figure 9a Spreading of M14#5 human melanoma cells (spreading increases as the shape factor gets smaller) on mixtures of looped RGD and RGE peptide amphiphiles.

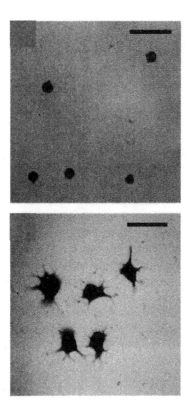

Figure 9b   Video-enhanced images of M14#5 human melanoma cells on surfaces of the looped RGE peptide amphiphile (top) or the looped RGD amphiphile (bottom). (From Ref. 48. Reproduced with permission from © 1999 Elsevier Science Ltd.)

RGD amphiphiles, the terminal amino acid in the respective monolayers contained an active side chain. In the amino-coupled RGD amphiphiles, the terminal group was aspartic acid; thus, the acidic side chain may have inhibited cell adhesion through electrostratic repulsion. In the case of carboxy-coupled RGD, the terminal arginine may have supported nonspecific adhesion through hydrophobic interactions between the terminal and ε-amino groups. In summary, a looped conformation of RGD specifically engaged cells, but the linear peptide amhiphiles were incapable of supporting specific cell–substrate interactions.

Conceptually similar amphiphiles were synthesized by Oku et al. (50). They coupled RGDS through the amino terminus to monoalkyl chains and through the carboxy terminus to natural and synthetic dialkyl tails. The bioactivity of the RGDS amphiphiles was evaluated by incorporating them into vesicles and evaluating the ability of the vesicles to inhibit lung metastases. An additional amphiphile that they synthesized using solution phase chemistry coupled monoalkyl tails to both termini of RGDS; however, this looped construct was ineffective at inhibiting tumor colonization of murine lungs. A hypothesis to explain the inactivity of the looped presentation could be that the loop, consisting of only four amino acids, may have been too tight to allow both tails to insert into the vesicle bilayer. The activity of the RGD amphiphiles synthesized by our group (48) and Oku et al. (50) differ, yet may be indicative of the subtle influence that immobilization methods have on peptide activity. While both groups used similar peptide head groups (RGD and RGDS, respectively), the hydrocarbon tails differed, as did the crystallinity of the amphiphilic bilayer (solid-like regime in the deposited LB film versus fluid-like regime in the liposome). These observations are a reflection of a global concern in the field of peptide-functionalized surfaces—namely, that the bioactivity of a peptide is affected not only by its presentation at an interface but by how it is tethered to that interface.

C. GRGDSP Peptide Amphiphiles

Beer et al. demonstrated that integrin engagement results from an optimal separation distance between the surface and the immobilized RGD peptide (i.e., distance that the peptide extends from its tethered surface) (55). Our subsequent research took into account this variable to aid in the design of additional RGD peptide amphiphiles that could probe further the effect of RGD conformation and presentation on cellular responses. A longer peptide sequence was used to increase the separation distance between the RGD peptide and the supported bilayer. We synthesized a second generation of "RGD" amphiphiles, this time incorporating the decamer KAbu**GRGDSP**AbuK, where GRGDSP is derived from the type III_{10} repeat of human fibronectin (47,57). These amphiphiles were synthesized by modifying our protocol (34) to attach dialkyl tails to the N-α-amine of the N-terminal lysine, yielding a linear structure similar to that in Fig. 10a, and to attach dialkyl tails to both the N-α-amine of the N-terminal lysine and the N-ε-amine of the C-terminal lysine, yielding the looped peptide shown in Fig. 10b. The aminobutyric residues (Abu) were inserted to hold the place for cysteine residues, which once incorporated would form cyclic RGD peptide amphiphiles.

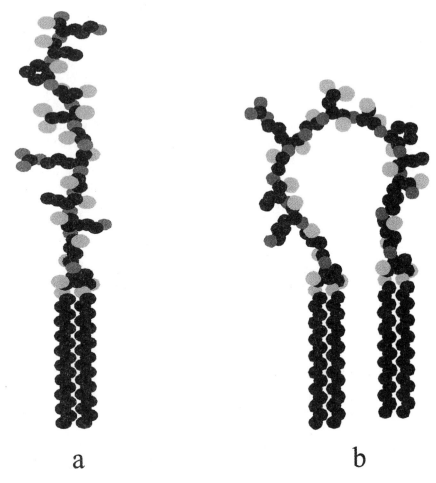

a   b

Figure 10 Schematic of the linear GRGDSP (a) and looped GRGDSP (b) peptide amphiphiles.

D. Cell Assays on GRGDSP Amphiphiles

Whereas the N- and C-coupled tripeptide RGD amphiphiles used above (48) did not support specific cell adhesion, LB films of linear and looped GRGDSP amphiphiles mediated human umbilical vein endothelial cell (HUVEC) adhesion and spreading in a dose-dependent and specific manner.

Mixing the selected GRGDSP amphiphiles with a polyethylene glycol 120 (PEG-120) amphiphile controlled peptide surface density. A monolayer of pure PEG-120 served as a negative control as even three repeats of PEG are sufficient to inhibit protein adsorption to a surface (58). Scrambled GRGDSP peptide amphiphiles were synthesized and incorporated into LB films. These scrambled amphiphiles did not support HUVEC adhesion, confirming the specificity of the cellular adhesion to the original GRGDSP peptides.

While cell adhesion and spreading are two of the most common means to assess the bioactivity of a biomimetic surface, these can be gross measurements of subtle signals transmitted from the RGD–integrin interaction to the cell cytoplasm. Integrin-blocking inhibition assays demonstrated that while LB films of the linear GRGDSP amphiphile engaged $\alpha_v\beta_3$ and the β_1 subunit, LB films of the looped GRGDSP amphiphiles preferentially engaged $\alpha_v\beta_3$. Collectively, the adhesion assays of the RGD tripeptides and the GRGDSP decamers (48) demonstrate that peptide sequence and presentation influences receptor engagement, which makes peptide amphiphiles an effective tool to target specific cell surface receptors.

Engagement of the $\alpha_v\beta_3$ integrin by GRGDSP amphiphiles was not surprising since $\alpha_v\beta_3$ exhibits a higher tolerance for RGD peptide heterogeneity than other integrins (59); yet this served as an inspiration for engineering a different integrin preference into the LB film using multiple peptide amphiphiles. The RGD peptide from the III_{10} repeat of fibronectin and the synergy peptide, PHSRN, from the III_9 repeat preferentially engage the classic fibronectin integrin, $\alpha_5\beta_1$ (60). Accordingly, we synthesized N-coupled PHSRN peptide amphiphiles, mixed GRGDSP and PHSRN amphiphiles in a native 1:1 molar ratio, and diluted the mixture using inert PEG-120 amphiphiles. Using deposited LB films, no change in integrin engagement for adhesion was noted at surface concentrations of 10 mol % GRGDSP/10 mol % PHSRN/80 mol % PEG-120 amphiphiles, regardless of whether the linear or looped GRGDSP amphiphiles were used. (As each dialkyl tail occupies about 40 Å^2, the surface density of total ligands is about 400 pmol/cm^2.) However, HUVEC spreading significantly increases when PHSRN was incorporated into GRGDSP/PEG deposited monolayers, which echoes the observations of Yamada and coworkers (60). A surface coverage of 50 mol % peptide amphiphiles—whether that was 50 mol % linear GRGDSP or 25 mol % GRGDSP/25 mol % PHSRN—yielded maximal spreading. These results demonstrated that LB films composed of multiple peptide amphiphiles mimic the noncontiguous signals presented by the microenvironment of a cell.

E. JKR Measurements of Adhesion Between GRGDSP/
PHSRN Amphiphiles and $\alpha_5\beta_1$ Integrins

The success of bioactive LB films in modulating the adhesion and spreading of intact cells suggested that these biomimetic films were ideal for the study of isolated ligand–receptor interactions. To measure the adhesion between our fibronectin-mimetic surfaces and individual integrin receptors, we used a classic contact mechanical approach, the JKR (Johnson, Kendall, and Roberts) method (61), to measure adhesion (62). In the modified JKR apparatus, two opposing surfaces are brought into contact in an aqueous environment under an applied load. The contact area formed between the two surfaces is measured as a function of the normal load, as shown in Fig. 11a. An energy balance is used to calculate the adhesion energy (G) as a function of the normal load, contact area, radius of curvature, and elastic moduli of the surfaces. Differences in the measured adhesion as the surfaces are brought together (advancing) and then pulled apart (receding) provide information about adhesion resulting from the interaction between the integrin and ligand(s) surfaces. Detailed explanation of the apparatus, measurements, and analysis of the JKR method can be found in the literature (63–65).

The effectiveness of the peptide (GRGDSP/PHSRN/PEG) amphiphile surfaces to mimic native fibronectin was evaluated by their ability to adhere to purified, activated $\alpha_5\beta_1$ integrin receptors that were immobilized on an opposing surface (Fig. 11b). Activity of immobilized integrins was verified by the measured concentration-dependent binding to fibronectin using enzyme-linked immunosorbent assay (ELISA). The effects of surface amphiphile composition, density, fluidity, and peptide conformation on adhesion to activated integrins were determined. For two-component systems of linear GRGDSP and PEG amphiphiles, maximal adhesion occurred at intermediate compositions. Dilution using the PEG amphiphile may have enhanced the accessibility of the GRGDSP ligand because the relative lengths of the two headgroups are approximately 3:1 (from unpublished neutron reflectivity data), which could allow the peptide to expose its binding site by folding over the shorter PEG brush (Fig. 12).

When an equimolar concentration of GRGDSP and PHSRN amphiphiles is diluted with PEG amphiphiles, maximal adhesion occurs at intermediate concentrations, again demonstrating that a balance between the number of binding sites and the accessibility of receptor to the binding site is required. The presence of the synergy site (PHSRN) greatly enhances the adhesion between $\alpha_5\beta_1$ and the biomimetic LB surfaces (Fig. 13). Adhesion of mixtures of GRGDSP/PHSRN and PEG amphiphiles to the integrin surface exceeds that of a similar two-component mixture of

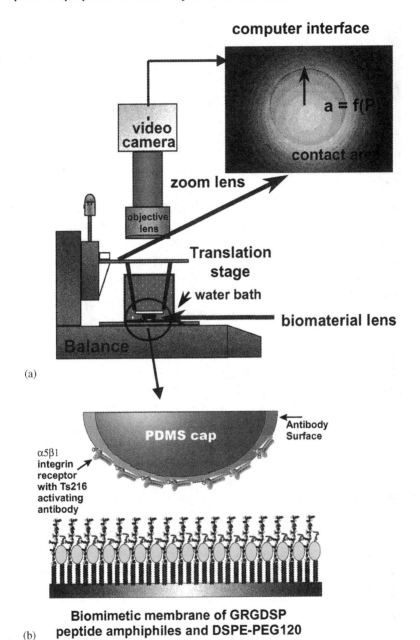

(a)

(b)

Figure 11 (a) Schematic diagram of JKR apparatus and (b) biomimetic bilayers in contact with integrin-immobilized lens.

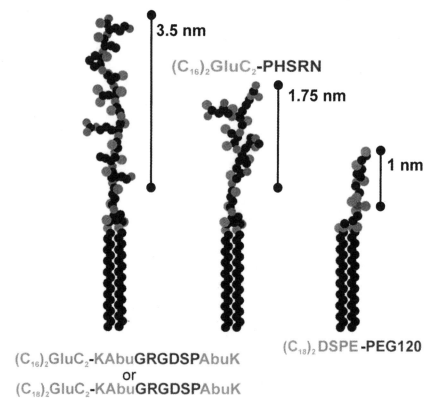

Figure 12 Schematic diagram and relative lengths of the linear GRGDSP, PHSRN, and PEG-120 amphiphiles.

GRGDSP and PEG. An increase in the temperature of the amphiphile surface also resulted in significant increases in adhesion at lower amphiphile concentrations in both the two- and three-component systems. Here we hypothesize that at lower peptide concentration and elevated temperature, the appropriate ligands can readily move about the surface to present themselves optimally to the integrin receptor. This provided additional evidence that accessibility of the ligand to the cell surface receptor is paramount for good adhesion.

Use of the modified JKR approach provided strong evidence for the inclusion of multiple ligands in the design of biomimetic materials. Clearly

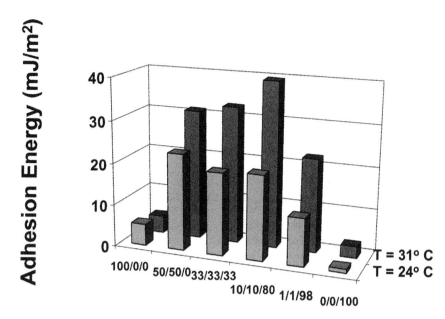

mol % RGD / PHSRN / PEG-120

Figure 13 Summary of average adhesion energy (G) for unloading of $\alpha_5\beta_1$ immobilized surfaces in contact with biomimetic surfaces constructed from mixtures of GRGDSP and PHSRN peptide amphiphiles with DSPE-PEG-120. All surfaces were deposited at 41 mN/m^2 and measurements were made in 1 mmol Mn^{2+}, pH = 6, and $T = 24\,°C$ or $31\,°C$.

multiple ligands create more authentic biomaterials, yet techniques such as the modified JKR technique are necessary to quantify how manipulating the microenvironment of the cell impacts cellular responses.

Recent work extending this type of force measurement to small contact areas and a few intermolecular interactions using atomic force microscopy (AFM) is in progress. The AFM and JKR experiments provide means to quantify interactions that have been impossible to isolate using classical techniques in molecular biology and encompass innovative methods that can be used to quantify biomimetic materials interactions with their desired targets.

F. Conclusions for Fibronectin Mimetic Materials

In the cell adhesion assays, JKR measurements, and AFM force curves, maximal interactions were observed at less than maximal surface densities of GRGDSP amphiphiles. This observation may relate to the native microenvironment of a cell. In fibronectin, an unusually small rotation between the ninth and tenth type III repeats places the PHSRN and RGD binding sites on same face of the fibronectin fragment, having a separation of only 30–40 Å (53). The average peptide amphiphile occupies about 40 Å^2 per dialkyl tail, which if a cylindrical model is used yields a diameter of 8 Å. To mimic the spacing within the fibronectin binding pocket (40 Å), four PEG-120 amphiphiles would need to separate a GRGDSP and PHSRN amphiphile. This surface organization corresponds to molar percentages of 17% GRGDSP/17% PHSRN/66% PEG-120. The simplistic, theoretical mixture is similar to the solution compositions at which maximal interactions were observed in the various techniques, which adds support to the hypothesis that mimicking the cellular microenvironment optimizes cellular adhesion.

G. Summary

Collectively, peptide amphiphiles are effective means to study fundamental aspects of cell–matrix interactions because model surfaces and interfaces can be constructed using these synthetic bioactive molecules. Using the LB technique, monolayers of amphiphiles can be deposited onto solid substrates, where the composition of ligands at the interface is easily controlled and modified. The LB-supported films have been used in cell adhesion assays and form the basis for new devices to measure biological phenomena. In summary, collagen-derived peptide amphiphiles demonstrated that lipidation induces formation of a bioactive triple helix, whereas fibronectin-derived peptide amphiphiles demonstrated that peptide sequence and presentation influence receptor engagement and multiple amphiphiles act synergistically to influence cell signaling. The bioactivity of each peptide can be sequentially masked using PEG amphiphiles, which provides a means to discriminate between peptide functions. Finally, new and modified techniques using biomimetic films of oriented peptide amphiphiles provide insights into fundamental ligand–receptor interactions.

Any peptide or nucleic acid sequence identified by biologists can be attached to lipid tails in order to characterize and modulate its three-dimensional structure, aggregation state, interaction with other proteins such as receptors, contribution to the microenvironment of the cell, and relationship to cell signaling. Such discoveries are possible because amphiphiles allow strict control over the number of components in the system, the surface density and accessibility of each ligand, the orientation and conformation of the immobilized peptide, and inducement of native and potentially novel secondary structures within the peptide headgroups. Control of secondary structure and accessibility are important for creating functional and efficacious drug delivery vehicles, of which vesicles are a leading technology. Peptide amphiphiles can be seamlessly incorporated into liposomes as a means of targeting the vehicle to a specific cell type or organ; thus, while cell–matrix interactions continue to be explored using deposited LB films, new research avenues continue to emerge for the development of intelligent biomaterials for use in both the drug delivery and tissue regeneration/replacement fields.

ACKNOWLEDGMENTS

This work was supported by the MRSEC Program of the National Science Foundation under Award No. DMR-98-09364 at the University of Minnesota and Award No. DMR00-80034 at UCSB, and by the National Institutes of Health Grant HL 62427-01.

REFERENCES

1. RO Hynes. Integrins: versatility, modulation, and signaling in cell adhesion. Cell 69:11–25, 1992.
2. E Ruoslahti, JC Reed. Anchorage dependence, integrins and apoptosis. Cell 77:477–478, 1994.
3. P Huhtala, MJ Humphries, JB McCarthy, PM Tremble, Z Werb, CH Damsky. Cooperative signaling by $\alpha_5\beta_1$ and $\alpha_4\beta_1$ integrins regulates metalloproteinase gene expression in fibroblasts adhering to fibroblasts. J Cell Biol 129:867–879, 1995.
4. H Bayley. Self-assembling biomolecular materials in medicine. J Cell Biochem 56(2):168–170, 1994.
5. SP Massia, JA Hubbell. Covalent surface immobilization of Arg-Gly-Asp- and Tyr-Ile-Gly-Ser-Arg-containing peptides to obtain well-defined cell-adhesive substrates. Anal Biochem 187(2):292–301, 1990.
6. SP Massia, JA Hubbell. An RGD spacing of 440 nm is sufficient for integrin $\alpha_v\beta_3$-mediated fibroblast spreading and 140 nm for focal contact and stress fiber formation. J Cell Biol 114(5):1089–1100, 1991.
7. T Matsuda, T Sugawara. Photochemical surface derivatization of a peptide containing Arg-Gly-Asp (RGD). J Biomed Mater Res 29(9):1047–1052, 1995.

8. Y Xiao, GA Truskey. Effect of receptor-ligand affinity on the strength of endothelial cell adhesion. Biophys J 71(5):2869–2884, 1996.

9. KC Olbrich, TT Andersen, FA Blumenstock, R Bizios. Surfaces modified with covalently-immobilized adhesive peptides affect fibroblast population motility. Biomaterials 17(8):759–764, 1996.

10. A Renzania, CH Thomas, AB Branger, CM Waters, KE Healy. The detachment strength and morphology of bone cells contacting materials modified with a peptide sequence found within bone sialoprotein. J Biomed Mater Res 37(1):9–19, 1997.

11. YW Tong, MS Shoichet. Peptide surface modification of poly(tetrafluoroethylene-co-hexafluoropropylene) enhances its interaction with central nervous system neurons. J Biomed Mater Res 42(1):85–95, 1998.

12. KC Dee, TT Anderson, R Bizios. Osteoblast population migration characteristics on substrates modified with immobilized adhesive peptides. Biomaterials 20(3):221–227, 1999.

13. G Maheshwari, G Brown, DA Lauffenburger, A Wells, LG Griffith. Cell adhesion and motility depend on nanoscale RGD clustering. J Cell Sci 113(10):1677–1686, 2000.

14. M Mrksich, GM Whitesides. Using self-assembled monolayers to understand the interactions of man-made surfaces with proteins and cells. Annual Rev Biophys Biomol Struct 25:55–78, 1996.

15. ME McGovern, KMR Kallury, M Thompson. Role of solvent on the silanization of glass with octadecyltrichlorosilane. Langmuir 10:3607–3614, 1994.

16. AS Blawas, WM Reichert. Protein patterning. Biomaterials 19(7–9):595–609, 1998.

17. Y Ito. Surface micropatterning to regulate cell functions. Biomaterials. 20:2333–2342, 1999.

18. LA Kung, L Kam, JA Hovis, SG Boxer. Patterning hybrid surfaces of proteins and supported lipid bilayers. Langmuir 16:6773–6776, 2000.

19. HB Lin, ZC Zhao, C Garcia-Echeverria, DH Rich, SL Cooper. Synthesis of a novel polyurethane co-polymer containing covalently attached RGD peptide. J Biomater Sci Polym Ed 3(3):217–227, 1992.

20. DA Barrera, E Zylstra, PT Lansbury, R Langer. Synthesis and RGD peptide modification of a new biodegradable copolymer: Poly(lactic acid-co-lysine). J Am Chem Soc 115:11010–11011, 1993.

21. JS Hrkach, J Ou, N Lotan, R Langer. Synthesis of poly(L-lactic acid-co-L-lysine) graft copolymers. Macromolecules 28(13):4736–4739, 1995.

22. PD Drumheller, JA Hubbell. Polymer networks with grafted cell adhesion peptides for highly biospecific cell adhesive substrates. Anal Biochem 222(2):380–388, 1994.

23. DL Hern, JA Hubbell. Incorporation of adhesion peptides into nonadhesive hydrogels useful for tissue resurfacing. J Biomed Mater Res 39(2):266–276, 1998.

24. DW Urry, A Pattanaik, J Xu, TC Woods, DT McPherson, TM Parker. Elastic protein-based polymers in soft tissue augmentation and generation. J Biomat Sci Polym Ed 9(10):1015–1048, 1998.

25. WJ Kao. Evaluation of protein-modulated macrophage behavior on biomaterials: designing biomimetic materials for cellular engineering. Biomaterials 20(23–24):2213–2221, 1999.

26. SE Sakiyama, JC Schense, JA Hubbell. Incorporation of heparin-binding peptides into fibrin gels enhances neurite extension: an example of designer matrices in tissue engineering. FASEB J 13(15):2214–22124, 1999.

27. JC Schense, JA Hubbell. Three-dimensional migration of neuritis is mediated by adhesion site density and affinity. J Biol Chem 275(100):6813–6818.

28. RJ Tressler, PN Belloni, GL Nicolson. Correlation of inhibition of adhesion of large cell lymphoma and hepatic sinusoidal endothelia cells by RGD-containing peptide polymers with metastatic potential: role of integrin-dependent and -independent adhesion mechanisms. Cancer Commun 1(1):55–63, 1989.

29. W Dai, J Belt, WM Saltzman. Cell-binding peptides conjugated to poly(-ethylene glycol) promote cell aggregation. Biotechnology (NY) 12(8):797–801, 1994.

30. K Kawasaki, M Namikawa, Y Yamashiro, Y Iwai, T Hama, Y Tsutsumi, S Yamamoto, S Nakagawa, T Mayumi. Amino acids and peptides. XXV. Preparation of fibronectin-related peptide poly(ethylene glycol) hybrids and their inhibitory effect on experimental metastasis. Chem Pharm Bull (Tokyo) 43(12):133–138, 1995.

31. M Maeda, K Kawasaki, T Mayumi, M Takahashi, H Kaneto. Amino acids and peptides. XXII. Preparation and antinociceptive effect of [D-Ala2]Leu-enkephalin-poly(ethylene glycol) hybrid. Biol Pharm Bull 17(6):823–825, 1994.

32. I Saiki. Antiadhesion peptides in the prevention of tumour metastasis. Clin Immunother 1(4):307–318, 1994.

33. S Hart. Use of adhesion molecules for gene delivery. Exp Nephrol 7(2):193–199, 1999.

34. P Berndt, GB Fields, M Tirrell. Synthetic lipidation of peptides and amino acids—monolayer structure and properties. J Am Chem Soc 117(37):9515–9522, 1995.

35. MB Chelber, JB McCarthy, AP Skubitz, LT Furcht, EC Tsilibary. Characterization of a synthetic peptide from type IV collagen that promotes melanoma cell adhesion, spreading, and motility. J Cell Biol 111(1):261–270, 1990.

36. GN Ramachandran. Stereochemistry of collagen. Int J Peptide Protein Res 31(1):1–16, 1988.

37. B Brodsky, NK Shah. Protein motifs. 8. The triple-helixmotif in proteins. FASEB J 9(15):1537–1546, 1995.

38. YC Yu, P Berndt, M Tirrell, GB Fields. Self-assembling amphiphiles for construction of protein molecular architecture. J Am Chem Soc 118(50):12515–12520, 1996.

39. B Alberts, D Bray, J Lewis, M Raff, K Roberts, JD Watson. Molecular Biology of the Cell, 3rd ed. New York: London: Garland Publishing, 1994.

40. B Brodsky, MH Li, CG Long, J Apigo, J Baum. NMR and CD studies of triple-helical peptides. Biopolymers 32(4):447–451, 1992.

41. YC Yu, V Roontga, VA Daragan, KH Mayo, M Tirrell, GB Fields. Structure and dynamics of peptide-amphiphiles incorporating triple-helical proteinlike molecular architecture. Biochemistry 38(5):1659–1668, 1999.

42. GB Fields, JL Lauer, Y Dori, P Forns, YC Yu, M Tirrell. Proteinlike molecular architecture: biomaterial applications for inducing cellular receptor binding and signal transduction. Bipolymers 47:143–151, 1998.

43. Y Dori, H Bianco-Peled, SK Satija, GB Fields, JB McCarthy, M Tirrell. Ligand accessibility as means to control cell response to bioactive bilayers membranes. J Biomed Mater Res 50(1):75–81, 2000.

44. YC Yu, T Pakalns, Y Dori, JB McCarthy, M Tirrell, GB Fields. Construction of biologically active protein molecular architecture using self-assembling peptide-amphihphiles. Methods Enzym 289:571–587, 1997.

45. Y Dori. Characterization and cell adhesion properties of supported bioactive Langmuir-Blodgett bilayer membranes. PhD dissertation, University of Minnesota, Minneapolis, 1999.

46. SP Palecek, JC Loftus, MH Ginsberg, DA Lauffenburger, AF Horwitz. Integrin-ligand binding properties govern cell migration speed through cell-substratum adhesiveness [published erratum appears in Nature 388(6638):210, 1997] Nature 385(6616):537–540, 1997.

47. MD Pierschbacher, E Ruoslahti. Cell attachment activity of fibronectin can be duplicated by small synthetic fragments of the molecule. Nature 309(5963):30–33, 1984.

48. T Pakalns, KL Haverstick, GB Fields, JB McCarthy, DL Mooradian, M Tirrell. Cellular recognition of synthetic peptide amphiphiles in self-assembled monolayer films. Biomaterials 20:2265–2276, 1999.

49. TM Winger, PJ Ludovice, EL Chaikof. Lipopeptide conjugates: biomolecular building blocks for receptor activating membrane-mimetic structures. Biomaterials 17(4):437–441, 1996.

50. N Oku, C Koike, Y Tokudome, S Okada, N Nishidawa, H Tsukada, M Kiso, A Hasegawa, H Fujii, J Murata, I Saiki. Application of liposomes for cancer metastasis. Adv Drug Del Rev 24(2-3):215–223, 1997.

51. B Hu, D Finsinger, K Peter, Z Guttenberg, M Barmann, H Kessler, A Escherich, L Moroder, J Bohm W Baumeister, SF Sui, E Sackmann. Intervesicle cross-linking with integrin $\alpha_{IIb}\beta_3$ and cyclic-RGD-lipopeptide. A model of cell-adhesion processes. Biochem 39(40):12284–12294, 2000.

52. TM Winger, EL Chaikof. Behavior of lipid-modified peptides in membrane-mimetic monolayers at the air/water interface. Langmuir 13(12):3256–3259, 1997.

53. DJ Leahy, I Aukhil, HP Erickson. 2.0 A crystal structure of a four-domain segment of human fibronectin encompassing the RGD loop and synergy region. Cell 84(1):155–164, 1996.

54. C Marcinkiewicz, S Vijay-Kumar, MA McLane, S Niewiarowski. Significance of RGD loop and C-terminal domain of echistatin for recognition of $\alpha_{IIb}\beta_3$ and $\alpha_v\beta_3$ integrins and expression of ligand-induced binding site. Blood 90(4):1565–1575, 1997.

55. JH Beer, KT Springer, BS Coller. Immobilized Arg-Gly-Asp (RGD) peptides of varying lengths as structural probes of the platelet glycoprotein IIb/IIIA receptor. Blood 79(1):117–128, 1992.
56. N Patel, R Bhandari, KM Shakesheff, SM Cannizzaro, MC Davies, R Langer, CJ Roberts, SJ Tendler, PM Williams. Printing patterns of biospecifically-adsorbed protein. J Biomater Sci Polym Ed 11(3):319–331, 2000.
57. A Hautanen, J Gailit, DM Mann, E Ruoslahti. Effects of modifications of the RGD sequence and its context on recognition by the fibronectin receptor. J Biol Chem 264(3):1437–1442, 1989.
58. M Mrksich, CS Chen, Y Xia, LE Dike, DE Ingber, GM Whitesides. Controlling cell attachment on contoured surfaces with self-assembled monolayers of alkanethiolates on gold. Proc Natl Acad Sci 93(20):10775–10778, 1996.
59. JM Healy, O Murayama, T Maeda, K Yoshino, K Sekiguchi, M Kikuchi. Peptide ligands for integrin $\alpha_v\beta_3$ selected from random phage display libraries. Biochemistry 34(12):3948–3955, 1995.
60. S Aota, M Nomizu, KM Yamada. The short amino acid sequence Pro-His-Ser-Arg-Asn in human fibronectin enhances cell-adhesive function. J Biol Chem 269(40):24756–24761, 1994.
61. KL Johnson, K Kendall, AD Roberts. Surface energy and the contact of elastic solids. Proc R Soc London Ser A A324:301–313, 1971.
62. AK Dillow, SE Ochsenhirt, GB Fields, JB McCarthy, M Tirrell. Adhesion of $\alpha_5\beta_1$ receptors to biomimetic substrates constructed from peptide amphiphiles. Biomaterials 22:1493–1505, 2001.
63. VS Mangipudi, M Tirrell. Contact-mechanics-based studies of adhesion between polymers. Rubber Chem Technol 71:407–448, 1998.
64. MK Chaudhury, GM Whitesides. Direct measurement of interfacial interactions between semispherical lenses and flat sheets of poly(dimethylsiloxane) and their chemical derivatives. Langmuir 7:1013–1025, 1991.
65. DA Hammer, M Tirrell. Biological adhesion at interfaces. Annu Rev Mater Sci 26:651–691, 1996.
66. Personal communication.

2

Engineering of Integrin-Specific Biomimetic Surfaces to Control Cell Adhesion and Function

Andrés J. García, David M. Collard, Benjamin G. Keselowsky, Sarah M. Cutler, Nathan D. Gallant, Benjamin A. Byers, and Sean N. Stephansson
Georgia Institute of Technology, Atlanta, Georgia

I. INTRODUCTION

Cell adhesion to extracellular matrices (ECMs) through integrin receptors plays a central role in numerous physiological and pathological processes. Moreover, cell attachment to proteins adsorbed onto material surfaces is important to many biomedical and biotechnological applications. In addition to anchoring cells, integrin binding triggers signals that direct cell proliferation and differentiation. In this chapter, we describe a recently developed experimental framework to analyze integrin binding to the ECM protein fibronectin (FN) in terms of binding strength, affinity, and intracellular signaling. Based on the insights obtained from these quantitative analyses, we present two biomolecular strategies for the engineering of surfaces to control integrin binding and cell adhesion in order to direct cell function. The first approach focuses on surfaces presenting well-defined chemistries to control the conformation of adsorbed FN to modulate integrin binding, focal adhesion formation, and gene expression. In a second approach, we have engineered nonadhesive surfaces presenting well-defined ligand densities of recombinant FN fragments to promote the binding of specific integrin receptors. Micropatterning of these surfaces provides control over cell spreading and focal adhesion formation.

These surface engineering strategies to control integrin binding and cell function are relevant to basic science studies as well as biomedical and biotechnological applications.

II.   CELL ADHESION TO EXTRACELLULAR MATRICES

A.   Significance of Cell Adhesion to Biotechnological and Biomedical Applications

Cell adhesion to ECM proteins is essential to development, organogenesis, wound healing, and tissue homeostasis. In addition to anchoring cells, supporting cell migration, and providing tissue structure, adhesion activates signaling pathways that regulate survival, proliferation, and differentiation in a variety of cellular systems (1–5). Many pathological conditions, including blood clotting defects and tumor invasion and metastasis, involve abnormal adhesion processes (6).

Cell adhesion considerations are also critical to numerous biomedical and biotechnological applications (7–9). Adhesion to proteins adsorbed onto material surfaces is particularly important to host–implant interactions in biomaterial and tissue engineering applications. Immediately upon contacting physiological fluids, many proteins, including albumin, immunoglobulins, fibrinogen, and FN, adsorb onto implant surfaces and modulate subsequent inflammatory responses (10–12). For instance, FN interacts with fibrin and activated platelets in clot formation and mediates the attachment and activation of neutrophils, macrophages, and other inflammatory cells. Cell–ECM interactions also have a central role in clot retraction, matrix contraction, and wound healing (13). For in vitro applications, such as tissue-engineered constructs, bioreactors, and cell culture supports, adhesion to proteins absorbed from serum-containing media or deposited by the cells themselves provides mechanical coupling to the underlying substrate and activates signaling pathways that control cell migration, proliferation, and differentiation (14).

Development of bioactive surfaces to direct cell function is central to biomaterials and tissue engineering scaffolds for enhanced repair. For instance, engineering of surfaces to promote bone cell differentiation and matrix mineralization is important to the osseointegration of orthopedic and dental implants and bone grafting scaffolds [more than 1.5 million procedures per year in the United States (15)]. In addition, the ability of bioactive surfaces to promote expression of differentiated phenotypes in vitro is critical to basic studies focusing on tissue-specific gene expression and drug efficacy and toxicity in differentiated cell types. Finally, engineering of surfaces that control adhesive interactions is important to fundamental studies of cell adhesion, such as the roles of receptor clustering and cytoskeletal assembly in adhesion strengthening.

B. Integrin Adhesion Receptors and Fibronectin

Cell adhesion to ECM components, such as FN and laminin, is primarily mediated by integrins, a widely expressed family of transmembrane receptors (16). Integrins are heterodimeric receptors, consisting of α and β subunits that are non-covalently associated and interact to bind specific amino acid sequences in the ligand. In many instances, integrin binding to its ligand is mediated by the arginine-glycine-aspartic acid (RGD) recognition sequence present in several ECM proteins, including FN, vitronectin, and thrombospondin (17). Integrin-mediated adhesion is a highly regulated, complex process involving receptor–ligand interactions and subsequent adhesion strengthening and cell spreading. For example, integrin binding to FN involves a conformational change (activation) in the receptor that results in mechanical coupling to the ligand (18,19). Bound receptors rapidly associate with the actin cytoskeleton and cluster together giving rise to focal adhesions, discrete complexes that contain cytoplasmic structural proteins, such as vinculin, talin, and α-actinin, and signaling molecules, including src, focal adhesion kinase (FAK) and paxillin, as well as transmembrane proteoglycans (20). Focal adhesions are central elements of the adhesion process, functioning as structural links between the cytoskeleton and the ECM and triggering signaling pathways (e.g., mitogen-activated protein kinase and protein kinase C) that direct growth and differentiation (21,22).

ECMs comprise a complex network of glycosaminoglycans/proteoglycans and structural (collagen, elastin) and adhesive (FN, laminin) proteins that provide tissue structure and signals that regulate development and the biochemical functions of matrix-associated cells. FN is one of the most intensively studied ECM components, particularly in terms of its effects on cells. FN, whether adsorbed from serum-containing solutions or secreted by cells, plays a central role in the adhesion of many cell types to ECM and artificial substrata (14). It is an essential component for normal development, as evidenced by the failure of FN knockout mice to develop beyond embryonic day 10–11 (23).

The FN molecule consists of a series of homologous repeats of three types (I, II, III) that are folded into globular domains specialized for particular functions, such as binding to integrins, collagen, heparan sulfate, and itself to form fibrils (24–27). The RGD sequence in the tenth type III repeat is the major integrin binding site, and it mediates the adhesion of most cell types (28). Although the RGD site is essential for adhesion, sequences in adjacent domains, like the PHSRN synergy site localized in the ninth type III domain, are also critical to the binding of some integrins, such as $\alpha_5\beta_1$ and $\alpha_{IIb}\beta_3$ (29,30). This domain often modulates integrin-mediated processes, such as cell spreading and matrix assembly (29,30).

C. Engineering Surfaces to Control Cell Adhesion

Because of the fundamental importance of adhesion in directing cell function, engineering of surfaces that either prevent or enhance protein adsorption and cell adhesion represents an extremely active area of biomaterials research. Numerous studies have shown that surface chemistry influences the type, quantity, and conformation of adsorbed proteins (11,31). For example, hydrophilic ethylene glycol–derivatized surfaces resist protein adsorption and cell adhesion, whereas hydrophobic substrates support protein adsorption, cell adhesion, and spreading (32,33). This principle of altering surface chemistry to control protein adsorption has been widely used to modulate cell adhesion (34–43).

The identification of recognition sequences, such as RGD for FN and YIGSR for laminin, that mediate cell adhesion to ECM has led to the development of bioadhesive synthetic surfaces. Several groups have shown that incorporation of short peptides containing these sequences into synthetic substrates results in enhanced cell adhesion (34,44–47). Although this approach provides substrates that support cell adhesion, the biological activity of these peptides is significantly lower than that of the complete protein (44). The loss in activity most likely results from conformation-dependent effects and the absence of crucial modulatory domains present in the intact protein. Moreover, as pointed out previously, many integrin-mediated processes, including signaling, cell spreading, and matrix assembly, require regions adjacent to these short recognition sequences that are not present in most bioadhesive synthetic surfaces. Nonetheless, biospecific surfaces remain one of the most promising approaches to the development of surfaces that control cell adhesion and function.

III. QUANTITATIVE ANALYSES OF INTEGRIN– FIBRONECTIN BINDING

We have developed an experimental framework to analyze integrin–FN binding in terms of adhesion strength and binding affinity—fundamental parameters of this receptor–ligand interaction (19,48). This mechanochemical framework has been applied to the analysis of structure–function relationships in cell adhesion and the investigation of integrin–FN interactions at the cell–biomaterial interface (19,48–51). In addition, these mechanistic studies provide design principles for the engineering of surfaces that elicit directed cellular responses.

A. Adhesion Strength

We have developed a spinning-disk device that applies a range of hydrodynamic forces to adherent cells and provides sensitive and reproducible measurements of adhesion strength (Fig. 1) (19,52). The applied shear stress τ (force/area) at any point on the surface of the disk varies linearly with radial position and is given by:

$$\tau = 0.800\, r \sqrt{\rho \mu \omega^3} \tag{1}$$

where r is radial position from the disk center, ρ and μ are fluid density and viscosity, and ω is angular speed. Following uniform cell seeding and spinning, cells are fixed, stained, and counted at specific radial positions. The fraction of adherent cells (cell counts normalized to counts at the center of the disk [no applied force]) decreases nonlinearly with shear stress (Fig. 1) and is accurately described by a sigmoid curve in which the shear stress for 50% detachment (τ_{50}) represents the mean adhesion strength. Thus, for a single disk, a linear range of forces is applied to a large cell population

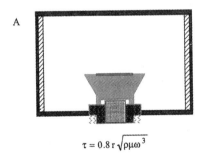
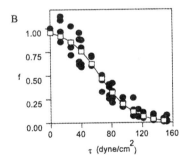

Figure 1 (A) Spinning-disk device for measuring adhesion strength. Substrate spins in fluid-filled chamber and the resulting shear stress (τ) depends on radial position (r), speed (ω), and fluid density (ρ) and viscosity (μ). (B) Detachment profile for K562 cells adhering to FN. Experimental points ($\bullet$) are fitted to a sigmoid ($\square$) to obtain values for the shear stress for 50% detachment, which represents the mean adhesion strength. (Adapted from Ref. 19.)

producing a cell detachment profile that permits calculation of a mean detachment force defined as the adhesion strength.

We have used this system to analyze the initial binding of integrin to FN and, in particular, the functional dependence of initial adhesion strength on receptor and ligand densities and binding affinity (19). These studies were performed on human K562 erythroleukemia cells, which remain spherical, even when plated on FN-coated surfaces. This allows direct calculation of the applied detachment force. From a biochemical perspective, this cell line provides an ideal model because it provides for the examination of a single class of receptor–ligand interactions. These cells express a single FN receptor, $\alpha_5\beta_1$ integrin. This receptor is expressed in a constitutively inactive binding state and can be activated to an FN-binding form using specific monoclonal antibodies, providing a model with uniform activation of the receptor. Furthermore, under the conditions of the assay, these cells do not increase their adhesion to FN over time, allowing isolation of the integrin–ligand interaction from subsequent adhesion strengthening events, such as focal adhesion assembly, cytoskeleton recruitment, and cell spreading (19).

Our functional analysis is based on the theoretical work of Hammer and Lauffenburger (53). The adhesion model considers a spherical cell with a single class of receptors attaching to a surface through uniformly distributed receptor–ligand bonds. The shear stress for detachment, τ_d, is given by:

$$\tau_d = G\psi N_R N_L + \lambda \qquad (2)$$

where G is a geometrical parameter related to the contact area and cell shape; N_R and N_L are the receptor and ligand densities, respectively; and λ represents the nonspecific adhesion between the cell and the surface. The adhesion constant ψ is a novel experimental parameter specific to the receptor–ligand interaction. ψ is related to the bond strength and receptor–ligand affinity, and is independent of geometry and ligand and receptor densities. Although ψ has no direct biophysical correlate, we have found that this parameter is characteristic of a particular receptor–ligand interaction. We have shown that changes in either receptor or ligand conformation, both of which alter adhesion strength, are manifested as changes in ψ (49,50).

This experimental analysis revealed that cell adhesion strength increases linearly with both FN and integrin densities as predicted by the model [Eq. (2)] (Fig. 2) (19). We have also shown linear increases in initial adhesion strength as a function of ligand density for normal fibroblasts and osteoblasts, cells that cluster integrins, recruit cytoskeleton, and spread on FN (49,50). The linear increases in adhesion strength suggest that initial

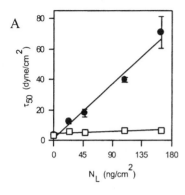 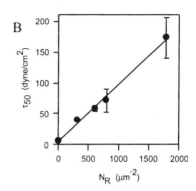

Figure 2 Cell adhesion strength (τ_{50}) increases linearly with (A) ligand (FN) and (B) receptor (integrin $\alpha_5\beta_1$) densities as predicted by Eq. (2). Adhesion strength is dependent on receptor activation: ●, TS2/16-antibody activation, □, control (inactive). (From Ref. 19.)

adhesion strength is directly proportional to the number of integrin–FN bonds. Furthermore, this linear relationship indicates that modulation of the receptor–ligand interaction is the dominant mechanism for adhesion during the initial stages of adhesion and suggests that cooperative binding contributes minimally to initial adhesion strength. In addition, we have shown the existence of three distinct activation states for $\alpha_5\beta_1$ integrin binding to FN (50). These multiple binding states reflect distinct interactions between $\alpha_5\beta_1$ and specific binding sites in FN. Multiple activation states for $\alpha_5\beta_1$ suggest the existence of distinct stages in adhesion signaling and strengthening and may provide a versatile mechanism for the regulation of adhesive interactions.

We have applied this experimental framework to examine adhesion strengthening in normal fibroblasts. Consistent with previous studies (54,55), our experiments indicate that cell adhesion strength increases over time, reaching values approximately 10 times higher than the attachment strength at 15 min (see Fig. 15). These increases in adhesion strength reflect changes in overall cell morphology, evolution of close attachment contacts from a small central zone to nonuniformly distributed discrete focal adhesions, clustering of integrin receptors, focal adhesion assembly, and reorganization of the underlying ECM. We have expanded this approach to analyze adhesion strengthening for cells adhering to micropatterned surfaces (see Section V) in order to examine the functional dependence of adhesion strength on integrin clustering and focal adhesion assembly (56).

B.   Binding Affinity and Bond Density

Bond formation and dissociation are fundamental properties of receptor–ligand interactions and determination of the number of bound receptors is critical for a quantitative analysis of cell adhesion. We have previously shown that, for initial adhesion to FN, $\alpha_5\beta_1$ is the dominant integrin and that the integrin–FN interaction can be modeled as simple monovalent binding (48). From chemical kinetics principles, the time rate of change in bond number (B) is given by Eq. (3), where R and L are the free receptor number and free ligand density and k_f and k_r are the forward and reverse rate constants (Fig. 3). Equation (3) simply states that the rate of accumulation of bonds equals the rate of bond formation minus the rate of bond dissociation.

$$\frac{dB}{dt} = k_f R \cdot L - k_r B \qquad (3)$$

At equilibrium, the rates of formation and dissociation are equal and the equilibrium bond number (B_{eq}) is given by:

$$B_{eq} = \frac{R_T L}{L + K_D} \qquad (4)$$

where R_T is the total number of receptors ($R_T = R + B$) and K_D is the dissociation constant ($K_D = 1/K_A = k_r/k_f$), where K_A is the equilibrium affinity constant. For conditions where $K_D \gg L$, this expression reduces to Eq. 5, which predicts that the number of bonds is proportional to the product of the total receptor number and ligand density:

$$B_{eq} = K_A R_T L \qquad (5)$$

We have developed a biochemical cross-linking/extraction/reversal method to quantify integrin binding to ECM proteins (48,51) (Fig. 4). Bound integrins are chemically cross-linked to their ligand using sulfo-BSOCOES, a cleavable, homobifunctional, cell-impermeable cross-linker. Taking advantage of the fact that most matrix proteins, including FN, are resistant

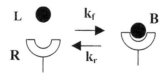

Figure 3   Simple monovalent receptor–ligand interaction.

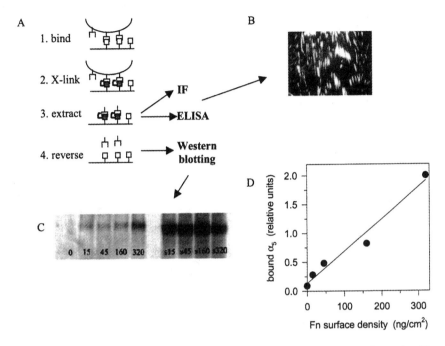

Figure 4 Biochemical procedure to quantify integrin binding. (A) Schematic: (1) integrins bind FN; (2) bound integrins are X-linked to FN using sulfo-BSOCOES; (3) cellular components are extracted, leaving behind FN-bound integrins; (4) X-linking is reversed and integrins are recovered. Samples can be analyzed by (B) immunofluorescence staining, ELISA, or (C,D) Western blotting. Analysis of initial integrin binding to FN. (C) Representative Western blot for recovered α_5 subunit for different FN surface densities (left) and soluble fractions of extracted cells (right) showing increases in bound integrins as a function of ligand density. (D) Quantification of fluorescent intensity bound $\alpha_5(b - \alpha_5)$ as a function of FN surface density. Linear regression: $b - \alpha_5 = 5.6 \times 10^{-3} FN + 0.13$, $R^2 = 0.97$. (Adapted from Ref. 48.)

to detergent extraction, the bulk of cell components (including unbound receptors) is then extracted with 0.1% sodium dodecyl sulfate (SDS), leaving behind matrix proteins bound to the dish and their associated integrins. Bound integrins can then be visualized by immunofluorescence staining or quantified by enzyme-linked immunosorbent assay (ELISA) (51). Alternatively, bound integrins can be recovered by cleaving the cross-linker following cell extraction and quantified by Western blotting (48,51). Extensive control experiments have indicated that this method is specific for ligated integrins.

We have used this methodology to quantify initial as well as long-term integrin binding to FN (48,51). For quantification of initial integrin binding, human fibroblasts were plated on different FN surface densities for 15 min and bound integrins were cross-linked and recovered. The amount of recovered α_5 (Fig. 4) and β_1 integrin subunits increases with FN surface density, indicating increases in bound $\alpha_5\beta_1$ integrin as a function of FN surface density. Regression analyses revealed that binding of $\alpha_5\beta_1$ integrin to FN increases linearly with FN surface density (Fig. 4), as predicted by the simple monovalent model [Eq. (5)]. A 30-fold increase in FN surface density results in a 7-fold increase in integrin binding, and this result is consistent with the relatively low affinity ($K_A \approx 10^{-7} M^{-1}$) of $\alpha_5\beta_1$ integrin for soluble FN (19). Moreover, the linear increases in the number of $\alpha_5\beta_1$ integrin–FN bonds with FN surface density are consistent with the linear increases in adhesion strength (Fig. 2).

Tyrosine phosphorylation of FAK has also been analyzed to examine the relationship between number of bonds and integrin-mediated signaling (48). FAK phosphorylation is one of the earliest signaling events associated with integrin binding (57,58). FAK was recovered by immunoprecipitation from samples analyzed for integrin binding, and the levels of phosphorylation were quantified on samples that contained equal amounts of FAK by Western blotting. FAK phosphorylation increases linearly with bound α_5, suggesting the absence of cooperative effects on intracellular signaling during the initial stages of the adhesion process. We have further analyzed intracellular signaling to examine the role of integrin binding in gene expression (see Section IV.A).

IV.   ENGINEERED SURFACES TO CONTROL INTEGRIN BINDING AND DIRECT CELL FUNCTION

The insights obtained from these structure–function studies provide rational design principles for the engineering of surfaces to modulate integrin receptor binding in order to control cell adhesion, proliferation, and differentiation. We describe two biomolecular strategies for the engineering of proactive surfaces to control cell function. These approaches are relevant to numerous biomedical and biotechnological applications, including the engineering of biomaterial surfaces, tissue engineering scaffolds, and cell growth supports.

A. Strategy I: Surfaces That Modulate Conformation of Adsorbed Fibronectin and Direct Integrin Binding and Cell Function

1. Principle

The binding of integrin $\alpha_5\beta_1$ to FN mediates the adhesion of many cell types and has a central role in the differentiation of myoblasts, osteoblasts, and chondrocytes (51,59,60). As previously discussed, binding of $\alpha_5\beta_1$ integrin requires both the PHSRN amino acid sequence in the ninth type III repeat and the RGD motif in the tenth type III repeat of FN (61). This interaction is controlled by the structural orientation of these two domains (about 3–4 nm apart), i.e., the nanoscale of operation. Each domain independently contributes little to binding, but in combination they synergistically bind to the receptor to produce significant (10-fold) increases in adhesion strength (Fig. 5) (62). In addition, the relative nanoscale orientation of these two binding domains is essential to the synergistic effects as incremental extensions in the interdomain link significantly reduce $\alpha_5\beta_1$ binding, cell spreading, and integrin-mediated signaling (63). Moreover, interdomain interactions are critical in the context of FN adsorption onto natural and synthetic substrates. We have demonstrated that, upon adsorption to surfaces, FN undergoes changes in conformation (three-dimensional

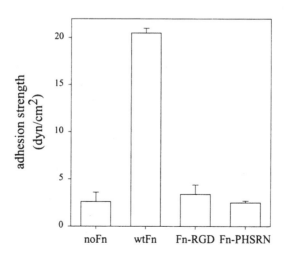

Figure 5 Integrin $\alpha_5\beta_1$-mediated adhesion strength to recombinant FNs: wild-type (wtFn), FN with deleted RGD site (Fn-RGD), and FN with mutated PHSRN site (Fn-PHSRN). (Adapted from Ref. 62.)

structure) that modify $\alpha_5\beta_1$ binding and signaling and modulate cell proliferation and differentiation (51).

We have examined changes in FN structure upon adsorption onto three commonly used surfaces: hydrophobic (untreated) bacteriological polystyrene, tissue culture-treated polystyrene, and type I collagen-coated polystyrene (FN binds to type I collagen). The conformation of adsorbed FN was examined in an antibody binding assay using monoclonal antibodies directed against specific structural epitopes in FN (51). This analysis revealed that the binding affinity of antibodies specific for the central cell binding domain in FN, which contains the PHSRN and RGD integrin binding sites, is particularly sensitive to adsorption onto different substrates, suggesting that the conformation of this domain is influenced by the adsorption process. These changes in conformation alter the binding of $\alpha_5\beta_1$, but not $\alpha_v\beta_3$ which binds only to the RGD and not the PHSRN site. These substrate-dependent differences in integrin binding modulate switching between proliferation and differentiation in muscle cells (Fig. 6) (51). Differentiation is controlled by the levels of $\alpha_5\beta_1$ bound to FN and is inhibited by either anti-FN or anti-α_5, but not anti-α_v, antibodies. We have recently demonstrated similar substrate-dependent differences in expression of the osteoblast phenotype for immature osteoblasts grown on these FN-coated surfaces (Fig. 7) (64).

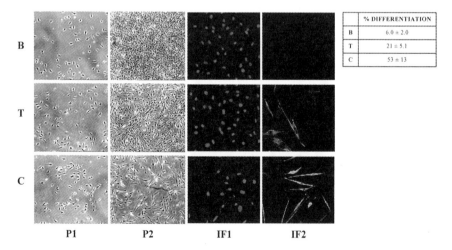

	% DIFFERENTIATION
B	6.0 ± 2.0
T	21 ± 5.1
C	53 ± 13

Figure 6 Substrate-dependent changes in FN conformation control cell proliferation and differentiation. Phase contrast micrographs showing C2C12 myoblast density at 16 h (P1) and 3 days (P2). Immunofluorescent staining at 3 days for DNA (IF1) and sarcomeric myosin (IF2), a specific marker of myogenic differentiation.

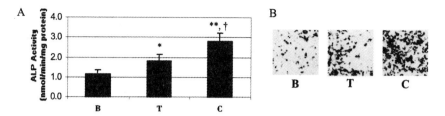

Figure 7 Enhanced MC3T3-E1 osteoblast differentiation on substrates that modulate FN conformation. (A) Alkaline phosphatase (ALP) activity at 7 days $[^* T > B (p < 0.05);\ ^{**} C > B (p < 0.0005);\ ^\dagger C > T (p < 0.005)]$. (B) Von Kossa staining for matrix mineralization at 21 days in culture. (From Ref. 64.)

2. Model Surfaces Presenting Well-Defined Chemistries to Modulate Fibronectin Conformation and Integrin Binding

We are actively engineering surfaces to control FN adsorption/conformation and target specific integrin receptors in order to direct cell adhesion and gene expression (56,65). Our model surfaces consist of self-assembled monolayers (SAMs) of alkanethiols on gold. This system has been extensively characterized and exhibits well-defined surface properties and flexibility in generating mixed compositions and introducing complex functionality. Long-chain alkanethiols (HS-$[CH_2]_n$-X, where $n \geq 10$ and X is the tail group), adsorb from solution onto gold surfaces to form stable, well-packed, and ordered monolayers (Fig. 8). (66–68). The sulfur on the chain head coordinates strongly to the gold and the trans-extended alkyl chain presents the tail group X at the SAM–solution interface. The tail group controls the physicochemical properties of the SAM, allowing the tailoring of specific surface chemistries, such as groups that resist protein adsorption or moieties that can be modified to immobilize peptides and proteins (69). Furthermore, surfaces of mixed composition can be engineered by coadsorption of different alkanethiols, providing a simple and robust system to generate multicomponent surfaces (68).

We have analyzed the interactions of FN with four functional chemistries: CH_3 (hydrophobic), OH (neutral hydrophilic), COOH (negatively charged at physiological pH), and NH_2 (positively charged at physiological pH) (65). Antibody binding measurements using monoclonal antibodies directed against the cell binding domain of FN reveal differences in antibody affinity for FN adsorbed onto the different surface chemistries (Fig. 9). The antibody binding profile is analyzed in terms of adsorbed FN density and provides estimates of antibody binding affinity. Shifts in the

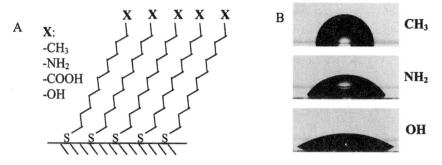

Figure 8 Functionalized SAMs. (A) Schematic of alkanethiol SAM on Au presenting tail group X which controls surface chemistry as demonstrated by wettability (B).

antibody binding profile reflect substrate-dependent differences in the conformation of the cell binding domain of FN. These conformational changes in FN result in significant differences in $\alpha_5\beta_1$ binding (Fig. 10). Extensive differences in bound receptor density and distribution as well as localization of focal adhesion components have been observed by

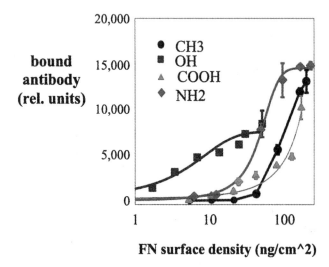

Figure 9 Substrate-dependent changes in FN conformation upon adsorption to SAMs as determined by changes in antibody binding to the central integrin-binding domains in FN. (From Ref. 65.)

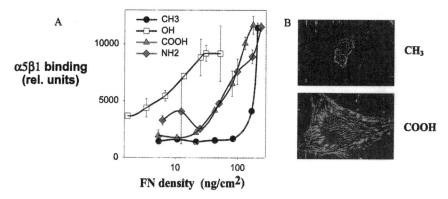

Figure 10 Integrin $\alpha_5\beta_1$ binding to FN adsorbed onto SAMs showing differences in bound density and distribution. (A) Quantification of integrin binding using biochemical assay. Experimental data is accurately described by Eq. (4). (B) Immunofluorescence staining for α_5. (Adapted from Ref. 65.)

immunofluorescence staining and our biochemical assay for integrin binding (OH > COOH, NH_2 > CH_3; Figure 10) (65). These differences in integrin binding and focal adhesion assembly modulate integrin signaling and expression of osteoblast-specific genes in immature osteoblast-like cells grown on these FN-coated surfaces (Fig. 11) (56).

These studies indicate that the structural orientation of synergistic integrin binding domains (PHSRN and RGD) is modulated upon adsorption onto different surfaces. These nanoscale structural changes are critical to $\alpha_5\beta_1$ integrin binding and signaling and subsequent activation of

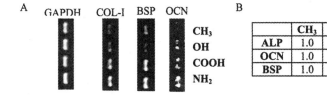

	CH₃	OH	COOH	NH₂
ALP	1.0	1.4	1.2	1.5
OCN	1.0	0.9	1.0	1.8
BSP	1.0	1.5	4.7	3.1

Figure 11 Differential expression of osteoblast-specific genes [COL-1: type I collagen; ALP: alkaline phosphatase; OCN: osteocalcin; BSP: bone sialoprotein; GAPDH (control)] in MC3T3-E1 osteoblast-like cells grown on SAMs coated with equal FN densities at 3 days. (A) Conventional RT-PCR results analyzed by gel electrophoresis. (B) Quantification of gene expression by real-time PCR (normalized to expression on CH_3). (Adapted from Ref. 56.)

gene expression programs. Control of cell fate through substrate-dependent changes in the structure of adsorbed ECM proteins represents a versatile approach for the engineering of surfaces to elicit specific cellular responses.

B. Strategy II: Bioadhesive Surfaces Presenting Recombinant Fibronectin Fragments to Target Specific Integrins

1. Principle

A common biomolecular strategy in the engineering of adhesive surfaces is to present small peptides encoding the recognition sequences, such as RGD and YIGSR, of several extracellular ligands. While this strategy supports integrin-mediated cell adhesion, several integrins, including $\alpha_5\beta_1$ and $\alpha_{IIb}\beta_3$, require additional binding domains in FN. Targeting of specific integrins is critical to control of cell function since different integrins trigger diverse signaling cascades (51). Therefore, biomolecular approaches to develop bioadhesive surfaces should not be limited to the RGD site but should extend to additional domains of FN required for full activity, such as the PHSRN synergy site. However, given the sensitivity of $\alpha_5\beta_1$ integrin binding to small perturbations to the orientation of these domains (51,63), reconstitution of the proper structural orientation using small synthetic peptides is a challenging task. To address these limitations, we have focused on engineering surfaces presenting a recombinant FN fragment that spans the central cell binding domain and contains both PHSRN and RGD binding sites to enhance integrin specificity (71). The use of recombinant fragments, rather than the complete FN molecule, has several advantages, including reduced antigenicity, elimination of domains that may elicit adverse reactions, and enhanced cost efficiency. Furthermore, recombinant fragments provide for the engineering of specific anchoring sites in the fragment to control the orientation of the protein on the surface.

2. Functionalized Surfaces That Support $\alpha_5\beta_1$ Integrin Binding and Cell Adhesion

We have engineered nonadhesive surfaces presenting controlled densities of recombinant FN7-10, a 39-kDa fragment of human FN spanning the seventh through tenth type III repeats (Fig. 12). The fragment is expressed in *Escherichia coli*, purified by precipitation, anion exchange chromatography, and crystallization (70). FN7-10 is biologically active and supports $\alpha_5\beta_1$ integrin–mediated adhesion and spreading as demonstrated by blocking experiments with integrin-specific antibodies (71).

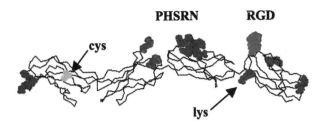

Figure 12 Backbone model of FN7-10 showing RGD and PHSRN binding sites and cysteine (cys) and lysine (lys) residues available for immobilization. (Adapted from Ref. 71.)

Model hybrid surfaces have been engineered by immobilizing FN7-10 onto nonadhesive, passively adsorbed serum albumin via conventional peptide chemistry methods (71). Homo- and heterobifunctional cross-linkers targeting either the cysteine or lysine residues in FN7-10 have been examined to optimize immobilized density and conformation (Fig. 13). Immobilization of the bioactive fragment onto a nonadhesive/nonfouling background results in surfaces with well-defined ligand densities that target specific integrin receptors while significantly reducing background effects arising from nonspecific protein adsorption. These hybrid surfaces support $\alpha_5\beta_1$-mediated adhesion, spreading, and assembly of focal adhesions containing $\alpha_5\beta_1$ and vinculin (Fig. 13). Furthermore, the immobilized fragment retains significant biological activity in comparison with passively adsorbed proteins, which lose biological activity as a result of changes in conformation upon adsorption. This approach can be extended to immobilize FN7-10 onto nonadhesive synthetic substrates to investigate the effects of ligand density and specific integrin binding on cell differentiation.

V. MICROPATTERNED SURFACES TO ENGINEER FOCAL ADHESION ASSEMBLY

Micropatterning approaches can be applied to engineer surfaces that control adhesive area and cell spreading/shape (33). These approaches generally involve creating cell adhesive domains that readily adsorb proteins and are surrounded by a protein adsorption–resistant, nonadhesive background. We have applied micropatterning techniques to engineer surfaces that control

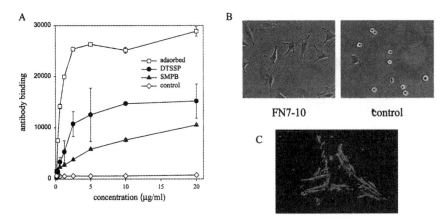

Figure 13 Functionalized nonadhesive surfaces. (A) Immobilization of FN7-10 onto nonadhesive surfaces using DTSSP and SMPB cross-linkers as a function of FN7-10 concentration. Also shown is FN7-10 passive adsorption onto untreated (adsorbed) and nonadhesive surfaces without cross-linker (control). (B) Immobilized FN7-10 supports efficient cell adhesion and spreading (4 h) compared to nonadhesive surfaces (control). (C) Immunofluorescence staining for α_5 integrin subunit on immobilized FN7-10. (Adapted from Ref. 71.)

available adhesive area, cell spreading, and the position and size of focal adhesions (56). Micropatterned surfaces consisting of cell adhesive circular islands in a nonadhesive background have been created using microcontact printing of alkanethiol SAMs (33). Standard photolithography techniques are used to manufacture templates of different island diameters (2, 5, 10, 20 µm) on Si wafers. A PDMS stamp having the desired features is then cast from the Si mold. To create micropatterns, the stamp is inked with "adhesive" (CH_3- or COOH-terminated) alkanethiols and pressed onto Au-coated surfaces. The remaining area is derivatized with triethylene glycol–terminated alkanethiols, which resist protein adsorption and cell adhesion.

Micropatterning provides precise control over FN adhesive area, cell spreading/shape, and position and size of focal adhesions (Fig. 14) (56). This approach allows decoupling of cell shape/spreading from focal adhesion formation. We have used micropatterned substrates to examine the relative contributions of receptor clustering and focal adhesion assembly to adhesion strength (56). For similar contact areas (5-µm patterns), integrin clustering, focal adhesion formation, and cytoskeletal recruitment result in

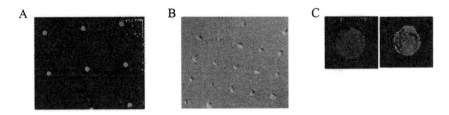

Figure 14 Micropatterned surfaces (10 μm diam) that control protein adsorption, cell spreading, and focal adhesion assembly. (A) Immunofluorescence staining for FN shows protein adsorption limited to adhesive islands. (B) Fibroblast cell adhesion and spreading at 2 days showing cells constrained to adhesive islands. (C) Immunofluorescence staining for $\alpha_5\beta_1$ (left) and vinculin (right) showing robust formation of focal adhesions localized to micropatterned islands. (Adapted from Ref. 56.)

five-fold increases in adhesion strength (Fig. 15). This surface engineering approach can be used to examine the effects of cell shape in cell differentiation. Recent studies have indicated that cell shape provides complementary signals that regulate cell survival, proliferation, and differentiation in several cell types (72–74).

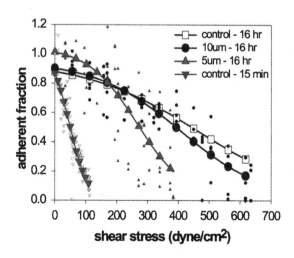

Figure 15 Cell adhesion strength profiles for FN-coated micropatterns showing increases in adhesion strength with available spreading area. (Adapted from Ref. 56.)

VI. CONCLUSIONS AND FUTURE DIRECTIONS

Because of the fundamental role of integrin-mediated cell adhesion to ECM proteins in cell function, the engineering of surfaces to control adhesive interactions holds tremendous promise for numerous biotechnological and biomedical applications. Driven by insights obtained from structure–function analyses, we focus on biomolecular engineering strategies to control integrin binding and cell adhesion in order to direct cell function. In the coming years, we anticipate that integration of advances in surface engineering technologies, especially in self-assembly and biomimetics, with enhanced understanding of the molecular and cell biology of adhesion will lead to the rational design of robust biospecific surfaces that tailor adhesive interactions and elicit specific cellular responses. In particular, elucidation of integrin-mediated signaling pathways and activation of specific gene expression programs will provide rational targets for the engineering of bioactive surfaces. Furthermore, biomolecular approaches focusing on growth factors and structural components of ECM will complement these bioadhesive surface strategies to produce bioinspired, engineered matrices.

ACKNOWLEDGMENTS

This work was funded by the National Science Foundation (BES-9986549), Whitaker Foundation, Arthritis Foundation, and the Georgia Tech/Emory NSF ERC on Engineering of the Living Tissues (EEC-9731643). B.G.K. was supported by an NSF Graduate Research Fellowship. The authors thank H. P. Erickson (Duke Univ.) for providing bacteria expressing FN7-10 and A. B. Frazier (Georgia Inst. Technology) for assistance in the creation of the Si micropatterning molds.

REFERENCES

1. AS Menko, D Boettiger. Occupation of the extracellular matrix receptor integrin is a control point for myogenic differentiation. Cell 51:51–57, 1987.
2. Z Werb, PM Tremble, O Behrendtsen, E Crowley, CH Damsky. Signal transduction through the fibronectin receptor induces collagenase and stromelysin gene expression. J Cell Biol 109:877–889, 1989.
3. JC Adams, FM Watt. Changes in keratinocyte adhesion during terminal differentiation: reduction in fibronectin binding precedes $\alpha_5\beta_1$ integrin loss from the cell surface. Cell 63:425–435, 1990.

4. CH Streuli, N Bailey, MJ Bissell. Control of mammary epithelial differentiation: Basement membrane induced tissue-specific gene expression in the absence of cell–cell interaction and morphological polarity. J Cell Biol 115:1383–1395, 1991.

5. X Zhu, M Ohtsubo, RM Bohmer, JM Roberts, RK Assoian. Adhesion-dependent cell cycle progression linked to the expression of cyclin D1, activation of cyclin E-cdk2, and phosphorylation of the retinoblastoma protein. J Cell Biol 133:391–403, 1996.

6. SM Albelda. Role of integrins and other cell adhesion molecules in tumor progression and metastasis. Lab Invest 68:4–17, 1993.

7. PK Park, BE Jarrell, SK Williams, TL Carter, DG Rose, A Martinez-Hernandez, RA Carabasi. III. Thrombus-free, human endothelial surface in the midregion of a Dacron vascular graft in the splanchnic venous circuit—observations after nine months of implantation. J Vasc Surg 11:468–475, 1990.

8. SK Sharma, PP Mahendroo. Affinity chromatography of cells and cell membranes. J Chromatogr 184:471–499, 1980.

9. R Langer, JP Vacanti. Tissue engineering. Science 260:920–926, 1993.

10. RE Baier. The role of surface energy in thrombosis. Bull N Y Acad Med 48:257–272, 1972.

11. JD Andrade, V Hlady. Protein adsorption and materials biocompatibility: A tutorial review and suggested hypotheses. Adv Polym Sci 79:1–63, 1986.

12. JL Brash. Protein adsorption at the solid-solution interface in relation to blood-material interactions. In: TA Horbett, JL Brash, eds, Proteins at Interfaces. American Chemical Society, Washington, DC, 1987, pp. 490–506.

13. F Grinnell. Fibroblast-collagen-matrix contraction: growth-factor signalling and mechanical loading. Trends Cell Biol 10:362–365, 2000.

14. RO Hynes. Fibronectins. Springer-Verlag, New York 1990.

15. A Praemer, S Furner, D Rice. Musculoskeletal Conditions in the United States. 1992.

16. RO Hynes. Integrins: versatility, modulation, and signaling in cell adhesion. Cell 69:11–25, 1992.

17. E Ruoslahti, MD Pierschbacher. New perspectives in cell adhesion: RGD and integrins. Science 238:491–497, 1987.

18. RJ Faull, NL Kovach, J Harlan, MH Ginsberg. Affinity modulation of integrin $\alpha_5\beta_1$: regulation of the functional response to fibronectin. J Cell Biol 121:155–162, 1993.

19. AJ García, F Huber, D Boettiger. Force required to break $\alpha_5\beta_1$ integrin-fibronectin bonds in intact adherent cells is sensitive to integrin activation state. J Biol Chem 273:10988–10993, 1998.

20. BM Jockusch, P Bubeck, K Giehl, M Kroemker, J Moschner, M Rothkegel, M Rudiger, K Schluter, G Stanke, J Winkler. The molecular architecture of focal adhesions. Annu Rev Cell Dev Biol 11:379–416, 1995.

21. EA Clark, JS Brugge. Integrins and signal transduction pathways: the road taken. Science 268:233–239, 1995.

22. K Burridge, M Chrzanowska-Wodnicka. Focal adhesions, contractility, and signaling. Annu Rev Cell Dev Biol 12:463–518, 1996.
23. EL George, EN Georges-Labouesse, RS Patel-King, H Rayburn, RO Hynes. Defects in mesoderm, neural tube and vascular development in mouse embryos lacking fibronectin. Development 119:1079–1091, 1993.
24. E Engvall, E Ruoslahti. Binding of soluble form of fibroblast surface protein, fibronectin to collagen. Int J Cancer 20:1–5, 1977.
25. EG Hayman, A Oldberg, GR Martin, E Ruoslahti. Codistribution of heparin sulfate proteoglycan, laminin and fibronectin in the extracellular matrix of normal rat kidney cells and their coordinate absence in transformed cells. J Cell Biol 94:28–35, 1982.
26. J Laterra, JE Silbert, LA Culp. Cell surface heparan sulfate mediates some adhesive responses to glycosaminoglycan-binding matrices, including fibronectin. J Cell Biol 96:113–123, 1983.
27. A Morla, E Ruoslahti. A fibronectin self-assembly site involved in matrix assembly: reconstruction in a synthetic peptide. J Cell Biol 118:421–429, 1992.
28. MD Pierschbacher, EG Hayman, E Ruoslahti. Location of the cell-attachment site in fibronectin with monoclonal antibodies and proteolytic fragments of the molecule. Cell 26:259–267, 1981.
29. M Obara, MS Kang, KM Yamada. Site-directed mutagenesis of the cell-binding domain of human fibronectin: separable, synergistic sites mediate adhesive function. Cell 53:649–657, 1988.
30. JL Sechler, SA Corbett, JE Schwarzbauer. Modulatory roles for integrin activation and the synergy site of fibronectin during matrix assembly. Mol Biol Cell 8:2563–2573, 1998.
31. BD Ratner. Surface modification of polymers: chemical, biological and surface analytical challenges. Biosens Bioelectron 10:797–804, 1995.
32. KL Prime, GM Whitesides. Self-assembled organic monolayers: model systems for studying adsorption of proteins at surfaces. Science 252:1164–1167, 1991.
33. M Mrksich, LE Dike, J Tien, DE Ingber, GM Whitesides. Using microcontact printing to pattern the attachment of mammalian cells to self-assembled monolayers of alkanethiolates on transparent films of gold and silver. Exp Cell Res 235:305–313, 1997.
34. SP Massia, JA Hubbell. Covalent surface immobilization of Arg-Gly-Asp- and Tyr-Ile-Gly-Ser-Arg- containing peptides to obtain well-defined cell-adhesive substrates. Anal Biochem 187:292–301, 1990.
35. KE Healy, CH Thomas, A Rezania, JE Kim, PJ McKeown, B Lom, PL Hockberger. Kinetics of bone cell organization and mineralization on materials with patterned surface chemistry. Biomaterials 17:195–208, 1996.
36. K Webb, V Hlady, PA Tresco. Relative importance of surface wettability and charged functional groups on NIH 3T3 fibroblast attachment, spreading, and cytoskeletal organization. J Biomed Mater Res 41:422–430, 1998.
37. R Singhvi, A Kumar, GP Lopez, GN Stephanopoulos, DI Wang, GM Whitesides, DE Ingber. Engineering cell shape and function. Science 264:696–698, 1994.

38. SN Bhatia, M Toner, RG Tompkins, ML Yarmush. Selective adhesion of hepatocytes on patterned surfaces. Ann N Y Acad Sci 745:187–209: 1994.
39. BJ Spargo, MA Testoff, TB Nielsen, DA Stenger, JJ Hickman, AS Rudolph. Spatially controlled adhesion, spreading, and differentiation of endothelial cells on self-assembled molecular monolayers. Proc Natl Acad Sci USA 91:11070–11074, 1994.
40. D Kleinfeld, KH Kahler, PE Hockberger. Controlled outgrowth of dissociated neurons on patterned substrates. J Neurosci 8:4098–4120, 1988.
41. P Clark, P Connolly, GR Moores. Cell guidance by micropatterned adhesiveness in vitro. J Cell Sci 103:287–292, 1992.
42. JP Ranieri, R Bellamkonda, J Jacob, TG Vargo, JA Gardella, P Aebischer. Selective neuronal cell attachment to a covalently patterned monoamine on fluorinated ethylene propylene films. J Biomed Mater Res 27:917–925, 1993.
43. CD Tidwell, SI Ertel, BD Ratner, B Tarasevich, S Atre, DL Allara. Endothelial cell growth and serum protein adsorption on terminally functionalized, self-assembled monolayers of alkanethiolates on gold. Langmuir 13:3404–3413, 1997.
44. MD Pierschbacher, E Ruoslahti. Cell attachment activity of fibronectin can be duplicated by small synthetic fragments of the molecule. Nature 309:30–33, 1984.
45. KC Dee, DC Rueger, TT Andersen, R Bizios. Conditions which promote mineralization at the bone-implant interface: a model in vitro study. Biomaterials 17:209–215, 1996.
46. A Rezania, CH Thomas, AB Branger, CM Waters, KE Healy. The detachment strength and morphology of bone cells contacting materials modified with a peptide sequence found within bone sialoprotein. J Biomed Mater Res 37:9–19, 1997.
47. JA Neff, KD Caldwell, PA Tresco. A novel method for surface modification to promote cell attachment to hydrophobic substrates. J Biomed Mater Res 40:511–519, 1998.
48. AJ García, D Boettiger. Integrin-fibronectin interactions at the cell-material interface: initial integrin binding and signaling. Biomaterials 20:2427–2433, 1999.
49. AJ García, P Ducheyne, D Boettiger. The effect of surface reaction stage on fibronectin-mediated adhesion of osteoblast-like cells to bioactive glass. J Biomed Mater Res 40:48–56, 1998.
50. AJ García, J Takagi, D Boettiger. Two-stage activation for $\alpha_5\beta_1$ integrin binding to surface-adsorbed fibronectin. J Biol Chem 273:34710–34715, 1998.
51. AJ García, MD Vega, D Boettiger. Modulation of cell proliferation and differentiation through substrate-dependent changes in fibronectin conformation. Mol Biol Cell 10:785–798, 1999.
52. AJ García, P Ducheyne, D Boettiger. Quantification of cell adhesion using a spinning disk device and application to surface-reactive materials. Biomaterials 18:1091–1098, 1997.

53. DA Hammer, DA Lauffenburger. A dynamical model for receptor-mediated cell adhesion to surfaces. Biophys J 52:475–487, 1987.
54. MM Lotz, CA Burdsal, HP Erickson, DR McClay. Cell adhesion to fibronectin and tenascin: Quantitative measurements of initial binding and subsequent strengthening response. J Cell Biol 109:1795–1805, 1989.
55. D Choquet, DP Felsenfield, MP Sheetz. Extracellular matrix rigidity causes strengthening of integrin-cytoskeletal linkages. Cell 88:39–48, 1997.
56. BG Keselowsky, ND Gallant, DM Collard, AJ García. Model surfaces to control integrin binding, cell adhesion, and gene expression. 2001 ASME Bioengineering Conference. BED 50:629–630, 2001.
57. MD Schaller, CA Borgman, BS Cobb, RR Vines, AB Reynolds, JT Parsons. pp125FAK, a structurally distinctive protein-tyrosine kinase associated with focal adhesions. Proc Natl Acad Sci USA 89:5192–5196, 1992.
58. L Kornberg, HS Earp, JT Parsons, M Schaller, RL Juliano. Cell adhesion or integrin clustering increases phosphorylation of a focal adhesion-associated tyrosine kinase. J Biol Chem 267:23439–23442, 1992.
59. AM Moursi, RK Globus, CH Damsky. Interactions between integrin receptors and fibronectin are required for calvarial osteoblast differentiation in vitro. J Cell Sci 110:2187–2196, 1997.
60. M Enomoto-Iwamoto, M Iwamoto, K Nakashima, Y Mukudai, D Boettiger, M Pacifici, K Kurisu, F Suzuki. Involvement of alpha5beta1 integrin in matrix interactions and proliferation of chondrocytes. J Bone Miner Res 12:1124–1132, 1997.
61. EH Danen, S Aota, AA van Kraats, KM Yamada, DJ Ruiter, GN van Muijen. Requirement for the synergy site for cell adhesion to fibronectin depends on the activation state of integrin alpha 5 beta 1. J Biol Chem 270:21612–21618, 1995.
62. AJ García, JE Schwarzbauer, D Boettiger. Distinct activation states of $\alpha_5\beta_1$ integrin show differential binding to RGD and synergy domains of fibronectin (submitted).
63. RP Grant, C Spitzfaden, H Altroff, ID Campbell, HJ Mardon. Structural requirements for biological activity of the ninth and tenth FIII domains of human fibronectin. J Biol Chem 272:6159–6166, 1997.
64. SN Stephansson, BA Byers, AJ García. Expression of the osteoblastic phenotype on substrates that modulate fibronectin conformation and integrin receptor binding. Biomaterials 23:2527–2534, 2002.
65. BG Keselowsky, DM Collard, AJ García. Surface chemistry alters adsorbed fibronectin conformation and modulates integrin binding and focal adhesion formation. 27th Annu Meet Soc Biomater 10, 2001.
66. A Ulman, JE Eilers, N Tillman. Packing and molecular orientation of alkanethiol monolayers on gold surfaces. Langmuir 5:1147–1152, 1989.
67. CD Bain, EB Troughton, Y-T Tao, J Evall, GM Whitesides, RG Nuzzo. Formation of monolayer films by the spontaneous assembly of organic thiols from solution onto gold. J Am Chem Soc 111:321–335, 1989.

68. CD Bain, J Evall, GM Whitesides. Formation of monolayers by the coadsorption of thiols on gold: Variation in the head group, tail group, and solvent. J Am Chem Soc 111:7155–7164, 1989.

69. M Mrksich, GM Whitesides. Patterning self-assembled monolayers using microcontact printing: a new technology for biosensors? Trends Biotechnol 13:228–235, 1995.

70. SD Redick, DL Settles, G Briscoe, HP Erickson. Defining fibronectin's cell adhesion synergy site by site-directed mutagenesis. J Cell Biol 149:521–527, 2000.

71. SM Cutler, AJ García. Immobilization of a recombinant fragment of fibronectin to engineer cell adhesive hybrid surfaces. 27th Annu Meet Soc Biomater 264, 2001.

72. PV Moghe, F Berthiaume, RM Ezzell, M Toner, RG Tompkins, ML Yarmush. Culture matrix configuration and composition in the maintenance of hepatocyte polarity and function. Biomaterials 17:373–385, 1996.

73. CS Chen, M Mrksich, S Huang, G Whitesides, DE Ingber. Geometric control of cell life and death. Science 276:1425–1428, 1997.

74. J Lincks, BD Boyan, CR Blanchard, CH Lohmann, Y Liu, DL Cochran, DD Dean, Z Schwartz. Response of MG63 osteoblast-like cells to titanium and titanium alloy is dependent on surface roughness and composition. Biomaterials 19:2219–2232, 1998.

3

Mimetic Peptide-Modified Materials for Control of Cell Differentiation

Gregory M. Harbers
University of California–Berkeley, Berkeley, California, and Northwestern University, Evanston, Illinois

Thomas A. Barber and Kevin E. Healy
University of California–Berkeley, Berkeley, California

Ranee A. Stile
Northwestern University, Evanston, Illinois

Dale R. Sumner
Rush Medical College, Chicago, Illinois

I. INTRODUCTION

Each year, millions of devices are implanted into the human body at a cost of billions of dollars to restore normal body function that has been diminished due to age, disease, or trauma (1,2). When these devices come in contact with the physiological environment, a series of initial events occur that are dominated by protein adsorption, and subsequent platelet and inflammatory cell adhesion. This native or nonspecific response to the device is not considered to be the optimal behavior between the materials from which the device is made and the host environment (3). Since the properties of the initial interfacial layer are determined by the surface chemistry of the material, the acceptance, durability, and integration of an implant are ultimately dependent on the surface characteristics of the material and the events at the material–tissue interface (4,5).

Several different approaches are being explored to develop the next generation of biomaterials and medical devices that interact with the host in a controlled and predictable manner, and ultimately replace diseased or damaged tissue and organs. These approaches range from incorporating biomacromolecules, such as peptides, proteins, enzymes, and plasmid DNA, either directly into or onto the surface of the material (6–17). Of these approaches, the use of peptides to exploit bimolecular engagement between the material and receptors on the surface of a mammalian cell has gained wide acceptance and appears to have great potential due to the simplicity of modifying a large range of implant materials (Table 1). Often the peptides used are designed to mimic a small domain found in proteins of the extracellular matrix (ECM), thereby recapitulating the biological activity of the whole protein without the ancillary drawbacks of protein modification of materials (see Section III). By modifying the surface prior to implantation, the material is ensured to interact through designed biomolecular recognition events with specific cell types in lieu of the aforementioned nonspecific interactions (Fig. 1). Potentially, such control could accelerate healing by recruiting targeted cells that generate an ECM consistent with the tissue of interest. This level of specific cell recruitment and native tissue growth ultimately reduces the recuperation time post procedure. For example, for orthopedic, dental, or craniofacial applications, good interfacial bonding or osseointegration is critical for short-term initial stability and long-term success of the implant, since loosening remains a common failure mode and often results in painful and difficult revision surgeries. By accelerating the healing process, less time is required before an implant can be tested under normal load by the patient. A similar analysis can be made for rapid endothelial cell coverage of implants functioning in blood-contacting environments. For example, peptide modification of stainless steels (316L and 304L) used to fabricate intravascular stents could benefit from improved initial blood compatibility associated with rapid endothelialization of the stent surface.

Ordered control of peptides at the interface not only may lead to precise control of the interaction between a biological system and an implant, but may also serve as the basis for cell-based sensing or drug screening devices. An underlying theme between implants and cell-based sensors is that the biological–synthetic interface must be controlled to achieve a precise response from the cell. A key aspect in designing such an interface is understanding that cells receive input signals when cell surface receptors interact with ligands, such as an immobilized peptide. That signal is then transduced via intracellular signaling and feedback pathways to create an output, such as protein or DNA synthesis, that is consistent with

Table 1 Representation of Different Materials That Have Been Modified with Peptide Ligands to Promote Direct Engagement with Cell-Surface Receptors[a]

Construct	Surface/material	Peptide signal	Ref.
Two dimensional surface treatment	Poly(ethylene terephthalate) (PET)	RGD, FN-C/H-V	100,127–129
	Fluorinated ethylene propylene copolymers	RGD, IKVAV, YIGSR, collagen mimetic (GP-Nleu)$_{10}$GP	130,131
	Glycophase glass	RGD, YIGSR, VAPG, KQAGDV	7,132–135
	Glass	KRSR	44
	Glassy carbon	IKVAV, CDPGYIGSR, PDSGR, YFQRYLI, RNIAEIIKDA	136
	Quartz	RGD, FHRRIKA	13,30,45
	Polyvinylalcohols	RGD	137,138
	Polyurethanes	RGD	139–141
	Polyacrylamide gels	RGD	69
	Polytetrafluoroethylene (PTFE)	RGD, YIGSR	8,100,133,134
	Acrylic acid–based copolymers	RGD, YIGSR, PHSRN, REDV, PRRARV	31,84,142–146
	Langmuir-Blodgett films (self-assembly)	RGD amphiphiles	147
	Polystyrene	FN-C/H-V, RGD, BSA-RGD	70,94,129
	Titanium	RGD, FHRRIKA	32,107,148,149
	Self-assembly on gold coatings	RGD, GVKGDKGN-PGTPGAP, YIGSR, IKVAV	85,150,151
	Stainless steel	RGD	99

Table 1 Continued

Construct	Surface/material	Peptide signal	Ref.
	Alginate	RGD	152
	Bovine anorganic bone mineral	P-15 (collagen-derived peptide)	153
	Silk-based materials	RGD	154
Three-dimensional matrices	Acrylamide based copolymers	RGD, FHRRIKA	14,119
	Alginate	BMP-2-derived peptide	120
	Agarose	RGD, YIGSR, IKVAV	17
	Collagen/ glycosamino-glycan matrices	RGD	101

[a]References are organized according to the mode of modification, either two-dimensional surface treatments or peptide modification of a material in three dimensions.

the phenotype of the cell (Fig. 1). This output ultimately governs how the cells interact with the underlying substrate and thus determines the success of the device or implant.

In this chapter we seek to point out the parameters that are important in the fabrication of mimetic peptide materials capable of controlling cell differentiation both in vitro and in vivo. We invoke themes from our own work that have general applicability for peptide modification of materials. The chapter first introduces the selection criteria for a particular peptide and then addresses the importance of ligand density and accessibility, surface treatments that prevent protein adsorption but enhance specific cell–material interactions, and, finally, three-dimensional matrices for tissue regeneration.

II. RATIONAL DESIGN OF MIMETIC SURFACES

The existence of a divergent range of biomimetic design strategies has prompted the search for application-specific design parameters useful for predicting the biological performance of these engineered surfaces a priori. The quest for such parameters has been complicated by the complex nature of ligand–receptor engagement and associated intracellular signaling and

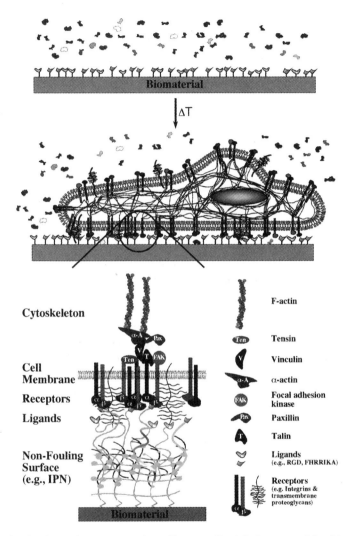

Figure 1 A schematic representation of how a cell might interact with a biomimetic material. To control the host–biomaterial response, a biomaterial should first be made nonfouling to prevent nonspecific protein adsorption and then further modified to ensure that the material interacts with specific cell types. Such specific interactions can be designed into the material by coupling bioactive ligands, such as peptides (e.g., -RGD- and -FHRRIKA-), that mimic proteins found within the ECM and are recognized by, and bind to, specific cell surface receptors (e.g., integrins and transmembrane proteoglycans). By using ligands present in the ECM of the tissue of interest, the cellular machinery can be activated, leading to proper phenotypic expression, cell proliferation, differentiation, and ultimately tissue regeneration.

dynamic feedback. However, as a guideline to identifying useful design rules, a previously developed receptor–ligand adhesion model is applicable for simplifying the complicated synergistic mechanisms that govern these events (18–20). The model incorporates three important aspects of receptor–ligand interactions and combines them into a single parameter: cell shear detachment strength (τ_d, dyne/cm^2). These parameters include cell surface receptor number (N, cm^{-2}), surface ligand density (Γ, cm^{-2}), and the receptor-ligand dissociation constant (ψ, dyne/cm^2). The relationship takes the form:

$$\tau_d = G\psi N\Gamma + \lambda \tag{1}$$

where (G) is a geometrical shape factor (assumed to be constant for short adhesion times) and (λ, dyne/cm^2) is a nonspecific cell adhesion constant. The justification that a single parameter, such as τ_d, can be used to establish design rules for cell–material interactions stems from observations made when correlating short-term mean cell–substratum detachment strength ($\bar{\tau}$) (τ_d required for 50% cell detachment) with either cell migration speed or intracellular ERK2 (extracellular signal–regulated kinase) expression (18,21). In both cases the relationship was biphasic in nature, increasing to an optimal level followed by a subsequent decrease. Thus, from a surface engineering standpoint, one can easily alter the ψ and Γ parameters by modification of a material with peptide ligands. The former (ψ) can be adjusted by selecting peptides with different binding affinity to specific receptors, such as peptide–integrin engagement. The later (Γ) can easily be adjusted during the synthesis protocol. In addition to ψ and Γ, the accessibility of the ligand at the surface is critical, and the ability to minimize nonspecific interactions, as identified by the parameter λ, is crucial. First, this chapter addresses ψ by demonstrating the selection process of peptides for interaction with bone-producing cells (i.e., osteoblasts). Second, the chapter discusses the experiments supporting a critical surface density (Γ) for cell adhesion and the requirement that λ must be minimized in the performance environment for the peptide surface modification to be successful.

III. MIMETIC PEPTIDES FOR SURFACE ENGINEERING: IMPORTANT ISSUES FOR PEPTIDE SELECTION

The use of peptides at interfaces holds many advantages over whole-protein immobilization or physisorption. Whole proteins (e.g., fibronectin, vitro-nectin) or protein fragments have been immobilized or physisorbed to surfaces to help develop improved materials (22–25). A major limitation of simple physisorption is that the adsorbed protein can denature, causing a significant conformational change and hence a greatly reduced affinity for a particular cell. In addition, the protein can adsorb in an orientation that makes the cell binding domains inaccessible to cell surface receptors. This is keenly demonstrated by surface protein densities necessary to elicit a favorable cellular response when physisorbed, compared with densities required when short protein fragments, or peptides, are grafted to a surface (26). Furthermore, protein–material interactions due to physisorption can mask the underlying mechanisms responsible for the observed behavior, thus making it difficult to draw absolute conclusions. Consequently, identifying minimal sequences within parent proteins responsible for cell binding or biological activity has gained considerable attention. The pioneering work of Pierschbacher and Ruoslahti (27), which identified the ubiquitous Arg-Gly-Asp (RGD) cell binding domain in fibronectin, set the foundation for modification of materials with peptide ligands. Since this initial discovery, the resources devoted to the identification of new peptide domains with greater specificity for specific cell surface receptors have been enormous. The use of peptides that possess binding affinities similar to that of the parent protein is an attractive approach, since both the surface density and orientation can be controlled more simply. In addition, compared to proteins, peptides are easily synthesized and purified, are relatively inexpensive, do not rely on tertiary structure for bioactivity, are less susceptible to enzymatic degradation, are less likely to elicit an immunogenic response, and do not denature.

In order to engineer a controlled biomaterial–host response to a peptide-modified surface, one must first consider which receptors on the surface of the cell can engage with the peptide ligands on the surface of the material. A popular method exploits cell–substratum adhesion mechanisms by incorporating peptides derived from ECM proteins that interact with either the integrin family of cell surface receptors or cell surface proteoglycans (6,7,13,26,28–32). The ECM is an intricate network of macromolecules composed of polysaccharides and a variety of proteins (collagenous and noncollagenous) that are secreted locally by the cells and assembled into an organized network surrounding the cells within tissues (24,33). Domains on these proteins are used by cells for attachment, migration, and differentiation, and therefore serve as ideal candidates to incorporate into the structure of synthetic materials. Cells interact with these domains on ECM proteins through transmembrane receptors, such as the integrin class of receptors. Integrins are heterodimer receptors, containing α and β subunits, that play a key role in various biological phenomena and disorders, including embryonic development, thrombosis, blood clotting, would healing, inflammation, osteoporosis, and cancer (27,34,35). Integrins interact with cell binding domains on ECM proteins, such as the ubiquitous arginine-glycine-aspartic acid (RGD) tripeptide sequence, through a binding site created by the dimeric, noncovalent interaction between α and β subunits (34,36,37). In contrast to integrin binding, cell surface proteoglycans (e.g., heparan sulfate) bind to ligands via purely electrostatic interactions. This binding is highly dependent on the spacial location of the charges within the ligand. For example, the negatively charged carboxyl and sulfate groups present in heparin interact with the positively charged heparin binding domains present in ECM proteins through consensus amino acid sequences such as [X-B-B-X-B-X] (X, hydrophobic; B, positive basic residue) (6,38,39).

In selecting a specific peptide sequence to engage with a particular cell surface receptor (e.g., integrin), one must understand the potential ECM proteins that the cell will typically encounter. For example, in osseous tissue, the ECM is composed of about 90% collagenous and about 10% noncollagenous proteins. Some of the noncollagenous proteins include osteopontin (OPN), bone sialoprotein (BSP), fibronectin (FN), vitronectin (VN), osteonectin (OSN), and thrombospondin (TS) (24,40). Many of these ECM proteins contain the ubiquitous RGD sequence, which has been incorporated into various peptides to enhance cell adhesion and interaction on biomaterial surfaces (see Refs. (6) and (41) for reviews). In addition to the cell binding domains, various heparin binding domains (42,43), such as Lys-Arg-Ser-Arg (-KRSR-) (44) and Phe-His-Arg-Arg-Ile-Lys-Ala (-FHRRIKA-) (13,30,45), have been used in a synergistic fashion with RGD to promote cell adhesion and spreading. By providing the cell with both the cell binding and heparin binding domains, the cellular response to the material becomes more "complete" (e.g., cell attachment, spreading, formation of discrete focal contacts, and organized assembly of the cytoskeleton) (13,42,44,46), which is critical to developing a truly biomimetic material and fostering cell differentiation.

When choosing sequences to ellicit specific receptor–ligand interactions, it is also important to consider the amino acids flanking the signal (e.g., RGD), which are specific for different ECM proteins and therefore tissues. Many studies have illustrated the importance of the flanking amino acids in determining the activity and specificity of RGD and other binding sites, where slight changes in or around the binding site result in diminished or abolished cell binding activity (27,47–51). For example, changing Asp to Glu in the RGD binding site (i.e., an addition of a methylene group) abolishes cell binding activity.

The work by Rezania et al. (13) demonstrates how these themes can be incorporated into the design of mimetic peptide surfaces containing different ratios of cell binding (-RGD-) and heparin binding (-FHRRIKA-) peptides derived from bone sialoprotein (BSP). It has been hypothesized that specific attachment of osteoblasts to the bone ECM resides within enzymatically generated fragments of BSP and that signals embedded in these fragments modulate osteoblast attachment and differentiation. Therefore, grafting short peptide fragments containing these signals to implant materials should promote osteogenic cell adhesion and function at an osseous implant interface to ensure better interfacial bonding with bone. BSP is ideal for endosseous applications since it is mainly specific to mature bone cells, is the major noncollagenous ECM protein secreted by osteoblasts (52–54), is primarily localized in mineralized connective tissues, and is up-regulated during bone formation (55). First isolated by Herring in 1972 from fetal bone, BSP was determined to be a highly glycosylated, acidic protein rich in glutamic acid (56,57). Rezania et al. (13) developed mimetic peptide surfaces (MPSs) by mixing different ratios of the -RGD- and -FHRRIKA- signals identified in BSP to examine the effect of ligand density and signal on primary osteoblast-like cell morphology, degree of spreading, number and strength of adhesions, focal contract formation, cytoskeletal organization, and degree of matrix mineralization (-RGD-:-FHRRIKA-, 25:75 MPS I, 75:25 MPS II, and 50:50 MPS III) (13,45,58,59). MPS II and III promoted greater spreading, strength of adhesion, focal contact and cytoskeletal organization, and mineralization of the deposited matrix compared with other surfaces (control and homogeneous). In addition, mature focal contact formation and cytoskeletal organization were examined using fluorescent staining of vinculin (focal contacts; indirect immunofluorescence) and F-actin (cytoskeleton; rhodamine-conjugated phalloidin) (Fig. 2) to examine rat calvarial osteoblast (RCO) behavior on different mimetic surfaces. It was determined that -RGD (either homogeneous or on MPS) was required for extensive focal contact formation and cytoskeletal organization. Although homogeneous -FHRRIKA- surfaces were shown to support cell adhesion and spreading (13), these substrates were insufficient in promoting focal contact formation or cytoskeletal organization. Since these surfaces were developed to enhance cell adhesion, the strength of cell adhesion via receptor–ligand interactions was examined using a radial flow apparatus (RFA). The RFA permitted controlled shear of cells from surfaces via an axisymmetric laminar flow (about 10–85 dyne/cm^2) (58). Data from these experiments suggest that integrin- and proteoglycan-mediated cell adhesion (homogeneous -RGD- and -FHRRIKA- surfaces, respectively) was similar under the applied hydrodynamic forces. In addition, the RFA and a panel of monolclonal anti-integrin antibodies were used to examine integrin-mediated adhesion events. These results suggested that initial adhesion events (< 30 min) of human

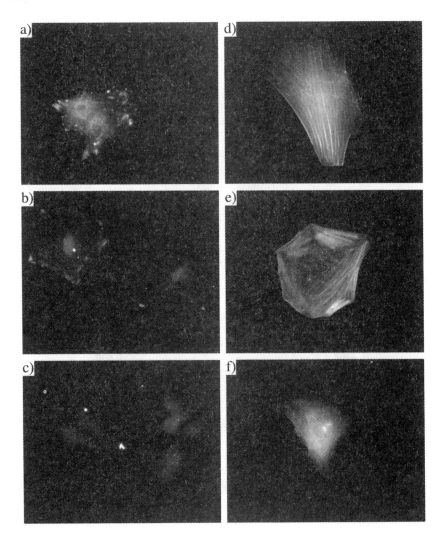

Figure 2 Representative images of cytoskeletal (d, e, f) and focal contact formation (a, b, c) on -RGD- (a, d), 50:50 -RGD-:-FHRRIKA- mix (MPS III) (b, e) and -FHRRIKA- (c, f) modified metal oxide substrates. Note the cytoskeletal organization on -RGD- and MPS III surfaces but not on homogeneous -FHRRIKA- grafted surfaces. Similarly, homogeneous -FHRRIKA- grafted surfaces were incapable of supporting mature focal contact formation unlike -RGD- and MPS III modified surfaces, which showed focal contacts localized to the periphery of the cell. In both respects, -FHRRIKA- surfaces behaved similarly to negative controls (-RGE- and -RFHARIK- surfaces), with the exception that these surfaces promoted cell spreading (13).

trabecular osteoblast-like cells (HTO cells) were governed by both the collagen ($\alpha_2\beta_1$) and vitronectin integrin receptors ($\alpha_v\beta_3$), where as longer term events ($> 30\,\text{min}$) were governed primarily by the vitronectin receptor (45).

Given the synergistic effect of the two ligands, surfaces with both cell binding and heparin binding domains (MPS II and MPS III) were shown to be more biologically relevant and specific for RCO cell function than those with homogeneous -RGD- and -FHRRIKA- modified surfaces. The temporal dependence on different ligands in mediating bone cell attachment to modified surfaces represents a useful strategy for developing materials with specificity to cell adhesion (45). By developing surfaces with the proper ratios of the different peptides, cells are presented with signals that allow both integrin- and proteoglycan-mediated adhesion and subsequently a more complete or biological signal (42,46). This strategy has been shown to result in enhanced cellular function and expression of mineralized tissue in vitro and provides an ideal strategy to elicit biological responses in other types of tissue.

IV. MIMETIC PEPTIDE SURFACES AND SCAFFOLDS TO MODULATE CELL BEHAVIOR

A. Molecular Modeling

Ideally, computer modeling could be employed to examine possible surface modifications and peptide sequence perturbations prior to material fabrication in a laboratory, which can be both expensive and time consuming. As previously stated, RGD-containing peptides are important in modulating cell surface adhesion and spreading either in solid-phase assays in which peptides have been immobilized onto solid substrates or in solution, where the peptides act as antagonists to cell adhesion. Since slight changes around or within the RGD binding region leads to diminished or abolished activity, the conformation of this region is crucial for ligand–receptor interactions (60). For this reason it is critical to relate structural conformation of this region to activity in order to develop potent adhesion peptides for use on biomimetic surfaces or in pharmaceutical development. Therefore, many authors have studied this region using molecular modeling, solution nuclear magnetic resonance (NMR) and X-ray crystallography (51,61–68). If simple models can be developed to predict structure–function relationships pertaining to various surfaces and active domains, then considerable progress would be made toward the rapid engineering of biocompatible and biologically active materials.

To this end, a robust molecular model was developed to study the interactions of bioactive peptides covalently coupled to model implant surfaces (rutile TiO_2/Ti) and to help develop criteria to assess structure–function relationships of peptide regions such as the RGD domain (66). The model allowed the investigation of the effect of both solvent (H_2O) and substrate on peptide structure and orientation. Of particular interest was the conformation of the -RGD- region within a 15-amino-acid peptide derived from BSP (Ac-Cys-Gly-Gly-Asn-Gly-Glu-Pro-Arg-Gly-Asp-Thr-Tyr-Arg-Ala-Tyr-NH_2 (-RGD-). Molecular mechanic and dynamic simulations suggested that the layer thickness was dependent on the crystal face and lattice spacing, the extent of monolayer coverage (packing density), and the underlying substrate (SiO_2 or TiO_2). The models representing the organosilane, cross-linker, and peptide layers closely predicted layer thicknesses observed experimentally with spectroscopic ellipsometry (30). Results indicated that the inactive -RGE- domain was not as broad or solvent accessible as the active -RGD- domain (Fig. 3). On average the distances between charge centers $(C+/C-)$ for -RGD- and -RGE- were $13.06\,\text{Å}$ and $10.1\,\text{Å}$, respectively. In addition, it was concluded that the substrate had minimal effect on the conformation of the -RGD- region when a sufficient distance between the surface and the peptide was present (i.e., the length of the spacer arm is sufficient). The distance between the substrate and the active binding site is an important issue because the availability of the ligand to interact with cell surface receptors is critical for control of cell behavior. To further address this issue, Section IV.B.2 examines the effect of spacer chains and coupling distances.

B. Ligand Surface Density and Accessibility Effects

1. Ligand Surface Density

To fully develop materials that interact with cells in a predictable manner, it is necessary to obtain a clear understanding of the effects of peptide ligand density (Γ) on the kinetics of cell function and attachment. Recent studies by Massia and Hubbell (7,26), Brandley et al. (69), Danilov et al. (70), and Rezania and Healy (59) examined the minimal number of adhesive ligands required for short-term (cell attachment, spreading, focal contact formation, and cell migration) and long-term (e.g., cell differentiation) cellular events on model biomaterials, thus contributing to this understanding. In particular, Massia and Hubbell (26) showed that ligand density controlled cell adhesion, spreading, and focal contact formation. Using fibroblasts, their results suggest that cell spreading required a minimal RGD ligand density of 1 fmol/cm^2, while cell spreading *and* focal contact formation required a minimum

a)   b)

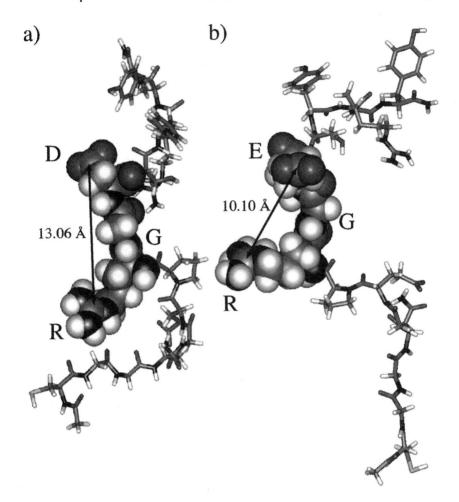

Figure 3 Representative peptide structures for (a) -RGD- (ac-CGGNGEP**RGD**-TYRAY-NH$_2$) and (b) -RGE- (ac-CGGNGEP**RGE**TYRAY-NH$_2$) showing that the active -RGD- binding site is broader and more solvent accessible than the inactive -RGE- binding site. For -RGD- C+/C− = 13.06 Å and for RGE- C+/C− = 10.10 Å. (Figure adapted from Ref. 155 with permission.)

density of 10 fmol/cm^2. In general, these data were supported by observations from another cell type, e.g., osteoblasts, and a different RGD-based peptide, indicating the potential universal nature of this response. Rezania et al. (30) showed that RCO cell adhesion and spreading were significantly enhanced at higher ligand densities (> 0.6 pmol/cm^2) compared with lower densities $(0.01\,\text{pmol/cm}^2)$ (Fig. 4) on quartz substrates modified with an -RGD- peptide from BSP. This universal observation of ligand density effect may be due to the saturation of a specific type of integrin (i.e., receptor) present on the cell surface $(N, \sim 10^5/\text{cell})$.

Various mathematical models have also been developed to study ligand–density effects. For example, Ward et al. (71,72) showed that at high ligand densities $(\sim 10^{12}/\text{cm}^2)$, the critical stress necessary to peel a cell from a surface was independent of ligand density and logarithmically dependent on receptor number $(N, \sim 10^5/\text{cell})$. However, at low ligand densities $(\sim 10^6/\text{cm}^2)$, the critical stress was logarithmically dependent on ligand density but independent of receptor number (N). Kuo et al. (73) have provided experimental evidence to support these findings.

In addition to cell spreading and focal contact formation, cell migration and the strength of attachment have been correlated to ligand density, as well as integrin-ligand binding affinity and the degree of integrin expression (i.e., number of receptors, N) (21,74,75). At low ligand density cell motility is limited due to too few available binding sites, but at high ligand density cell locomotion is severely restricted by a surface that is too adhesive. For example, DiMilla et al. (74,75) showed that smooth muscle cell attachment strength increased linearly with the concentration of fibronectin physisorbed to glass and that a biphasic relationship existed for cell migration speed due to density effects (surface adhesiveness). In addition, at high ligand densities, the rate of cell spreading and the strength of cell detachment have been shown to plateau (72,76,77), and Zygourakis et al. (78,79) have shown that migration may directly influence proliferation. In fact, Lauffenburger and Horwitz have theorized that an optimal ligand density exists for cell migration and ultimately for phenotypic expression (80).

Long-term events, such as matrix mineralization, are also affected by surface ligand density. Rezania et al. (30,59) demonstrated the density effect of an immobilized peptide containing the cell-binding -RGD- motif on osteoblast-like cell adhesion, spreading, and matrix mineralization in vitro. Data show that higher ligand densities $(> 0.6\,\text{pmol/cm}^2)$, compared with lower densities $(0.01\,\text{pmol/cm}^2)$, were necessary for RCO matrix mineralization (Fig. 5) (59). For example, peptide-modified surfaces (-RGD-, $\Gamma > 0.6\,\text{pmol/cm}^2$) supported $\sim 85\%$ mineral coverage compared to surfaces with adsorbed protein $(\sim 27\%)$ or surfaces at lower densities $(0.01\,\text{pmol/cm}^2 \sim 1\%)$. In general, these matrix mineralization results are similar to what Zhou et al. (81) reported for MC3T3-E1 cells (osteoblast-like) on surfaces preadsorbed with different concentrations of BSP. However, a major limitation associated with studies in which cellular activities are characterized on surfaces defined by adsorbed proteins is that the surface density of

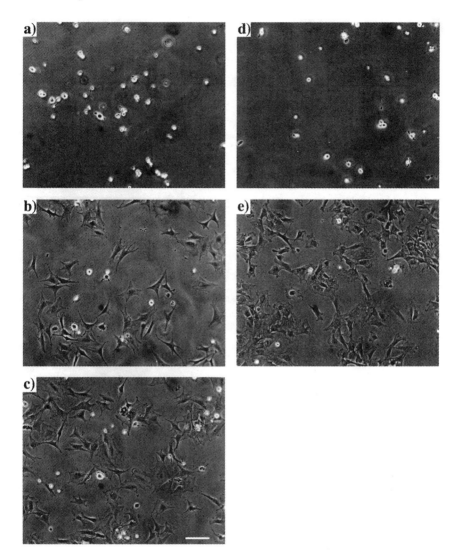

Figure 4 Phase contrast microscopy images of rat calvarial osteoblasts seeded on peptide-modified quartz substrates following 4 h of incubation in the presence of 1% BSA in DMEM, (a) 0.01 pmol/cm² -RGD-, (b) 0.62 pmol/cm² -RGD, (c) 4 pmol/cm² -RGD-, (d) -RGE-, (e) TCPS with 15% FBS. TCPS and -RGD- grafted substrates with ligand densities $\geqslant 0.62$ pmol/cm² showed the highest degree of cell attachment and spreading. Scale bar, 100 μm. (Figure adapted from Ref. 30 with permission.)

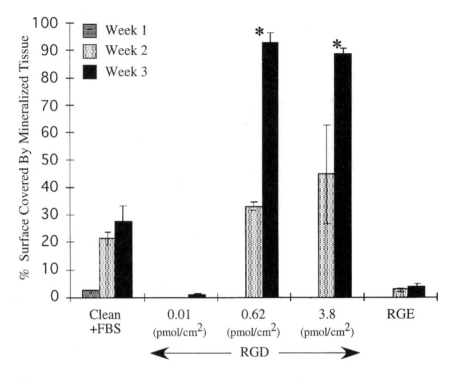

Figure 5 Homogeneous -RGD- surface density effect on mineralized tissue formation. Peptide-modified quartz disks were seeded with rat calvarial osteoblasts, the cells were allowed to reach confluence, and the substrates were stained for calcified tissue using Von Kossa stain following 1, 2, and 3 weeks of incubation in mineralization media (post confluency). -RGD- surface densities equal to or greater than $0.62 \, \text{pmol/cm}^2$ showed significantly greater ($p < 0.05$) mineralized matrix formation than other surfaces [$0.01 \, \text{pmol/cm}^2$ -RGD-, and controls (-RGE- ($\sim 4 \, \text{pmol/cm}^2$) and clean + adsorbed serum proteins)]. (Adapted from Ref. 59 with permission.)

the active ligand is unknown and is difficult to quantify. Therefore, it is difficult to use these surfaces to fully characterize cell–material interactions for developing new materials. One means for circumventing this effect is to use engineered surfaces that are nonfouling (Section IV.C.), and have a defined available ligand density and orientation.

2. Ligand Accessibility

In addition to ligand density, ligand accessibility is crucial for developing biomimetic materials for tissue engineering. Therefore, work has been done to study the effect of using different cross-linkers and chain lengths (82–85) to bind the active ligand (i.e., protein or peptide) to model surfaces or pharmaceuticals. For example, Houseman and Mrksich (85) created nonfouling bioactive self-assembled monolayers on gold substrates using RGD grafted to different oligo(ethylene glycol) units (i.e., tri-, tetra-, penta-, and hexa-). Results demonstrated that the attachment and spreading of 3T3 fibroblast to these monolayers presenting the same peptide density decreased as glycol chain length increased. In accordance with these results, the strength of cell–substrate interaction decreased as chain length increased. In a complementary study, Dori et al. (83) created Langmuir-Blodgett lipid membranes on mica using either pure poly(ethylene glycol) (PEG) lipids with headgroups of different lengths or a 50 mol% binary mixture of the PEG lipids and a collagen-like peptide amphiphile. Results showed that human melanoma cell adhesion and spreading depended on the length of the head group. On mixed surfaces in which the head group was shorter than the amphiphile, cells adhered and spread. In contrast, on surfaces in which the PEG headgroup was approximately the same length as the amphiphile, cells adhered but did not spread. Finally, on mixed surfaces where the PEG lipid was approximately twice the length as the amphiphile (e.g., amphiphile not accessible), cells neither adhered nor spread, consistent with results observed on the nonfouling surfaces with only the PEG lipids. In another study, Hern and Hubbell (84) demonstrated the effect of a PEG spacer arm on RGD binding activity. In this study, an RGD peptide, with or without a 3400 MW PEG spacer arm, was incorporated into a photopolymerized cross-linked hydrogel network of PEG diacrylate. Without peptide, modified substrates permitted spreading of only 5% of seeded human foreskin fibroblasts after 24 h. With no spacer arm, RGD and RDG (inactive control) supported spreading of about 50% and 15% of cells, respectively, in serum-containing media. However, when the 3400 MW spacer arm was incorporated into the network, RGD surfaces with the same ligand density supported 70% spreading, whereas RDG surfaces supported no spreading. Therefore, without the 3400 MW spacer, substrates supported nonspecific cell spreading but specificity was reintroduced by incorporating the spacer. These results clearly demonstrate the effect of ligand accessibility on cell adhesion and illustrate the extreme importance in developing well-defined surfaces for controlled and specific cell–material interactions.

C. Development and Bioactivation of Nonfouling Surfaces

Several nonfouling surface treatments have been developed to minimize nonspecific interactions (e.g., protein adsorption) between a material and biological environments. Many of these surfaces are amenable to functionalization with a wide range of macromolecules (e.g., peptides and growth factors), which makes them ideal to fully examine the *receptor–ligand adhesion model* (see Section II). Specifically, as λ is minimized [see Eq. (1)], the biological performance of a peptide-modified material can be modulated by manipulating Γ and ψ, without interfering nonspecific macromolecular (e.g., protein) adsorption. The prevention of protein adsorption is critical for developing peptide-modified materials for use in complex biological environments since protein adsorption can mask the specific signal and any subsequent analysis. The following section discusses the development of these "nonfouling" platforms and how they have been used to engineer biospecific surfaces for various applications.

To develop nonfouling materials, the unique properties of PEG, which has demonstrated low protein, cell, and bacterial adhesion due to its unique interaction with water, have been exploited (29). When a PEG-enriched region comes into contact with water, a protective hydration shell forms around the PEG molecules. When other molecules, such as proteins, encounter this hydrated water shell, protein adsorption is unfavorable, and cell and bacterial adhesion are unlikely due to a combination of water structure, entropic repulsion, and osmotic pressure effects (86–88). Given these beneficial properties, PEG is an excellent candidate for modifying materials with nonfouling coatings. However, as discussed in Section IV.B.2, PEG chain length can have a significant effect on the nonfouling character and therefore must be considered when developing these materials (84,89). In addition, other materials have been examined for their nonfouling properties. For example, Massia et al. (90) investigated dextran as an alternative surface modification to PEG. In this study, glass and PET surfaces modified with a 70-kDa MW dextran resisted fouling when exposed to 3T3 fibroblasts in a serum-containing environment. Similar to PEG, dextran modifications allow for high-density immobilization of bioactive molecules and provide another possible nonfouling surface with the propensity for control of Γ and ψ.

Various methodologies have been utilized to modify materials with PEG for numerous applications. PEG-based materials have been studied for use as blood-contacting materials for cardiovascular applications, as bone-contacting materials to enhance osseointegration, in pharmaceuticals to promote greater solubility, and have been proposed as coatings to prevent postoperative adhesions or to encourage tissue resurfacing. Some modification methodologies include self-assembly or chemisorption (85,91–94), plasma deposition (95), and photochemical grafting (29,31,84,96,97). Examples of applications resulting from chemisorption and grafting can be found in Section IV.B.2.

Due to their greater stability and consistency, coatings that are covalently bonded to the underlying material have an advantage over chemisorbed modifications. An adaptation on this theme is the development of materials that are physically cross-linked. One such technology is the formation of interpenetrating polymer networks (IPNs), composed of two or more cross-linked, intertwined networks that typically demonstrate improved mechanical properties and strength due to the forced compatibility of the components. Bearinger et al. (31,96) developed an IPN using photoinitiated free-radical polymerization on metal oxides (e.g., quartz, glass, and silicon wafers). After modifying the metal oxide with an unsaturated organosilane, an IPN of poly(acrylamide-*co*-ethylene glycol/acrylic acid) [P(AAm-*co*-EG/AAc)] was formed with a nominal thickness of about 20 nm using a two-stage discontinuous solution photopolymerization of AAm and EG/AAc. The acrylic acid in the network makes the IPN amenable to surface grafting of biological molecules (e.g., -RGD- and -FHRRIKA-) through the carboxylic acid sites, allowing for control of Γ (~ 0.1 to $10\,\text{pmol/cm}^2$) and ψ. X-ray photoelectron spectroscopy (XPS) results indicated the formation of the IPN, as well as the near-surface peptide functionality. The IPN prevented protein adsorption in complex serum-containing environments (e.g., in vivo), and when grafted with the -RGD- bioactive peptide from BSP ($\Gamma \sim 10\,\text{pmol/cm}^2$) using a 3400 MW PEG spacer chain, these IPNs promoted osteoblast adhesion and phenotypic expression (i.e., membrane-bound alkaline phosphatase and mineralized matrix formation) (31).

In addition to Si-based materials, the IPN has been transferred to polystyrene for rapid screening on functionalized nonadhesive surfaces (manuscript in preparation), as well as to clinically relevant titanium (98) and 316L stainless steel (99). Following IPN modification and functionalization with -RGD-, TiO_2/Ti disks showed enhanced RCO matrix mineralization compared with untreated titanium in vitro (98), and peptide-functionalized IPN-modified titanium intramedullary rods showed promising results in vivo (Section IV.D.2). For use in cardiovascular applications (e.g., intravascular stents), 316L stainless steel was modified with the IPN and prevented human coronary artery endothelial cell (HCAEC) adhesion compared with controls and unmodified material, which supported substantial adhesion and proliferation (manuscript in progress). Since the IPN can be functionalized with various macromolecules, different EC-specific peptides could be identified and then coupled to the IPN-modified stent to encourage endothelialization and improve initial blood compatibility. Such EC-specific attachment, migration, and proliferation would generate a native tissue layer on the stent that could arrest the cascade of events that can lead to neointimal hyperplasia, restenosis, and subsequent device failure, and therefore prove to be a valuable biomimetic surface treatment. The nonfouling treatment of surfaces with subsequent reintroduction of biospecificity through ligands derived from ECM proteins is an attractive approach to developing new biomaterials and therefore will continue to receive substantial research attention.

D. Biomimetic Surfaces In Vivo

1. In Vivo Studies on Peptide-Modified Materials

Although in vitro studies are essential for the development of new biomaterials, a material that has shown promise in vitro must ultimately be tested in vivo to demonstrate the effect of the various surface treatments or material constructs. To date, few studies have been published which demonstrate the effects of peptide or growth factor modified materials in vivo. Tweden et al. (100) modified cardiovascular devices (polytetrafluoroethylene vascular patches and polyethyleneterephthalate cardiac valves) with a peptide containing RGD (PepTite) and assessed their biological response using vascular and cardiac valve models in the dog. In the vascular model, modified materials enhanced endothelial-like cell attachment and layer formation compared to unmodified controls. In addition, a reduced neointima formed on the polyethyleneterephthalate-modified material compared with controls. This latter result was similar to what was reported using the valve model. The coated materials produced a thinner neointima and resulted in less thrombus formation. Peptide modified materials have also been shown to be beneficial in the enhancement of dermal and corneal wound healing. Grzesiak et al. (101) reported that a viscous gel of hylauronic acid modified with an RGD-containing peptide improved dermal wound healing. When this same peptide was combined with chondroitin sulfate for use in clinical studies, the composite material aided in restructuring the architecture of the normal eye surface, which had reduced tear volume due to aging and autoimmune diseases (102). Acceleration of the healing process can both improve the quality of the regenerated tissue and limit the fibrous encapsulation that occurs with many implants by quickly generating a native tissue layer.

With orthopedic and dental implants, accelerated healing and recruitment of osteogenic cells is critical to ensure osteointegration and good bone-material apposition. Over the last few decades, in vivo studies to improve orthopedic and dental implants have mainly examined the ability of surface macro- and microarchitectures to stimulate bone growth and ensure implant fixation. One such treatment is the use of plasma sprayed coatings of hydroxyapaetite and tricalcium phosphate (i.e., bioceramics). Although bioceramics (see Refs. 103 and 104 for review) can be remodeled to produce osseous tissue, there remains a problem with degradation and delamination of the ceramic coating due to poor metal–ceramic bonding. In addition, these coatings and treatments remain non-biospecific and appear to interact via receptor-mediated interactions only through nonspecifically adsorbed serum proteins. Surface modification of these materials with biospecific macromolecules therefore remains an attractive solution. For example, titanium implants treated with a transforming growth factor β stimulated bone in-growth in large defects and were able to bridge bone implant gaps of 3 mm (105,106). However, the use of growth factors in large-scale implant production is limited by availability, stability, and expense. Therefore, small synthetic peptides provide a viable solution due to the aforementioned benefits (Section III). The following section discusses two recent in vivo pilot studies using peptide-modified titanium intramedullary rods.

2. Preliminary In Vivo Experiments with Peptide-Modified Titanium Intramedullary Rods

Few in vivo results have been reported for implants modified with peptides to enhance bone–implant interactions in osseous tissue. The ultimate goal is to effect short-term events to stimulate rapid bone growth and osseointegration of orthopedic and dental implants and thus enhance the rate of healing. Ferris et al. (107) modified titanium implants by first coating the implant with 500 Å of gold and then using well-established self-assembly gold-thiol techniques to form a monolayer of self-assembled bioactive peptide (Arg-Gly-Asp-Cys). Following 2 and 4 weeks of implantation in a rat femoral model, the implant–bone interface was tested for mechanical strength using a standard pull-out test and examined for new bone growth using histology. This pilot study reported encouraging results. After 2 and 4 weeks, a significantly thicker shell of new bone was reported around the RGDC-modified implants compared with the unmodified gold-coated controls. In addition, there was a significant increase in bone thickness between the second and fourth week on RGDC-modified implants, but no significant increase on unmodified implants. As Ferris et al. (107) discuss, results may not be directly related to RGD–receptor interactions but to nonspecific interactions between adsorbed proteins to the modified implant. One way of addressing the latter issue is to use peptide-inactive controls (i.e., RGE) with similar surface energies to allow direct comparison between active and inactive surfaces. Ideally, the implant surface would be nonfouling to prevent nonspecific protein adsorption and then have specific functionality reintroduced to control receptor–ligand interactions. A recent pilot study (unpublished) explores the feasibility of the latter case.

Previous data from our group demonstrated the effectiveness of the peptide grafted IPN in vitro in promoting the osteogenic phenotype (Section IV.C). To test the IPN and the efficacy of biomimetic surface modifications to enhance the bone–implant interface in vivo, titanium rods (+99.99% purity, 1 mm diameter; Goodfellow, PA) were cut to 15-mm lengths, polished, cleaned (Kroll's reagent), and passivated (nitric acid). Modification of the rods with the IPN was confirmed using XPS. IPN-TiO_2/Ti rods were then modified with a 50:50 mixture of -RGD-:-FHRRIKA- and sterilized (70% EtOH) using previously published methods (30,31). In this pilot study, unmodified and modified titanium rods were implanted bilaterally into the femurs of eight animals following

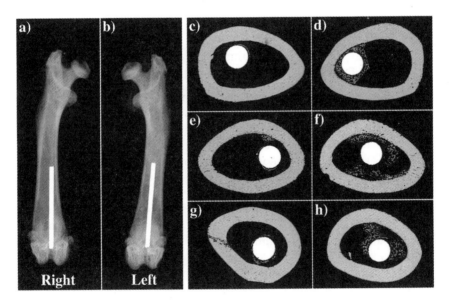

Figure 6 In vivo results of peptide-grafted, IPN-modified titanium rods. Panels a and b are contact radiographs of intact femora following 7 days. Panels c–h are representative cross-sectional scanning electron micrographs, taken in the backscattering mode, for different implants. Control implants (c, e, g) and 50:50 -RGD-: -FHRRIKA- modified implants (d, f, h) from the right and left femur of three rats. Note the increased bone formation and trabecular morphology of the bone around the peptide-modified implants.

a marrow ablation model in the rat (Fig. 6a, b) (108,109). The implant placed in the right femur was unmodified and served as a control while that placed in the left femur had been modified with the peptide coating. Following 7 days post operation, animals were sacrificed and the femurs were collected and sectioned. Sections were imaged using back-scattered scanning electron microscopy, and new bone that formed adjacent to the implant was quantified using digital analysis. Two methods were utilized to measure new-bone formation. In the first method, five of the eight animals showed higher mean values of new bone in the femur with the peptide-modified implant compared with the unmodified one. In the second method, six of the eight animals showed higher mean values for the modified implant (Fig. 6c–h). In terms of appearance, the newly formed bone was intramembranous with no evident endochondral phase. In addition, new bone either formed mostly in the vicinity of the implant (Fig. 6d) or filled more of the medullary cavity (Fig. 6f, h). Although the peptide-modified implants resulted in higher mean values of quantified new bone, the differences were not statistical. This is probably due to the variance in response due to placement of the implants and will be addressed in future studies. In addition, to fully examine the effectiveness of the IPN peptide surfaces, mechanical pull-out tests should be performed and are currently planned (110). The results from this pilot study and that of Ferris et al. (107) are encouraging and therefore warrant further investigation to prove the efficacy of using peptide-modified implants to enhance osseous tissue formation in vivo. This technology could easily be combined with a current paradigm of using implants with porous surface macroarchitectures (i.e., sintered beads). This would enhance the mechanical pull-out strength due to tissue in-growth as well as the bone–biomaterial apposition due to the bioactive chemical treatment.

E. Functionalized Polymer Matrices for Tissue Regeneration

As discussed in this chapter, the modification of material surfaces is an attractive route to develop new and improved "smart" biomaterials. A natural extension of this technology is to move from two-dimensional surfaces to three-dimensional (3D) polymer matrices, or scaffolds, to accelerate tissue regeneration by fabrication with various bioactive molecules (e.g., peptides, growth factors). 3D polymer matrices have been studied extensively in numerous tissue engineering initiatives, including the regeneration of bone (111,112), cartilage (113,114), blood vessels (115), and peripheral nerves (116). When isolated cells are seeded into the scaffolds, the 3D structures guide the cells' organization and development into tissue both in vitro and in vivo (117,118). Scaffolds act as artificial 3D templates and serve to mimic the in vivo environment of the native ECM, providing a milieu in which the cells can proliferate, differentiate, maintain their natural phenotype, and ultimately function as a tissue. Both natural (113,114,116) and synthetic (111,115) polymers have been used to construct scaffolds, and various fabrication methods and implantation procedures have been reported (111,113–116). In addition, several studies have described the modification of scaffolds with biomolecules to promote interactions between the matrices and the biological environment (i.e., cells and ECM components) (14,17,119,120).

Stile et al. reported the development of injectable 3D polymer scaffolds for use in tissue engineering applications (121). The scaffolds, which consisted of loosely cross-linked networks of *N*-isopropylacrylamide (NIPAAm) and acrylic acid (AAc), i.e., P(NIPAAm-*co*-AAc) hydrogels, were injectable through a small-diameter aperture at 22°C. Due to the unique phase behavior of P(NIPAAm) in aqueous media (122–126), the injectable P(NIPAAm-*co*-AAc) hydrogels demonstrated a significant increase in rigidity when heated from 22°C to body temperature (i.e., 37°C), without exhibiting a significant change in volume or water content (121). Furthermore, the hydrogels supported bovine articular chondrocyte viability and promoted articular cartilage-like tissue formation in vitro.

In order to induce interactions between the injectable P(NIPAAm-*co*-AAc) hydrogels and the biological system, the AAc groups in the matrix were functionalized with peptides containing relevant sequences found in ECM macromolecules, such as BSP (14). The peptide conjugation scheme was similar to that used to modify 2D substrates, as described in Ref. 31. Chemical modification of the AAc groups with peptides, verified using a number of different techniques, significantly affected the phase behavior of the P(NIPAAm-*co*-AAc) hydrogels (14). Rat calvarial osteoblasts (RCOs) seeded into the peptide-modified hydrogels were viable for at least 21 days of in vitro culture. In addition, the RCOs spread more and demonstrated significantly greater proliferation, as compared to RCOs seeded into control hydrogels. Thus, these peptide-modified P(NIPAAm-*co*-AAc) hydrogels serve as useful tools for studying cell–material interactions in 3D and show promise for use as injectable scaffolds in tissue engineering applications.

V. CONCLUDING REMARKS

In this chapter, we have attempted to identify the salient aspects of current considerations in the field of biomimetic surface and materials engineering. Important factors include signal selection, density, and accessibility.

Furthermore, careful presentation of mimetic ECM-derived peptides has been demonstrated to be a sound approach for modulating desirable phenotypic expression in complex physiological environments, particularly when applied in conjunction with nonfouling surface engineering. Although the underlying concepts of this approach have been validated, future efforts are needed to establish a set of robust criteria with which to direct the design of these advanced materials. Continuing innovation in these areas promises to significantly impact the biological performance of materials in a wide range of diagnostic and clinical applications.

REFERENCES

1. LL Hench. Biomaterials. Science 208(23):826, 1980.
2. CM Agrawal. Reconstructing the human body using biomaterials. J Mat 50(1):31–35, 1998.
3. KE Healy, A Rezania, RA Stile. Designing biomaterials to direct biological responses. Ann N Y Acad Sci 875:24–35, 1999.
4. JS Hanker, BL Giammara. Biomaterials and biomedical devices. Science 242:885, 1988.
5. B Kasemo, J Lausmaa. Biomaterial and implant surfaces: a surface science approach. Int J Oral Maxillofac Implants 3(4):247–259, 1988.
6. JA Hubbell. Biomaterials in tissue engineering. Biotechnology 13(6):565–576, 1995.
7. SP Massia, JA Hubbell. Covalent surface immobilization of Arg-Gly-Asp- and Tyr-Ile-Gly-Ser-Arg-containing peptides to obtain well-defined cell-adhesive substrates. Anal Biochem 187:292–301, 1990.
8. SP Massia, JA Hubbell. Covalently attached GRGD on polymer surfaces promotes biospecific adhesion of mammalian cells. Ann N Y Acad Sci 589:261–270, 1990.
9. J Bonadio. Tissue engineering via local gene delivery: update and future prospects for enhancing the technology. Adv Drug Deliv Rev 44(2–3):185–194, 2000.
10. JO Hollinger, S Winn, J Bonadio. Options for tissue engineering to address challenges of the aging skeleton. Tissue Eng 6(4):341–350, 2000.
11. ZL Ding, GH Chen, AS Hoffman. Unusual properties of thermally sensitive oligomer-enzyme conjugates of poly(n-isopropylacrylamide)-trypsin. J Biomed Mater Res 39(3):498–505, 1998.
12. AS Hoffman. Bioconjugates of intelligent polymers and recognition proteins for use in diagnostics and affinity separations. Clin Chem 46(9):1478–1486, 2000.
13. A Rezania, KE Healy. Biomimetic peptide surfaces that regulate adhesion, spreading, cytoskeletal organization, and mineralization of the matrix deposited by osteoblast-like cells. Biotechnol Prog 15(1):19–32, 1999.

14. RA Stile, KE Healy. Thermo-responsive peptide-modified hydrogels for tissue regeneration. Biomacromolecules 2:185–194, 2001.

15. Y Tabata, K Yamada, S Miyamoto, I Nagata, H Kikuchi, I Aoyama, M Tamura, Y Ikada. Bone regeneration by basic fibroblast growth factor complexed with biodegradable hydrogels. Biomaterials 19(7–9):807–815, 1998.

16. H Uludag, B Norrie, N Kousinioris, TJ Gao. Engineering temperature-sensitive poly(n-isopropylacrylamide) polymers as carriers of therapeutic proteins. Biotechnol Bioeng 73(6):510–521, 2001.

17. R Bellamkonda, JP Ranieri, P Aebischer. Laminin oligopeptide derivatized agarose gels allow three-dimensional neurite extension in vitro. J Neurosci Res 41(4):501–509, 1995.

18. AR Asthagiri, CM Nelson, AF Horwitz, DA Lauffenburger. Quantitative relationship among integrin-ligand binding, adhesion, and signaling via focal adhesion kinase and extracellular signal–regulated kinase 2. J Biolog Chem 274(38):27119–27127, 1999.

19. AJ García, F Huber, D Boettiger. Force required to break alpha5beta1 integrin-fibronectin bonds in intact adherent cells is sensitive to integrin activation state. J Biol Chem 273(18):10988–10993, 1998.

20. DA Hammer, DA Lauffenburger. A dynamical model for receptor-mediated cell adhesion to surfaces. Biophys J 52:475–487, 1987.

21. SP Palecek, JC Loftus, MH Ginsberg, DA Lauffenburger, AF Horwitz. Integrin-ligand binding properties govern cell migration speed through cell-substratum adhesiveness. Nature 385:537–540, 1997.

22. SK Bhatia, LC Shriver-Lake, KJ Prior, JH Georger, JM Calvert, R Bredehorst, FS Ligler. Use of thiol-terminal silanes and heterobifunctional crosslinkers for immobilization of antibodies on silica surfaces. Anal Biochem 178(2):408–413, 1989.

23. E Delamarche, G Sundarababu, H Biebuyck, B Michel, C Gerber, H Sigrist, H Wolf, H Ringsdorf, N Xanthopoulos, HJ Mathieu. Immobilization of antibodies on a photoactive self-assembled monolayer on gold. Langmuir 12:1997–2006, 1996.

24. WJ Grzesik, PG Robey. Bone matrix RGD glycoproteins: Immunolocalization and interaction with human primary osteoblastic bone cells in vitro. J Bone Miner Res 9(4):487–495, 1994.

25. HG Hong, M Jiang, SG Sligar, PW Bohn. Cysteine-specific surface tethering of genetically engineered cytochromes for fabrication of metalloprotein nanostructures. Langmuir 10:153–158, 1994.

26. SP Massia, JA Hubbell. An RGD spacing of 440 nm is sufficient for integrin $\alpha_v\beta_3$-mediated fibroblast spreading and 140 nm for focal contact and stress fiber formation. J Cell Biol 114(5):1089–1100, 1991.

27. MD Pierschbacher, E Ruoslahti. Cell attachment activity of fibronectin can be duplicated by small synthetic fragments of the molecule. Nature 309:30–33, 1984.

28. SP Massia, JA Hubbell. Biomaterials Which Selectively Support the Attachment of Vascular Endothelial Cells Via a New Adhesion Receptor. Society for Biomaterials, Scottsdale, AZ, 1991, p 238.

29. PD Drumheller, DL Elbert, JA Hubbell. Multifunctional poly(ethylene glycol) semi-interpenetrating networks as highly selective adhesive substrates for bioadhesive peptide grafting. Biotechnol Bioeng 43:772–780, 1994.

30. A Rezania, R Johnson, AR Lefkow, KE Healy. Bioactivation of metal oxide surfaces: I. Surface characterization and cell reponse. Langmuir 15(20):6931–6939, 1999.

31. JP Bearinger, DG Castner, KE Healy. Biomolecular modification of p(AAm-co-EG/AA) IPNs supports osteoblast adhesion and phenotypic expression. J Biomater Sci Polym Ed 9(7):629–652, 1998.

32. SJ Xiao, M Textor, ND Spencer, M Wieland, B Keller, H Sigrist. Immobilization of the cell-adhesive peptide Arg-Gly-Asp-Cys (RGDC) on titanium surfaces by covalent chemical attachment. J Mat Sci, Mat Med 8(12):867–872, 1997.

33. B Alberts, D Bray, J Lewis, M Raff, K Roberts, JD Watson. Cell junctions, cell adhesion, and the extracellular matrix. Molecular biology of the cell. New York: Garland Publishing, 1994, pp 971–1000.

34. RO Hynes. Integrins: Versatility, modulation, and signaling in cell adhesion, Cell 69:11–25, 1992.

35. AF Horwitz. Integrins and health. Sci Am 276(5):68–75, 1997.

36. RO Hynes. Integrins: A family of cell surface receptors. Cell 48:549–554, 1987.

37. CH Damsky. Extracellular matrix–integrin interactions in osteoblast function and tissue remodeling. Bone 25(1):95–96, 1999.

38. FJ Bober Barkalow, JE Schwarzbauer. Localization of the major heprin-binding site in fibronectin. J Biol Chem 266:7812–7818, 1991.

39. AD Cardin, HJR Weintraub. Molecular modeling of protein–glycosamino-glycan interactions. Arteriosclerosis 9:21–32, 1989.

40. MF Young, JM Kerr, K Ibaraki, A Heegard, PG Robey. Structure, expression, and regulation of the major noncollagenous matrix proteins of bone. Clin Orthop Rel Res 281:275–294, 1992.

41. KE Healy. Molecular engineering of materials for bioreactivity. Curr Opin Solid State Mater Sci 4(4):381–387, 1999.

42. BA Dalton, CD McFarland, PA Underwood, JG Steele. Role of the heparin binding domain of fibronectin in attachment and spreading of human bone–derived cells. J Cell Sci 108(5):2083–2092, 1995.

43. J Laterra, JE Silbert, LA Culp. Cell surface heparan sulfate mediates some adhesive responses to glycosaminoglycan-binding matrices, including fibronectin. J Cell Biol 96(1):112–123, 1983.

44. KC Dee, TT Anderson, R Bizios. Design and function of novel osteoblast-adhesive peptides for chemical modification of biomaterials. J Biomed Mater Res 40(3):371–377, 1998.

45. A Rezania, KE Healy. Integrin subunits responsible for adhesion of human osteoblast–like cells to biomimetic peptide surfaces. J Orthop Res 17(4):615–623, 1999.

46. A Woods, JR Couchman, S Johansson, M Hook. Adhesion and cytoskeletal organisation of fibroblasts in response to fibronectin fragments. EMBO J 5(4):665–670, 1986.

47. M Sato, V Garsky, RJ Majeska, TA Einhorn, J Murray, AH Tashjian Jr., RJ Gould. Structure–activity studies of s-echistatin inhibition of bone resorption. J Bone Miner Res 9(9):1441–1449, 1994.

48. T Maeda, K Hashino, R Oyama, K Titani, K Sekiguchi. Artificial cell adhesive proteins engineered by grafting the Arg-Gly-Asp cell recognition signal: factors modulating the cell adhesive activity of the grafted signal. J Biochem (Tokyo) 110:381–387, 1991.

49. A Hautanen, J Gailit, DM Mann, E Ruoslahti. Effects of modification of the RGD sequence and its context on recognition by the fibronectin receptor. J Biol Chem 264(3):1437–1442, 1989.

50. MA Horton, EL Dorey, SA Nesbit, J Samanen, FE Ali, JM Stadel, A Nichols, R Greig, MH Helfrich. Modulation of vitronectin receptor–mediated osteoclast adhesion by Arg-Gly-Asp peptide analogs: a structure–function analysis. J Bone Miner Res 8(2):239–247, 1993.

51. MJ Bogusky, AM Naylor, SM Pitzenberger, RF Nutt, SF Brady, CD Colton, JT Sisko, PS Anderson, DF Veber. NMR and molecular modeling characterization of RGD containing peptides. Int J Pept Protein Res 39(1):63–76, 1992.

52. T Nagata, HA Goldberg, Q Zhang, C Domenicucci, J Sodek. Biosynthesis of bone proteins by fetal porcine calvariae in vitro. Rapid association of sulfated sialoproteins (secreted phosphoprotein-1 and bone sialoprotein) and chondroitin sulfate proteoglycan (CS-PGIII) with bone mineral. Matrix 11:86–100, 1991.

53. T Nagata, CG Bellows, S Kasugai, WT Butler, J Sodek. Biosynthesis of bone proteins, spp-1(secreted phophoprotein 1, osteopontin), BSP (bone sialoprotein) and SPARC (osteonectin) in association with mineralized tissue formation by fetal rat calvarial cells in culture. Biochem J 274:513–520, 1991.

54. S Kasugai, RJ Todescan, T Nagata, K-L Yao, WT Butler, J Sodek. Expression of bone matrix proteins associated with mineralized tissue formation by adult rat bone marrow cells in vitro: inductive effects of dexamethasone on the osteoblastic phenotype. J Cell Physiol 147:111–120, 1991.

55. A Oldberg, A Franzen, D Heinegard. Cloning and sequence analysis of rat bone sialoprotein (osteopontin) cDNA reveals an Arg-Gly-Asp cell-binding sequence. Proc Natl Acad Sci USA 83:8819–8823, 1986.

56. GM Herring. The organic matrix of bone. In: GH Bourne, ed. The Biochemistry and Physiology of Bone. New York: Academic Press, 1972, pp 127–189.

57. HS Shapiro, J Chen, JL Wrana, Q Zhang, M Blum, J Sodek. Characterization of porcine bone sialoprotein: primary structure and cellular expression. Matrix 13:431–440, 1993.

58. A Rezania, CH Thomas, AB Branger, CM Waters, KE Healy. The detachment strength and morphology of bone cells contacting materials modified with a peptide derived from bone sialoprotein. J Biomed Mater Res 37:81–90, 1997.

59. A Rezania, KE Healy. The effect of peptide surface density on the mineralization of matrix deposited by osteogenic cells. J Biomed Mater Res 52(4):595–600, 2000.

60. MJ Bogusky, AM Naylor, SM Pitzenberger, RF Nutt, SF Brady, CD Colton, JT Sisko, PS Anderson, DF Veber. NMR and molecular modeling characterization of RGD containing peptides. Int J Pept Protein Res 39(1):63–76, 1992.

61. SN Rao. Bioactive conformation of Arg-Gly-Asp by X-ray data analyses and molecular mechanics. Pept Res 5(3):148–155, 1992.

62. T Yamada, A Uyeda, A Kidera, M Kikuchi. Functional analysis and modeling of a conformationally constrained Arg-Gly-Asp sequence inserted into human lysozyme. Biochemistry 33(39):11678–11683, 1994.

63. WS Craig, S Cheng, DG Mullen, J Blevitt, MD Pierschbacher. Concept and progress in the development of RGD-containing peptide pharmaceuticals. Biopolymers 37:157–175, 1995.

64. PP Mager. Interactive multivariate modeling of ArgGlyAsp (RGD) derivatives [review]. Med Res Rev 14:75–126, 1994.

65. PM Cardarelli, RR Cobb, DM Nowlin, W Scholz, F Gorcsan, M Moscinski, M Yasuhara, SL Chiang, TJ Lobl. Cyclic RGD peptide inhibits alpha-4 beta-1 interaction with connecting segment 1 and vascular cell adhesion molecule. J Biol Chem 269(28):18668–18673, 1994.

66. GM Harbers, KE Healy. Bioactivation of metal oxide surfaces: II. Computer modeling of a bioactive peptide in the presence and absence of an oxide substrate. Langmuir, in preparation, 2002.

67. GM Harbers. Computer-aided biomolecular surface engineering of peptide modified materials, Masters of Science thesis, Northwestern University, Evanston, IL, 1998.

68. V Copie, Y Tomita, SK Akiyama, S Aota, KM Yamada, RM Venable, RW Pastor, S Krueger, DA Torchia. Solution structure and dynamics of linked cell attachment modules of mouse fibronectin containing the RGD and synergy regions: comparison with the human fibronectin crystal structure. J Mol Biol 277(3):663–682, 1998.

69. BK Brandley, RL Schnaar. Covalent attachment of an Arg-Gly-Asp sequence peptide to derivatizable polyacrylamide surfaces: support of fibroblast adhesion and long-term growth. Anal Biochem 172:270–278, 1988.

70. YN Danilov, RL Juliano. (Arg-Gly-Asp)n-albumin conjugates as a model substratum for integrin-mediated cell adhesion. Exp Cell Res 182(1):186–196, 1989.

71. MD Ward, M Dembo, DA Hammer. Kinetics of cell detachment: peeling of discrete receptor clusters. Biophys J 67(6):2522–2534, 1994.
72. MD Ward, M Dembo, DA Hammer. Kinetics of cell detachment—effect of ligand density. Ann Biomed Eng 23(3):322–331, 1995.
73. SC Kuo, DA Hammer, DA Lauffenburger. Simulation of detachment of specifically bound particles from surfaces by shear flow. Biophys J 73(1):517–531, 1997.
74. PA DiMilla, JA Stone. SM Albelda, DA Lauffenburger, JA Quinn. Measurement of cell adhesion and migration on protein-coated surfaces. Mater Res Soc Symp Proc 252:205–212, 1992.
75. PA DiMilla, JA Stone, JA Quinn, SM Albelda, DA Lauffenburger. Maximal migration of human smooth muscle cells on fibronectin and type IV collagen occurs at an intermediate attachment strength. J Cell Biol 122(3):729–737, 1993.
76. DJ Mooney, R Langer, DE Ingber. Cytoskeletal filament assembly and the control of cell spreading and function by extracellular matrix. J Cell Sci 108(Pt 6)(5):2311–2320, 1995.
77. A Saterbak, DA Lauffenburger. Adhesion mediated by bonds in series. Biotechnol Prog 12(5):682–699, 1996.
78. K Zygourakis, P Markenscoff, R Bizios. Proliferation of anchorage-dependent contact-inhibited cells: III. Experimental results and validation of the theoretical models. Biotechnol Bioeng 38(5):471–479, 1991.
79. K Zygourakis, R Bizios, P Markenscoff. Proliferation of anchorage-dependent contact-inhibited cells: I. Development of theoretical models based on cellular automata. Biotechnol Bioeng 38(5):459–470, 1991.
80. DA Lauffenberger, AF Horwitz. Cell, migration: A physically integrated molecular process. Cell 84:359–369, 1996.
81. HY Zhou, H Takita, R Fujisawa, M Mizuno, Y Kuboki. Stimulation by bone sialoprotein of calcification in osteoblast-like MC3T3-El cells. Calcif Tissue Int 56(5):403–407, 1995.
82. GE Francis, D Fisher, C Delgado, F Malik, A Gardiner, D Neale. Pegylation of cytokines and other therapeutic proteins and peptides: The importance of biological optimisation of coupling techniques. Int J Hematol 68(1):1–18, 1998.
83. Y Dori, H Bianco-Peled, SK Satija, GB Fields, JB McCarthy, M Tirrell. Ligand accessibility as means to control cell response to bioactive bilayer membranes. J Biomed Mater Res 50(1):75–81, 2000.
84. DL Hern, JA Hubbell. Incorporation of adhesion peptides into nonadhesive hydrogels useful for tissue resurfacing. J Biomed Mater Res 39(2):266–276, 1998.
85. BT Houseman, M Mrksich. The microenvironment of immobilized Arg-Gly-Asp peptides is an important determinant of cell adhesion. Biomaterials 22(9):943–955, 2001.
86. JD Andrade. Surface and interfacial aspects of biomedical polymers. Surface chemistry and physics. New York: Plenum Publishers, 1985.

87. J Israelachvili, H Wennerstrom. Role of hydration and water structure in biological and colloidal interactions. Nature 379(6562):219–225, 1996.

88. SI Jeon, JH Lee, JD Andrade, PG De Gennes. Protein–surface interactions in the presence of polyethylene oxide. I. Simplified theory. J Colloid Interf Sci 142(1):149–158, 1991.

89. NP Desai, JA Hubbell. Biological responses to polyethylene oxide modified polyethylene terephthalate surfaces. J Biomed Mater Res 25(7):829–843, 1991.

90. SP Massia, J Stark, DS Letbetter. Surface-immobilized dextran limits cell adhesion and spreading. Biomaterials 21(22):2253–2261, 2000.

91. H Otsuka, Y Nagasaki, K Kataoka. Self-assembly of poly(ethylene glycol)-based block copolymers for biomedical applications. Curr Opin Colloid Interf Sci 6(1):3–10, 2001.

92. C Pale-Grosdemange, ES Simon, KL Prime, GM Whitesides. Formation of self-assembled monolayers by chemisorption of derivatives of oligo(ethylene glycol) of structure HS(CH2)11(OCH2CH2)meta-OH on gold. J Am Chem Soc 113(1):12–20, 1991.

93. GB Fields, JL Lauer, Y Dori, P Forns, YC Yu, M Tirrell. Protein-like molecular architecture: biomaterial applications for inducing cellular receptor binding and signal transduction. Biopolymers 47(2):143–151, 1998.

94. JA Neff, KD Caldwell, PA Tresco. A novel method for surface modification to promote cell attachment to hydrophobic substrates. J Biomed Mater Res 40(4):511–519, 1998.

95. SK Hendricks, C Kwok, MC Shen, TA Horbett, BD Ratner, JD Bryers. Plasma-deposited membranes for controlled release of antibiotic to prevent bacterial adhesion and biofilm formation. J Biomed Mater Res 50(2):160–170, 2000.

96. JP Bearinger, DG Castner, SL Golledge, A Rezania, S Hubchak, KE Healy. P(AAm-co-EG) interpenetrating polymer networks grafted to oxide surfaces: surface characterization, protein adsorption, and cell detachment studies. Langmuir 13:5175–5183, 1997.

97. AS Sawhney, CP Pathak, JA Hubbell. Bioerodible hydrogels based on photopolymerized poly(ethylene glycol)-co-poly(α-hydroxy acid) diacrylate macromers. Macromolecules 26(4):581–587, 1993.

98. TA Barber, SL Golledge, DG Castner, KE Healy. Peptide-modified p(AAm-co-EG/AAC) IPNs grafted to bulk titanium modulate osteoblast behavior in vitro. J Biomed Mat Res, accepted 2002.

99. GM Harbers, TA Barber, ME Yanez, HB Larman, KE Healy. IPN Modified 316L SS: Surface Characterization and HCAEC Adhesion Studies. Society for Biomaterials, St. Paul, MN, 2001, p 275.

100. KS Tweden, H Harasaki, M Jones, JM Blevitt, WS Craig, M Pierschbacher, MN Helmus. Accelerated healing of cardiovascular textiles promoted by an RGD peptide. J Heart Valve Dis 4(1):S90–97, 1995.

101. JJ Grzesiak, MD Pierschbacher, MF Amodeo, TI Malaney, JR Glass. Enhancement of cell interactions with collagen/glycosaminoglycan matrices by RGD derivatization. Biomaterials 18(24):1625–1632, 1997.

102. MD Pierschbacher, JW Polarek, WS Craig, JF Tschopp, NJ Sipes, JR Harper. Manipulation of cellular interactions with biomaterials toward a therapeutic outcome: a perspective. J Cell Biochem 56(2):150–154, 1994.

103. P Ducheyne, Q Qiu. Bioactive ceramics: The effect of surface reactivity on bone formation and bone cell function. Biomaterials 20(23–24):2287–2303, 1999.

104. HM Kim. Bioactive ceramics: challenges and perspectives. J Ceram Soc Jpn 109(4):S49–S57, 2001.

105. DR Sumner, TM Turner, AF Purchio, WR Gombotz, RM Urban, JO Galante. Enhancement of bone ingrowth by transforming growth factor-beta. J Bone Joint Surg Am 77(8):1135–1147, 1995.

106. M Lund, S Overgaard, B Ongpipaittanakul, T Nguyen, C Bunger, K Soballe. Transforming growth factor-b1 stimulates bone in-growth to weight-loaded tricalcium phosphate coated implates. Soc Bone Joint Surg 78B:377–382, 1996.

107. DM Ferris, GD Moodie, PM Dimond, CW Gioranni, MG Ehrlich, RF Valentini. RGD-coated titanium implants stimulate increased bone formation in vivo. Biomaterials 20(23–24):2323–2331, 1999.

108. C Liang, J Barnes, JG Seedor, HA Quartuccio, M Bolander, JJ Jeffrey, GA Rodan. Impaired bone activity in aged rats: alterations at the cellular and molecular levels. Bone 13(6):435–441, 1992.

109. LJ Suva, JG Seedor, N Endo, HA Quartuccio, DD Thompson, I Bab, GA Rodan. Pattern of gene expression following rat tibial marrow ablation. J Bone Miner Res 8(3):379–388, 1993.

110. A Berzins, DR Sumner. Implant pushout and pullout tests. In: YH An, YH Draughn, eds. Mechanical Testing of Bone and the Bone–Implant Interface. Boca Raton, FL: CRC Press, 2000, pp 463–476.

111. K Whang, DC Tsai, EK Nam, M Aitken, SM Sprague, PK Patel, KE Healy. Ectopic bone formation via rhBMP-2 delivery from porous bioabsorbable polymer scaffolds. J Biomed Mater Res 42(4):491–499, 1998.

112. AS Breitbart, DA Grande, R Kessler, JT Ryaby, RJ Fitzsimmons, RT Grant. Tissue engineered bone repair of calvarial defects using cultured periosteal cells. Plast Reconstr Surg 101(3):567–574, 1998.

113. KT Paige, LG Cima, MJ Yaremchuk, JP Vacanti, CA Vacanti. Injectable cartilage. Plast Reconstr Surg 96(6):1390–1398, 1995.

114. S Kawamura, S Wakitani, T Kimura, A Maeda, AI Caplan, K Shino, T Ochi. Articular cartilage repair. Rabbit experiments with a collagen gel-biomatrix and chondrocytes cultured in it. Acta Orthop Scand 69(1):56–62, 1998.

115. T Shinoka, D Shum-Tim, PX Ma, RE Tanel, N Isogai, R Langer, JP Vacanti, JE Mayer Jr. Creation of viable pulmonary artery autografts through tissue engineering. J Thorac Cardiovasc Surg 115(3):536–545, 1998.

116. BR Seckel, D Jones, KJ Hekimian, K-K Wang, DP Chakalis, PD Costas. Hyaluronic acid through a new injectable nerve guide delivery system enhances peripheral nerve regeneration in the rat. J Neurosci Res 40:318–324, 1995.

117. LG Cima, JP Vacanti, C Vacanti, D Ingber, D Mooney, R Langer. Tissue engineering by cell transplantation using degradable polymer substrates. J Biomech Eng 113:143–151, 1991.
118. JA Hubbell, R Langer. Tissue engineering. Chem Eng News 73(11):42–53, 1995.
119. MJ Moghaddam, T Matsuda. Molecular design of three-dimensional artificial extracellular matrix: photosensitive polymers containing cell adhesive peptide. J Polym Sci A Polym Chem 31(6):1589–1597, 1993.
120. Y Suzuki, M Tanihara, K Suzuki, A Saitou, W Sufan, Y Nishimura. Alginate hydrogel linked with synthetic oligopeptide derived from BMP-2 allows ectopic osteoinduction in vivo. J Biomed Mater Res 50(3):405–409, 2000.
121. RA Stile, WR Burghardt, KE Healy. Synthesis and characterization of injectable poly(n-isopropylacrylamide)-based hydrogels that support tissue formation in vitro. Macromolecules 32:7370–7379, 1999.
122. M Heskins, JE Guillet. Solution properties of poly(n-isopropylacrylamide). J Macromol Sci Chem A2(8):1441–1455, 1968.
123. K Kamide. Thermodynamics of Polymer Solutions: Phase Equilibria and Critical Phenomena. New York: Elsevier, 1990.
124. EF Casassa. Phase equilibrium in polymer solutions. In: LH Tung, ed. Fractionation of Synthetic Polymers: Principles and Practices. New York: Marcel Dekker, 1977, pp 3–55.
125. HG Schild. Poly(n-isopropylacrylamide): experiment, theory, and application. Prog Polym Sci 17:163–249, 1992.
126. LD Taylor, LD Cerankowski. Preparation of films exhibiting a balanced temperature dependence to permeation by aqueous solutions—a study of lower consolute behavior. J Polym Sci, Polym Chem 13:2551–2570, 1975.
127. JA Chinn, JA Sauter, RE Phillips, Jr., WJ Kao, JM Anderson, SR Hanson, TR Ashton. Blood and tissue compatibility of modified polyester: thrombosis, inflammation, and healing. J Biomed Mater Res 39(1):130–140, 1998.
128. J Glass, J Blevitt, K Dickerson, M Pierschbacher, WS Craig. Cell attachment and motility on materials modified by surface-active RGD-containing peptides. Ann N Y Acad Sci 745(5):177–186, 1994.
129. JB Huebsch, GB Fields, TG Triebes, DL Mooradian. Photoreactive analog of peptide FN-C/H-V from the carboxy-terminal heparin-binding domains of fibronectin supports endothelial cell adhesion and spreading on biomaterial surfaces. J Biomed Mater Res 31(4):555–567, 1996.
130. G Johnson, M Jenkins, KM McLean, HJ Griesser, J Kwak, M Goodman, JG Steele. Peptoid-containing collagen mimetics with cell binding activity. J Biomed Mater Res 51(4):612–624, 2000.
131. YW Tong, MS Shoichet. Enhancing the interaction of central nervous system neurons with poly(tetrafluoroethylene-co-hexafluoro-propylene) via a novel surface amine-functionalization reaction followed by peptide modification. J Biomater Sci Polym Ed 9(7):713–729, 1998.
132. BK Mann, AT Tsai, T Scott-Burden, JL West. Modification of surfaces with cell adhesion peptides alters extracellular matrix deposition. Biomaterials 20(23–24):2281–2286, 1999.

133. JA Hubbell, SP Massia, PD Drumheller. Surface-grafted cell-binding peptides in tissue engineering of the vascular graft. Ann N Y Acad Sci 665(2):253–258, 1992.

134. SP Massia, JA Hubbell. Human endothelial cell interactions with surface-coupled adhesion peptides on a nonadhesive glass substrate and two polymeric biomaterials. J Biomed Mater Res 25(2):223–242, 1991.

135. Y Xiao, GA Truskey. Effect of receptor–ligand affinity on the strength of endothelial cell adhesion. Biophys J 71(5):2869–2884, 1996.

136. M Huber, P Heiduschka, S Kienle, C Pavlidis, J Mack, T Walk, G Jung, S Thanos. Modification of glassy carbon surfaces with synthetic laminin-derived peptides for nerve cell attachment and neurite growth. J Biomed Mater Res 41(2):278–288, 1998.

137. A Kondoh, K Makino, T Matsuda. Two-dimensional artificial extracellular-matrix—bioadhesive peptide-immobilized surface design. J Appl Polym Sci 47(11):1983–1988, 1993.

138. T Sugawara, T Matsuda. Photochemical surface derivatization of a peptide containing Arg-Gly-Asp (RGD). J Biomed Mater Res 29:1047–1052, 1995.

139. HB Lin, C García-Echeverría, S Asakura, W Sun, DF Mosher, SL Cooper. Endothelial cell adhesion on polyurethanes containing covalently attached RGD-peptides. Biomaterials 13(13):905–914, 1992.

140. M Sanchez, A Deffieux, L Bordenave, C Baquey, M Fontanille. Synthesis of hemocompatible materials. 1: Surface modification of polyurethanes based on poly(chloroalkylvinylether)s by RGD fragments. Clin Mater 15(4):253–258, 1994.

141. HB Lin, W Sun, DF Mosher, C García-Echeverría, K Schaufelberger, PI Lelkes, SL Cooper. Synthesis, surface, and cell-adhesion properties of polyurethanes containing covalently grafted RGD-peptides. J Biomed Mater Res 28(3):329–342, 1994.

142. PD Drumheller, JA Hubbell. Polymer networks with grafted cell adhesion peptides for highly biospecific cell adhesive substrates. Anal Biochem 222(2):380–388, 1994.

143. Y Hirano, Y Kando, T Hayashi, K Goto, A Nakajima. Synthesis and cell attachment activity of bioactive oligopeptides: RGD, RGDS, RGDV, and RGDT. J Biomed Mater Res 25(12):1523–1534, 1991.

144. Y Hirano, M Okuno, T Hayashi, K Goto, A Nakajima. Cell-attachment activities of surface immobilized oligopeptides RGD, RGDS, RGDV, RGDT, and YIGSR toward five cell lines. J Biomater Sci Polym Ed 4(3):235–243, 1993.

145. Y Ito, M Kajihara, Y Imanishi. Materials for enhancing cell adhesion by immobilization of cell-adhesive peptide. J Biomed Mater Res 25(11):1325–1338, 1991.

146. WJ Kao. Evaluation of protein-modulated macrophage behavior on biomaterials: designing biomimetic materials for cellular engineering. Biomaterials 20(23–24):2213–2221, 1999.

147. T Pakalns, KL Haverstick, GB Fields, JB McCarthy, DL Mooradian, M Tirrell. Cellular recognition of synthetic peptide amphiphiles in self-assembled monolayer films. Biomaterials 20(23–24):2265–2279, 1999.
148. TA Barber. Engineered titanium surfaces to modulate osteoblast behavior. Masters of Science thesis, Northwestern University, Evanston, IL, 2000.
149. E De Giglio, L Sabbatini, S Colucci, G Zambonin. Synthesis, analytical characterization, and osteoblast adhesion properties on RGD-grafted poly-pyrrole coatings on titanium substrates. J Biomater Sci Polym Ed 11(10):1073–1083, 2000.
150. C Roberts, CS Chen, M Mrksich, V Martichonok, DE Ingber, GM Whitesides. Using mixed self-assembled monolayers presenting RGD and (EG)(3)OH groups to characterize long-term attachment of bovine capillary endothelial cells to surfaces. J Am Chem Soc 120(26):6548–6555, 1998.
151. S Saneinejad, MS Shoichet. Patterned poly(chlorotrifluoroethylene) guides primary nerve cell adhesion and neurite outgrowth. J Biomed Mater Res 50(4):465–474, 2000.
152. JA Rowley, G Madlambayan, DJ Mooney. Alginate hydrogels as synthetic extracellular matrix materials. Biomaterials 20(1):45–53, 1999.
153. RS Bhatnagar, JJ Qian, A Wedrychowska, M Sadeghi, YM Wu, N Smith. Design of biomimetic habitats for tissue engineering with P-15, a synthetic peptide analogue of collagen. Tissue Eng 5(1):53–66, 1999.
154. S Sofia, MB McCarthy, G Gronowicz, DL Kaplan. Functionalized silk-based biomaterials for bone formation. J Biomed Mater Res 54(1):139–148, 2001.
155. KE Healy, GM Harbers, TA Barber, DA Sumner. Osteoblast interactions with engineered surfaces. In: JE Davies, ed. Bone Engineering. Toronto: Em Squared Inc., 2000, pp 268–281.

4

Effects of Substratum Topography on Cell Behavior

**George A. Abrams, Ana I. Teixeira, Paul F. Nealey, and
Christopher J. Murphy**
University of Wisconsin, Madison, Wisconsin

I. INTRODUCTION

An individual cell is exposed to a large number of environmental stimuli that initiate complex interconnecting intracellular signaling cascades, which in turn modulate a dynamic community of intracellular proteins. Stimuli may act through binding to specific receptors on the cell surface. Such ligand–receptor interactions include receptor binding of hormones, growth factors, neuropeptides, and specific amino acid sequences found in the extracellular matrix (e.g., arginine-glycine-aspartic acid, also termed RGD). Cells can also be greatly influenced through interaction with factors that are nonspecific in that they do not require membrane-associated receptors. An example of such a factor is provided by antimicrobial defense peptides that form multimeric pores in cell membranes and can serve as trophic factors over a narrow range of concentrations while inducing toxicity at high concentrations. Finally, cells are also impacted by numerous nonspecific environmental factors, such as pH, osmolality, temperature, ion concentrations, electrical fields, surface chemistry of the substratum, and biomechanical stressors. How a cell assimilates and responds to a multitude of simultaneous stimuli is still largely unknown.

The extracellular matrix (ECM) plays a dynamic role in modulating cell behaviors through interaction with specific receptors as well as through nonspecific mechanisms. The ECM provides the scaffolding for cell attachment that allows organization of cells into tissues and tissues into organs; contains specific ligands (e.g., RGD) that interact with integrin binding sequences; serves as a depot for a variety of cytoactive compounds (e.g., growth factors); serves as a filter through which elements of the extracellular milieu must percolate to reach the cell; transmits biomechanical stress to the cell membrane; and, by nature of its topography, directly imparts nonspecific biomechanical stimuli. The role of topography in modulating cell behavior is the focus of this chapter.

A. Cell–Substratum Interactions

There are a number of mechanisms that control how a cell perceives and responds to the ECM. These include integrin–ligand interactions, influences of surface chemistry, and the topographical effects of the matrix itself. Undoubtedly, all of these factors come into play to influence the community of intracellular proteins that, in turn, dictate cell behavior.

Integrins are a family of transmembrane glycoproteins that are composed of two subunits, α and β, which are covalently bound together. The $\alpha\beta$ heterodimer determines the specificity for ligands found in proteins located in the ECM. These ligands are amino acid sequences with the RGD sequence binding the largest number of integrin receptors. ECM-associated integrin-binding sequences include RGDS, LDV, and REDV sequences of fibronectin that bind $\alpha_5\beta_1$ and RGDV of vitronectin that binds $\alpha_v\beta_3$. By linking the actin cytoskeleton to the ECM, integrins provide bidirectional transmission of signals between the ECM and cytoplasm. This linkage occurs at sites of focal adhesions. Several proteins have been found to be concentrated around these sites and act as linking elements, including cytoplasmic proteins such as vinculin, talin, and α-actinin. Integrins participate in cell signaling by undergoing activation and deactivation as a result of ligand binding. Activation results in conformational changes in integrin extracellular domains, reorganization of intracytoplasmic connections, and redistribution of integrins on the cell surface. This redistribution of receptors leads to a series of events inside the cell, including changes in pH and calcium, tyrosine phosphorylation of proteins such as focal adhesion kinase (FAK), and activation of the RAS-ERK cascade. It is believed that providing stable cell attachment conditions, integrins also allow for growth factor receptors to be optimally activated. Integrin activation is also important for normal cell cycle function and the extension of lamellipodia, filiopodia, and stress fiber formation during cell movement (1–6).

The cytoskeleton of a cell also participates in mediating responses to the ECM through interactions with integrin receptors at sites of focal adhesions. The cytoskeleton is composed of three different types of molecular proteins known as microfilaments (actin), microtubules (tubulin), and intermediate filaments (keratin). Microfilaments range in diameter from 7 mm to 9 mm; microtubules average 24 mm, and intermediate filaments average 10 mm (7). The cytoskeleton not only provides mechanical support but also is directly involved in a large number of signaling pathways often in association with G proteins. Through these pathways, transduction of external forces through the cytoskeleton can induce phosphorylation of tyrosine kinases, recruitment of phospholipases and lipid kinases to the cytoskeleton, regulation of intracellular Ca^{2+} and transmembrane ion flux, and control of nuclear gene expression (8–10).

B. Basement Membranes

A variety of cell types anchor themselves to their underlying stroma through a unique specialization of the ECM, i.e., the basement membrane. The basement membrane is composed of a complex mixture of constituents including collagens, laminins, proteoglycans, and other glycoproteins. In addition to their structural roles in supporting attached cells, basement membranes serve as reservoirs for cytoactive compounds, such as growth factors. A universal characteristic of epithelial and endothelial cells is that they are associated with basement membranes through which they attach to the underlying stroma (11,12). The cornea has two basement membranes. These consist of the anterior basement membrane of the epithelium and the posterior basement membrane or Descemet's membrane associated with the endothelium or posterior epithelium of the cornea. Basement membranes of the cornea have been shown to affect corneal epithelial cell shape, growth, migration, differentiation, and endothelial proliferation through RGD–integrin interactions (13–15).

It is well documented that the presence of a basement membrane facilitates epithelial wound healing. In the absence of basement membrane, epithelial cells will resurface a stromal defect, albeit at a slower rate, using integrin binding sequences made available by other extracellular constituents including fibronectin, which typically coats the stromal surface subsequent to wounding. After reestablishment of epithelial continuity across the surface, a new basement membrane is produced but may take months until fully mature (16–18). Clearly, basement membranes are a vital element in maintaining homeostasis for many cell types, and maintaining the integrity of its structure is vital to cell dynamics.

C. Extracellular Matrix Topography

Basement membrane properties likely to influence cell behavior include the cell's native protein composition, which offers opportunities for specific ligand–receptor interaction in the case of integrin binding as well as determining general surface chemistry parameters such as relative surface charge and hydrophilicity, the presence of soluble cytoactive compounds for which it serves as a repository, and its native topography. In recent years, our laboratories have focused on the study of topographical features of basement membranes and the capacity of surface topography to modulate fundamental cell behaviors. We have completed morphological studies of the corneal basement membranes from the human, canine, Rhesus macaque, as well as Matrigel, a commercially available basement membrane complex (Fig. 1a–f) (19–21). Corneal basement membranes were chosen for study due to their convenient location and their proven significance for corneal epithelial wound healing. We chose to use three distinct but complementary methods (scanning electron microscopy, atomic force microscopy, and

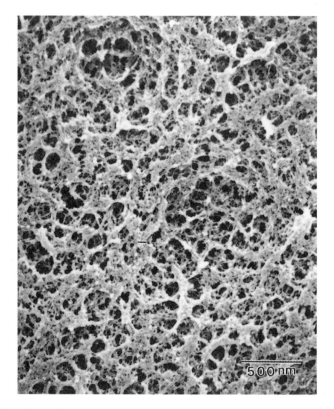

Figure 1a Scanning electron micrographs of the anterior corneal epithelial basement membrane of the human.

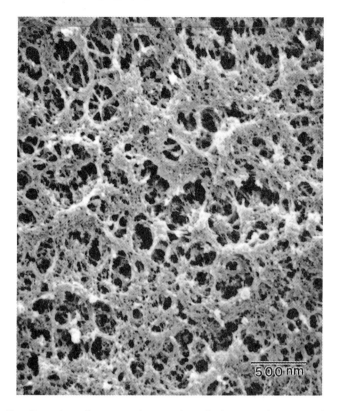

Figure 1b Scanning electron micrographs of the anterior corneal epithelial basement membrane of the Rhesus macaque.

transmission electron microscopy) for data acquisition and comparative analysis to minimize the impact of possible confounding variables, such as specimen processing and fixation artifacts. We found these basement membranes to be composed of a complex topography consisting of a felt-like intertwining of fibers mixed with elevations and pores of varying nanoscale dimensions (Table 1). Remarkably similar findings were found using all three imaging techniques from intact tissues and from tissues that were imaged after removal of the overlying epithelium. The topographical features were also found to be similar between all species examined and Matrigel. It should also be noted that the topographies described reflect the unique topography of the basement membranes as the topography of the underlying stromal elements of the cornea differ considerably (22). Earlier studies examining basement membranes from a variety of tissues also

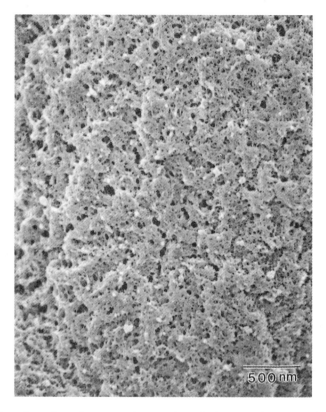

Figure 1c Scanning electron micrographs of the anterior corneal epithelial basement membrane of the canine.

describe surface topographical features similar to those found in the cornea and Matrigel. This implies that basement membranes have a conservative surface topography that may be important in directing cell behaviors beyond integrin–ligand interactions alone (23–29). The detailed description of the topography of basement membranes provides a logical starting point for the fabrication of biomaterials with biologically relevant topographical features.

II. SUBSTRATUM TOPOGRAPHY AND CELL BEHAVIOR

Flemming et al. (30) provided an extensive review of the effects of surface topography on cell behavior. We have updated the tables provided in

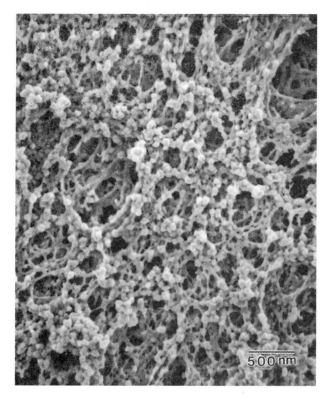

Figure 1d Scanning electron micrographs of the anterior corneal epithelial basement membrane of the Matrigel.

Flemming's publication to incorporate recent findings (Table 2). The impact of substratum topography on cytoskeletal orientation, focal adhesion formation, and vinculin localization has been investigated. Historically, the vast majority of studies examined surfaces with topographical features equal to or greater than 1 μm. The size range of topographical features investigated has been determined largely by the constraints in nanofabrication. It is only recently with advances in materials sciences that controlled fabrication of submicrometer surface features has become possible.

The reader is referred to Table 2 for a review of cellular consequences of large-scale features greater than or equal to 1 μm as the following discussion is limited to studies of the more biologically relevant features of less than 1 μm.

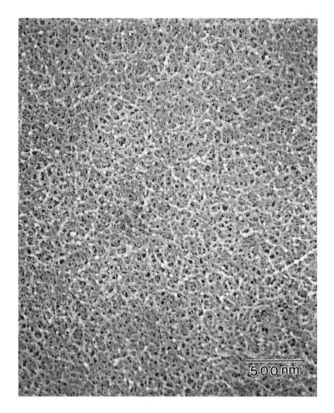

Figure 1e   Scanning electron micrographs of Descemet's membrane of the human.

We hypothesize that the topography of the ECM is important for proper cell signaling interactions to occur. The ability to fabricate and evaluate the effect of nanometer-size topographical features similar to the ECM allows investigators to more accurately represent the cells true in vivo environment (Fig. 2 and 3).

A.   Studies Utilizing Production of Random Topographic Features

Surfaces that have been studied generally fall into one of two categories, namely, those with well-defined and those with random topographical features. Investigators have used porous filters to evaluate the effect of substratum pores on cell behavior. The effects of porous filters with pore

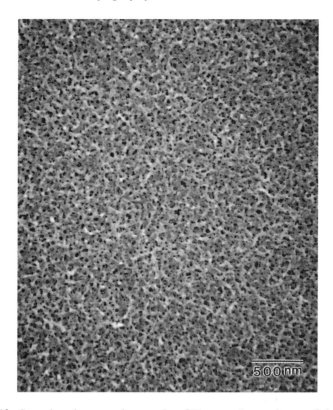

Figure 1f Scanning electron micrographs of Descemet's membrane of the canine. Note the complex topography of fibers, elevations, and pores. The basic topography varies very little between species. Features of Descemet's membrane are generally smaller and more tightly packed than the anterior corneal epithelial basement membrane. (Reprinted with permission from Refs. 19–22.)

sizes ranging from 100 nm to 3 µm and porosity ranging from 3.14% to 15.7% on corneal epithelial cells have been evaluated in vitro using bovine corneal buttons as the source of epithelial cells. This range of pore sizes and periodicities is comparable with that described for the native corneal basement membrane. It was demonstrated that migration of epithelial cells was improved on porous surfaces compared with smooth surfaces. However, epithelial tissue migration was increasingly inhibited by increasing pore sizes greater than 900 nm. Pores with diameters of 100–800 nm and porosities of 2.5–12% provided the best surface for tissue migration and differentiation of the epithelium (31–33). Similar results were obtained with

Table 1 Feature Dimensions (mean ± SD nm) of the Corneal Basement Membranes of the Human, Canine, Macaque, and Matrigel

	Epithelial basement membrane				Descemet's membrane	
Dimension	Human[a]	Canine[b]	Macaque[c]	Matrigel[c]	Human[a]	Canine[b]
SEM						
Elevations	182 ± 49	150 ± 41	190 ± 72	162 ± 52	131 ± 41	115 ± 30
Pores	92 ± 34	32 ± 18	71 ± 44	105 ± 70	38 ± 15	24 ± 8
Fibers	46 ± 16	18 ± 9	77 ± 39	69 ± 35	31 ± 9	15 ± 7
TEM						
Elevations	165 ± 78	119 ± 39	149 ± 60	N/A	107 ± 50	85 ± 21
AFM						
Elevations	243 ± 34	N/A	147 ± 42	196 ± 57	186 ± 45	N/A

Adapted from: [a](20); [b](21); [c](19).

Table 2 Effect of Textured Surfaces on Cell Behavior

Feature type	Fabrication technique	Material	Feature dimensions	Feature frequency	Cell type studied	Cellular effect	Ref.
Grooves	Photolithography and reactive ion etching, UV and glow discharge treatment	PDMS cast of silicon original	Square grooves 2, 5, 10 μm width 0.5 μm depth	Equal groove and ridge width	Rat dermal fibroblasts	2-, 5-μm grooves induced stronger orientation than 10-μm grooves; growth lower on UV-treated surface than on glow discharge treated surface	41
	Photolithography and reactive ion etching	Quartz	0.5, 5, 10, 25 μm width 0.5, 5 μm depth	Equal groove and ridge width	Murine P388-D1 macrophage	Cells spread faster on shallow grooves, but elongated faster on deeper grooves; more elongation on wider grooves; orientation dependent on depth during first 30 min; 60% more F-actin in cells in grooves; LPS-activation enhanced orientation	60
	Photolithography and reactive ion etching	Quartz	Square grooves 0.98–4.01 μm width 1.12–1.17 μm depth	Groove and ridge width similar	Mesenchymal tissue cells	Cells migrated along grooves; cells became highly polarized; highest alignment on widest repeat spacing	61
	Photolithography and anisotropic etching, glow discharge	Titanium-coated silicon	V-shaped 15 μm width 3 μm depth	Equal groove and ridge width	Porcine epithelial cells	Cells oriented in direction of grooves; actin filaments and microtubules aligned along walls and edges; single cells showed less variability of aligned cytoskeletal arrangements than cell clusters; no significant elliptical morphology	62
	Photolithography and reactive ion etching	Epoxy replica of silicon original	Square grooves 0.5 μm width 1 μm depth	Equal groove and ridge width	Human gingival fibroblasts	Cells showed strong alignment to topography; cells bridged or conformed to features	63

Table 2 Continued

Feature type	Fabrication technique	Material	Feature dimensions	Feature frequency	Cell type studied	Cellular effect	Ref.
	Photolithography and reactive ion etching	Epoxy replica of silicon original	Square grooves 0.5 µm width 1 µm depth	Equal groove and ridge width	Human gingival fibroblasts	Cells grew mostly in monolayers; some cells extended processes into grooves; inner corners of grooves not occupied by cellular processes; some cells bridged grooves; cytoskeletal elements oriented parallel to long axis of grooves	64
	Photolithography and anisotropic etching	Titanium-coated epoxy replica of silicon original	Square and V-shaped grooves, 30 µm repeat spacing with 3, 10, or 22 µm depth or 7 and 39 µm repeat spacing with 3 or 10 µm depth	Regular spacing, but unequal groove and ridge width	Rat parietal implant model grooves oriented horizontally or vertically to long axis of implant	Endothelial cell attachment observed on smooth and 3, 10 µm grooves; endothelial cells bridged 22-µm horizontal grooves; fibroblasts encapsulated smooth and 3-, 10-µm horizontal grooves; fibroblasts inserted obliquely into 22-µm horizontal grooves; epithelial downgrowth greatest on vertical and smooth surface while least on 10-, 22-µm horizontal grooves	65
	Photolithography and anisotropic etching	Titanium-coated silicon, epoxy replicas, photoresist	Square and V-shaped grooves 0.5–60 µm depth repeat spacing 30–220 µm	Regular spacing but groove and ridge width not listed	Porcine periodontal ligament epithelial cells	Cells oriented by all grooves; highest repeat orientation on smallest repeat spacing; some cells crossed ridges or descended into grooves; grooves directed migration of cells; 0.5-µm-deep grooves less effective than deeper grooves at directing cells; cell observed to have lamellae and filiopodia bending around edges	66

Method	Material	Dimensions	Spacing	Cell type	Observations	Ref.
Photolithography and reactive ion etching	Quartz	5, 10, 25 μm width 0.5, 1, 2, 5 μm depth	Spacing not listed	BHK cells	F-actin condensation observed at topographic discontinuities; condensations often at right angles to groove edge with periodicity of 0.6 μm; vinculin organization similar to that of actin; microtubules observed after 30 min; colcemid increased spreading and reduced orientation and elongation; cytochalasin D reduced spreading, elongation, and orientation, taxol reduced elongation	52
Cutting with diamond or tungsten	PS, epoxy replicas	2, 10 μm width, depth not listed	5–30 μm spacing	Chick heart fibroblasts, murine epithelial cells	75% of cells aligned on 5-μm grooves; 60% of cells aligned on 30-μm grooves; cytoplasmic extensions not related to surface features; alignment of cells not guided by lamellae or filopodia; cells bridged 2- and 10-μm grooves without touching surface	48
Photolithography and anisotropic etching	Silicon dioxide	0.5 μm width 1 μm depth	Equal groove and ridge width	Human fibroblasts, gingival keratinocytes, neutrophils, monocytes, macrophages	100% of fibroblasts and 20% of macrophages aligned; no orientation or alignment observed with keratinocytes or neutrophils; some macrophages extended processes parallel to long axis of grooves after 2 h	42
Photolithography and anisotropic etching	Titanium-coated silicon, epoxy replicas, photoresist	Square and V-shaped major grooves 5–120 μm deep (width not listed), minor grooves 2 μm deep on floor at 54° to major grooves	5–80 μm repeat spacing	Human gingival fibroblasts	Alignment observed in grooves and on flat ridges; cells oriented preferentially to major grooves; minor grooves caused orientation of cells in absence of major grooves or when discontinuity existed in major groove pattern	67

Table 2 Continued

Feature type	Fabrication technique	Material	Feature dimensions	Feature frequency	Cell type studied	Cellular effect	Ref.
	Photolithography followed by glow discharge	PDMS cast of silicon original	2.0, 5.0, 10.0 μm width 0.5 μm depth	Equal groove and ridge width	Rat dermal fibroblasts	Cells on 2- and 5-μm grooves were elongated and aligned parallel to grooves; cells on 10-μm grooves were similar to those on smooth substrate	68
	Photolithography and anisotropic etching, glow discharge	Titanium-coated silicon	V-shaped, 3 μm depth, width not listed	6–10 μm repeat spacing	Human gingival fibroblasts	Cells elongated and oriented along grooves; cell height 1.5-fold greater on grooves; fibronectin mRNA and secreted fibronectin increased in cells on grooves; GAPD mRNA not affected; half-lives of fibronectin mRNA altered; 2-fold increase in fibronectin mRNA assembled into ECM	69
	Photolithography and reactive ion etching	Quartz	1.65–8.96 μm width 0.69 μm depth	3.0–32.0 μm repeat spacing	Chick heart fibroblasts	Ridge width more important than groove width in determining cell alignment; alignment of cells inversely proportional to ridge width	70
	Photolithography and anisotropic etching	Epoxy replica of silicon original	V-shaped grooves 17 μm width, 10 μm depth	22 μm ridge width	Porcine periodontal ligament epithelial cells, rat parietal implant model	Epithelial cells attached to grooved surfaces more than to smooth surfaces and were oriented by grooves; shorter length epithelial attachment and longer connective tissue attachment in grooved parts of implant compared to smooth parts; grooves impeded epithelial downgrowth on implants	71

Fabrication method	Material	Feature dimensions	Spacing	Cells	Results	Ref.
Photolithography and anisotropic etching	Ti-coated silicon	V-shaped grooves 70, 130, 165 μm width	80, 140, 175 μm spacing	Human gingival cells, porcine epithelial cells	Cells from suspension aligned to long axis of grooves; epithelial cells did not bend around ridges between cells; grooves caused alignment of migration of explanted cells; multilayering of epithelial cells within and along grooves	72
Photolithography and anisotropic etching	Ti-coated silicon	V-shaped grooves 3 μm depth	6–10 μm repeat spacing	Human gingival fibroblasts	Cells oriented along grooves by 16 h; cells on grooves showed altered matrix metalloproteinase-2 mRNA time-course expression and levels compared to cells on smooth Ti or tissue culture plastic	73
Photolithography and anisotropic etching	Ti-coated silicon	15 μm width 3 μm depth, V-shaped	Groove and ridge width equal	Human gingival fibroblasts	Microtubules were the first element to become aligned; microtubules aligned at bottom of grooves after 20 min; actin observed first at wall-ridge edges after 40–60 min; after 3 h a majority of cells exhibited aligned focal contacts	74
Photolithography and reactive ion etching, glow discharge treatment	PDMS cast of silicon original	2, 5, 10 μm width 0.5 μm depth	Groove and ridge width equal	Rat dermal fibroblasts	Microfilaments and vinculin aggregates oriented along 2 μm grooves after 1, 3, 5, and 7 days, but was less oriented on 5- and 10-μm grooves; vinculin located primarily on surface ridges; bovine and endogenous fibronectin and vitronectin were oriented along grooves; groove-spanning filaments also observed	47
Electron beam lithography and wet etching, glow discharge treatment	PDMS cast of silicon original	Square grooves 1 μm width 1 μm depth	Grooves separated by 4-μm-wide ridges	Human gingival fibroblasts	Vinculin-positive attachment sites observed; cells aligned to grooves in PDMS, which had been made hydrophilic by glow discharge treatment; focal adhesion contacts also aligned to grooves	75

Table 2 Continued

Feature type	Fabrication technique	Material	Feature dimensions	Feature frequency	Cell type studied	Cellular effect	Ref.
	Photolithography and wet etching	PDMS cast of silicon original	2, 5, 10 μm width 0.5 μm depth	Groove and ridge width equal	Human skin fibroblasts	Cells on smooth PDMS entered S phase of cell cycle faster than cells on textured PDMS; cells on 10-μm texture proliferated less than those on 2- and 5-μm textures	76
	Cutting with diamond	Serum-coated glass	2 μm width 2 μm depth	Spacing not listed	Human neutrophil leukocytes	When cells moving across plane of glass encountered a groove, they were highly likely to migrate along groove rather than cross it	77
	Photolithography and reactive ion etching, glow discharge treatment	PDMS cast of silicon oxide original	Square grooves 1.0–10.0 μm width **0.45, 1.00 μm depth**	1.0–10.0 μm ridge width	Rat dermal fibroblasts	Cells oriented and elongated along grooves with ridge widths 4.0 μm or less; protrusions contacting ridges observed on oriented cells; cells randomly oriented and were more circular on grooves with ridges more than 4.0 μm wide; groove width and depth did not effect cell size, shape, or orientation	78
	Photolithography and reactive ion etching	PMMA	2, 3, 6, 12 μm width **0.2, 0.56, 1.10, 1.9 μm depth**	Equal groove and ridge width	BHK cells, MDCK cells, chick embryo cerebral neuron	Alignment of BHK cells increased with depth but decreased with increasing width; width had no effect on MDCK cells; alignment of MDCK cells increased with depth; response of MDCK cells depended on whether or not cells were isolated; alignment of chick embryo cerebral neurons also increased with depth	51

Technique	Substratum	Groove dimensions	Spacing	Cell types	Results	
Laser holographic technique used to define masks for X-ray lithography and reactive ion etching	Quartz and PLL coated quartz	**130 nm width 100, 210, 400 nm depth**	Equal groove and ridge width	BHK, MDCK, chick embryo cerebral neurons	BHK cells aligned on all groove patterns, but degree of alignment increased with increasing depth; MDCK aligned and elongated to grooves, but only elongation increased with depth; MDCK cells in groups and chick embryo cerebral neurons not affected by grooves	50
Laser holographic technique used to define masks for X-ray lithography and reactive ion etching	Poly-D-lysine-coated chrome-plated quartz	**0.13–4.01 μm width 0.1–1.17 μm depth**	**0.13–8.0 μm spacing**	Rat optic nerve oligodendrocytes, optic nerve astrocytes, hippocampal cerebellar neurons	Oligodendrocytes were highly aligned by features as small as 100 nm depth and 260 nm repeat spacing; astrocytes were also aligned while hippocampal and cerebellar neuron cells were not; oligodendrocytes showed little high order F-actin networks; aligned astrocytes showed extensive arrangement of actin stress fibers; maximum oligodendrocyte alignment induced by pattern corresponding to diameter of axon in 7-day optic nerve	43
Electron beam lithography, wet etching, and reactive ion etching	Quartz, PLL-coated quartz and PS replicas	Square grooves 1, 2, 4 μm width **14 to 1,100 nm depth**	Spacing not listed	Embryonic Xenopus spinal cord neurons, rat hippocampal neurons	*Xenopus* neurites grew parallel to all groove sizes; hippocampal neurites grew perpendicular to narrow, shallow grooves and parallel to wide, deep grooves; *Xenopus* neurites emerged from soma regions parallel to grooves; rat hippocampal presumptive axons emerged perpendicular to grooves, but presumptive dendrites emerged parallel to grooves; neurites turned to align to grooves	79

Table 2 Continued

Feature type	Fabrication technique	Material	Feature dimensions	Feature frequency	Cell type studied	Cellular effect	Ref.
	Photolithography, casting, radiofrequent glow discharge	PS or PLA cast of silicon	1, 2, 5, 10 μm width 0.5, 1, 1.5 μm depth	Equal groove and ridge width	Rat bone marrow cells	Microtopography did not influence proliferation or actin organization; focal adhesions occurred only on the ridge for 1- and 2-μm surfaces and also in grooves for 5- and 10-μm surfaces for PS but not on PLA where they were only found on the ridges; Calcium content was higher on PLA than PS.	80
	Electron beam lithography, wet etching, and reactive ion etching	Quartz, PLL-coated quartz and PS replicas	Square grooves 1, 2, 4 μm width **14 to 1,100 nm depth**	Spacing not listed	Embryonic Xenopus spinal cord neurons, rat hippocampal neurons	Orientation of Xenopus and hippocampal neurites was unaffected by cytochalasin B, which eliminated filopodia; taxol and nocodazole disrupted hippocampal microtubules, but did not affect orientation or turning toward grooves; perpendicular alignment of hippocampal neurites was not inhibited by several calcium channel, G protein, protein kinase, protein tyrosine kinase inhibitors; some calcium channel and protein kinase inhibitors did inhibit alignment	56
	Photolithography, casting, radiofrequent glow discharge	PS cast of silicon	1, 2, 5, 10 μm width 0.5 μm depth	Equal groove and ridge width	Rat bone marrow cells	Up to 1 hour, cell attachment on grooved substrate was impaired; orientation to microgrooves was fastest on the narrow grooves; well-formed actin filaments were not present in cell body before 4 h, concluded that well-formed cellular actin cytoskeleton is not a prerequisite for occurrence of contact guidance	81

	Method	Material	Dimensions	Groove/ridge	Cell type	Results	Ref.
	Photolithography, casting, radiofrequency glow discharge	PS, PLA, silicon, or titanium casts of silicon	1, 2, 5, 10 μm width 0.5 μm depth	Equal groove and ridge width	Rat dermal fibroblasts	Production process more accurate for PS and PLA; cells proliferated better on RFGD surfaces. PLL showed highest proliferation; even if no sharp discontinuities present, microtextures still induce contact guidance implying that preferential absorbtion of protein at surface discontinuities is unlikely explanation for contact guidance; definite influence on cell morphology and behavior based on surface used.	82
	Photolithography, casting, radiofrequency glow discharge	PS cast of silicon	1–20 μm width 0.5–5.4 μm depth	Equal groove and ridge width	Rat dermal fibroblasts	Orientation was increased by increase of groove depth; confluency on microgrooves were able to support greater numbers of cells; largest cell numbers were not found on the narrowest and deepest microgrooves even though these had largest surface area and strongest alignment. RDF's follow contour of shallow and wide microgrooves but bridge deeper, narrower ones. Absence of contact between cells and bottom of grooves is important factor for establishing contact guidance.	83
Grooves and pits	Photolithography and anisotropic etching	Titanium-coated epoxy replicas of silicon original	V-shaped grooves 35–165 μm width, 30, 60, and 120 μm depth V-shaped pits 35–270 μm width and 30, 60, 120 μm depth	Repeat spacing 40–175 μm for grooves and 40–280 μm for pits, unequal groove and ridge width	Rat parietal bone implant model	Mineralization occurred often on grooved or pitted surfaces, but rarely on smooth control surfaces; frequency of formation of bone-like foci increased decreased as groove depth increased; frequency of mineralization increased as depth of pit increased; bone-like foci oriented along long axis of grooves	63

Table 2 Continued

Feature type	Fabrication technique	Material	Feature dimensions	Feature frequency	Cell type studied	Cellular effect	Ref.
Grooves and chemical pattern	Photolithography and reactive ion etching, silanization	Aminosilane and methyl-silane-coated quartz	Square grooves 2.5, 6, 12.5, 25, 50 μm width **0.1, 0.5, 1.0, 3.0, 6.0 μm depth**	Groove and ridge width equal, silane tracks equal	BHK cells	Cells aligned most to 25-μm aminosilane tracks and 5-μm-wide, 6-μm-deep grooves; stress fibers and vinculin aligned with adhesive tracks and grooves and ridges; alignment increased when adhesive tracks and grooves parallel; cells aligned to adhesive tracks which were perpendicular to grooves; F-actin oriented to both adhesive cues and topographic cues within same cell on the substrates with 3 and 6 μm depth; adhesive cues dominant	49
	Photolithography, anisotropic etching, polymer micromolding, treatment with alkanethiols	Ti, Au-coated polyurethane treated with fibronectin alkane thiols	V-shaped grooves, 25, 50 μm width, depth not listed	Groove and ridge width equal	Bovine capillary endothelial cells	Cells adhered to regions coated with fibronectin, which adsorbed to regions silanized with methyl- but not tri(ethylene glycol)-terminated silanes; cells attached to either grooves or ridges, depending on which possessed the methyl-terminated silane and fibronectin coatings	84
Ridges	Photolithography and reactive ion etching	PS cast of silicon original	0.5–100.0 μm width **0.03–5.0 μm height**	0.5–62 μm between ridges	*Uromyces appendiculatus* fungus	Maximum cell differentiation observed for ridges or plateaux 0.5 μm high; ridges higher than 1.0 μm or smaller than 0.25 μm were not effective signals; ridge spacing of 0.5–6.7 μm caused high degree of orientation of the fungus	85

Type	Method	Material	Dimensions	Pattern	Cells	Results	Ref
	Evaporative coating	Silicon oxide on PS	4 μm width **50 nm height**	Radial array	Murine neuroblastoma cells	Cells adhered to lines and processes aligned along the lines; processes grew in bipolar manner	86
	Excimer laser etching, casting replica, membrane replica	PDMS cast of polyamide, collagen 1 or gelatin cast of PDMS	40–200 μm width 40–200 μm height	Equal ridge width	Human epidermal keratinocytes	Keratinocytes differentiated to form stratified epidermis conforming to features of the membranes; stratification enhanced in deeper channels, infolds of epidermis increased as channel depth increased.	87
Steps	Photolithography/oxygen plasma etching	PMMA	1–18 μm steps	Blanket etching	BHK cells, chick embryonic neural, chick heart fibroblast, rabbit neutrophils	Cells exhibited decrease in frequency of crossing steps and increased alignment at steps with increasing step height regardless of direction of approach; rabbit neutrophils showed twice the crossing frequency over 5-μm step as did the other cells; presence of adhesive difference resulted in decrease in frequency of ascent only for step heights of 1 and 3 μm	45
Waves	Solution polymerization	PDMS gels of varying softness	Softer gels had smaller waves while hard gel had larger waves	3, 4, 15 μm periodicity	Human dermal fibroblasts and keratinocytes	Fibroblasts proliferated equally on all substrates; keratinocytes spread more and secreted more ECM on soft gels than on hard gel	88
Wells and nodes	Photolithography and etching	PDMS replicas of silicon original	2, 5 μm diameter round nodes, **0.38 and 0.46 μm high,** respectively 8 μm round well, 0.57 μm deep	4, 10, 19 μm center-to-center spacing for the 2, 5, 8 μm features, respectively	Rabbit implant model murine macrophages	2- and 5-μm textured implants had fewer mononuclear cells and thinner fibrous capsules than did smooth and 8-μm textured implants; cells on smooth PDMS were round with few pseudopods, but cells on 2- and 5-μm textures were elongated with pseudopods	89

Table 2 Continued

Feature type	Fabrication technique	Material	Feature dimensions	Feature frequency	Cell type studied	Cellular effect	Ref.
	Photolithography and etching	PDMS cast of silicon original	2, 5, 8 µm diameter variable spacing 2, 5, 10 µm constant spacing	Variable spacing or constant spacing of 20.4 µm	Murine peritoneal macrophages	Cells on 5-µm textures had smallest dimensions while cells on smooth silicone and glass had largest dimensions; mitochondrial activity highest on cells on 5- and 8-µm variable pitch surfaces and on polystyrene; PMA-stimulated cells on smaller textures were less active than unstimulated cells	90
	Photolithography and etching	PDMS cast of silicon original	Square nodes or wells 2, 5, 10 µm diameter	Depth or height of 0.5 µm	ATCC human abdomen fibroblasts	Cells on 2- and 5-µm nodes showed increased rate of proliferation and increased cell density than cells on 2- and 5-µm wells; 10-µm nodes and wells did not differ statistically from smooth surfaces	91
	Laser modification	Polycarbonate, polyetherimide	Square nodes 7, 25, or 50 µm wide 0.5, 1.5, 2.5 µm height	Uniform square array	Human neutrophils, fibroblasts	None of the textured surfaces significantly stimulated neutrophil movement compared to chemical stimulators, although neutrophil movement was greater on some of the textured surfaces than on an untextured surface; no effects on fibroblast orientation, spreading, or elongation	92

Pillars and pores	Laser ablation used in conjunction with masks made by electron beam lithography, reactive ion etching	PMMA, PET, PS	Circular pillars and pores 1, 5, 10, 50 μm diameter	Uniform array	Human osteoblasts and amniotic epithelial cells	Cells engulfed pillars or stretched between adjacent 1- and 5-μm pillars; cells attached to edges of pores, especially on 10-μm pores; texture caused increase in cell adhesion on all materials but PMMA; greatest increase in adhesion was on 50-μm PET pillars; 10-μm pores caused 5% increase in resistance to shear force	93
	Photolithography	Single-crystal silicon	Pillars: 0.5–2.0 μm width, 1 μm height Wells: 0.5 μm width, 1.0 μm depth	1–5 μm spacing for pillars, 0.5–2 μm spacing for wells	LRM55 astroglial cells	75% preference for cell attachment on pillars over smooth surface and 40% for wells over smooth surface; actin and vinculin highly polarized on pillars; cells made contact with tops of pillars but not into spaces	94
Pores	Microporous filter, nylon dip-coated with PVC/PAN copolymer	Uncoated and silicon-coated filters	0.2–10 μm diameter, depth not listed	Spacing not listed	In vivo canine model	Nonadherent, contracting capsules around implants with pores smaller than 0.5 μm implants with pores of 1.4–1.9 μm showed adherent capsules but no inflammatory cells; pores bigger than 3.3 μm were infiltrated with inflammatory tissue; pores 1–2 μm allowed for fibroblast attachment	95
	Microporous filter, corona treated for wettability	Polycarbonate	0.2–8.0 μm diameter, depth not listed	Spacing not listed	NIH 3T3 mouse embryo fibroblasts	Cells adhered and grew better on hydrophilic positions of the membranes vs hydrophobic positions regardless of pore size; Cell adhesion and growth were progressively inhibited with increasing micropore size.	34

Table 2 Continued

Feature type	Fabrication technique	Material	Feature dimensions	Feature frequency	Cell type studied	Cellular effect	Ref.
	Liquid–liquid phase separation	Glass coverslips coated with PGLA ± collagen	0.92–3.68 µm diameter	Surface roughness 0.277 ± 0.023 µm	Human hepatoma (HepG2)	200% increase in adhesion strength on microtopography vs. smooth surfaces; with the addition of collagen, 420% increase in adhesion over smooth surface; demonstrated that equivalent levels of cell motility were achieved with lower ligand density on microtextured vs. smooth surfaces.	96
	Microporous filters trabecular or columnar pores	Cellulose acetate/nitrate or polycarbonate	Trabecular: 0.22–3 µm pore size; Columnar: 0.1–3 µm pore sizes	Varying porosity	Bovine corneal button	Corneal epithelial tissue out-growth was increasingly inhibited by increased pore sizes of diameters greater than 0.9 µm. Porosity of columnar pore membranes at which outgrowth is inhibited is less than porosity of trabecular membranes. Pore topography is less restrictive on the migration of monolayers vs. tissue outgrowth; topography predominated over adhesiveness of substrate	31

Microporous filters	Polycarbonate	Columnar 0.1–3.0 μm pore sizes	0–16% porosity	Bovine corneal button	Continuous basement membrane and a regular pattern of hemidesmosomal plaque occurred only on the 0.1-μm surface likely due to both small pores and total surface area covered by pores; Adhesive structure formation on 0.4 to 2.0-μm pore surfaces was restricted to regions with no pores; No adhesive structures assembled on the nonporous or on the 3.0-μm surface	35
Miroporous filters	Polycarbonate	Columnar 0.1–3.0 μm pore sizes	0–16% porosity	Bovine corneal button	Surfaces with 0.1–0.8 μm pores supported superior stratification; Cytoplasmic processes penetrated 2- and 3-μm pores; Nonporous surfaces had a lower level of stratification	33
Microporous filters radio-frequency gas deposition	Microporous filters radio-frequency gas deposition	0.1 μm	Varying porosity	Bovine corneal button	Increase in tissue migration with increased hydrophilicity of the surface; migration was increased by 1.5 to 3-fold by the presence of pores; Collagen deposition enhanced migration on both nonporous and porous tissue with maximal migration on collagen coated porous substrates.	32
Spheres Particle settling	Poly(NI-PAM) particles on PS surface	0.86 to 0.63 μm diameter when temperature raised from 25°C to 37°C	2D hexagonal lattice, 0.96 μm avg. distance between sphere centers	Neutrophil-like induced HL-60 cells	Cells loosely adhered but did not spread on sphere-coated surface and could roll easily; excess active oxygen released when temperature was increased on sphere-coated surface, but not on poly(NIPAM) grafted surface	97

Table 2 Continued

Feature type	Fabrication technique	Material	Feature dimensions	Feature frequency	Cell type studied	Cellular effect	Ref.
Cylinders	Fiberoptic light conduit-fused quartz cylindrical fibers placed on agarose-covered coverslips	Fused quartz	12–13 or 25 μm radii	Spacing not listed	Primary mouse embryo fibroblasts and rat epithelial cell lines	Cells in the polarization stage of spreading with straight actin bundles became elongated, oriented along cylinder, and resisted bending around cylinders; cells in the radial stage of spreading with circular actin bundles or cells with no actin bundles tended to bend around cylinder and exhibited less elongation and orientation to long axis of cylinder	98
General roughness	Industrial polishing, sandblasting, plasma spraying with Ti-6Al-4V	Titanium/ aluminum/ vanadium alloy	Smooth, rough, porous-coated surfaces 100–1,000 μm pores on porous-coated surfaces	Random	Chick embryonic calvarial osteoblasts	Cells adhered to surfaces, using cellular processes to bridge uneven areas; ECM synthesis and mineralization were enhanced on rough and porous titanium surfaces	99
	Scratching with glass rod	PS and H2SO4-treated PS	Dimensions not listed	Random	Murine peritoneal macrophages Fibroblasts	Macrophages accumulated preferentially on roughened surfaces while fibroblasts preferred smooth surfaces	100
	Plasma pulse discharge	Carbon-coated polyethylene	Bare PE (10 pulses), globular 0.5 μm (50 pulses), fibrillar 3–4 μm (100 pulses)	Random	Human platelets	All coated surfaces demonstrated weaker platelet activation than uncoated PE; 50 pulse was the least suitable for contact with platelets	101

Treatment	Material	Topography/Feature dimensions	Type	Cell type	Observations	Ref.
Reactive ion etching followed by photolithography and isotropic wet etching	Areas of rougher, reactive ion etched silicon and smoother, wet-etched silicon	Reactive ion etched features: 57 nm avg. diameter, 230 nm height Wet etched features: 115 nm peak-to-valley roughness, depressions 100–250 nm in width	Reactive ion etched features: 137/μm² surface density Wet etched features: 27/μm² surface density	Transformed rat astrocytes, primary rat cortical astrocytes	Transformed cells attached preferentially to wet-etched regions rather than reactive ion–etched columnar structures; transformed cells on wet-etched areas spread in epithelial-like manner and were smooth; transformed cells on columnar regions were rounded, loosely attached, and exhibited complex surface projections; transformed cells preferred areas exposed to increasing amounts of wet etching; primary cells preferred columnar structures of reactive ion etched areas and did not spread on wet-etched areas	102
Acid washing, electropolishing, sandblasting, plasma-sprayed Ti	Titanium	1–2 μm pits 1 μm pits, 10 μm craters 10–20 μm globules and sharp features of < 0.1 μm	Random	MG63 osteoblast	Electropolished surface had more cells while TI-plasma-sprayed had less than TCPS; sandblasted surfaces had the same as TCPS; thymidine incorporation inversely related to roughness; proteoglycan synthesis decreased on all surfaces; alkaline phosphatase production decreased with increasing roughness except on coarse blasted Ti; correlation observed between roughness and RNA and CDP production	103
Alumina emulsion polishing, grinding with SiC paper	Ti, Ti/Al/V alloy, TiTa alloy	0.04, 0.36, and 1.36 μm peak-to-valley heights	Random	Human gingival fibroblasts	Cells aligned to grinding marks: 10% of cells oriented on surface with 0.04 μm roughness, 60% on 0.36 μm roughness, and 72% on 1.36 μm roughness	104

Table 2 Continued

Feature type	Fabrication technique	Material	Feature dimensions	Feature frequency	Cell type studied	Cellular effect	Ref.
	Electropolishing, sandblasting, acid etching	Titanium	0.14 μm, 0.41 μm, and 0.80 μm peak-to-valley heights for electropolished, etched, and sandblasted Ti, respectively	Random	Human gingival fibroblasts	Cells on smooth, electropolished surfaces showed flat morphology and grew in layers; cells on etched Ti migrated along irregular grooves; cells on sandblasted Ti grew in clusters; round and flat cells found on etched and sandblasted Ti; actin bundles and vinculin-containing focal adhesions observed in spreading cells on electropolished and etched Ti, but not in spreading cells on sandblasted Ti	40
	Sandblasting with different grain sizes and air pressures	PMMA	Sand grain sizes of 50, 125, and 250 μm produced peak-to-valley heights from 0.07 to 3.34 μm	Random	Chick embryo vascular and corneal cells	Surface roughness was highest for surfaces sandblasted with largest grains; migration area of cells increased 2-fold for vascular cells and 3-fold for corneal cells on rough surfaces compared to smooth; cell adhesion increased with surface roughness	39
	Sandblasting	Ti6A 14V alloy	Sand grain sizes of 500 μm or 3 mm alumina produced surface roughness measures of 0.16–3.4 μm	Random	Mouse osteoblast cells, and primary human osteoblast cells	Cells more spread on smooth surfaces; decreased proliferation and adhesion on rough surfaces; found ALOx rich layer on surface after sandblasting that may have influenced osteoblast behavior	105

Polymer solution casting	Nitrocellulose, PVDF	Smooth and rough surfaces, feature size not listed	Random	Rat sciatic nerve implant model	Tissue strips bridged nerve stumps in all of the rough and in some of the smooth nitrocellulose and PVDF tube implants; bell-shaped tissue adhered to rough tube implants; free-floating nerve cables, containing myelinated and unmyelinated axons and Schwann cells grouped in microfascicles and surrounded by an epineurial layer observed in smooth tubes; macrophages comprised initial cell layer on rough polymers; epinurial layer thinner on rough PVDF than on rough nitrocellulose; smooth PVDF showed more myelinated axons than did smooth nitrocellulose	106
Titania ceramic coating of substrates	Glass, alumina, titania	Surface features with roughness ranging from **6 nm to 813 nm**	Random	Rat ventricular cardiomyocytes	Favored formation of focal adhesion complexes; promoted cellular expression of vinculin, promoted preservation and maintenance of cardiomyocyte differentiated phenotype in long-term primary culture	37
Nanophase sintering of ceramics	Alumina, titania, hydroxyapatite	Grain size **24**–4520 nm; surface roughness 10–32 nm; pore diameters 6.6–233 Å	Random	Rat osteoblasts, fibroblasts, bovine endothelial	After 4 h: significantly increased osteoblast adhesion, decreased fibroblast adhesion, decreased endothelial adhesion on alumina and titania but equal on HA.	36

Table 2 Continued

Feature type	Fabrication technique	Material	Feature dimensions	Feature frequency	Cell type studied	Cellular effect	Ref.
	Anodization and hydrothermal treatment	Hydroxyapatite on titanium	Surface roughness 0.62 ± - μm 0.0–0.03 μm	Random	Rat bone marrow stromal cells	Increased cell adhesion over titanium surface alone; cell morphology was more spread with filopodia intimately adapted to the HA microcrystals. Actin filaments were localized to the filopodia	107
Protein tracks	Photolithography followed by silanization and laminin coating	Quartz, hydrophobic silane, laminin	2, 3, 6, 12, 25 μm width thickness not listed	Feature and spacing equal, also 2-μm tracks separated by 50 μm	Chick embryo neurons, murine dorsal root ganglia neurons	Smaller spacing caused decreased guidance; isolated 2-μm tracks strongly guided neurite extension while 2-μm repeat tracks did not; growth cones bridged narrow nonadhesive tracks; growth cone morphology simpler on narrower single tracks; growth cones spanned many tracks on narrow repeats; neurite branching reduced on 25-μm tracks	108
	Photolithography followed by silanization and laminin coating	Quartz, hydrophobic silane, laminin	25 μm width, thickness not listed	Feature and spacing equal	Embryonic Xenopus laevis neuritis	Neuritogenesis not affected; 65% of neurites aligned to tracks after 5 h; after an orthogonally opposed 100–140 DC field was applied; majority of cells remained aligned; some cells responded to both cues	109

Photolithography alternating strips of silanization	Quartz	50 μm or 100 μm widths	Not specified	Human bone-derived cells	HBDC cells localized preferentially to the EDS regions mediated by adsorption on vitronectin onto the EDS region; fibronectin was unable to absorb in the face of competition from other serum components; cell spreading constrained on EDS domains with lack of integrin receptor clustering and focal adhesion formation	110
Fibronectin coating	Glass coated with fibronectin	**0.2–5 μm width**	Spacing not listed	BHK cells, rat tendon fibroblasts, rat dorsal root ganglia cells, P388D1 macrophages	Fibers increased spreading and alignment in direction of fiber; actin aligned in fibroblasts; alignment of focal contacts in fibroblasts and macrophages; increased polymerization of F-actin, fibers increased speed and persistence of cell movement and rate of neurite outgrowth; macrophages had actin-rich microspikes and became polarized and migratory	111
Coating glass with protein and with- drawing liq- uid to orient protein	Oriented collagen or fibrin	Size of fibers not listed	Spacing of fibers not listed	Human neutrophil leaukocytes	Cells tended to move in direction of fiber axis alignment; movement was bidirectional; no chemotaxis evident	77

Table 2 Continued

Feature type	Fabrication technique	Material	Feature dimensions	Feature frequency	Cell type studied	Cellular effect	Ref.
Micro-textured surface	ECM replication-PMMA polymerization followed by polyurethane solution casting	Polyurethane positive cast of PMMA negative	**Micrometer and nanometer scale topography**	Similar to ECM not listed	Bovine aortic endothelial cells	Cells grown on replicas of ECM spread faster and had three dimensional appearance and spread areas at confluence which appeared more like cells in their native arteries than cells grown on untextured control surfaces	112
	Monomers and polymers of collagen	Polymerization of collagen I on coverslips	Homogeneous and dense network of collagen fibrils	Size not listed	Human skin fibroblasts	Collagen polymers induced a looser organization of the actin network and linear clustering of integrins, talin, vinculin, and phosphotyrosine-containing proteins.	113

Polymers: NIPAM: *N*-isopropylacrylamide; PAN: poly(acrylonitrile); PDMS: poly(dimethyl siloxane); PET: poly(ethylene terephthalate); PLA: poly-*l*-lactic acid; PMMA: poly(methyl methacrylate); PS: polystyrene; PVC: poly(vinyl chloride); PVDF: poly(vinylidene fluoride); TCPS: tissue culture polystyrene; *Other*: BHK: baby hamster kidney; CDP: collagenase digestable protein; ECM: extracellular matrix; GAPD: glyceraldehyde-3-dehydrogenase; LPS: lipopolysaccharide; MDCK: Madin Darby canine kidney; PLL: poly-L-lysine; PMA: phorbol 12-mystrate 13-acetate. Modified after Flemming et al., 1999 (30).
Bold type indicates nanometer size range features.

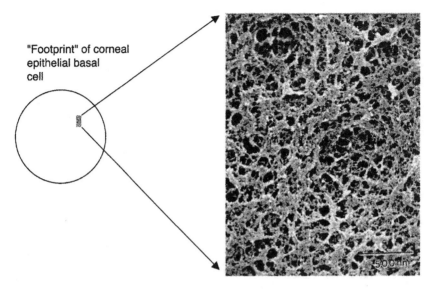

"Footprint" of corneal
epithelial basal
cell

Figure 2   Diagrammatic representation of the surface topography in contact with a corneal epithelial basal cell. The circle depicts a "footprint" of the epithelial cell. The insert is a scanning electron micrograph of the surface of the basement membrane underlying a small section of the epithelial cell. This demonstrates the large amount of nanoscale topography that the cell contacts.

National Institutes of Health 3T3 fibroblasts in cell culture (34). The formation of a continuous basement membrane and hemidesmosomal plaques were noted only on filters with pore sizes of 100 nm. On filters with large pore sizes, adhesive structures were noted only on smooth areas between the pores. Curiously, no adhesive structures were noted on control smooth surfaces, thus raising questions about the overall effect of porosity and pore size in this model system (35).

A number of studies have also evaluated random nanoscale surface features defined in terms of surface roughness. Cellular responses reported on these surfaces vary depending on the material and cell type investigated, making it difficult to determine trends. It is also difficult to compare the effect of topography based on comparing surface roughness value (R_a). R_a can be the same for two surfaces with very different topographical features. Nanophase ceramics created by sintering of alumina, titiania, and hydroxyapatite were used to investigate rat osteoblast, fibroblast, and bovine arterial endothelial cell behaviors (36). R_a values ranged between 10 and 32 nm. Osteoblast adhesion was improved on all nanoceramics, whereas

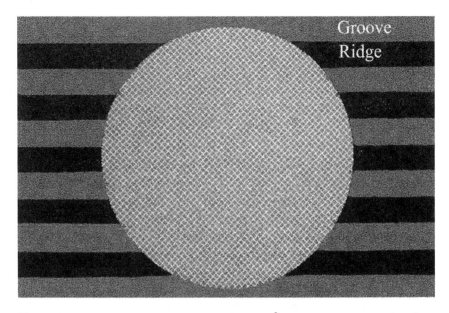

Figure 3 Diagrammatic representation of a 10-cm² cell on a 1-µm textured surface. A majority of previous investigations have used large surface features to evaluate cell behavior. Nanoscale features have also been shown to effect cell behavior and more accurately represent the true external environmental features in contact with cells.

fibroblast adhesion was reduced on all surfaces. Endothelial cell adhesion was decreased on alumina and titiania but was similar on both the nanophase and conventional hydroxyapaptite. There was increased vitronectin absorption to the surface of all nanoceramics, however, laminin was absorbed in high concentrations on control ceramic surfaces. The differences in protein absorption may explain the differences in cell behavior between cell lines. Sol-gel-derived titanium coating of ceramics with R_a values ranging from 6 to 813 nm maintained the structural organization of rat ventricular cardiomyoctyes in vitro (37). This surface favored the formation and even distribution of focal adhesion complexes and expression of vinculin over the entire area of cell surface contact when compared with ceramics without titanium coatings. Sandblasting has allowed the creation of surfaces with nanometer peak-to-valley heights. The percentage of oriented human gingival fibroblasts increased with increasing surface roughness from 40 nm to 1360 nm; increased migration was detected with chick vascular and corneal cells on rough versus smooth surfaces; human gingival fibroblasts had actin bundles and vinculin containing focal

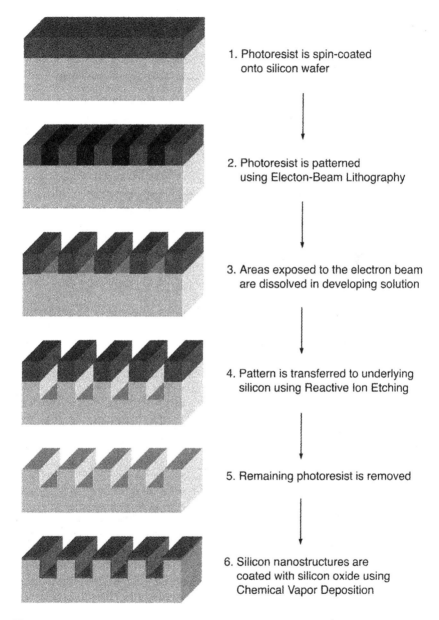

1. Photoresist is spin-coated onto silicon wafer

2. Photoresist is patterned using Electon-Beam Lithography

3. Areas exposed to the electron beam are dissolved in developing solution

4. Pattern is transferred to underlying silicon using Reactive Ion Etching

5. Remaining photoresist is removed

6. Silicon nanostructures are coated with silicon oxide using Chemical Vapor Deposition

Figure 4 Fabrication of surfaces with well-defined topographies through the sequential use of electron beam writing, reactive ion etching, and low-pressure chemical vapor deposition.

adhesions on electropolished and etched surfaces but not on sandblasted surfaces (38–40).

B. Studies Utilizing Controlled Fabrication of Topographic Features

The majority of the surfaces that have been investigated to date use techniques to create well-defined patterned topographies. Due to recent advances in fabrication techniques, surface features in the nanometer range are now obtainable. We have used electron beam lithography and reactive ion etching to pattern grooves and ridges with sizes down to 70 nm (Fig. 4). We have modeled our nanostructured surfaces after those feature types and sizes found in the basement membrane of the cornea (Fig. 5). These surfaces offer several advantages in that the features can be adequately described through a few parameters and are easily reproducible. Since they allow a variety of single feature types, sizes, and periodicities to be evaluated individually, interpretation of a cell's response to a single feature or a combination of features is possible.

When cultured on substrates presenting topographical anisotropies, most cell types elongate and align along the anisotropies. This phenomenon

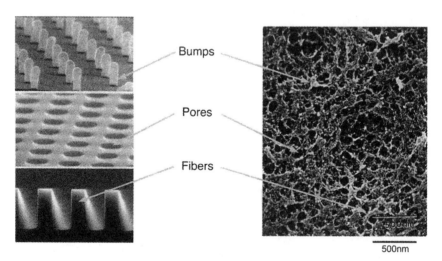

500nm

Figure 5 Surfaces with well-defined topographies can be used to investigate the effects of individual types of features (bumps, pores, and fibers) present in the basement membrane on cell behavior. This model is valid when the length scale of the fabricated features is similar to the sizes of the features found in the basement membrane.

is called "contact guidance" and has been reported in such disparate cell types as epithelial, macrophage, neuronal, and fibroblastic (Table 2). Anisotropic substrates can consist of orderly arrays of grooves and ridges precisely fabricated using microelectronics patterning methods or can be made by simple scratching of a tissue culture surface.

The chemical nature of the substrate plays a secondary role relative to that of topography in eliciting contact guidance. Similar cellular responses to topography were observed on substrates with vastly different chemical compositions (Table 2). Moreover, contact guidance was shown to be independent of surface chemistry in systems where cell proliferation was affected by the chemical nature of the substrate (41). A few cell lines have been found to be refractory to contact guidance; these include neutrophils (42) and cerebellar neurons (43).

Different explanations for contact guidance have been proposed depending on the length scale of the topographical features of the cell culture substrates that cause it. Glass fibers with diameters less than 100 µm were shown to align fibroblasts (44). The inability of certain linear microfilament bundles to conform to the substrate curvature was deemed responsible for preventing other cell orientations. The stiffness of microfilament bundles also explains why cell orientation along single steps correlates with step height in the range of 1–18 µm (45). This theory does not apply when more than one substrate feature is in contact with a single cell.

When a single cell encompasses several ridges and deep grooves it forms contacts preferentially with the top of the ridges (46–48). Contact guidance in these systems has been proposed to occur as a result of geometrical constraints imposed on the orientation of focal adhesions at the top of the ridges. Focal adhesions are ellipsoid structures approximately 2–10 µm long and 250–500 nm wide (48). Therefore, on narrow ridges only focal adhesions oriented along the ridges can have maximal area. Orientation of focal adhesions is thought to then drive orientation of the cell as a whole. It has indeed been observed that decreasing the ridge width from 10 µm to 2 µm results in stronger cell alignment (49) and that focal adhesions increasingly orient along the ridges. The orientation of microfilaments correlates with that of focal adhesions (47). All of the aforementioned work was conducted on grooves and ridges of micrometer dimensions. However, some cell lines have been shown to respond to features as small as 130 nm (43,50). This theory does not explain the impact of topographical features with lateral dimensions smaller than the width of focal contacts.

We have tested the response of human corneal epithelial cells to substrates with ridges 70 nm wide (unpublished observations). Cells elongated and oriented along these substrates to the same degree as cells cultured on 1-μm-wide ridges. The fact these 70-nm-wide ridges are much narrower than the reported width of focal adhesions raises the interesting possibility that the mechanism of cell orientation on these substrates differs from those previously described. As mentioned previously, cellular alignment on patterned substrates has been widely recognized to be inversely proportional to the groove/ridge width (49). This is contrary to our observations of the response of epithelial cells to features of submicrometer dimensions, where alignment was found to be independent of ridge dimensions smaller than 2 μm. This, in our opinion, reaffirms the need to study cell response to substrate features with dimensions in the more biologically relevant submicrometer range.

Even though in our studies cell orientation was insensitive to groove widths ranging from 70 nm to 1 μm, orientation increased with depth, as observed previously with other cell lines (49–52). Orientation was significantly greater on grooves that were 600 nm deep than 150 nm deep. We have gathered preliminary data using scanning electron microscopy that indicates that at least in the narrower grooves, cells are unable to extend cytoplasmic processes into the grooves. The reaction to groove depth was shown to be dependent on the presence of an intact microtubule system in baby hamster kidney fibroblasts (52). The degree of cell orientation is not dictated exclusively by the topographical characteristics of the substrate. In our investigations, cells cultured in the presence of serum aligned to the substrate topographical patterns to a greater degree than cells cultured in the same basal medium not supplemented with serum. Serum provides cells with an array of growth factors that initiate cell signaling pathways that are interrelated to pathways stimulated by cell attachment to substrate and may therefore act in concert to amplify the effect of the topographical stimuli. The serum also contains adhesive and nonadhesive proteins that adsorb onto the surface before cells adhere. Therefore, the chemistry of the surface that cells encounter during initial adhesion is vastly different when serum is present than when no serum has been added to the medium. The fact that proteins might be preferentially adsorbed on the groove and ridge boundaries has been proposed to contribute cell orientation on these substrates (47). Patterns of proteins would then be formed presenting areas of higher density of ligands for specific cell binding, leading to spatially segregated areas for focal adhesion formation and actin cytoskeleton organization. We have coated our substrates with a conformal layer of silicon oxide using low-pressure chemical vapor deposition to ensure that the chemistry of the patterned surfaces is uniform.

Cytoskeletal reorganization in response to substrate topography has been reported by several groups. In this respect, the use of cytoskeletal poisons to selectively alter the actin or microtubule cytoskeleton is particularly informative. In systems with patterned grooves and ridges of micrometer dimensions, it has been shown that only one of these systems (actin or microtubules) must function for contact guidance to occur (52,53). Moreover, even when both actin and microtubules were disrupted, cell reaction to substrate topography was not totally inhibited (52). Surprisingly, when submicrometer features were used, a functional microtubule system was found to be necessary to elicit contact guidance (53).

The study of cellular mechanotransduction would broadly include the modulation of cell behaviors by surface topography. In addition to focal adhesions, stretch-activated ion channels have been proposed to mediate mechanotransduction (54–56). The theory of tensegrity views cells as prestressed systems dependent on tensional continuity provided by contractile microfilaments to maintain their stability. External ECM adhesions, intracellular microtubules, and rigid microfilament bundles act as compression-resistant elements (57). Increased axial tension between two adhesion points to proteins adsorbed onto a rigid substrate leads to remodeling of the cytoskeleton and the formation of microfilament bundles between them, a phenomenon called *tension molding* (58). The observed alignment of microfilament bundles on patterned substrates is consistent with a form of anisotropic tension molding. However, it doesn't seem possible in the framework of this theory to explain contact guidance observed in the absence of a microfilament system (52,53).

C. Significance of Cell Shape

Chen et al. (59) have established that cell shape dictates cell fate. They used micropatterned substrates containing adhesive islands of ECM proteins of different sizes separated by nonadhesive areas. These substrates were used to control the shape of capillary endothelial cells. As cell spreading was allowed the cells would grow, and when cell size was decreased the cell would enter apoptosis. Next, by making the adhesive islands smaller so that the area of total integrin–ligand contact was similar to cells that were rounder but keeping them spread apart so the cell remained spread out, the cell continued to function and grow. This suggests that shape is very important in regulating cell function. Since a cell's shape can be controlled through cytoskeletal interactions with nanoscale topography, we can potentially control cell signaling pathways and therefore dictate the cell's fate.

III. SIGNIFICANCE AND CONCLUSIONS

As demonstrated here, surface topography has been documented to influence a variety of cell behaviors and undoubtedly has a role in how a cell responds to environmental stimuli. The vast majority of in vitro investigations have utilized cells that are grown on flat glass or plastic surfaces, a topography that is not found in nature. This fact may partially explain why discrepancies are often found in comparing results from in vitro and in vivo investigations. In addition, a better understanding of the effects of topographical features on cell behavior will likely impact the design of laboratory cell plasticware, cell reactors, and implantable prosthetic devices. Finally, the ability of topographical features of the substratum to influence diverse cell behaviors, such as orientation, adhesion, migration, proliferation, and differentiation, holds great significance for tissue engineering.

REFERENCES

1. LA Cary, DC Han, JL Guan. Integrin-mediated signal transduction pathways. Histol Histopathol 14:1001–1009, 1999.
2. FG Giangotti, E Ruoslahti. Integrin signaling. Science 285:1028–1032, 1999.
3. E Ruoslahti. Stretching is good for a cell. Science 276:1345–1346, 1997.
4. SA Mousa, DA Cheresh. Recent advances in cell adhesion molecules and extracellular matrix proteins: potential clinical applications. DDT 2:187–199, 1997.
5. E Ruoslahti. RGD and other recognition sequences for integrins. Annu Rev Cell Dev Biol 12:697–715, 1996.
6. RL Juliano, S Haskill. Signal transduction from the extracellular matrix. J Cell Biol 120:577–585, 1993.
7. H Lodish, A Berk, SL Zipursky, P Matsudaira, D Baltimore, J Darnell. Cell Motility and Shape. Vol. 1. Microfilaments, 4th ed. New York: WH Freeman and Co., 2000.
8. SM Schoenwaelder, K Burridge. Bidrectional signaling between the cytoskeleton and integrins. Curr Opin Cell Biol 11:274–286, 1999.
9. PA Janmey. Component localization and mechanical coupling. Physiol Rev 78:763–781, 1998.
10. K Burridge, M Chrzanowska-Wodnicka. Focal adhesions, contractility, and signaling. Annu Rev Cell Dev Biol 12:463–519, 1996.
11. R Timpl. Macromolecular organization of basement membranes. Curr Opin Cell Biol 8:618–624, 1996.
12. E Ekblom, R Timpl. Cell to cell contact and extracellular matrix, a multifaceted approach emerging. Curr Opin Cell Biol 8:599–601, 1996.

13. V Trinkaus-Randall, AW Newton, C Franzblau. The synthesis and role of integrins in corneal epithelial cells in culture. Invest Ophthalmol Vis Sci 31:440–447, 1990.

14. CH Streuli, MJ Bisell. Expression of extracellular matrix components is regulated by substratum. J Cell Biol 110:1406–1415, 1990.

15. DA Blake, H Yu, DL Young, DR Caldwell. Matrix stimulates the proliferation of human corneal endothelial cells in culture. Invest Ophthalmol Vis Sci 38:1119–1129, 1997.

16. HS Dua, JAP Gomes, A Singh. Corneal epithelial wound healing. Br J Ophthalmol 78:401–408, 1994.

17. IK Gibson, S Spurr-Michaud, A Tisdale, M Keough. Reassembly of the anchoring structures of the corneal epithelium during wound repair in the rabbit. Invest Ophthalmol Vis Sci 425–434, 1989.

18. M Berman. The pathogenesis of corneal epithelial defects. Acta Ophthalmol 67:66–64, 1989.

19. GA Abrams, SL Goodman, PF Nealey, M Franco, CJ Murphy. Nanoscale topography of the basement membrane underlying the corneal epithelium of the Rhesus Macaque. Cell Tissue Res 299:39–46, 2000.

20. GA Abrams, SS Schaus, SL Goodman, PF Nealey, CJ Murphy. Nanoscale topography of the corneal epithelial basement membrane and Descemet's membrane of the human. Cornea 19:57–64, 2000.

21. GA Abrams, E Bentley, PF Nealey, CJ Murphy. Electron microscopy of the canine corneal basement membranes. Cells Tissues Organs, in press, 2001.

22. E Bentley, GA Abrams, D Covitz, et al. Morphology and immunohistochemistry of spontaneous chronic corneal epithelial defects in dogs. Invest Ophthalmol Vis Sci, in press, 2001.

23. S Inoue. Basic structure of basement membranes is a fine network of cords, irregular anastomosing strands. Micros Res Techn 28:29–47, 1994.

24. H Kubosawa, Y Kondo. Quick-freeze, deep-etch studies of the renal basement membrane. Micros Res Techn 28:2–12, 1994.

25. HJ Merker. Morphology of the basement membrane. Micros Res Techn 28, 1994.

26. GC Ruben, PD Yurchenco. High resolution platinum-carbon replication of freeze dried basement membrane. Micros Res Techn 28:13–28, 1994.

27. Y Yamasake, H Makino, Z Ota. Meshwork structures in bovine glomerular and tubular basement membrane as revealed by ultra-high resolution scanning electron microscopy. Nephron 66:189–199, 1994.

28. K Hironaka, H Makino, Y Yamsaki, Z Ota. Renal basement membranes by ultrahigh resolution scanning electron microscopy. Kidney Int 43:334–345, 1993.

29. I Shirato, Y Tomino, H Koide, T Sakai. Fine structure of the glomerular basement membrane of the rat kidney visualized by high resolution scanning electron microscopy. Cell Tissue Res 266:1–10, 1991.

30. RG Flemming, CJ Murphy, GA Abrams, SL Goodman, PF Nealey. Effects of synthetic micro- and nano-structured surfaces on cell behavior. Biomaterials 20:573–588, 1999.

31. JH Fitton, BA Dalton, G Beumer, G Johnson, HJ Griesser, JG Steele. Surface topography can interfere with epithelial tissue migration. J Biomed Mater Res 42:245–257, 1998.

32. JG Steele, G Johnson, MK McLean, GJ Beumer, HJ Griesser. Effect of porosity and surface hydrophilicity on migration of epithelial tissue over synthetic polymer. J Biomed Mater Res 50:475–482, 2000.

33. BA Dalton, MDM Evans, GA McFarland, JG Steele. Modulation of corneal epithelial stratification by polymer surface topography. J Biomed Mater Res 45:384–394, 1999.

34. JH Lee, SH Lee, G Khang, HB Lee. Interaction of fibroblasts on polycarbonate membrane surfaces with different micropore sizes and hydrophilicity. Biomater Sci Polym Ed 10:283–294, 1999.

35. MD Evans, BA Dalton, JG Steele. Persistant adhesion of epithelial tissue is sensitive to polymer topography. J Biomed Mater Res 46:485–493, 2000.

36. TJ Webster, E Ergun, RH Doremus, RW Siegel, R Bizios. Specific proteins mediate enhanced osteoblast adhesion on nanophase ceramics. J Biomed Mater Res 51:475–483, 2000.

37. L Polonchuk, J Elbel, L Eckert, J Blum, E Wintermantel, HM Eppenberger. Titanium dioxide ceramics control the differentiated phenotype of cardiac muscle cells in culture. Biomaterials 21:539–550, 2000.

38. E Eisenbarth, J Meyle, W Nachtigail, J Breme. Influence of the structure of titanium materials on the adhesion of fibroblasts. Biomaterials 17:1399–1403, 1996.

39. M Lampin, R Warocquier-Clerout, C Legris, M Degrange, MF Sigot-Luizard. Correlation between substratum roughness and wettability, cell adhesion, and cell migration. J Biomed Mater Res 36:99–108, 1997.

40. M Kononen, M Hormia, J Kivilahti, J Hautaniemi, I Thesleff. Effect of surface processing on the attachment, orientation, and proliferation of human gingival fibroblasts on titanium. J Biomed Mater Res 26:1325–1341, 1992.

41. ET den Braber, JE de Ruijter, HTJ Smits, LA Ginsel, AF von Recum, JA Jansen. Effect of parallel surface microgrooves and surface energy on cell growth. J Biomed Mater Res 29:511–518, 1995.

42. J Meyle, K Gutlig, W Nisch. Variation in contact guidance by human cells on a microstructured surface. J Biomed Mater Res 29:81–88, 1995.

43. A Webb, P Clark, J Skepper, A Compston, A Wood. Guidance of oligodendrocytes and their progenitors by substratum topography. J Cell Sci 108:2747–2760, 1995.

44. GA Dunn, JP Health. A new hypothesis of contact guidance in tissue cells. Exp Cell Res 101:1–14, 1976.

45. P Clark, P Connolly, ASG Curtis, JAT Dow, CDW Wilkinson. Topographical control of cell behavior: I. Simple step cues. Development 99:439–448, 1987.

46. TG van Kooten, AF von Recum. Cell adhesion to textured silicon surfaces: The influence of time of adhesion and texture on focal contact and fibronectin formation. Tissue Eng 5:223–240, 1999.

47. ET den Braber, JE de Ruitjer, LA Ginsel, AF von Recum, JA Jansen. Orientation of ECM protein deposition, fibroblast cytoskeleton, and attachment complex components on silicone microgrooved surfaces. J Biomed Mater Res 40:291–300, 1998.

48. PT Ohara, RC Buck. Contact guidance in vitro: a light, transmission, and scanning electron microscopic study. Exp Cell Res 121:235–249, 1979.

49. S Britland, H Morgan, B Wojiak-Stodart, M Riehle, A Curtis, C Wilkinson. Synergistic and hierarchical adhesive and topographic guidance of BHK cells. Exp Cell Res 228:313–325, 1996.

50. P Clark, P Connolly, ASG Curtis, JAT Dow, CDW Wilkinson. Cell guidance by ultrafine topography in vitro. J Cell Sci 99:73–77, 1991.

51. P Clark, P Connolly, ASG Curtis, JAT Dow, CDW Wilkinsin. Topographical control of cell behavior: II. multiple grooved substrata. Development 108:635–644, 1990.

52. B Wojciak-Stothard, ASG Curtis, W Monaghan, M McGrath, I Sommer, CDW Wilkinson. Role of the cytoskeleton in the reaction of fibroblasts to multiple grooved substrata. Cell Motil Cytoskel 31:147–158, 1995.

53. C Oakley, AF Jaeger, DM Brunette. Sensitivity of fibroblasts and their cytoskeletons to substratum topographies: topographic guidance and topographic compensation by micromachined grooves of different dimensions. Exp Cell Res 234:413–424, 1997.

54. A Curtis, C Wilkinson. New depths in cell behavior: reactions of cells to nanotopography. Biochem Soc Symp 65:15–26, 1999.

55. A Curtis, C Wilkinson. Topographical control of cells. Biomaterials 18:1573–1583, 1997.

56. AM Rajnicek, CD McCraig. Guidance of CNS growth cones by substratum grooves and ridges: effects of inhibitors of the cytoskeleton, calcium channels and signal transduction pathways. J Cell Sci 110:2915–2924, 1997.

57. DE Ingber, L Dike, L Hansen, S Karp, L H., et al. Cellular tensegrity: exploring how mechanical changes in the cytoskeleton regulate cell growth, migration, and tissue pattern during morphogenesis. Int Rev Cytol 150:173–224, 1994.

58. DM Ingber. Cellular tensegrity: defining new rules of biological design that govern the cytoskeleton. J Cell Sci 104:613–627, 1993.

59. CS Chen, M Mrksich, S Huang, G Whitesides, DE Ingber. Geometric control of cell life and death. Science 276:1425–1428, 1997.

60. B Wojciak-Stothard, Z Madeja, W Korohoda, A Curtis, C Wilkinson. Activation of macrophage-like cells by multiple grooved substrata. Topographical control of cell behavior. Cell Biol Int 19:485–490, 1995.

61. A Wood. Contact guidance on microfabricated substrata: the response of teleost fin mesenchyme cells to repeating topographical patterns. J Cell Sci 90:667–681, 1988.

62. C Oakley, DM Brunette. Response of single, pairs, and clusters of epithelial cells to substratum topography. Biochem Cell Biol 73:473–489, 1995.
63. B Chehroudi, D McDonnell, DM Brunette. The effects of micromachined surfaces on formation of bonelike tissue on subcutaneous implants as assessed by radiography and computer image processing. J Biomed Mater Res 34:279–290, 1997.
64. J Meyle, K Gultig, H Wolburg, AF von Recum. Fibroblast anchorage to microtextured surfaces. J Biomed Mater Res 27:1553–1557, 1993.
65. B Chehroudi, TRL Gould, DM Brunette. Titanium-coated micromachined grooves of different dimensions affect epithelial and connective-tissue cells differently in vivo. J Biomed Mater Res 24:1203–1219, 1990.
66. DM Brunette. Spreading and orientation of epithelial cells on grooved substrata. Exp Cell Res 167:203–217, 1986.
67. DM Brunette. Fibroblasts on micromachined substrata orient hierarchically to grooves of different dimensions. Exp Cell Res 164:11–26, 1986.
68. ET den Braber, JE de Ruijter, HTJ Smits, LA Ginsel, AF von Recum, JA Jansen. Quantitative analysis of cell proliferation and orientation on substrata with uniform parallel surface micro-grooves. Biomaterials 17:1093–1099, 1996.
69. SY Chou, PR Krauss, PJ Renstrom. Imprint of sub-25 nm vias and trenches in polymers. Appl Phys Lett 67:3114–3116, 1995.
70. GA Dunn, AF Brown. Alignment of fibroblasts on grooved surfaces described by a simple geometric transformation. J Cell Sci 83:313–340, 1986.
71. B Chehroudi, TR Gould, DM Brunette. Effects of a grooved epoxy substratum on epithelial cell behavior in vitro and in vivo. J Biomed Mater Res 22:459–473, 1988.
72. DM Brunette, GS Kenner, TRL Gould. Grooved titanium surfaces orient growth and migration of cells from human gingival explants. J Dent Res 62:1045–1048, 1983.
73. L Chou, JD Firth, VJ Uitto, DM Brunette. Effects of titanium substratum and grooved surface topography on metalloproteinase-2 expression in human fibroblasts. J Biomed Mater Res 39:437–445, 1998.
74. C Oakley, DM Brunette. The sequence of alignment of microtubules, focal contacts and actin filaments in fibroblasts spreading on smooth and grooved titanium substrata. J Cell Sci 106:343–354, 1993.
75. J Meyle, K Gultig, M Brich, H Hammerle, W Nisch. Contact guidance of fibroblasts on biomaterial surfaces. J Mater Sci Mater Med 5:463–466, 1994.
76. TG van Kooten, JF Whitesides, AF von Recum. Influence of silicone (PDMS) surface texture on human skin fibroblast proliferation as determined by cell cycle analysis. J Biomed Mater Res (Appl Biomater) 43:1–14, 1998.
77. PC Wilkinson, JM Shields, WS Haston. Contact guidance of human neutrophil leukocytes. Exp Cell Res 140:55–62, 1982.
78. ET den Braber, JE de Ruijter, HTJ Smits, LA Ginsel, AF von Recum, JA Jansen. Quantitative analysis of fibroblast morphology on microgrooved

surfaces with various groove and ridge dimensions. Biomaterials 17:2037–2044, 1996.

79. AM Rajnicek, S Britland, CD McCraig. Contact guidance of CNS neurites on grooved quartz: influence of groove dimensions, neuronal age and cell type. J Cell Sci 110:2905–2913, 1997.

80. K Matsuzaka, F Walboomers, A de Ruijter, JA Jansen. Effect of microgrooved poly-l-lactic (PLA) surfaces on proliferation, cytoskeletal organization, and mineralized matrix formation of rat bone marrow cells. Clin Oral Impl Res 11:325–333, 2000.

81. XF Walboomers, LA Ginsel, JA Jansen. Early spreading events of fibroblasts on microgrooved substrates. J Biomed Mater Res 51:529–534, 2000.

82. XF Walboomers, HJE Croes, LA Gensel, JA Jansen. Contact guidance of rat fibroblasts on various implant materials. J Biomed Mater Res 47:204–212, 1999.

83. XF Walboomers, W Monaghan, ASG Curtis, JA Jansen. Attachment of fibroblasts on smooth and microgrooved polystyrene. J Biomed Mater Res 46:245–256, 1999.

84. M Mrksich, CS Chen, Y Xia, LE Dike, DE Ingber. Controlling cell attachment on contoured surfaces with self-assembled monolayers of alkanethiolates on gold. Proc Natl Acad Sci USA 93:10775–10778, 1996.

85. HC Hoch, RC Staples, B Whitehead, J Comeau, ED Wolf. Signaling for growth orientation and cell differentiation by surface topography in *Uromyces*. Science 235:1659–1662, 1997.

86. A Cooper, HR Munden, GL Brown. The growth of mouse neuroblastoma cells in controlled orientations on thin films of silicon monoxide. Exp Cell Res 103:435–439, 1976.

87. GD Pins, M Toner, JR Morgan. Microfabrication of an analog of the basal lamina: biocompatible membranes with complex topographies. FASEB J 14:593–602, 2000.

88. M Rosdy, B Grisoni, LC Clauss. Proliferation of normal human keratinocytes on silicone substrates. Biomaterials 12:511–517, 1991.

89. JA Schmidt, AF von Recum. Texturing of polymer surfaces at the cellular level. Biomaterials 12:385–389, 1991.

90. JA Schmidt, AF von Recum. Macrophage response to microtextured silicone. Biomaterials 13:1059–1069, 1992.

91. AM Green, JA Jansen, JPCM ven der Waerden, AF von Recum. Fibroblast response to microtextured silicone surfaces: texture orientation into or out of the surface. J Biomed Mater Res 28:647–653, 1994.

92. JA Hunt, RL Williams, SM Tavakoli, ST Riches. Laser surface modification of polymers to improve biocompatibility. J Mater Sci Mater Med 6:813–817, 1995.

93. SD Fewster, RRH Coombs, J Kitson, S Zhou. Precise ultrafine surface texturing of implant materials to improve cellular adhesion and biocompatibility. Nanobiology 3:201–214, 1994.

94. AMP Turner, N Dowell, SWP Turner, et al. Attachment of astroglial cells to microfabricated piller arrays of different geometries. J Biomed Mater Res 51:430–441, 2000.

95. CE Campbell, AF Von Recum. Microtopography and soft tissue response. J Invest Surgery 2:51–74, 1989.

96. CS Ranucci, PV Moghe. Substrate microtopography can enhance cell adhesive and migratory responsiveness to matrix ligand density. J Biomed Mater Res 54:149–161, 2001.

97. K Fujimoto, T Takahashi, M Miyaki, H Kawaguchi. Cell activation by the micropatterned surface with settling particles. J Biomater Sci Polym Ed 8:879–891, 1997.

98. YA Rovensky, VI Samoilov. Morphogenetic response of cultured normal and transformed fibroblasts, and epitheliocytes, to a cylindrical substratum surface. Possible role for the actin filament bundle pattern. J Cell Sci 107:1255–1263, 1994.

99. B Groessner-Screiber, RS Tuan. Enhanced extracellular matrix production and mineralization by osteoblasts cultured on titanium surfaces in vitro. J Cell Sci 101:209–217, 1992.

100. A Rich, AK Harris. Anomalous preferences of cultured macrophages for hydrophobic and roughened substrata. J Cell Sci 50:1–7, 1981.

101. IA Titushkin, SL Vasin, IB Rozanova, EN Pokidysheva, AP Alehhin, VI Sevastianov. Carbon coated polyethylene: effect of surface energetics and topography on human platelet activation. ASAIO 47:11–17, 2001.

102. S Turner, L Kam, M Isaacson, HG Craighead, W Shain, J Turner. Cell attachment on silicon nanostructures. J Vac Sci Technol B 15:2848–2854, 1997.

103. JY Martin, Z Schwartz, TW Hummert, et al. Effect of titanium surface roughness on proliferation, differentiation, and protein synthesis of human osteoblast-like cells (MG63). J Biomed Mater Res 29:389–401, 1995.

104. E Eisenbarth, J Meyle, W Nachtigail, J Breme. Influence of the surface structure of titanium materials on the adhesion of fibroblasts. Biomaterials 17:1399–1403, 1996.

105. K Anselme, P Linez, M Bigerelle, et al. The relative influence of topography and chemistry of TiA 16V4 surfaces on osteoblast cell behavior. Biomaterials 21:1567–1577, 2000.

106. V Geunard, RF Valenti, P Aebischer. Influence of surface texture of polymeric sheets on peripheral nerve regeneration in a two-compartment guidance system. Biomaterials 12:259–263, 1991.

107. J Takebe, S Itoh, J Okada, K Ishibashi. Anodic oxidation and hydrothermal treatment of titanium results in a surface that can cause increased attachment and altered cytoskeletal morphology of rat bone marrow stromal cells in vitro. J Biomed Mater Res 51:398–407, 2000.

108. P Clark, S Britland, P Connolly. Growth cone guidance and neuron morphology on micropatterned laminin surfaces. J Cell Sci 105:203–212, 1993.

109. S Britland, C McCraig. Embryonic *Xenopus* neurites integrate and respond to simultaneous electrical and adhesive guidance cues. Exp Cell Res 225:31–38, 1996.
110. CK McFarland, CH Thomas, C DeFilippis, JG Steele, KE Healy. Protein absorption and cell attachment to patterned surfaces. J Biomed Mater Res 2000:200–210, 2000.
111. B Wojciak-Stothard, M Denyer, M Mishra, RA Brown. Adhesion, orientation, and movement of cells cultured on ultrathin fibronectin fibers. In Vitro Cell Dev Biol Anim 33:110–117, 1997.
112. SL Goodman, PA Sims, RM Albrecht. Three-dimensional extracellular matrix textured biomaterials. Biomaterials 17:2087–2095, 1996.
113. I Mercier, JP Lechaire, A Desmouliere, F Gaill, M Aumailley. Interactions of human skin fibroblasts with monomeric or fibrillar collagens induce different organization of the cytoskeleton. Exp Cell Res 225:245–256, 1996.

5
Cytomimetic Biomaterials
Fabrication, Characterization, and Applications

Xue-Long Sun, Keith M. Faucher and Elliot L. Chaikof
Emory University, Atlanta, Georgia

I. INTRODUCTION

Supported lipid membranes can be produced by assembling a layer of closely packed hydrocarbon chains onto an underlying substrate, followed either by controlled dipping through an organic amphiphilic monolayer at an air–water interface or by exposure to a dilute solution of emulsified lipids or unilamellar lipid vesicles (1) (Fig. 1). In the process of membrane formation, the functional reconstitution of integral or membrane-anchored proteins can be readily achieved. As a consequence, supported lipid membranes have proven to be useful tools for characterizing both protein function and cell–cell interactions. Moreover, interest has been generated in the potential application of supported membranes as sensors or biofunctional coatings for artificial organs and other implanted medical devices (1,2).

A significant limitation in the widespread use of supported biomembranes remains their limited stability for most applications outside of a laboratory environment. In order to generate more robust systems, strategies have been developed to tether membranes to an underlying substrate, such as gold or glass with or without an intervening flexible spacer or polymer cushion. Characteristically, surface anchoring to gold has been achieved by thiol, methyl sulfide, or disulfide groups and by reactive silanes to glass (3–11). Recent reports have also described the use of a variety of membrane-inserting amphiphiles that have been covalently linked to the substrate through derivatization of either the surface, the amphiphile, or the

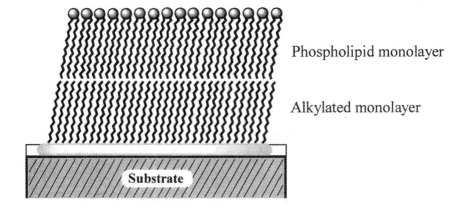

Phospholipid monolayer

Alkylated monolayer

Figure 1 Schematic representation of a supported phospholipid monolayer on a self-assembled monolayer of long chain alkanes.

intervening polymer cushion with reactive functionalities, such as maleimide (12), isocyanate (13), anhydride (14–16), or benzophenone groups (17). As an additional strategy, Stora et al. (18) have noted that surface-bound Ni ion chelators may serve to immobilize histidine-tagged amphiphiles. An objective of all of these approaches is the retention of lateral diffusion within the supported lipid membrane.

Membrane fluidity is critical for many of the functional responses of biological membranes. However, certain applications lend themselves to compromise in which a substantial increase in membrane stability may be achieved by in situ polymerization of the planar lipid assembly, admittedly at the expense of reducing lateral mobility. Utilizing this approach, surfaces that closely mimic living cells in their chemical heterogeneity and biological activity can be produced with increased physiochemical stability. As robust materials for biomedical applications, we term these systems *cytomimetic biomaterials.*

II. FORMATION OF ALKYLATED SUPPORTS ON SOLID AND HYDRATED SUBSTRATES

The formation of an underlying alkylated support is a critical initial step in the production of a substrate-supported biomembrane. In this regard, we have investigated the assembly and polymerization of phospholipids on self-assembled monolayers (SAMs) of long chain alkanes bound directly to gold and glass (2,19) and through an intervening polymer cushion to gold (20) and hydrogel substrates (21) (Fig. 2). A description of the formation of these alkylated supports follows.

A. Alkylated Glass Supports

Organosilanes, such as alkyltrichlorosilanes, bind to hydroxylated surfaces via the formation of a polysiloxane (Si-O-Si) network yielding robust SAMs (22–24). For example, octadecyltrichlorosilane, $CH_3(CH_2)_{17}SiCl_3$ (OTS), monolayers on glass or silicon can be easily prepared using a standard solution deposition technique (2). Characteristically, optimized OTS-coated substrates, even when prepared on commercially available glass coverslips, are topographically uniform with an average roughness of less than 2 Å/μm^2 and with associated advancing water contact angles of 110–113°.

We have used polarized external reflection spectroscopy to study the conformation and orientation of an OTS monolayer on silicon (Fig. 3). In both perpendicular (R_s) and parallel (R_p) polarized spectra, negative absorption bands due to the methylene (CH_2) stretching vibrations were observed. Significantly, the position of the methylene symmetrical (v_s CH_2) and antisymmetrical (v_a CH_2) stretching vibrations can be used as a qualitative indicator of hydrocarbon chain order (25–27). For example, the observed v_s and v_a CH_2 stretching vibrations at 2850.2 and 2917.5 cm^{-1}, respectively, suggest that the alkyl chains exist in a well-ordered, all-trans conformation. In applying quantitative methods, a molecular orientation of

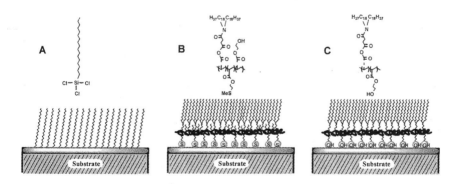

Figure 2 Schematic representation of an OTS self-assembled monolayer on glass (A), a sulfur-containing terpolymer self-assembled monolayer on Au (B), and a dialkyl-containing amphiphilic copolymer on alginate (C).

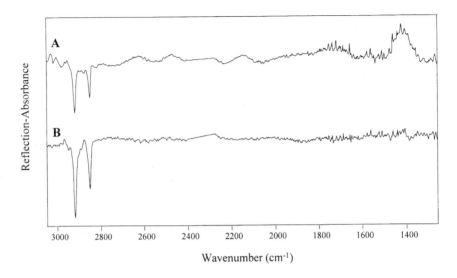

Figure 3 Polarized external reflectance infrared spectra of OTS monolayer on silicon (A) R_s polarized and (B) R_p polarized.

21.5° was determined (19,28–30). Additional descriptions of these systems, including the kinetics of monolayer formation and the characterization of these thin films using other vibrational spectroscopy techniques, as well as by atomic probe microscopy, can be found elsewhere (31–36).

B. Alkylated Metal Supports

In alkanethiol systems, the sulfur atom can form a coordinate covalent bond with noble metals such as gold, platinum, silver, and copper, yielding densely packed, oriented monolayer films (37,38). Notably, the binding sites of thiols on the substrate depend on the underlying lattice and, therefore, may be different depending on the metal type and structure. Gold has been the most widely studied surface for SAM formation because of its relative inertness and the ease with which it permits the formation of reproducibly ordered monolayers. Initial studies by Bain and Whitesides (39) on the formation of octadecanethiol monolayers on gold have been followed by extensive investigations by other groups. In an intriguing report by Spinke et al. (40), a molecularly mobile alkylated surface on a polymeric cushion was produced on gold through the design of a sulfur-containing terpolymer.

Specifically, the terpolymer consisted of 2-hydroxyethyl acrylate (HEA), 2-(methylthio)ethyl methacrylate (MTEM), and 3-acryloyl-3-

oxapropyl-3-(N,N-dioctadecylcarbamoyl)propionate (AOD). The methyl sulfide group of MTEM binds to gold as an anchor, with the hydrophilic HEA component acting as a "hydrophilic cushion," facilitating self-assembly of the alkyl chains of the hydrophobic monomer AOD. Optimal self-assembly of the dialkyl units at the solid–water interface occurs at a molar ratio of HEA AOD MTEM of 6:3:1. The resulting surface is hydrophobic, with average advancing and receding contact angles of 102° and 82°, respectively.

C. Alkylated Hydrogels

As an approach for generating a membrane-mimetic film on a hydrogel, we have described the synthesis of an amphiphilic copolymer composed of HEA and AOD (21). Alginate films were incubated in a copolymer/ tetrahydrofuran (THF) solution, followed by solvent desorption and resolution in water. Stable alkylation of the hydrogel surface was achieved, as determined by contact angle measurements and electron spectroscopy for chemical analysis (ESCA), with little change in wetting properties after 6 weeks of storage in an aqueous environment. We suspect that film stability is related to chain entanglement that likely occurs during the process of THF desorption and resolution in water.

D. Alkylated Polyelectrolyte Films

Recently, we have developed a convenient method for alkylation of a polyelectrolyte multilayer consisting of poly-L-lysine (PLL) and alginate (Fig. 4) (41). A necessary requirement was the preparation of a polyanionic amphiphilic terpolymer, composed of HEA, AOD, and sodium styrene sulfonate (SSS) [poly(HEA:AOD:SSS)]. The amphilic terpolymer is anchored to the polyelectrolyte multilayer by electrostatic interactions between oppositely charged sulfonate and amino groups. Contact angle analysis during the assembly process revealed that advancing contact angles were low for successive alginate ($\sim 5°$) and PLL ($\sim 10°$) mutilayers, but exceeded 100° after terpolymer coating. Ellipsometry revealed a film thickness of 28 Å for each PLL-alginate bilayer and 52 Å for the terpolymer coating. Unique infrared (IR) absorption bands included an amide I vibration for PLL ($1650\,\mathrm{cm}^{-1}$), antisymmetrical ($1550\,\mathrm{cm}^{-1}$) and symmetrical carboxylate stretches ($1400\,\mathrm{cm}^{-1}$) due to alginate, as well as methylene (3000–$2800\,\mathrm{cm}^{-1}$) and ester carbonyl ($1739\,\mathrm{cm}^{-1}$) stretching bands from the terpolymer (Fig. 5). Using the theoretical framework established in analyzing the polarized external reflection IR spectra of OTS/Si films (19), we concluded that the alkyl chains were tilted away from the surface normal.

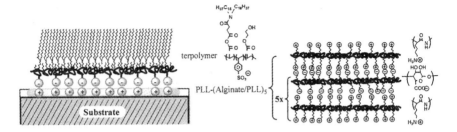

Figure 4 Schematic representation of the multilayer assemblies by consecutive adsorption of anionic and cationic polyelectrolytes on glass with the adsorbed polyanionic terpolymer assembly.

III. ASSEMBLY AND IN SITU POLYMERIZATION OF SUBSTRATE SUPPORTED PLANAR LIPID FILMS

An extensive literature exists on the two-dimensional polymerization of lipids in the form of vesicles; however, only a few studies have evaluated the feasibility of in situ polymerization of dialkyl amphiphiles at a solid–liquid

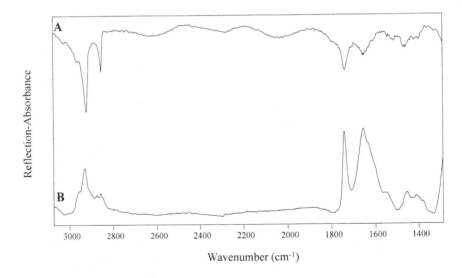

Figure 5 Polarized external reflectance IR spectra of terpolymer assembly on a PLL-alginate multiplayer (A) R_s polarized and (B) R_p polarized.

interface. For example, Regen et al. were the first to report the polymerization of bismethacrylate- and bisdiacetylene-containing phospholipids after vesicle fusion onto a polyethylene surface (42). Others have also polymerized bisdiacetylene containing phospholipids after Langmuir-Blodgett deposition onto a solid support (43,44). We have found that polymerization of acrylate-modified lipid assemblies on supporting SAMs can be readily achieved using both thermal and visible light–sensitive initiators and provides a convenient route for generating a supported membrane-mimetic surface assembly (Fig. 6). Notably, stable surfaces can be achieved without the need to form a cross-linked surface network.

A. Thermally Initiated Polymerization of Lipid Assemblies

O'Brien and coworkers were the first to study the polymerization of mono- and bissubstituted phosphatidylcholines containing acryloyl, methacryloyl, or sorbyl ester groups (45,46). While these investigations were largely conducted using lipid vesicles, they provided an important foundation for our own efforts focused on the polymerization of planar lipid assemblies (19,20,47). Typically, we prepare the monoacrylate phospholipid, 1-palmitoyl-2-[12-(acryloyloxy)dodecanoyl]-sn-glycero-3 phosphorylcholine (acryl PC), as unilamellar vesicles with a mean diameter of 600 nm and at an average concentration of 1.20 mM. A fusion time of 24 h is considered optimal and performed at 40°C, above the known T_m for the acrylate-functionalized phospholipid monomer. Thermally induced free-radical polymerization was performed using a water-soluble initiator 2,2′-azobis(2-methylpropionamidine)dihydrochloride (AAPD) at 70°C and at a monomer/initiator ratio of about 10:1.

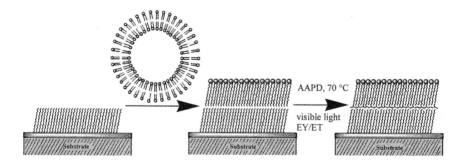

Figure 6 Vesicle fusion and in situ polymerization of a planar lipid assembly on an alkylated substrate by thermal or visible light–sensitive free-radical initiators.

Following polymerization of the planar lipid assembly, supported films displayed similar properties regardless of the underlying alkylated surface. Lipid films on $OTS/glass$ displayed advancing and receding water contact angles of 64° and 44°, respectively, and angle-dependent ESCA confirmed the presence of phosphorus and nitrogen. Likewise, advancing and receding contact angles of 58° and 31°, respectively, were observed for lipid assemblies on the *gold-anchored terpolymer system*, and the ratio of phosphorus to sulfur, as determined by angle-dependent ESCA, was in good agreement with anticipated results. The polymerization of a lipid assembly on *alkylated alginate* was performed in similar fashion, with advancing and receding water contact angles of 47° and 26°, respectively.

B. Visible Light–Mediated Photopolymerization of a Supported Lipid Assembly

A recognized limitation of a thermally initiated polymerization scheme is the inability to incorporate heat-sensitive biomolecules into this assembly. Toward this end, we found photopolymerization to be a useful technique, as the free-radical process can be initiated at room temperature. As an example, visible light–mediated photopolymerization has been successfully achieved at room temperature using the xanthine dye eosin Y (EY), which was initially characterized by Neckers and colleagues (48). The mechanism of initiation involves reductive electron transfer from a donor, commonly triethanolamine (TEA), to the dye. A proton is subsequently lost from the TEA radical cation, at the α position to the amine, to yield a radical species that serves as the initiator. In extending this strategy to the polymerization of a supported lipid film, we postulated that the TEA radical was small enough to diffuse into a lipid assembly and thereby initiate a polymerization reaction.

With these issues in mind, photopolymerization was investigated using visible light under physiologically benign conditions involving the EY/TEA initiating system. After vesicle fusion and in situ photopolymerization of deposited phospholipid layer on OTS/Si, an advancing contact angle of about 60° was observed, in good agreement with previous results using AAPD as the initiator. Additional confirmation of film structure was provided by ESCA.

Polarized external-reflectance IR spectroscopy revealed several distinct spectral changes and was particularly helpful in characterizing lipid alkyl chain orientation (19) (Fig. 7). Absorption bands that could be attributed uniquely to the lipid molecules included that of an ester carbonyl mode ($1739\,cm^{-1}$) and that of a methylene scissoring vibration ($1467\,cm^{-1}$). Significantly, a shift in the frequency positions of the v_s and v_a CH$_2$ modes

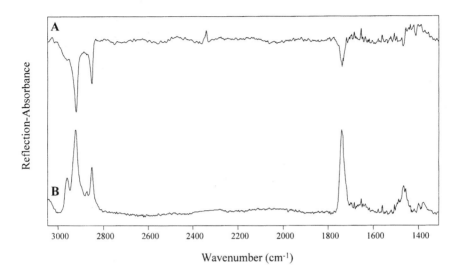

Figure 7   Polarized external reflectance IR spectra of a polymerized lipid assembly on OTS/Si (A) R_s polarized and (B) R_p polarized.

to 2920.2 and 2850.9 cm^{-1}, respectively, indicated a substantial increase in conformational disorder after lipid fusion. These frequency shifts were consistent with a calculated molecular orientation of 46.5° and suggests the possibility of multilayers or the presence of associated vesicles within the supported lipid film.

IV. CHARACTERIZATION OF FILM STABILITY, BLOOD COMPATIBILITY, AND THE IMPACT OF A MEMBRANE-MIMETIC FILM ON BARRIER PERMEABILITY

A. Stability of Polymerized Lipid Films

The relative stability of lipid films produced by thermal or photopolymerization strategies was characterized in two series of experiments. In the *first phase*, changes in contact angle were determined following sample incubation in deionized water at 23°C. Photopolymerized films demonstrated little change in contact angle over a 1-week incubation period in water. In contrast, the thermally initiated system exhibited an increase in advancing contact angle of greater than 10°, which may be due to the generation of a higher proportion of oligomers and/or low molecular weight polymer chains when a self-assembled lipid film is polymerized under these conditions. Paradoxically, others have reported high polymer molecular weights when lipid monomers are polymerized, in the form of lipid vesicles, at temperatures above the T_m of the monomer (49–58). This observation has been attributed to enhanced lateral diffusion of the lipid species as well as improved permeability of the lipid bilayer to the free radical initiator. Thus, our observations suggest that the assembly of lipids onto a planar support influences the effectiveness of polymerization.

We suspect that when the polymerization temperature exceeds the melting point of the acrylated lipid, monomer loss probably occurs throughout the polymerization process, which proceeds over a relatively long reaction period. Since the number average degree of polymerization of monoacrylated lipids in bilayers has been reported proportional to $[M]^2$, surface loss of lipid may have a profound impact on polymer molecular weight (49). Although a change in the phase state of the lipid monolayer does not establish a mechanism for lipid loss, several investigators have documented spontaneous thermodynamic rearrangement of phosphatidyl-choline molecules in favor of structures with smaller radii of curvature upon input of thermal (59,60), chemical (61), or mechanical energy (62–64). Therefore, with an increase in temperature, vesicles may be generated and subsequently lost from the lipid monolayer. We believe that visible light–mediated polymerization, which occurs at a temperature below monomer T_m, minimizes local monomer loss from the supporting substrate.

Polymer desorption occurs when a displacing moiety, such as a solvent, a solvent mixture, a surfactant, or some other polymer, replaces established polymer–surface contacts. Since high molecular weight polymer chains exhibit greater adsorption energy than their lower molecular weight analogs by virtue of increased surface contacts, it follows that the lower molecular weight polymers are more easily desorbed, all other factors being equal. In a *second phase of stability analysis*, octyl glucoside was used as a displacer molecule for the desorption of supported lipid films. A rapid increase in contact angle followed by a plateau region at longer incubation times was observed for both thermal and photopolymerized samples (Fig. 8). However, the rate of rise in contact angle and the final plateau values obtained for the heat-initiated system were indicative of accelerated lipid desorption, probably as a consequence of shorter polymer chains.

B. Blood-Contacting Properties of Polymerized Lipid Assemblies

An intriguing observation in the mid-1980s was the recognition that surfaces functionalized with the phosphorylcholine (PC) headgroup were associated with limited induction of blood clot formation (65,66). While not fully

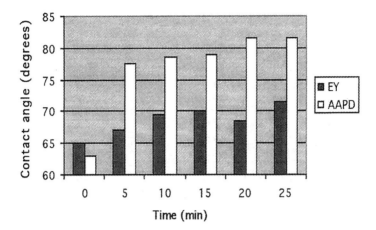

Figure 8 Change in advancing contact angle in the presence of octyl glucoside for thermal and photopolymerized lipid films.

understood, this biological property was attributed to surface bound water or, alternatively, the selective adsorption of specific plasma proteins, which inhibit the blood clotting process (67). In response to these observations, the PC functional group has been incorporated into a variety of copolymer systems, either as a pendant side group or, less frequently, into the polymer backbone itself (68–73). For example, in a series of studies from Nakabayashi's group, Kojima et al. (68) prepared a copolymer of 2-methacryloyloxyethylphosphorylcholine (MPC) and styrene, and Ueda et al. (69) prepared copolymers of MPC with various alkyl methacrylates, e.g., butyl-*co-n*-methacrylate (BMA). In a more recent report from this same group, Ishihara et al. (70) synthesized a copolymer of MPC, BMA, and a methacrylate with a urethane bond in the side chain, to facilitate polymer casting onto a segmented polyurethane. A similar strategy, in which a copolymer of MPC and lauryl methacrylate was synthesized and coated onto metal, glass, and polymer surfaces, has been reported by Campbell et al. (71). In an interesting variation of these approaches, Nakaya et al. (72,73) produced a polymer composed of PC groups in the main backbone chain. Most of these reports have confined their analysis of blood compatibility to short-term in vitro assays of protein or platelet adsorption.

We have used an external femoral arteriovenous shunt in a baboon model to assess the blood contacting properties of polymerized lipid films

(2). The baboon is considered the animal of choice for blood compatibility testing because its blood clotting system most closely resembles that of man (74). Our initial investigations have revealed minimal platelet deposition on polymerized phospholipid surfaces, in contrast to high levels of reactivity exhibited by uncoated glass surfaces (Fig. 9). Thus, we continue to believe that the biological membrane is a useful starting point for the generation of synthetic blood-compatible coatings for medical implants or biosensors.

C. Polymerized Lipid Films as a Modulator of Interfacial Permeability

Recent experiments have shown that non-covalently associated lipid bilayers can be deposited onto soft hydrated hydrophilic polymer cushions and in our view offers a route to barrier formation with enhanced control over both surface and transport properties (1,75). For example, Monshipouri et al. (76) have reported the encapsulation of alginate in lipid vesicles. Using standard extrusion techniques, particles were produced with an average diameter of 800 nm, and the presence of a nonpolymerized lipid membrane

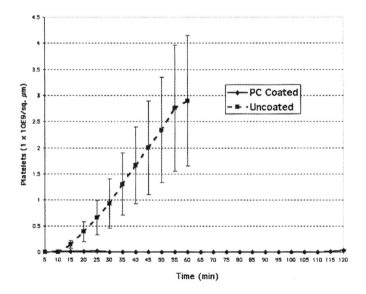

Figure 9 Platelet deposition on lipid-coated and uncoated glass surfaces in a balloon femoral arteriovenous shunt.

reduced the release of cytochrome c from the alginate core. Likewise, Kiser et al. (77) and Moya et al. (78) have noted that lipid assemblies adsorbed onto the surface of a polyelectrolyte can reduce the release of doxorubicin and 6-carboxyfluorescein, respectively. In principle, functional reconstitution of membrane proteins, including channels, transporters, and pores, could further enhance the selectivity of molecular transport across a membrane-mimetic film (4,5,79–82).

We have demonstrated that a polymerized lipid film can be formed on the surface of large alginate beads (diam. 2.3 mm) with an associated reduction in bovine serum albumin (BSA) diffusivity (47) (Fig. 10). Specifically, diffusivity of BSA through the alginate–aqueous interface was reduced from 3.42×10^{-4} cm^2/h to 2.25×10^{-16} cm^2/h by the addition of a membrane-mimetic coating. Similarly, the overall mass transfer coefficient for BSA through polymer-coated alginate beads was 4.71×10^{-9} cm/min, which was significantly less than that demonstrated by either Matthew et al. (83) for standard PLL-alginate capsules (1.5×10^4 cm/min) or by Crooks et al. (84) for microcapsules composed of a hydroxyethylmethacrylate–methyl methacrylate copolymer (4.21×10^{-6} cm/min).

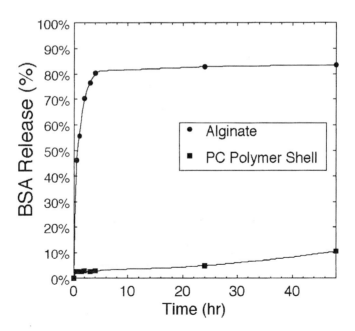

Figure 10   Release of BSA (MW 6.9×10^4) from alginate beads with or without a polymeric phospholipid membrane coating.

V. CREATING CHEMICALLY AND BIOLOGICALLY HETEROGENEOUS MEMBRANE-MIMETIC SURFACES

In order to enhance the capacity to create multifunctional membrane-mimetic surfaces, we recently designed a polymerizable lipid-acrylate functionalized phosphatidylethanolamine (mono acryl-PE) in which the amino function can serve as a handle for conjugation reactions (85). As shown in Fig. 11, terminal groups, such as biotin and N-(ε-maleimidoca-proyl) (EMC), can be introduced by acylation of the amine group of phosphotidylethanolamine. These linkers facilitate the incorporation of proteins or other target molecules via specific high-affinity (biotin) interaction (86–89) or by covalent (EMC) attachment (90,91). The utility of these polymerizable conjugates has been demonstrated on both flat surfaces and spherical microbeads using vesicles doped with 1 mol % of mono fluorescein isothiocyanate acryl-PE-FITC (Fig. 12).

VI. FUTURE PERSPECTIVES

Scientists and engineers are recognizing with increasing frequency that paradigms established in nature offer new approaches to the design of biomaterials with selective and specific enhancement of structural and/or functional properties. In this regard, membrane-mimetic systems appears to be an ideal starting point for the generation of coatings for biosensors,

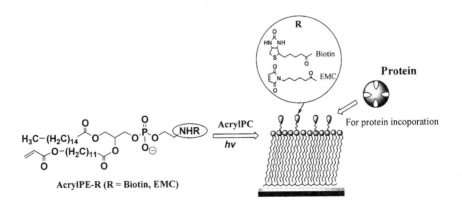

Figure 11 Structure of bifunctional phospholipid conjugates and their incorporation into a polymerized phospholipid surface.

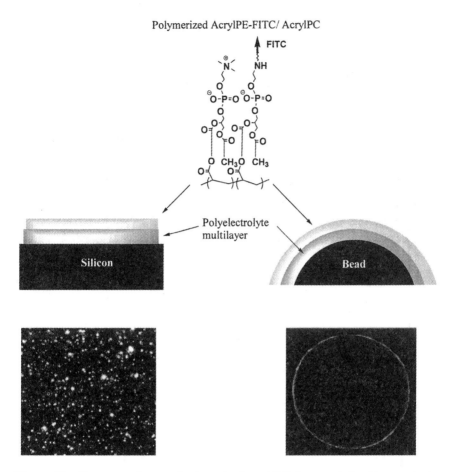

Figure 12 Fluorescent image of polymerized acryl-PE–fluorescein isothiocyanate–/ Acryl-PC surface on polyanionic terpolymer assemblies on glass (left) and on an alginate microbead (right).

large-scale arrays for high-throughput screening based on microfluidic technology, as well as implanted medical devices. We have demonstrated that in situ polymerization of a monoacrylated phospholipid is a convenient means for stabilizing a lipid film at a solid–liquid interface. In the process, both surface and interfacial transport properties may be modulated. Importantly, this approach offers a number of potential advantages over conventional PC-polymer-based surface modification strategies, including enhanced control over surface physiochemical properties and the capacity to incorporate diverse biomolecular functional groups into the membrane-mimetic surface.

REFERENCES

1. E Sackmann. Science 271:43–48, 1996.
2. KC Marra, TM Winger, SR Hanson, EL Chaikof. Macromolecules 30:6483–6487, 1997.
3. JY Spinke, H Wolf, M Liley, H Ringsdorf, W Knoll. Biophys J 63:1667–1671, 1992.
4. E-L Florin, HE Gaub. Biophys J 64:375–383, 1993.
5. AL Plant. Langmuir 9:2764–2767, 1993.
6. H Lang, C Duschl, H Vogel. Langmuir 10:197–210, 1994.
7. C Duschl, M Liley, H Lang, A Ghandi, SM Zakeeruddin, H Stahlberg J Dubochet, A Nemetz, W Knoll, H Vogel. Mater Sci Eng C 4:7–18, 1996.
8. B Raguse, V Braach-Maksvytis, BA Cornell, LG King, PDJ Osman, RJ Pace, L Wieczorek. Langmuir 14:648–659, 1998.
9. M Hausch, D Beyer, W Knoll, R Zentel. Langmuir 14:7213–7216, 1998.
10. CW Meuse, S Krueger, CF Majkrzak, JA Dura, J Fu, JT Connor, AL Plant. Biophys J 74:1388–1398, 1998.
11. A Toby, A Jenkins, R Boden, RJ Bushby, SD Evans, PF Knowles, RE Miles, SD Ogier, H Schönherr, GJ Vancso. J Am Chem Soc 121:5274–5280, 1999.
12. S Heysel, H Vogel, M Sanger, H Sigrist. Protein Sci 4:2532–2544, 1995.
13. M Seitz, JY Wong, CK Park, NA Alcantar, J Israelachvili. Thin Solid Films 329:767–771, 1998.
14. G Brink, L Schmitt, R Tampe, E Sackmann. Biochim Biophys Acta 1196:227–230, 1994.
15. D Beyer, W Knoll, H Ringsdorf, G Elender, E Sackmann. Thin Solid Films 285:825–828, 1996.
16. J Lahiri, P Kalal, AG Frutos, ST Jonas, R Schaeffler. Langmuir 16:7805–7810, 2000.
17. WW Shen, SG Boxer, W Knoll, CW Frank. Biomacromolecules 2:70–79, 2001.
18. T Stora, Z Dienes, H Vogel, C Duschl. Langmuir 16:5471–5478, 2000.
19. J Orban, K Faucher, RA Dluhy, EL Chaikof. Macromolecules 33:4205–4212, 2000.
20. KC Marra, DDA Kiddani, EL Chaikof. Langmuir 13:5697–5701, 1997.
21. JH Chon, KG Marra, EL Chaikof. J Biomat Sci Polym Ed 10:95–108, 1999.
22. DQ Li, MA Rater, TJ Marks, CH Zhang, J Yang, GK Wong. J Am Chem Soc 112:7389–7390, 1990.
23. K Bierbaum, M Grunze, AA Basaki, LF Chi, W Schrepp, H Fuches. Langmuir 11:2143–2150, 1995.
24. M Calistri-Yeh, EJ Kramer, R Sharma, W Zhao, MH Rafailovich, J Sokolov, JD Brock. Langmuir 11:2747–2755, 1996.
25. RG Snyder, SL Hsu, S Krimm. Spectrochim. Acta, Part A 34A:395–406, 1978.

26. RG Snyder, HL Strauss, CA Elliger. J Phys Chem 86:5145–5150, 1982.
27. RA MacPhail, HL Strauss, RG Snyder, CA Elliger. J Phys Chem 88:334–341, 1984.
28. T Hasegawa, S Takeda, A Kawaguchi, J Umemura. Langmuir 11:1236–1243, 1995.
29. H Sakai, J Umemura. Bull Chem Soc Jpn 70:1027–1032, 1997.
30. H Sakai, J Umemura. Langmuir 14:6249–6255, 1998.
31. A Ulman. An Introduction to Ultrathin Organic Films from Langmuir-Blodgett to Self-Assembly. New York: Academic Press, 1991.
32. A Ulman, ed. Characterization of Organic Thin Films, Stoneham, MA: Butterworth-Heinemann, 1995.
33. MN Jones. Micelles, Monolayers and Biomembranes. New York: Wiley-Liss: 1995.
34. MC Petty. Langmuir-Blodgett Films: An Introduction. Cambridge, UK: Cambridge University Press, 1996.
35. RA Dluhy, SM Stephens, S Widayati, AD Williams. Spectrochim Acta 51A:1413–1447, 1995.
36. R Mendelsohn, JW Brauner, A Gericke. Annu Rev Phys Chem 46:305–334, 1995.
37. PE Laibinis, GM Whitesides, DL Allara, Y-T Tao, AN Parikh, RG Nuzzo. J Am Chem Soc 113:7152–7167, 1991.
38. H Keller, W Schrepp, H Fuches. Thin Solid Films 210/211:799–802, 1992.
39. CD Bain, T E.B, Y-T Tao, J Evall, GM Whitesides, N R.G. J Am Chem Soc 111:321–335, 1989.
40. J Spinke, J Yang, H Wolf, M Liley, H Ringsdorf, W Knoll. Biophys J 63:1667–1671, 1992.
41. H Liu, KM Faucher, X-L Sun, J Feng, TL Johnson, JM Orban, RP Apkarian, RA Dluhy, EL Chaikof. Langmuir 18:1332–1339, 2002.
42. SLKP Regen, A Singh. Macromolecules 16:335–338, 1983.
43. LR McLean, AA Durrani, MA Whittam, DS Johnson, D Chapman. Thin Solid Films 99:127–131, 1983.
44. JA Hayward, D Chapman. Biomaterials 5:135–142, 1984.
45. DF O'Brien, V Ramaswami. Encyl Polym Sci Eng 17:108–135, 1989.
46. DF O'Brien, B Armitage, A Benedicto, DE Bennett, HG Lamparski, Y-S Lee, W Srisir, TM Sisson. Acc Chem Res 31:861–868, 1998.
47. JH Chon, AD Vizena, BM Rock, EL Chaikof. Anal Biochem 252:246–254, 1997.
48. O Valdes-Aguilers, CP Pathak, J Shi, D Watson, DC Neckers. Macromolecules 25:541–547, 1992.
49. TD Sells, DF O'Brien. Macromolecules 27:226–233, 1994.
50. PJ Clapp, BA Armitage, DF O'Brien. Macromolecules 30:32–41, 1997.
51. TMSW Sisson, DF O'Brien. J Am Chem Soc 120:2322–2329, 1998.
52. H-HKH Hub, H Ringsdorf. Angew Chem Int Ed Engl 19:938–940, 1980.
53. H Ringsdorf, B Schlarb, J Venzmer. Angew Chem Int Ed Engl 27:113–158, 1988.

54. DN Batchelder, SD Evans, TL Freeman, L Haussling, H Ringsdorf, H Wolf. J Am Chem Soc 116:1050–1053, 1994.
55. J Tsibouklis, JW Feast. Trends Polym Sci 1:16–19, 1993.
56. A Singh, MA Markowitz. In: J Singh, SM Copley, eds. Novel Techniques in Synthesis of Processing of Advanced Materials. 1995.
57. YSO Einaga, T Iyoda, A Fujishima, K Hashimoto. J Am Chem Soc 121:3745–3750, 1999.
58. JSTM Lei, HG Lamparski, DF O'Brien. Macromolecules 32:73–78, 1999.
59. RRC New. Liposomes: A Practical Approach. New York: Oxford University Press, 1992.
60. R Lipowsky. Curr Opin Struct Biol 5:531–540, 1995.
61. S Batzri, ED Korn. Biophys Acta 298:1015–1019, 1973.
62. F Olson, CA Hunt, FC Szoka, WJ Vail, D Papahadjopolous. Biochim. Biophys. Acta 557:9–23, 1979.
63. RC MacDonald, RI MacDonald, BPM Menco, K Takashita, NK Subbarao, L-R Hu. Biochem Biophys Acta 1061:297–303, 1991.
64. SG Clerc, TE Thompson. Biophys J 67:475–477, 1994.
65. RL Bird, B Hall, KE Hobbs, D Chapman. J Biomed Eng 11:231–234, 1989.
66. S Hunter, GD Angelini. Ann Thorac Surg 56:1339–1342, 1993.
67. D Chapman. Langmuir 9:39–45, 1993.
68. MIK Kojima, A Watanabe, N Nakabayashi. Biomaterials 12:121–124, 1991.
69. TOH Ueda, K Kurita, K Ishihara, N Nakabayashi. Polym J 24:1159–1269, 1992.
70. K Ishihara, H Hanyuda, N Nakabayashi. Biomaterials 16:873–879, 1995.
71. EJ Campbell, V O'Byrne, PW Stratford, I Quirk, TA Vick, MC Wiles, YP Yianni. ASAIO J 40:M853, 1994.
72. TM Chen, YF Wang, YJ Li, T Nakaya, I Sakurai. J Appl Polym Sci 60:455–464, 1996.
73. M Yamada, Y Li, T Nakaya. J Pure Appl Chem A32:1723–1733, 1995.
74. HM Feingold, LE Pivacek, AJ Melaragno, CR Valeri. Am J Vet Res 47:2197–2199, 1986.
75. M Monshipouri, AS Rudolph, J Microencapsulation 12:117–127, 1995.
76. PF Kiser, G Wilson, D Needham. Nature 394:459–462, 1998.
77. S Moya, E Donath, GB Sukhorukov, M Auch, H Baumler, H Lichtenfeld, H Mohwald. Macromolecules 33, 4538–4544, 2000.
78. M Stelzle, G Wissmuller, E Sackman. J Phys Chem 91:2974, 1993.
79. K Seifert, K Fendler, E Bamberg. Biophys J 64:384–391, 1993.
80. J-H Fuhrhop, U Liman, V Koesling. J Am Chem Soc 110:6840–6845, 1988.
81. TM Fyles, TD James, KC Kaye. J Am Chem Soc 115:12315–12321, 1993.
82. HW Matthew, SO Salley, WD Peterson, MD Klein. Biotechnol Prog 9:510–519, 1993.
83. CA Crooks, JA Douglas, RL Broughton, MV Sefton. J Biomed Mater Res 24:1241–1262, 1990.
84. X-L Sun, H Liu, JM Orban, L Sun, EL Chaikof. Bioconj Chem 12:673–677, 2001.

85. AL Plant, MV Brizyge, L Lacasio-Brown, RA Durst. Anal Biochem 176:420, 1989.
86. DH Kim, AL Klibanov, D Needham. Langmuir 16:2808–2817, 2000.
87. PJ Hergenrother, KM Depew, SL Schreiber. J Am Chem Soc 122:7849–7850, 2000.
88. DS Wilbur, M-K Chyan, PM Pathare, DK Hamlin, MB Frownfelter, BB Kegley. Bioconj Chem 11:569–583, 2000.
89. T Viitala, I Vikholm, J Peltonen. Langmuir 16:4953–4961, 2000.
90. JT Elliott, GD Prestwich. Bioconj Chem 11:832–841, 2000.

6

Micro- and Nanoscale Organizations of Proteins Modulate Cell-Extracellular Matrix Interactions
Lessons for the Design of Biomaterials

Jeffrey D. Carbeck and Jean E. Schwarzbauer
Princeton University, Princeton, New Jersey

I. INTRODUCTION

The interaction of cells with their extracellular matrix (ECM)—a network of biopolymers secreted by cells and assembled into a three-dimensional network—is a hierarchical process. Cell adhesion, the process of attachment to the ECM, starts at the nanoscale through specific receptor–ligand interactions; these interactions, in turn, result in the clustering of cell surface adhesion receptors into polyvalent focal adhesion complexes on submicrometer length scales. Focal adhesions act to organize the cytoskeleton over length scales of 1–10 µm. These interactions between cells and substrate guide the organization of cells into tissues on the length scale of millimeters to centimeters.

A general goal in the engineering of biomaterials is to integrate essential molecular elements of ECM into the biomaterial interface. Current efforts primarily focus on two objectives: (a) to pattern cell contact regions through control of protein patterning; and (b) to improve cell compatibility of surfaces by presenting small peptide fragments of ECM proteins that act as ligands for biospecific cell adhesion. These two strategies focus on the largest and smallest length scales over which cell–matrix interactions are modulated. The effects on cell behavior of protein organization on intermediate-length scales have largely been ignored in biomaterial design.

Protein organization in ECM on subcellular length scales plays an important role in determining cell behavior and should therefore be considered as a strategy for engineering materials with improved biocompatibility. This chapter therefore has three objectives:

To provide examples of ways in which ECM regulates cell behavior through the organization of proteins on multiple length scales;

To propose ways that synthetic materials might mimic some aspects of protein organization in ECM and, thereby, have improved bioactivity and biocompatibility;

To describe strategies for the processing and synthesis of synthetic materials that provide control over protein organization on multiple length scales.

II. CELLS INTERACT WITH NEIGHBORING SURFACES ON MULTIPLE LENGTH SCALES

Cell behavior is an integrated response to interactions with neighboring surfaces on multiple length scales. In vivo, most cell types adhere to the ECM, a protein- and carbohydrate-rich network that is both a framework for cell organization and a source of environmental information that directs tissue-specific cell activities (1). Cell adhesion to the ECM requires formation of productive connections over a range of length scales from the molecular to the cellular. Individual components of ECM or architectures derived from associations among several different molecular components induce distinct cellular responses. These cell–ECM interactions are mediated by cell surface transmembrane receptors that connect the ECM to the interior of cells through linkages with the cytoskeleton and interactions with a subset of intracellular signaling pathways. Therefore, examination of cell adhesion and multicellular organization over a broad size range is necessary to understand tissue development and regulation, and to translate this understanding into strategies for engineering the cell–materials interface.

A. Cell Adhesion Is Mediated by Specific Receptor–Ligand Interactions

Cells adhere to ECM and to each other through interactions with specific adhesion receptors on the cell surface. The primary receptors for binding to ECM belong to the integrin family (2,3). Integrins extend approximately 20 nm above the plasma membrane of cells, and the contact site between one integrin receptor and the major binding site on fibronectin, a major protein component of most extracellular matrices (4), spans about 5 nm (5). Integrins are heterodimeric transmembrane complexes consisting of one α and one β subunit. Humans have at least 26 different $\alpha\beta$ pairs, each with a unique specificity for a ligand and/or a distinct tissue distribution. At least 8 of these integrins recognize fibronectin; interactions between fibronectin and many of these 8 integrins require the Arg-Gly-Asp (RGD) cell-binding sequence. In most cases, the RGD sequence alone does not provide sufficient information for specificity or optimal cell binding. Other nearby sequences in fibronectin make significant contributions to cell–fibronectin interactions (6,7).

B. Cell Adhesion Molecules in the ECM Are Composed of Multiple Subunits and Multiple Functional Domains

ECM proteins come in a wide variety of shapes and sizes (8). Those ECM proteins that perform both structural and cell adhesive roles tend to be large (>100 kDa) with multiple subunits and binding sites. Some examples include fibronectin, laminin, collagen, and tenascin. Each of these ECM proteins has more than one cell binding site and is capable of interacting with more than one integrin heterodimer. In addition to cell binding domains, these proteins can interact with other ECM components, including themselves. For example, fibronectin is a dimeric protein composed of 250 kDa subunits. Each subunit has binding sites for cell receptors, collagen, tenascin, heparin, and other fibronectin molecules (Fig. 1). (4). Similarly, each tenascin subunit binds to cells, heparin, and fibronectin (Fig. 1) (9). The fibronectin dimer extends about 140 nm in length and the tenascin hexamer is about 170 nm across (10); individual domains and binding sites range in size from approximately 3 to 10 nm (5,11).

C. Molecules in the ECM Are Organized into Supramolecular Structures

The multimeric nature of these ECM proteins provides a way to link numerous components with each other and with cells to optimize cell–ECM interactions. Such a combinatorial approach provides significant pliability in the organization of the network. Light and electron microscopy (1,4,12) have revealed only limited types of gross organization. Long extended fibrils are a common ECM protein architecture. For fibronectin, these fibrils vary in width from 10 to more than 100 nm, with lengths extending well beyond 5–10 μm (Fig. 2). Much larger dimensions are found with certain types of collagen fibers. The assembly of ECM proteins into fibrils is orchestrated by

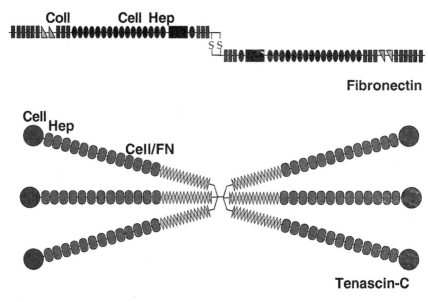

Figure 1 Fibronectin and tenascin-C are multimeric modular proteins. Both fibronectin and tenascin C are large multimeric proteins consisting of repeating modules (designated by ovals, rectangles, triangles, and diamonds). Sets of modules comprise domains that have binding activities for other extracellular molecules. Domains for interacting with cell receptors (Cell), collagen (Coll), heparin (Hep), and fibronectin (FN) are indicated. Dimeric fibronectin is formed through a pair of disulfide bonds at the carboxy terminus of each subunit (SS). The tenascin-C hexamer is held together by a disulfide knot containing the amino termini of six identical subunits.

cells (13); interactions with specific cell receptors lead to conversion of soluble proteins to insoluble fibrils, which are further stabilized and strengthened by additional protein–protein interactions, both covalent and non-covalent.

D. ECM Protein Binding Induces Integrin Receptor Clustering on the Cell Surface

Multimeric ECM proteins bind to integrins and thereby stimulate receptor movement into clusters; a very small initial contact area between a single receptor–ligand pair is rapidly converted to a multivalent structure, called a focal adhesion (Fig. 3). (14). The dimensions of focal adhesions usually

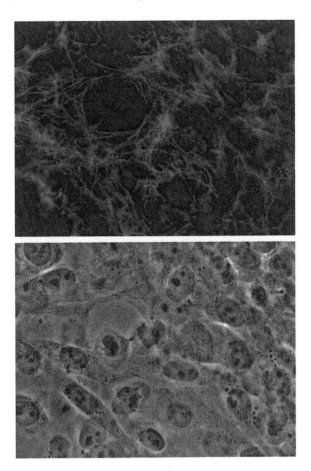

Figure 2   Cells surround themselves with fibrillar fibronectin matrix. CHO cells use integrin receptors to bind and assemble fibronectin into a fibrillar network. Fibrils are detected by immunofluorescence using an antifibronectin monoclonal antibody (top). The dense cell monolayer can be seen in the phase image (bottom).

range from 20 to 100 nm. The specific composition and organization of this protein-rich complex depends on the cell type, ECM substrate, and specific integrins involved in its formation. On the inner membrane face of focal adhesions, integrin cytoplasmic domains serve as anchoring points for the actin cytoskeleton (Fig. 3); integrins within focal adhesions are physical links between ECM fibrils and actin filaments. In this way, cytoskeletal organization reflects the architecture of proteins in the ECM, and

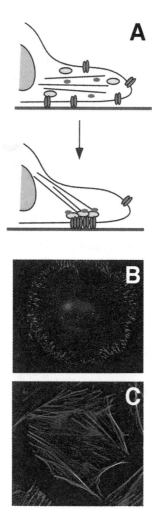

Figure 3 Cell–ECM interactions induce formation of focal adhesions and stress fibers. (A) Cell adhesion is promoted by binding of cell surface integrins (ovals) to fibronectin matrix. Integrins cluster at sites of receptor–ligand contact and are activated to bind cytoskeletal-associated proteins. These proteins link integrins to actin filaments (black lines), which are then organized into stress fibers. Focal adhesions also recruit components of intracellular signaling pathways. (B) The cytoskeletal-associated protein vinculin localizes to focal adhesions at the periphery of a fibroblast cell spreading on fibronectin as detected by immunofluorescence with an antivinculin antibody. (C) Cell spreading on fibronectin also induces formation of actin stress fibers as detected with rhodamine-conjugated phalloidin. The stress fibers terminate at focal adhesions.

information within the ECM structure can be interpreted by cells through rearrangements of the cytoskeleton. Thus, integrin binding on the nanoscale controls cytoskeletal structure on the micrometer scale and, ultimately, tissue organization on the millimeter scale. In addition to this role of anchoring the cytoskeleton to the underlying substrate, focal adhesions are also initiation sites for intracellular signaling.

E. Cell–ECM and Cell–Cell Contacts Determine the Architectures of Tissues and Organs

Cells establish the ECM network and then reorganize themselves within that framework to optimize contacts with other cells and connections to their protein environments. In this way, small clusters of cells with surrounding ECM develop into larger multicompartment tissues. Cell functions develop concomitantly, induced by specific tissue structures and components. This propagation of structure then expands the size range of interactions to the multicellular scale: for example, from 20 μm for an individual cell to 500 μm for a hepatic lobule, up to centimeters for a full-sized liver. The information that leads to these macroscopic structures initiates at the molecular scale.

III. EXTRACELLULAR MATRIX REGULATES CELL BEHAVIOR

In the ECM, multiple components combine to provide a unique environment for cell organization and function. The molecular organization of ECM varies between different tissues and with the stage of development in a specific tissue; organization of ECM also changes in response to many pathological processes. These changes in organization at the molecular level regulate cell–ECM interactions and have important roles in embryogenesis, wound healing, tumor growth, and normal tissue homeostasis (1,15). At the cellular level, ECM structure and composition modulate cell morphology, cytoskeletal organization, intracellular signaling, cell cycle progression, and rates of cell migration. To be able to mimic or control these cellular processes in the context of synthetic materials requires an understanding of the mechanisms that underlie control of cell behavior via the ECM. Although we lack a detailed understanding of how the individual components of the ECM combine to help regulate and direct cell function, some general mechanisms by which this complex network controls and activates specific cellular responses have been identified. Below are described some of these mechanisms.

A. Cell Binding of Matrix Proteins Activates Intracellular Signaling Pathways

In general, the matrix alters cell behavior through the activation of intracellular signaling pathways. However, the specific pathways activated by the presence of distinct proteins within ECM vary with ligand presentation and density, cell surface receptor repertoire, and availability of essential intracellular intermediates. Thus, different cell types can respond quite differently to the same matrix. For one cell type, a particular ECM may induce cell adhesion, whereas another cell type will respond by migrating or proliferating.

Binding of an ECM protein like fibronectin to its integrin receptors has been shown to activate a number of different intracellular pathways that control cellular processes. Examples of specific proteins involved in these pathways include Ras and ERK/MAP kinases, focal adhesion kinase, Src family kinases, adapter proteins like Cas and paxillin, and members of the Rho GTPase family (2,16). It is becoming clear that signals initiated by integrin ligation synergize with signals from other types of receptor–ligand interactions including growth factors and chemokines (17). The cell then alters its physiological state in response to the combined signals.

One example of such synergy lies in the regulation of cell signaling and cytoskeletal organization by Rho GTPases. This family of small GTP-binding proteins consists of Rho, Rac, and Cdc42, all of which are activated by GTP binding and lead to distinct rearrangements of the actin cytoskeleton (18). Active Rho induces formation of focal adhesions and actin stress fibers—stable actin filaments that exist under tension in the cytoplasm and are indicative of cell adhesion (Fig. 3). Stimulation of Rac or Cdc42 induces extension of lamellipodia or filopodia, respectively (membrane projections associated with cell migration). Multiple routes exist for in vivo activation of these GTPases. For example, binding of the soluble factor lysophosphatidic acid (LPA) to its cell surface receptor leads to downstream activation of Rho, which in turn initiates a cascade of events culminating in actin reorganization into stress fibers. Integrin-mediated adhesion on fibronectin also activates Rho via a process that is independent of LPA but results in a similar cell response. Concomitant assembly of focal adhesions, however, requires dual activation of receptors for both LPA and fibronectin (19); this requirement for dual activation provides a clear demonstration that signals from these two stimuli are coordinated to regulate Rho activity. ECM and soluble factors affect other signaling pathways in a similar way.

B. Density of Cell Binding Sites Affects Adhesion and Migration

Traditionally, cell adhesion has been studied using in vitro assays where pure proteins are coated onto planar surfaces. In the simplest system, various concentrations of fibronectin are coated, and the number of cells attached over time and the area of cell spreading are monitored. Using this type of approach, it has been demonstrated that cells show increased attachment and spreading with increasing fibronectin concentrations. These results show that the number of cell–fibronectin interactions and thus the availability of cell binding sites determines the specific cell responses to fibronectin.

A more quantitative example of the effects of ECM variation on cell behavior comes from the analysis of cell migration speed by Palecek et al. (20). Using cells expressing integrin receptors of known activity and number with substrates coated with varying concentrations of fibronectin, they showed that maximal cell migration speed was attained at intermediate adhesive strength. Strong adhesion, which could be attained by increasing either the amount of fibronectin on the substrate or the number of integrin receptors on the cells, reduced migration speed. Likewise, weak adhesion on low fibronectin substrates or with low numbers of integrins slowed migration rates.

C. Organization of Matrix Contact Sites Regulates Cell Proliferation

In a classic study by Folkman and Moscona (21), the extent of spreading of fibroblasts and endothelial cells was shown to be proportional to the amount of DNA synthesis and thus to progression through the cell cycle. Using two approaches to modulate cell shape—substrate adhesivity and cell confluence—they also showed that shape played a critical role, with rounder cells showing less DNA synthesis than flatter cells. In a more detailed analysis of the correlations between cell shape and growth, Chen et al. (22) considered the potential contributions from integrin–fibronectin binding. Micropatterned fibronectin substrates were used to provide a constant number of cell contact areas distributed over different total surface areas. Their results showed that patterns that produce more highly spread cells stimulate cell proliferation and suppress cell death. Therefore, the balance between cell growth and death is not solely dependent on the number of integrin–fibronectin interactions; the shape of the cell makes a major contribution.

The architecture of matrix fibrils also contributes to regulation of cell growth. Small-molecule inhibitors and fibronectin-null cells have been used to show that fibronectin fibril formation can have a dramatic stimulatory effect on cell proliferation (23–25). Furthermore, changes in matrix structure affect cell growth. For example, certain mutant recombinant fibronectins assemble into a fibrillar matrix that is structurally distinct from a native fibronectin matrix (26). The fibrils show less uniformity in thickness and length and are less evenly distributed over the cell surface. The mutant matrix actually inhibits cell cycle progression relative to native fibronectin matrix, indicating that fibril organization provides positional information that affects intracellular processes. Taken together, there appears to be interplay between cell shape, integrin engagement, and matrix architecture in the control of cell growth and probably other cell functions.

Simple systems in which one ECM protein is provided as a substrate for cells with defined types of receptors show us what the ECM can do. What do these in vitro studies tell us about the role of the matrix in vivo? Manipulations of ECM components in amphibian embryos have provided a unique model system to determine the matrix requirements for cell migration and early developmental processes such as gastrulation during which cells on the outside of the embryo move inward to establish the main body plan. Embryonic cells move inside over a fibronectin matrix (27–29). Inhibition of matrix formation prevents further development of *Xenopus* and *Pleurodeles* embryos, showing an early requirement for this structure. Perturbation of fibronectin fibril organization by incorporation of mutant fibronectins also results in dramatic defects in embryo morphology by reducing cell adhesion and migration (30). Together these amphibian embryo studies show that similar ECM defects can be obtained in cell culture as well as in embryos and that these defects have dire consequences in vivo. Furthermore, the similar effects of matrix organization on cells in culture and in embryos serve to validate cell culture as a useful model for dissecting ECM structure and function.

D. Combinations of ECM Proteins Modulate Cell Functions

The composition of the ECM is dynamic; protein deposition and degradation occur continuously and are up-regulated in situations where significant changes in matrix organization are required, such as at sites of injury or disease. In these situations, cell movement and growth is required and depends in large part on the constitution of the ECM. One way to generate a matrix that is conducive to cell migration is by depositing proteins that modulate the adhesive nature of the matrix. The presence of proteins like tenascin-C and thrombospondin-1 correlates with cell movement in vivo (9,31). These two proteins belong to a class of proteins shown to modulate cell adhesion in culture. Each of these proteins can support cell adhesion on its own; however, such proteins also have contradictory effects on cell interactions when mixed with other adhesion proteins. Chick embryo fibroblasts fail to adhere to fibronectin in the presence of tenascin-C or tenascin fragments containing certain domains (32,33). Some cell types respond to thrombospondin-1 by formation of fascin-rich actin microspikes that are indicative of a motile cell phenotype (34). The mechanisms by which these proteins modulate cell morphology have been recently identified. Using a three-dimensional matrix composed of fibronectin, fibrin, and tenascin-C, similar to the wound provisional matrix, Wenk et al. (35) showed that the presence of tenascin-C suppresses activation of Rho and prevents fibronectin-induced actin stress fiber formation. The inability to form stress fibers changes the way cells spread on fibronectin. Thrombospondin-1-induced fascin microspike formation is dependent on activation of the other members of the Rho family, Rac and Cdc42, and cell spreading on this ECM protein can be prevented by blocking these two GTPases (36). Both tenascin-C and thrombospondin-1 therefore act to change cell–ECM interactions by modulating intracellular pathways required for cytoskeletal reorganization.

New components within the matrix can also be generated by changing the isoforms of existing matrix proteins through new-gene expression, in the case of laminin and collagen, or through alternative splicing for fibronectin and tenascin. Distinct functions have been attributed to different isoforms of fibronectin (37). Dimer secretion, cell adhesion, and incorporation into blood clot and tissue matrices are all affected by alternative splicing. In this way, new cell binding sites and new orientations within the matrix can develop by deposition of a new fibronectin isoform. This idea probably also holds for tenascin and other alternatively spliced matrix proteins, but specific functions have yet to be determined.

E. The ECM Acts as a Reservoir for Soluble Growth Factors

ECM proteins not only bind to cell receptors and to other ECM proteins, but many of them also interact with a range of growth factors. Thus, the ECM becomes a reservoir for deposition of soluble factors that can induce specific cell functions. Although growth factors such as transforming growth factor β and tumour necrosis factor α can bind directly to major matrix glycoproteins (38,39), the major sites of growth factor interaction in the ECM reside on proteoglycans, in particular on their glycosaminoglycan side chains (40). Both large structural proteoglycans like perlecan (41) and smaller matrix–associated proteoglycans such as decorin (42) perform growth factor binding functions within the matrix and play significant roles in sequestration and presentation of these otherwise soluble molecules.

F. Cells Actively Remodel the ECM

It has been known for some time that matrix protein fragments possess functions that are not present in the intact protein. Increased chemotactic activity and exposure of novel binding sites in certain fibronectin fragments are examples of this property (43). It appears that matrix proteins contain cryptic sites that become active when exposed through matrix remodeling. The ECM protein network can be remodeled by removal and release of proteins through controlled proteolysis or by rearrangement of protein organization by cell-mediated manipulations. Cells secrete matrix proteases in an inactive form and their activity is regulated outside the cell by specific protease inhibitors and activators (44). Changes in the balance of these molecules allow regulated levels of extracellular proteolysis. Furthermore, protease expression and regulation is cell type specific, so that different cells will vary in the ways in which they alter the matrix through proteolysis. Knowledge of the cell type variation in protease isoforms and specificities will allow some control over how synthetic matrices are remodeled in vitro. Controlled proteolysis may also represent a novel post assembly mechanism for generating distinct matrix organizations and compositions in synthetic biomaterials.

Cells also have the ability to rearrange the distribution of proteins within the ECM network. Receptor binding and generation of cell-based tension lead to formation of novel structures in the matrix. The simplest example of this idea is in rearrangement of substrate-bound fibronectin fragments by primary fibroblasts. Woods et al. (45) showed that proteins immobilized in a homogeneous layer could be rearranged into fibrils by cells. Cell interactions with synthetic materials would be expected to result in reorganizations through tension or proteolysis. In some situations, it will be beneficial to inhibit these changes and maintain matrix organization. Remodeling by cells may also provide a novel mechanism by which to generate new materials with novel properties via cell-based manipulations.

From this brief description, we conclude that ECM modulates cell behavior through an array of biophysical and biochemical mechanisms. ECM components are adjusted continuously by cells to provide a specific set of complementary functions from structural to cell adhesive to modulatory.

IV. REGULATION OF CELL FUNCTIONS THROUGH ENGINEERED BIOMATERIALS

There are clearly a large number of potential design strategies for the production of synthetic materials that mimic certain properties of ECM in tissues. These strategies must take into consideration the lessons learned from the study of functional ECM and provide the requisite balance of ECM components and complementary functions. In this section, we consider ways to regulate cell organizations and functions through design of synthetic materials.

A. Cell Patterning

The ability to pattern cell adhesion proteins and peptide ligands on length scales that range from 5 to 100 μm allows the controlled placement of single cells on synthetic substrates (46–48). This controlled placement is important in the development of cell-based sensors (e.g., where arrays of cells in well-defined locations are necessary for accurate readout) and in tissue engineering (e.g., for the controlled growth of neurons and microcapillaries). Bhatia et al. (49,50) have shown the importance of patterning multiple cell types in cocultures. Their work showed that micropatterned cocultures of hepatocytes and fibroblasts produce albumin and urea (biochemical indicators that hepatocytes are in their differentiated state) for much longer periods of time, relative to random cocultures (50). The ability to pattern multiple cell types in well-defined locations will clearly play an important role in the development of culture models of complex tissues.

B. Control of Cell Migration

The use of complex three-dimensional scaffolds in the engineering of tissues requires cells seeded on the outside of these scaffolds to rapidly migrate into the interior of the scaffolds. Also, the need for a supporting vasculature requires the coordinated ingrowth of multiple cell types. Control over the relative rates of migration of different cell types into these scaffolds would therefore be a useful strategy for the production of engineered tissues. One way in which this type of control may be achieved is through the organization of multiple proteins and peptides that modulate cell adhesion and migration within the scaffold. In particular, the formation of gradients of increasing or decreasing adhesiveness within a scaffold could produce variations in the density of different cell types within the engineered tissue. Implementation of this strategy in biomaterials design requires two things: (a) a better understanding of ways in which the presence and spatial organization of multiple proteins in the ECM modulate cell adhesion and migration; and (b) processing strategies for the production of interfaces that mimic the organization of multiple proteins and functional subdomains in the ECM.

C. Selective Adhesion of Specific Cell Types

Another approach to tissue engineering involves the direct implanting of a scaffold that is then infiltrated by the desired cell type in vivo. This strategy requires the directed adhesion, spreading, and proliferation of specific cells in a competitive environment (i.e., one in which multiple cells potentially compete for attachment). One example of this strategy comes from orthopedic implants, where the desired implant interface is one that is intimately integrated with the surrounding bone. To achieve this integration, the implant interface must promote the adhesion and proliferation of bone cells (osteoblasts and osteoclasts) while controlling the adhesion and function of other cells found in bone and surrounding tissues such as fibroblasts, myoblasts, or chondrocytes. The selective adhesion and proliferation of specific cell types in the formation of new tissue in vivo is the integrated result of cell interactions with the substrate, neighboring cells, and soluble growth factors. Replicating this process with synthetic materials will likely require the organization of multiple proteins on the surface of the scaffold, as well as the controlled release of specific growth factors from the scaffold.

D. Long-Term Cell Viability and Maintenance of Differentiated States

The formation of engineered tissues through cell interactions with synthetic scaffolds requires that these cells remain viable and maintain a differentiated state for long periods (weeks to months). Differentiated states have been maintained successfully in relatively simple engineered tissues, such as skin. Loss of differentiated states is a problem in the engineering of more complex tissues, such as liver. Maintenance of differentiated states in these tissues may require the engineering of substrates that provide organization of different cell types, organization of multiple ECM components at subcellular length scales, and controlled release of growth factors.

E. Cell-Based Processing and Functionalization of Materials

In tissues, the interplay between cells and the ECM is dynamic: cells secrete and organize the macromolecules that form the ECM; specific organizations of ECM provide environmental cues for cells, which alter their physiology in response to these cues. Part of this physiological response is to remodel the surrounding ECM and, thereby, provide a new set of environmental cues to neighboring cells. This continuous processing of ECM by cells is a paradigm that may be translated to biomaterial design (51). The next generation of biomaterials will consist of materials in which the synthesis and processing is a hybrid effort, i.e., synthetic materials will act as templates that direct the further processing of materials by cells. This cellular processing of materials will occur in vivo, for applications such as implants and tissue engineering, or in vitro, where the goal is to use cells to introduce biological functions (sensing, catalysis, self-healing) into synthetic materials and devices.

V. PROCESSING STRATEGIES FOR THE PRODUCTION OF BIOMATERIAL INTERFACES THAT MIMIC THE TISSUE ECM

Attempts to engineer optimal biomaterials generally focus on either interface composition or interface topology. It is almost certain that both topology and composition play an important role in regulating cell behavior at biomaterial interfaces. There may also be important synergistic effects that arise through the combination of specific compositions and topologies. Effects of surface topology have been reviewed recently (52) and will not be covered in this chapter; we focus specifically on the role of interface composition.

A. Surface Deposition of Proteins

Two common ways to deposit proteins or peptides onto surfaces are adsorption from solution and covalent surface modification. In the simplest method, surface adsorption, a solution of protein(s) is incubated with a surface and nonspecific interactions (primarily hydrophobic and electrostatic) lead to immobilization of the protein. With multiprotein mixtures, the surface composition may not reflect the relative amount of protein in solution due to differences in rates of adsorption and affinity of a surface for particular proteins. In vivo, the amounts of different proteins adsorbed on a synthetic surface often correlate with their concentration in the biological fluids with which they make contact, implying that nonspecific protein adsorption is often controlled by rates of mass transport and not by the relative affinity or energetics of adsorption (53).

Instead of working with large adhesion proteins, there has been interest in modifying the surfaces of synthetic materials—either covalently or non-covalently—with small fragments of these proteins called *adhesion peptides* (53). The hypothesis that underlies this approach is that some of the cell adhesive properties of large-matrix proteins like fibronectin, laminin, and others are manifested in short peptide sequences. These sequences are often found in loop regions of matrix proteins and are known to bind to specific integrins on the surface of cells. One aspect of these peptides that makes them desirable to the biomaterials scientist is their ease of production (synthetic rather than recombinant) and incorporation into synthetic materials. Mechanisms for presentation of adhesive peptides on synthetic materials include the following: as polymer side chains (53–55); on self-assembled monolayers (SAMs) (56,57), and as components of a lipid bilayer (58,59). Often the amount of peptide required for cell adhesion varies dramatically depending on the mode of presentation (i.e., as polymer side chain, lipid headgroup, or terminal group on a SAM). We infer that the spatial organization of adhesive peptides may play an important role in modulating cell behavior. We emphasize that these peptides never recapitulate the full activity of the native protein from which they are derived.

The macroscopic orientation of protein fibers has also been used to direct cell behavior. The orientation of collagen fibers can orient the direction of growth and migration of cells. As an example, Tranquillo aligned fibers within three-dimensional collagen gels over macroscopic dimensions using an applied magnetic field and observed a positive correlation between cell orientation of fibroblasts and collagen fibril orientation (60). This effect of fiber alignment, referred to as contact guidance, occurs in the absence of specific interactions between collagen fibers and receptors on the cell surface. The mechanism by which oriented fibers in a gel orient cell growth and migration is not clear.

Control over the directional alignment of other fibrillar proteins, such as fibronectin, may also play an important role in controlling the behavior of cells. There are several techniques that have been shown to produce stretched and aligned arrays of DNA (61–63). These techniques generally involve the end attachment of DNA to substrate and the subsequent stretching and aligning of these molecules through the motion of an air–water interface or meniscus. As the meniscus passes over the end-attached DNA, individual molecules are stretched in a direction perpendicular to the interface. Similar techniques may be used to produce arrays of oriented fibronectin fibrils. It is expected that such an alignment of adhesion proteins could have an impact on the organization of cytoskeleton and intracellular signaling.

B. Substrate Patterning of Proteins and Cells

Current efforts to control the position and function of cells are focused on the synthesis of interfaces with well-defined cell contact regions. These efforts generally involve the patterning of proteins and cells on length scales greater than 1 micrometer. Approaches to patterning cell contact regions fall into two classes. The first approach involves the patterning of cell adhesion proteins and peptides in such a way that cells only attach through biospecific interactions to patterned proteins (46–48). Regions that do not present specific proteins or peptides are rendered nonadhesive to cells through modifications, such as the attachment of hydrophilic polymers (e.g., polyethylene glycol), that result in surfaces that resist nonspecific protein adsorption. The second approach involves physically constraining cells so that they only have access to specific regions of the surface (64).

The main approaches to synthesizing material interfaces with well-defined cell contact regions come from the techniques of soft lithography (65,66). Soft lithography describes a collection of techniques that use soft, polymeric materials to fabricate stamps, channels, or membranes, often with micrometer-sized features; these constructs, in turn, are used for the transfer of patterns or modification of surfaces. The use of soft lithography to pattern proteins and cells has been reviewed recently (46–48), and we will describe these different approaches only briefly.

There are three basic ways of patterning proteins with soft lithography (Fig. 4): microcontact printing with elastomeric stamps (47,67); the flow of liquids through microfluidic channels (68,69); and physically constraining access to surfaces through elastomeric membranes (64). All three of these approaches have been used to pattern proteins and, thereby, the adhesion of cells. Flow through microfluidic channels (68,69) and elastomeric membranes (64) have also been used to pattern cells directly. The use of soft lithography is clearly a powerful and flexible strategy for patterning cell contact regions.

Microcontact printing has been used to pattern cells in three ways: by patterning of SAMs into regions that either adsorb proteins (i.e., with SAMs terminated in a hydrophobic methyl group) or resist protein adsorption (i.e., with SAMs terminated in a hydrophilic oligoethylene glycol group) (70); by patterning directly SAMs that present ligands for cell adhesion (i.e., with SAMs terminated in an RGD containing peptide) (57); and by the direct patterning of proteins (67). Microcontact printing can produce patterns of

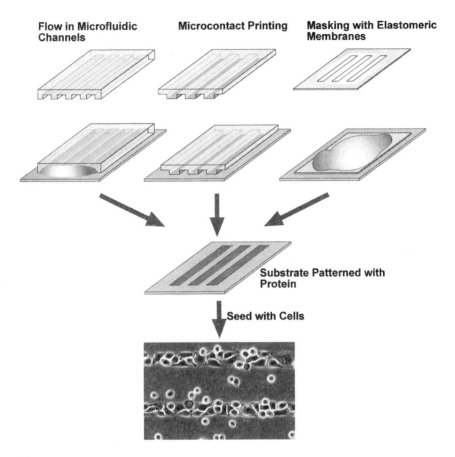

Figure 4   Soft lithography patterns proteins and cells. The flow of fluids in microchannels, printing with stamps, and masking with membranes can all be used to form micropatterns of cell adhesion proteins, such as fibronectin. The seeding of fibroblasts on these surfaces results in the patterned adhesion of cells.

proteins that are either continuous (e.g., lines) or discrete (e.g., circles) on a variety of substrates, both flat and curved. This soft lithographic technique has not been used to pattern cells directly; the physical process of stamping would likely kill most cells.

The flow of liquids through microfluidic channels (69) and physical masking of substrates with an elastomeric membrane (64) have both been used to pattern adhesion proteins and cells on adhesive substrates. Deposition of cells and proteins with microfluidics initially required the patterns to be continuous, reflecting the topology of the channels. Recently, Anderson et al. demonstrated the fabrication of microchannels three dimensionally (71); Chiu et al. used these 3D microchannels to produce discrete patterns of both proteins and cells (68). Physical masking of substrates with elastomeric membranes can also produce continuous and discrete patterns of proteins or cells.

C. Patterning of Proteins on Subcellular Length Scales

The goals of protein patterning at these length scales are twofold. The first goal is to pattern regions composed of a single protein on length scales less than 1 μm. This goal is nothing more than an extension of techniques to control cell contact regions to smaller length scales. Patterning a single protein on submicrometer length scales may allow control over the location of focal adhesions and the organization of cytoskeleton within cells. It may also set constraints on the way in which cells can remodel the matrix and provide directional guidance to the growth of axons.

The second goal is to control the spatial distribution of multiple proteins on length scales less than 1 μm. This goal reflects the fact that cell behavior in vivo is an integrated response to multiple components of ECM in tissues. For example, the combined presence of fibronectin and tenascin in the ECM in vivo plays a role in modulating the strengths of adhesive interactions between the cell and the ECM (35); this modulation, in turn, is thought to play a role in the control of cell migration rates in tissues. This strategy for modulating cell adhesion and migration has not been replicated through the adsorption of mixtures of these two proteins onto synthetic surfaces. A more successful strategy may involve introducing each of these proteins in separate microdomains; that is, control over both average surface composition of these two proteins as well as their spatial distribution on subcellular length scales may be important for modulation of cell adhesion and migration. The fact that different functional domains are distributed spatially on large ECM proteins, such as fibronectin and tenascin, also implies that spatial distribution of components on the length scale of 10–100 nm may be important in regulating cell behavior. The use of multiple synthetic peptides (like RGD) that mimic the function of some of these different domains may be most effective when there is spatial control over the distribution of these peptides on a synthetic substrate.

The goal of patterning a single type of protein at length scales smaller than 1 μm may be addressed using current techniques in soft lithography. The feature sizes obtainable with these techniques are limited by the resolution of the lithography used to produce the master from which the soft material constructs (stamps, channels, and membranes) are cast. Since these masters are most often made using photolithography, the limit in feature size that these techniques have produced reflects the limitation of optical photolithography and not soft lithography itself. For example, nanoscale features produced by e-beam lithography may be easily replicated in soft elastomeric materials (72). Feature sizes much smaller than the characteristic size of the soft lithographic construct may also be realized, for example, by the hydrodynamic focusing of fluidic flow in microchannels (69,73), by the compression of elastomeric stamps (72), or through the use of optical interference patterns (74,75). The use of soft lithography to create patterns of multiple proteins is a challenge; most approaches would require careful alignment and multiple applications of the elastomeric construct.

Dip-pen nanolithography allows the direct writing of alkanethiols on gold with linewidths on the order of 30 nm (76–78). This technique has not yet been used to pattern protein on these length scales. It could be easily adapted to do so, either by the writing of lines of alkanethiols that will adsorb proteins nonspecifically (e.g., through hydrophobic interactions), or by the writing of alkanethiols that present specific ligands for protein attachment, such as biotin. In either case, a subsequent filling in of the background with an ethylene glycol–terminated alkanethiol would be necessary to block nonspecific protein adhesion. Writing with multiple inks, each of which contains a separate ligand for attaching a specific protein or peptide, is one way this approach could be used to pattern multiple proteins.

The directed assembly of microscopic and nanoscopic particles that present specific biomolecules on their surfaces may be a general way of controlling the organization of proteins at interfaces. Griffith has developed techniques to control the spatial distribution of the YGRGD peptide on the 50 nm length scale by presenting this peptide on polymer "stars" (55). The number of peptides per star, and the relative density of stars with and without peptides, can be independently varied to control both the average composition of protein as well as the local density and spatial arrangements of peptides. Using this system, they showed that, in contrast to randomly distributed peptides, peptide clusters increased fibroblast adhesion strength and actin stress fiber formation.

We have begun to use polymer colloids in a similar way. These colloids provide some advantages relative to the polymer stars in that their diameter can be varied from 20 nm to many micrometers. In this way, a broader range of length scales may be studied. Also, there is a developed body of work on how to control the assembly and organization of colloidal particles.

We believe that the approach of using assemblies of functionalized micro- or nanoparticles to produce biofunctional surfaces will be most powerful when combined with other patterning techniques to obtain control over protein organizations at multiple length scales. Colloidal particles have been directed to assemble into well-defined and tunable micropatterns using a combination of electric fields and light (79). Using this approach, one can control the spatial distribution of proteins or peptides on two length scales: the size of the micropatterns and the size of the individual particles. There is also an intermediate length scale of spatial control that can arise from interactions between particles that have different surface properties. Matsushita showed that particles of the same size but with different surface properties pack into 2D arrays; the organization of the two different particles within the array was shown to depend on the strength of interaction between particles (80). Depending on this strength of interaction, particles can either separate into large domains or be evenly dispersed. The length scale of domains was described by a fractal dimension that varied continuously with the strength of interactions between particles. This type of "phase segregation" may provide another length scale for the control of protein composition.

D. Materials That Release Growth Factors and Support Remodeling

Growth factors and adhesion peptides, such as RGD, have been incorporated into biodegradable polymer matrix materials (51,81–84). This approach is based on the physical entrapment of these molecules in a polymer matrix and subsequent release when the matrix is degraded. The rate of release is controlled by the rate of degradation of the matrix (usually determined by the rate of hydrolysis of covalent bonds in the polymer backbone) and not by a particular physiological process. This approach is in contrast to the way ECM in tissues provides a reservoir of growth factors, i.e., through the reversible binding of these proteins with components in the ECM.

Processing of synthetic matrix materials that may be remodeled by cells represents a significant challenge (51). One strategy that has been demonstrated recently by Hubbell's group is to synthesize 3D synthetic polymer gels, the cross-links of which are composed of specific sequences of peptides that are recognized by specific proteases associated with the remodeling of ECM by cells. In one particular example, West and Hubbell synthesized PEG hydrogels where the cross-links were composed of the peptide sequence Val-Arg-Asn, a target sequence for the cleavage of fibrinogen by plasmin (85). These gels were degraded in the presence of plasmin but not in the presence of collagenase. Growth factors and other soluble proteins and peptides could be incorporated into these gels and then released upon cleavage of the peptide cross-links. In this way, the release of growth factors may be linked with specific physiological responses, such as wound healing.

VI. CONCLUSIONS

Cell adhesion to the ECM is a hierarchical process with control occurring through the interaction and organization of proteins on multiple length scales. The focus of biomaterial science has been on two length scales: micropatterning of cell contact regions (10–100 μm) and the use of small peptide fragments (about 1 nm) as ligands for cell adhesion. There is a collection of mechanisms by which cell–ECM interactions operate at length scales between those of a cell and a single receptor to modulate cell function. New strategies for processing biomaterials are needed to take advantage of mechanisms that operate at these length scales. Doing so will open new opportunities for controlling the behavior of cells and their interactions with and biocompatability of synthetic materials.

REFERENCES

1. ED Hay, ed. Cell Biology of Extracellular Matrix. New York: Plenum Press, 1991.
2. FG Giancotti, E Ruoslahti. Integrin signaling. Science 285:1028–1032, 1999.
3. RO Hynes. Integrins: versatility, modulation and signaling in cell adhesion. Cell 69:11–25, 1992.
4. RO Hynes. Fibronectins. New York: Springer-Verlag, 1990.
5. DJ Leahy, I Aukhil, HP Erickson. 2.0 A crystal structure of a four-domain segment of human fibronectin encompassing the RGD loop and synergy region. Cell 84:155–164, 1996.
6. S Aota, M Nomizu, K Yamada. The short amino acid sequence pro-his-ser-arg-asn in human fibronectin enhances cell adhesive function. J Biol Chem 269:24756–24761, 1994.
7. RD Bowditch, M Hariharan, EF Tominna, JW Smith, KM Yamada, ED Getzoff, MH Ginsberg. Identification of a novel integrin binding site in fibronectin: differential utilization by $\beta 3$ integrins. J Biol Chem 269:10856–10863, 1994.
8. J Engel. Common structural motifs in proteins of the extracellular matrix. Curr Opin Cell Biol 3:779–785, 1991.
9. FS Jones, PL Jones. The tenascin family of ECM glycoproteins: structure, function, and regulation during embryonic development and tissue remodeling. Dev Dyn 218:235–259, 2000.

10. HP Erickson, JL Inglesias. A six-armed oligomer isolated from cell surface fibronectin preparations. Nature 311:267–269, 1984.
11. AL Main, TS Harvey, M Baron, J Boyd, ID Campbell. The three-dimensional structure of the tenth type III module of fibronectin: an insight into RGD-mediated interactions. Cell 71:671–678, 1992.
12. LB Chen, A Murray, RA Segal, A Bushnell, ML Walsh. Studies on intercellular LETS glycoprotein matrices. Cell 14:377–391, 1978.
13. JE Schwarzbauer, JL Sechler. Fibronectin fibrillogenesis: a paradigm for extracellular matrix assembly. Curr Opin Cell Biol 11:622–627, 1999.
14. K Burridge, M Chrzanowska-Wodnicka, C Zhong. Focal adhesion assembly. Trends Cell Biol 7:342–347, 1997.
15. S Huang, DE Ingber. The structural and mechanical complexity of cell-growth control. Nat Cell Biol 1:E131–E138, 1999.
16. NJ Boudreau, PL Jones. Extracellular matrix and integrin signalling: the shape of things to come. Biochem J 339:481–488, 1999.
17. AE Aplin, AK Howe, RL Juliano. Cell adhesion molecules, signal transduction and cell growth. Curr Opin Cell Biol 11:737–744, 1999.
18. A Hall. Rho GTPases and the actin cytoskeleton. Science 279:509–514, 1998.
19. NA Hotchin, A Hall. The assembly of integrin adhesion complexes requires both extracellular matrix and intracellular rho/rac GTPases. J Cell Biol 131:1857–1865, 1995.
20. SP Palecek, JC Loftus, MH Ginsberg, DA Lauffenburger, AF Horwitz. Integrin-ligand binding properties govern cell-substratum adhesiveness. Nature 385:537–540, 1997.
21. J Folkman, A Moscona. Role of cell shape in growth control. Nature 273:345–349, 1978.
22. CS Chen, M Mrksich, S Huang, GM Whitesides, DE Ingber. Geometric control of cell life and death. Science 276:1425–1428, 1997.
23. S Bourdoulous, G Orend, DA MacKenna, R Pasqualini, E Ruoslahti. Fibronectin matrix regulates activation of Rho and CDC42 GTPases and cell cycle progression. J Cell Biol 143:267–276, 1998.
24. KO Mercurius, AO Morla. Inhibition of vascular smooth muscle cell growth by inhibition of fibronectin matrix assembly. Circ Res 82:548–556, 1998.
25. J Sottile, DC Hocking, PJ Swiatek. Fibronectin matrix assembly enhances adhesion-dependent cell growth. J Cell Sci 111:2933–2943, 1998.
26. JL Sechler, JE Schwarzbauer. Control of cell cycle progression by fibronectin matrix architecture. J Biol Chem 273:25533–25536, 1998.
27. R Winklbauer, M Nagel. Directional mesoderm cell migration in the Xenopus gastrula. Dev Biol 14:573–589, 1991.
28. JW Ramos, DW DeSimone. Xenopus embryonic cell adhesion to fibronectin: position-specific activation of RGD/synergy site-dependent migratory behavior at gastrulation. J Cell Biol 134:227–240, 1996.
29. J-C Boucaut, T Darribere, TJ Poole, H Aoyama, KM Yamada, JP Thiery. Biologically active synthetic peptides as probes of embryonic development: a competitive peptide inhibitor of fibronectin function inhibits gastrulation in

amphibian embryos and neural crest cell migration in avian embryos. J Cell Biol 99:1822–1830, 1984.

30. T Darribere, JE Schwarzbauer. Fibronectin matrix composition and organization can regulate cell migration during amphibian development. Mech Dev 92:239–250, 2000.
31. JC Adams, RP Tucker. The thrombospondin type 1 repeat superfamily: diverse proteins with related roles in neuronal development. Dev Dyn 218:280–299, 2000.
32. J Spring, K Beck, R Chiquet-Ehrismann. Two contrary functions of tenascin: dissection of the active sites by recombinant tenascin fragments. Cell 59:325–334, 1989.
33. CY Chung, JE Murphy-Ullrich, HP Erickson. Mitogenesis, cell migration, and loss of focal adhesions induced by tenascin-C interacting with its cell surface receptor, annexin II. Mol Biol Cell 7:883–892, 1996.
34. JC Adams. Characterization of cell-matrix adhesion requirements for the formation of fascin microspikes. Mol Biol Cell 8:2345–2363, 1997.
35. MB Wenk, KS Midwood, JE Schwarzbauer. Tenascin-C suppresses Rho activation. J Cell Biol 150:913–920, 2000.
36. JC Adams, MA Schwartz. Stimulation of fascin spikes by thrombospondin-1 is mediated by the GTPases Rac and Cdc42. J Cell Biol 150:807–822, 2000.
37. JE Schwarzbauer. Alternative splicing of fibronectin: three variants, three functions. Bioessays 13:527–533, 1991.
38. JE Murphy-Ullrich, M Poczatek. Activation of latent TGF-beta by thrombospondin-1: mechanisms and physiology. Cytokine Growth Factor Rev 11:59–69, 2000.
39. RAF Clark. The Molecular and Cellular Biology of Wound Repair. New York: Plenum Press, 1996.
40. N Perrimon, M Bernfield. Specificities of heparan sulphate proteoglycans in developmental processes. Nature 404:725–728, 2000.
41. D Aviezer, D Hecht, M Safran, M Eisinger, G David, A Yayon. Perlecan, basal lamina proteoglycan, promotes basic fibroblast growth factor-receptor binding, mitogenesis, and angiogenesis. Cell 79:1005–1013, 1994.
42. Y Yamaguchi, DM Mann, E Ruoslahti. Negative regulation of transforming growth factor-β by the proteoglycan decorin. Nature 346:281–284, 1990.
43. DF Mosher. Fibronectin. New York: Academic Press, 1989.
44. Z Werb. ECM and cell surface proteolysis: regulating cellular ecology. Cell 91:439–442, 1997.
45. A Woods, JR Couchman, S Johansson, M Höök. Adhesion and cytoskeletal organisation of fibroblasts in response to fibronectin fragments. EMBO J 5:665–670, 1986.
46. RS Kane, S Takayama, E Ostuni, DE Ingber, GM Whitesides. Patterning proteins and cells using soft lithography. Biomaterials 20:2363–2376, 1999.
47. E Ostuni, L Yan, GM Whitesides. The interaction of proteins and cells with self-assembled monolayers of alkanethiolates on gold and silver. Colloids Surf B Biointerf 15:3–30, 1999.

48. A Folch, M Toner. Microengineering of cellular interactions. Annu Rev Biomed Eng 2:227–256, 2000.
49. SN Bhatia, UJ Balis, ML Yarmush, M Toner. Microfabrication of hepatocyte/ fibroblast co-cultures: role of homotypic cell interactions. Biotechnol Prog 14:378–387, 1998.
50. SN Bhatia, UJ Balis, ML Yarmush, M Toner. Effect of cell–cell interactions in preservation of cellular phenotype: cocultivation of hepatocytes and nonparenchymal cells. FASEB J 13:1883–1900, 1999.
51. JA Hubbell. Bioactive biomaterials. Curr Opin Biotechnol 10:123–129, 1999.
52. RG Flemming, CJ Murphy, GA Abrams, SL Goodman, PF Nealey. Effects of synthetic micro- and nano-structured surfaces on cell behavior. Biomaterials 20:573–588, 1999.
53. DL Elbert, JA Hubbell. Surface treatments of polymers for biocompatibility. Annu Rev Mater Sci 26:365–394, 1996.
54. JC Schense, J Bloch, P Aebischer, JA Hubbell. Enzymatic incorporation of bioactive peptides into fibrin matrices enhances neurite extension. Nat Biotechnol 18:415–419, 2000.
55. G Maheshwari, G Brown, DA Lauffenburger, A Wells, LG Griffith. Cell adhesion and motility depend on nanoscale RGD clustering. J Cell Sci 113:1677–1686, 2000.
56. M Mrksich. A surface chemistry approach to studying cell adhesion. Chem Soc Rev 29:267–273, 2000.
57. C Roberts, CS Chen, M Mrksich, V Martichonok, DE Ingber, GM Whitesides. Using mixed self-assembled monolayers presenting RGD and (EG)(3)OH groups to characterize long-term attachment of bovine capillary endothelial cells to surfaces. J Am Chem Soc 120:6548–6555, 1998.
58. T Pakalns, KL Haverstick, GB Fields, JB McCarthy, DL Mooradian, M Tirrell. Cellular recognition of synthetic peptide amphiphiles in self-assembled monolayer films. Biomaterials 20:2265–2279, 1999.
59. DA Hammer, M Tirrell. Biological adhesion at interfaces. Annu Rev Mater Sci 26:651–691, 1996.
60. S Guido, RT Tranquillo. A methodology for the systematic and quantitative study of cell contact guidance in oriented collagen gels. J Cell Sci 105:317–331, 1993.
61. JF Allemand, D Bensimon, L Jullien, A Bensimon, V Croquette. pH-dependent specific binding and combing of DNA. Biophys J 73:2064–2070, 1997.
62. X Michalet, R Ekong, F Fougerousse, S Rousseaux, C Schurra, N Hornigold, M vanSlegtenhorst, J Wolfe, S Povey, JS Beckmann, A Bensimon. Dynamic molecular combing: Stretching the whole human genome for high-resolution studies. Science 277:1518–1523, 1997.
63. A Bensimon, A Simon, A Chiffaudel, V Croquette, F Heslot, D Bensimon. Alignment and Sensitive Detection of DNA By a Moving Interface. Science 265:2096–2098, 1994.
64. E Ostuni, R Kane, CS Chen, DE Ingber, GM Whitesides. Patterning mammalian cells using elastomeric membranes. Langmuir 16:7811–7819, 2000.

65. YN Xia, GM Whitesides. Soft lithography. Annu Rev Mater Sci 28:153–184, 1998.
66. YN Xia, GM Whitesides. Soft lithography. Angewandte Chemie Int Ed 37:551–575, 1998.
67. A Bernard, JP Renault, B Michel, HR Bosshard, E Delamarche. Microcontact printing of proteins. Adv Mater 12:1067–1070, 2000.
68. DT Chiu, NL Jeon, S Huang, RS Kane, CJ Wargo, IS Choi, DE Ingber, GM Whitesides. Patterned deposition of cells and proteins onto surfaces by using three-dimensional microfluidic systems. Proc Natl Acad Sci USA 97:2408–2413, 2000.
69. S Takayama, JC McDonald, E Ostuni, MN Liang, PJA Kenis, RF Ismagilov, GM Whitesides. Patterning cells and their environments using multiple laminar fluid flows in capillary networks. Proc Nat Acad Sci USA 96:5545–5548, 1999.
70. M Mrksich, CS Chen, YN Xia, LE Dike, DE Ingber, GM Whitesides. Controlling cell attachment on contoured surfaces with self-assembled monolayers of alkanethiolates on gold. Proc Natl Acad Sci USA 93:10775–10778, 1996.
71. JR Anderson, DT Chiu, RJ Jackman, O Cherniavskaya, JC McDonald, HK Wu, SH Whitesides, GM Whitesides. Fabrication of topologically complex three-dimensional microfluidic systems in PDMS by rapid prototyping. Anal Chem 72:3158–3164, 2000.
72. XM Zhao, YN Xia, GM Whitesides. Soft lithographic methods for nanofabrication. J Mater Chem 7:1069–1074, 1997.
73. JB Knight, A Vishwanath, JP Brody, RH Austin. Hydrodynamic focusing on a silicon chip: mixing nanoliters in microseconds. Phys Rev Lett 80:3863–3866, 1998.
74. JA Rogers, KE Paul, RJ Jackman, GM Whitesides. Generating similar to 90 nanometer features using near-field contact-mode photolithography with an elastomeric phase mask. J Vac Sci Technol B 16:59–68, 1998.
75. JA Rogers, Z Bao, M Meier, A Dodabalapur, OJA Schueller, GM Whitesides. Printing, molding, and near-field photolithographic methods for patterning organic lasers, smart pixels and simple circuits. Synth Me 115:5–11, 2000.
76. RD Piner, J Zhu, F Xu, SH Hong, CA Mirkin. "Dip-pen" nanolithography. Science 283:661–663, 1999.
77. SH Hong, J Zhu, CA Mirkin. Multiple ink nanolithography: toward a multiple-pen nano-plotter. Science 286:523–525, 1999.
78. SH Hang, CA Mirkin. A nanoplotter with both parallel and serial writing capabilities. Science 288:1808–1811, 2000.
79. RC Hayward, DA Saville, IA Aksay. Electrophoretic assembly of colloidal crystals with optically tunable micropatterns. Nature 404:56–59, 2000.
80. S Matsushita, T Miwa, A Fujishima. Distribution of components in composite two-dimensional arrays of latex particles and evaluation in terms of the fractal dimension. Langmuir 13:2582–2584, 1997.

81. YJ Park, YM Lee, JY Lee, YJ Seol, CP Chung, SJ Lee. Controlled release of platelet-derived growth factor-BB from chondroitin sulfate-chitosan sponge for guided bone regeneration. J Contr Rel 67:385–394, 2000.

82. MH Sheridan, LD Shea, MC Peters, DJ Mooney. Bioadsorbable polymer scaffolds for tissue engineering capable of sustained growth factor delivery. J Contr Rel 64:91–102, 2000.

83. MF Haller, WM Saltzman. Nerve growth factor delivery systems. J Contr Rel 53:1–6, 1998.

84. HD Kim, RF Valentini. Human osteoblast response in vitro to platelet-derived growth factor and transforming growth factor-beta delivered from controlled-release polymer rods. Biomaterials 18:1175–1184, 1997.

85. JL West, JA Hubbell. Polymeric biomaterials with degradation sites for proteases involved in cell migration. Macromolecules 32:241–244, 1999.

7
Cell Adhesion–Dependent Signaling Pathways on Biomaterials Surfaces

Andrea L. Koenig and David W. Grainger
Colorado State University, Fort Collins, Colorado

I. INTRODUCTION

One primary goal of current biomaterials research and development is to provide permanent or temporary scaffolding materials or implants for tissue functional regeneration. Approaches often require tissue–implant integration, with intimate cell–surface attachment, migration, and proliferation desired immediately upon implantation. This is not as simple as might be expected from a survey of the multitude of basic cell–surface adhesion studies that abound in the literature, showing cell–surface interactions. Four decades of cell culture work on various substrates (metals, ceramics, polymers) have provided a wealth of knowledge about how numerous cell types recognize, attach, and proliferate on surfaces. Proteins, surface chemistry, topology, culture conditions and cell lineages are well-studied components of classical quasi-planar, two-dimensional culture conditions. However, one look at "real" cell culture environments in vivo places the stark contrast of in vitro culture conditions versus physiological tissue- or organ-based cell culture into context. Cell adhesion, recognition, and proliferation in a physiological environment proceeds under conditions quite distinct from those typically supplied in vitro. While appreciation of these details is important, the true challenge relevant to the biomaterials field and to tissue engineering strategies in particular is associated with duplication, maintenance, and preservation of long-term cell behavior in a context of functional tissue regeneration and, typically, an array of biomaterials. Tissue engineering aspects of organ architecture, mass transport, and three-dimensional structure are coupled with preservation and control of cell phenotype, cell growth and motility, constant and dynamic cell–cell communication, coexistence of multiple cell types in coordinated spatial relationships, and, ultimately, consistent expression of distinct cell behaviors to facilitate duplication of tissue function over long-term periods—hopefully, a human lifetime.

Many cell phenotypes coexist naturally in spatial proximity, separated by surfaces (basement membranes, extracellular matrix) but bombarded by flow of soluble (e.g., cytokines, chemokines) and insoluble (cell adhesion molecules and matrix motifs) cues that constantly influence, guide, and alter cell behavior. Obviously, cell culture technology has not advanced sufficiently to address these somewhat daunting implant technology challenges successfully with synthetic or biologically derived materials that sufficiently duplicate many aspects of physiological environments. Nevertheless, the collective progress witnessed in stem cell research, tissue engineering, molecular bioscience, and cell biology appears to be on a collision course whereby coincidental research paths will provide new answers to key issues surrounding cell–biomaterial interactions and implant-associated healing.

Consideration of organ physiology from the cellular perspective indicates that the tissue-based cellular environment is constantly communicating. Active processing of both soluble and insoluble signals between organs, within tissues, between cells in each tissue compartment, and within cellular organelles is a critical feature of physiology to both understand and build into modern tissue engineering constructs. Recent and continuing advances in molecular biology of the cell have provided a wealth of information on cell-signaling molecules, mechanisms, and cascades directly relevant to exploitation in biomaterials research. Control and facilitation of these signal pathways in cell cultures, in bioreactors, and in tissue-engineered devices is a goal of current research in this direction. Thousands of these cell cascades continually operate in vivo simultaneously; understanding and assaying even a few of these selected paths in vitro is a continuing challenge. Predicted control of these pathways using biomaterials to promote specific cell responses remains a dream.

Cell signal transduction cascades continually process the flow of information transduced by cellular receptor families external to the cell membrane. These cascades serve to amplify, coordinate, and modulate cell functions in an appropriate manner such that the individual cell can benefit the organism as a whole. While the effects of such signaling cascades are generally favorable (i.e., resulting in normal cell growth, differentiation, and development), some consequences can be dire (e.g., intracellular signaling causing expression of a proto-oncogene, ultimately resulting in a transformed cancer phenotype). To complicate matters, where signaling prompts certain cell subtypes for either growth, cell cycle arrest, or programmed cell death (apoptosis) advantageous to these particular cell populations, other cell types in the same tissue or organism exposed to similar signals might experience completely different responses—and, in some cases, detrimental effects.

This chapter focuses on aspects of biomaterials surfaces that encourage cell attachment and proliferation, or that stimulate various cellular signaling pathways and are accessible to experimental interrogation. Examples of various surfaces used for promoting or studying cellular adhesion and resulting signaling are provided. Definitions and explanations of some current biomaterials used as biomimetic surfaces, a number of mammalian cell types that interact with these surfaces, and key signaling molecules identified to date—namely, cell surface receptors and the cytoplasmic components that act to sense receptor activation events and respond to them—are discussed. Continual progress correlating specific biomaterial surface chemistries in in vitro environments with cell signaling responses facilitates an understanding of how selection or design of a surface may target a particular cell type as well as activate a specific intracellular signaling cascade, producing a predictable response. Such research is only now beginning and represents enormous opportunity to enhance biomaterials performance.

Comprehensive review of the results of many important studies with polymers and/or biomaterials surfaces, cells and tissues, and extracellular and intracellular signaling molecules is outside the scope of this chapter. Some signaling substances that exhibit fairly well-understood cellular and molecular mechanisms are included. The purpose of this chapter is to familiarize the reader with (a) aspects of nonliving biomaterial surfaces used in vivo and in vitro; (b) the modification of these surfaces to enhance cell-to-material interactions, such as polymer surfaces grafted with extracellular matrix (ECM) peptide recognition sequences (1,2); (c) the various cell types and tissues interacting with these surfaces; (d) the cell membrane receptors involved in the outside-to-inside signaling; and (e) the intracellular signaling messengers that serve to modulate cell behavior, i.e., growth, proliferation, gene expression, apoptosis, and necrosis. Research has too often examined cell–surface interactions in static, quiescent culture conditions. However, little physiological cell proliferation occurs in the absence of stress, strain, shear, or other dynamic mechanical coupling. Recent movements away from static cell culture to dynamic fluid and mechanical influences on cell signaling are included as well.

II. BIOMATERIALS SURFACES RELEVANT TO CELL CULTURE AND SCAFFOLDING

Many materials have been used for in vivo and in vitro supports of cell and tissue growth, frequently exhibiting a spectrum of favorable characteristics: mechanical properties such as flexibility and strength, nontoxicity, low inflammatory responses, poor scaffolds for bacterial growth, and either acceptable implant longevity or a programmed, controlled, short half-life. Table 1 summarizes many current clinically tested biomaterials, including the cells/tissues of relevance and selected literature references. The point is that this compilation of materials represents a substantial body of clinically useful biomaterials empirically developed and applied without much knowledge of molecular or cellular signaling processes to date.

III. ABSORBED PROTEIN–CARBOHYDRATE INTERFACE: MOLECULE(S) MEDIATING CELL ATTACHMENT TO NONLIVING SURFACES

Cells often require adhesion molecule deposition on surfaces to facilitate their adhesion, motility, and proliferation. Adhesion molecules are supplied by the extracellular milieu (e.g., serum) or produced by the cell in situ. Probably the most studied class of cell-adhesive molecules comprises the soluble ECM proteins, including fibronectin (108–110), vitronectin (111), collagen families (112–115), thrombospondin (116), osteopontin (117), fibrinogen (118), von Willebrand factor (119), and laminin (66,67,120,121). Of these, classes of fibronectins ubiquitously found in virtually all physiological fluids as well as on cell surfaces have been most studied for cell adhesion (122). Collagens are a diverse family of ECMs, found generally cross-linked in vivo. However, recombinant soluble human collagen has been recently developed for cell/tissue work (123). Within the primary amino acid sequences of several of these ECM proteins are conserved peptide motifs—either RGDS, YIGSR, DGEA, or IKVAV domains— known to support cell–surface adhesion mediated through the integrin family of cell surface receptors (2,124). Truncated soluble and tethered forms of these peptides, in particular RGD, can be utilized as cell adhesion inhibitors and promoters, respectively (1,125). Commercial sources of these ECM-derived soluble peptides are numerous (126,127). Because these small, sufficiently enabling peptide molecules are now readily available, less than 100 times as massive as their ECM parent molecules, and effective as adhesion promoters when immobilized, their applications in various biomedical and biotechnology device settings are now widespread (1,2).

Table 1   Selected Biomaterials Used In Vivo and In Vitro

Biomaterial	Purpose	Cell type	Ref.
Tissue culture polystyrene (TCPS)	Oxidized surface for in vitro culturing of cells	Many	3–8
Bacteriological polystyrene (BPS)	Hydrophobic surface for in vitro culturing of bacteria	Many (bacterial cells)	3–9
Polymethyl methacrylate (PMMA)	Bone cement, ophthalmic lenses	Bone, cartilage	10–16
Poly-L-lactide; Poly-D,L-lactide; Polyglycolide	Sutures, bone plates, bone scaffolds, tissue scaffolds, delivery matrix for bone morphogenetic protein (BMP), growth factors	Epithelium, endothelium, blood, bone	17–19
Ti, TiO$_2$, and alloys with Mo/V/Fe	Bone/dental replacement, joint replacement; solid and coated metallic forms	Bone, joint function, blood and tissue contact	20–28
Self-assembled monolayers (SAMs)	Organic film surface application with highly controlled surface-exposed functional groups	Many (for in vitro cell culture; less practical for in vivo use)	29–33
Hydroxyapatite	Bone/dental replacement material	Bone	34–38
Polyethylene glycol/ polyethylene oxide (PEG/PEO)	Hydrophilic polymer used for tagging proteins and making hydrogels. Little protein adsorption and therefore little inflammatory response in vivo.	Many	39–54
Polycarbonate	In vitro tissue culture plastic	Many	55,56

Table 1 Continued

Biomaterial	Purpose	Cell type	Ref.
Polyurethane	Catheters, diaphragms, sensor/ microelectronics insulation, pump membranes, vessel conduits, latex rubber substitute	Epithelium, endothelium, blood	57–63
Dacron/polyester	Vascular graft materials	Endothelium, blood, smooth muscle cells (heart)	64,65
Polytetrafluoroethylene (PTFE)/Gore-Tex	Vascular graft materials, abdominal mesh	Endothelium, blood, smooth muscle cells	66–68; 372–376
Ultrahigh molecular weight polyethylene (UHMWPE)	Orthopedic total joint replacements	Bone, cartilage	69–72
Poly(hydroxyethylmethacrylate) [Poly(HEMA)]	Bioencapsulation, drug delivery devices, contact lenses	Ocular, liver, Islet cells	73,74
Polyvinyl acetate (PVA)	Hydrogels, tissue engineering scaffolds, drug delivery devices, contact lenses	Epithelium	75–79
Hyaluronic acid (HA)	Naturally occurring glycosaminoglycan used for surface coatings and hydrogels. Advantageous physical (hydrophobicity, lubricity, abrasion resistance, and flexibility) and biological properties (nonthrombogenicity, resistance to bacterial attachment and enzyme degradation)	Cartilage, blood	80–86

Table 1 Continued

Biomaterial	Purpose	Cell type	Ref.
Collagen	Naturally occurring ECM protein family used for hydrogels and wound-healing scaffolds.	Epithelium	87–91
Polypropylene fumarate	Degradable bone scaffolds, drug delivery devices		50,51,92
Calcium phosphate	Ceramic material that promotes bone growth in vivo	Bone	93–96
Polyvinyl chloride (PVC)	Blood bags, tubing	Blood and bone	97–99
Poly-L-lysine	Polymer of a naturally occurring amino acid used in tissue culture coatings to enhance cell adhesion.	Many	100–102
Gelatin	Soluble collagen	Many (bone)	93,103
Stainless steel	Bone, total joints, dental fixation	Bone	104–107

Although RDG immobilization to promote cell attachment has received the most attention as a cell-targeting moiety, new classes of biomaterials have been designed that seek to adsorb specific adhesive protein classes (40,128), immobilize specific adhesive peptides (126,129–132) and carbohydrates (133–137), and mimic phospholipid membranes (138). For example, a cardiovascular stent coating product in clinical trials (Cardiovasc, Menlo Park, CA) uses a surface activation process that covalently bonds synthetic fibronectin-derived adhesion peptide, P-15, to attract and anchor host vascular endothelial cells. The catheter-delivered stent, coated with the peptide, is designed to encourage complete endothelialization by attracting host endothelial cells to cover its surface.

IV. INTEGRINS AS CELL MEMBRANE SIGNAL TRANSDUCERS (OUTSIDE-TO-INSIDE SIGNALING)

Integrin receptors are found on most cell surfaces and are involved in regulating cell functions and behavior (139,140). Table 2 shows the known integrin transmembrane heterodimeric (containing non-covalently linked α and β subunits) receptors and the ECM proteins with the amino acid sequences therein that integrins recognize. Some examples of integrin involvement with cell functions include (a) replication of adherent cells on solid substratum (141,142); (b) synergy with antigen receptors to promote cell cycle progression (143,144); (c) apoptosis (145–147); (d) cell differentiation and gene expression based upon integrin interaction with ECM proteins (148–151); (e) cell migration (152,153). All of these interactions are significant to cell–surface behavior in the context of biomaterials. Regulation of cell spreading by contact with surfaces coated with fibronectin or other ECM proteins and subsequent integrin engagement induces a number of cell transmembrane signaling events. These include the release of arachidonic acid by phospholipase A_2 (154); production of diacylglycerol (DAG) with subsequent activation of protein kinase C (PKC) (155); activation of the GTP-binding protein Rho with subsequent activation of a phosphatidylinositol phosphate 5-kinase (156); and activation of protein tyrosine kinases, including pp125[FAK]. Inhibitors of integrin clustering, a common phenomenon that occurs upon integrin activation, also tend to invoke activation of intracellular secondary messengers to produce cell spreading.

Table 2 The Cell Integrin Adhesion Receptor Family

Subunits	Ligands	Protein recognition motif
$\alpha_1\beta_1$	Collagens, laminin	DGEA
$\alpha_2\beta_1$	Collagens, laminin	RGD
$\alpha_3\beta_1$	Fibronectin, laminin, collagens	EILDV
$\alpha_4\beta_1$	Fibronectin (V25), VCAM-1	RGD
$\alpha_5\beta_1$	Fibronectin (RGD)	
$\alpha_6\beta_1$	Laminin	
$\alpha_7\beta_1$	Laminin	
$\alpha_8\beta_1$	?	
$\alpha_V\beta_1$	Vitronectin, fibronectin (?)	RGD
$\alpha_L\beta_2$	ICAM-1, ICAM-2	
$\alpha_M\beta_2$	C3b component of complement (inactivated), fibrinogen, factor X, ICAM-1	
$\alpha_X\beta_2$	Fibrinogen, C3b component of complement (inactivated?)	GPRP
$\alpha_{II}b\beta_3$	Fibrinogen, fibronectin, von Willebrand factor, vitronectin, thrombospondin	RGD, KQAGDV
$\alpha_V\beta_3$	Vitronectin, fibrinogen, von Willebrand factor, thrombospondin, fibronectin, osteopontin, collagen	RGD
$\alpha_6\beta_4$	Laminin??	
$\alpha_V\beta_5$	Vitronectin	RGD
$\alpha_V\beta_6$	Fibronectin	RGD
$\alpha_4\beta_7$	Fibronectin (V25), VCAM-1	EILDV
$\alpha_{IEL}\beta_7$	?	
$\alpha_V\beta_8$	?	

Adapted from Ref. 157.

V. ADSORBED ECM PROTEINS ON BIOMATERIALS FACILITATE CELL ATTACHMENT

Cell attachment strategies attempt to specifically target and regulate certain cell types using biomaterial surfaces. Primarily, successful integrating biomaterials substrates are shown to adsorb ECM proteins at densities sufficient to readily interact with and engage cell receptors. Biomaterial surface chemistries currently exhibit only two classes of generic interfacial protein behaviors, either (a) nonselective interaction with many or all soluble proteins, or (b) nonselective rejection of most or all proteins. Little graded surface response or control over specific families of adsorbed proteins has been shown to date. As serum contains more than 200 soluble proteins, each with their own surface behavior and bioactivity, nonselective multicomponent protein uptake by surfaces truly limits subsequent control over or understanding of cell–surface events. Nonselective protein adsorption onto biomaterials from serum passively or indirectly determines which ECMs deposit on surfaces while limiting other non-ECM protein attachment. This passive solution adsorption approach remains the current state of the art to biomaterial protein conditioning. Precoating of biomaterials surfaces with selected ECM proteins from pure prepared solutions (e.g., collagens, vitronectin, or fibronectin) eliminates the ambiguity of serum multicomponent adsorption. Most synthetic surfaces better facilitate cell integrin receptors by direct coating/attaching biomaterial surfaces with pure ligands specific for these receptors, such as fibronectin, vitronectin, collagen, fibrinogen, or their specific short amino acid sequences known to be integrin ligands (Table 2) without interference or competition from other non-ECM protein adsorption. Thus, ECM-modified surfaces often invoke a desired cellular response (i.e., adhesion of the particular cell type to a surface in vivo, with resulting cell activation and proliferation) that would ideally benefit the particular tissue of interest (1,2).

For example, laminin ECM peptide-grafted polymer surfaces have facilitated regeneration of nerve cells on surfaces that mimic the basal cell lamina (66,67). Peptides derived from collagen (RGD and DGEA) have been used as biomaterials scaffolds for dermal wound repair (158). Titanium rods coated with RGDC and transplanted into rat femurs exhibited a significant increase in bone formation observed around the peptide-modified titanium implants versus unmodified implants (129). RGDS-grafted polyethylene glycol (PEG) networks caused an unfavorable formation of foreign body giant cell (FBGC) response upon initial interaction with cultured human macrophages (159). The literature is replete with examples of peptide-grafted surfaces (1,2). Where modified surfaces activate or inhibit specific tissue growth, intracellular signals resulting from cell–surface interaction play a major role in the long-term response. Understanding the connections between biomaterials surface chemistry, ECM adhesion, ligand presentation, cell response via signal transduction and resulting cell behavior is critical in predicting and controlling such response. For example, the fate of surface-immobilized ECM peptides in serum and their availability to integrin recognition after substantial serum adsorption has not been well studied. Biomaterials that adsorb little protein from serum nonspecifically, e.g., polysaccharide, PEG, or polyvinylpyrrolidone (PVP) hydrogels, provide an alternative method of eliminating all cell and protein interactions except when grafted with ECM cell–specific adhesion peptides (160–168). This strategy eliminates the "noise" from nonspecific serum protein adsorption while selectively presenting requisite cell adhesion motifs, thus facilitating biomaterial control over cell attachment.

VI. CELL SIGNALING CASCADES: SOLUBLE AND INSOLUBLE TRIGGERS

Cells within a living organism continually use regulatory control both within and between tissues to maintain homeostasis in a normal, healthy individual. This regulation begins with a diverse array of extracellular receptor–mediated binding events. Extracellular binding triggers specific biochemical cascades inside the cell. These cascades are effectively controlled by the cell's active inhibitors (negative feedback) at each sequential step, or amplified by positive feedback mechanisms and branch points in the cascade, producing a versatile, tailored, dynamic range of responses to receptor adhesion stimuli. Figure 1 presents a limited overview of several classes of outside-in signal transduction mechanisms on a model cell. The assessment of these cascades is complicated by their multiplicity, redundancy, and complexity. Clearly, a divide-and-conquer strategy to isolate different signal pathways and analyze their individual effects is an attractive experimental approach. However, such a strategy neglects pathway synergies and redundancies that, across an entire cell, a collection of cells, a tissue organ, or a physiological system, might lead to false conclusions about the impact or importance of any one isolated mechanism. As in blood coagulation, endocrine regulation, and hormonal cascades, appreciation of any one cascade should be couched within its influence on all other feedback loops. The intractable nature shown in Fig. 1 begins, then, to hint at the complexity of the challenge facing studies intending to use biomaterials to understand, promote, or alter cell signaling.

Outside-to-inside signaling mechanisms can also be disturbed by various outside influences (e.g., chronic situations caused by infectious

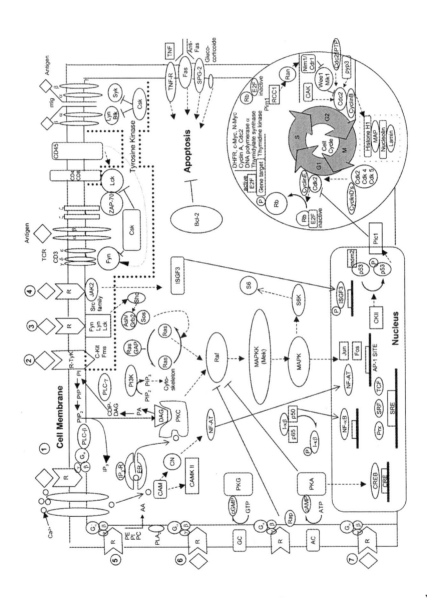

Figure 1

bacterial or viral pathogens or abnormal mechanical stress) that have both short- and long-term effects. Furthermore, some signals may initiate a long-term detrimental effect, such as in disease states, cancer pathogenesis, viral or bacterial infection, or genetic disorders that increase the extent of cell death or adherent cell behavior. Other signals may be short term, including synaptic transmission in nerves, transient nitric oxide bursts from endothelial cells, and contractile activation by smooth muscle cells. Such signals may also produce host physiological responses, e.g., eating of a hot pepper causing perspiration due to activation of the vanilloid-1 receptor in peripheral neurons; inflammatory responses ranging from activation of eisonophils due to anaphalaxis; allergic reaction to antigens such as pollens, pet dander, or other sensitizing chemicals; or signals that control cell cycles coinciding with aging and/or cell turnover.

However, an understanding of cycle triggers, events, and consequences should improve the ability to design new biomaterials that help modulate

---

Figure 1 Overview of the complex signal transduction mechanisms responsible for cell regulation. Dashed arrows (- - - ▶) indicate the activation of a molecule; (|) indicates the inhibition of a molecule; (→) indicates the movement of a molecule. In addition, circled numbers indicate known receptor-binding ligands as shown. ① Angiotensin II; α1 adrenaline; bombesin; IL-8; M1, M3, M5, muscarin; PAF; serotonin (5-HT2); substance P; thrombin; and TRH. ② EGF; insulin; M-CSF; NGF; PDGF; and SCF. ③ IL-2; IL-3; and IL-7. ④ Erythropoietin; IL-3; GM-CSF; and G-CSF. ⑤ Epinephrine and norepinephrine. ⑥ Leukotriene D4, C4. ⑦ A2 Adenosine; FSH; M2, muscarin; parathyroid hormone; somatostatin; TSH; and VIP. *Abbreviations*: AA, arachidonic acid; AC, adenylate cyclase; CAM, calmodulin; CAMK, calmodulin-dependent kinase; CDP-DG, cytidine diphosphate diacylglycerol; CK II, casein kinase II; CN, calcineurin; DAG, diacylglycerol; EGF, epidermal growth factor; ER, endoplasmic reticulum; G, G protein; GAP, GTPase-activating protein; GC, guanylate cyclase; G-CSF, granulocyte-macrophage colony-stimulating factor; IP_3, inositol 1,4,5-triphosphate; MAPK, mitogen-activated protein (MAP) kinase; MAPKK, MAP kinase kinase; mlg, membrane-localized immunoglobulin; NGF, nerve growth factor; PA, phosphatidic acid; PAF, platelet-activating factor; PC, phosphatidylcholine; PDGF, platelet-derived growth factor; PE, phosphatidylethanolamine; PI, phosphatidylinositol; PI3K, phosphatidylinositol 3-kinase; PIP, phosphatidylinositol 4-phosphate; PIP_2, phosphatidylinositol 4,5-biphosphate; PIP_3, phosphatidylinositol 3,4,5-triphosphate; PKA, cAMP-dependent protein kinase; PKC, protein kinase C; PKG, cGMP-dependent protein kinase; PLA_2, phospholipase A_2; PLC, phospholipase C; R, receptor; Rb, retinoblastoma gene product; SCF, stem cell factor; SGP2, sulfated glycoprotein 2; TCR, T-cell receptor; TNF, tumor necrosis factor; TRH, thyrotropin-releasing hormone; TSH, thyrotropin-stimulating hormone; TyK, tyrosine kinase; VIP, vasoactive intestinal polypeptide. (Adapted from PanVera Corp., Madison, WI.)

such responses. Overall, tissue engineering challenges aim to regulate cell growth, phenotype, senescence, apoptosis, and necrosis by using soluble and insoluble stimuli that contact cell membrane receptors or penetrate through the cell membrane to initiate deterministic cascades. The use of biomaterial surfaces with subsequent control over protein/carbohydrate signal attachment is a potentially productive area of study because these adsorbed components can be selected and tailored to allow cellular recognition, attachment, division, and other effects that are mechanisms of cellular control on biomaterials surfaces. Biomaterials improvement strategies should take into account eliminating the noise (nonspecific protein adsorption) while reliably presenting signal (soluble or insoluble biochemical cues) in order to exert some control over cell-integrating responses. Figure 2 schematically depicts the influence of a biomaterial on ECM deposition and, thereby, subsequent cell recognition and signaling responses. Information "flow" in this scenario from the biomaterial protein–covered surface to cell receptors through the membrane and into possible nuclear signaling of the genome can now be interrogated experimentally at various points. Elucidation of biomaterials influences and possible control features on these signal cascades should prove a fertile area of research.

VII. OUTSIDE–INSIDE SIGNALING

Because this chapter focuses on the role biomaterial surfaces as cell attachment signaling stimuli, outside-to-inside signaling cascades, as opposed to inside-to-outside cascades, are the limited pathways of interest. Typically, the two systems naturally interact to maintain and regulate one another. External factors interacting with cell receptors activate soluble secondary messengers within the cytosol of the cell. If this cascade continues into the cell nucleus, genetic transcription factors frequently get activated, regulating gene expression. Up-regulation of a particular gene, in part, permits its cytosolic transcription into mRNA, translation into its protein product, and possible transport for presentation at the cell surface (e.g., the expression of E-selectin upon activation of endothelial cells) or extracellular release (growth factors or hormones) into the cell's extracellular environment. Hence, initially recognized extracellular signals are presented internally to provide new feedback signals that can result in release of new extracellular signals. Regulation of this loop is just beginning to be appreciated by the tissue engineering community.

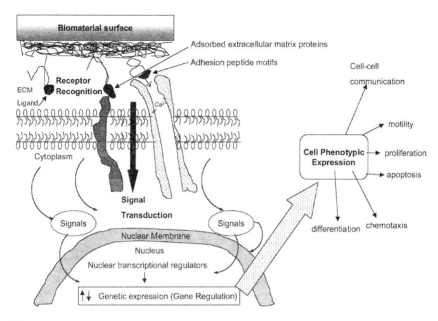

Figure 2 Outside-in cell signal transduction: attachment-dependent cells on biomaterials. Many cell-signaling mechanisms and necessary attachment-dependent behaviors are activated by cell–surface attachment. These attachment mechanisms and their resulting signaling phenomena are influenced by adsorbed or insoluble receptor-mediated stimuli on biomaterials surfaces. Soluble protein surface deposition from both extracellular matrix and other serum proteins is known to be influenced by biomaterial surface chemistry. Composition and conformation of the adsorbed protein layer are influenced by surface chemistry and directly affect cell attachment mechanisms, receptor activation, and resulting signaling pathways through the membrane receptors. Ultimately, cell genetic regulation and phenotypic expression are altered by this mechanism. Hence, some aspects of biomaterials surface chemistry are conveyed through these indirect receptor-mediated pathways, and translated ultimately to genetic regulation and message expression.

VIII. MECHANISMS OF SIGNAL TRANSDUCTION THROUGH RECEPTORS

Outside-to-inside signal transduction at the cellular level refers to the movement of signals from outside the cell to inside across the cell membrane via specific receptor processing, ultimately ending up in nuclear signaling. Signal movement can be direct, like that associated with receptor molecules of the acetylcholine (nicotinic) class: receptors that constitute ligand-

dependent ion channels which, upon external ligand interaction, allow
signals to be passed in the form of small ion currents (such as Na^+ and K^+),
either into or out of the cell through the membrane. These ion movements
result in changes in the electrical potential of the cells, which in turn
stimulates additional cytosolic and/or nuclear events and propagates the
signal along the cell.

More often, however, the relationship between extracellular ligand
binding and opening or closing of ion channels and many other receptor
types is indirect, mediated through coupled messenger cascades. This more
complex signal transduction involves the coupling of ligand–receptor
interactions to many intracellular events via cascades of enzymatically
controlled soluble signals within the cell. These events frequently include
protein phosphorylation by tyrosine kinase and/or serine/threonine kinase
enzymes. Specific protein phosphorylation changes target protein net
charge, bioactivities, and protein conformations, providing a level of
cascade control. For example, phosphorylation usually reduces receptor
activity, particularly when it is coupled to a G protein (see below), so that
higher hormone concentrations are required to generate physiological
responses. The eventual outcome is the programmed alteration in cellular
activity that changes cell behavior at the genetic level within the responding
cells.

In most cases, transmembrane receptors with domains exposed on
both the extracellular and cytosolic cell surfaces act to fish out signal
molecules, both soluble and insoluble, from the extracellular milieu. Specific
receptor recognition of these ligands (binding) prompts conformational
changes in the receptor across the membrane, triggering cytosolic cascades,
enzyme activation, and Ca^{2+} ion transients. Therefore, transduction of
binding events outside the cell to response events inside the cell is produced
both conformationally and via ionic fluxes using cell membrane receptors.

IX. RECEPTOR TYROSINE KINASES

Numerous intracellular protein tyrosine kinase enzymes are responsible for
propagating signal cascades by phosphorylating a variety of intracellular
proteins on tyrosine residues following activation of cellular growth and
proliferation signals through membrane (i.e., integrin) receptors. However,
some cell membrane receptors have their own intrinsic kinase activity
triggered by ligand binding. One common family, receptor tyrosine kinase,
contains four major domains: (a) an extracellular ligand binding domain; (b)
a transmembrane domain; (c) an intracellular tyrosine kinase domain; and
(d) an intracellular regulatory domain. Protein tyrosine kinases can be

classified into different subfamilies based on the structure of their extracellular domains. These 10 receptor subcategories include (a) epidermal growth factor (EGF) receptors, NEU/HER2 and HER3 containing cysteine-rich sequences (169); (b) insulin receptors (170) and IGF-I receptor containing cysteine-rich sequences and characterized by disulfide-linked heterotetramers (171); (c) platelet-derived growth factor (PDGF) receptors, c-Kit, CSF-1 receptors containing five immunoglobulin-like domains and also the kinase insert (172); (d) fibroblast growth factor (FGF) receptors containing three immunoglobulin-like domains as well as the kinase insert (173); (e) vascular endothelial growth factor (VEGF) receptors, Flt-1, Flt-1/KDR, and Flt-4 containing seven immunoglobulin-like domains extracellularly as well as the kinase insert domain intracellularly (174); (f) hepatocyte growth factor (HGF) receptor and scatter factor (SC) receptor (heterodimeric receptors where one of the two protein subunits is completely extracellular). In addition, they undergo proteolytic cleavage which, for HGF-R, is necessary for ligand binding (175). The HGF receptor is a proto-oncogene product originally identified from the Met oncogene (176); (g) the neurotrophin receptor family (TrkA, TrkB, TkC) and neurotrophin growth factor receptor (NGF-R) containing no or few cysteine-rich domains; NGF-R has leucine-rich domains (177); (h) the Eph-like receptor family—the largest of the receptor family—containing an N-terminal immunoglobulin-like domain, followed by a cysteine-rich domain and two fibronectin type III–like domains (178); (i) the Axl/Ark/Ufo receptor family characterized by two immunoglobulin-like domains and two fibronectin type III–like extracellular domains (179). These receptors help mediate reactions with the coagulation factor, protein S, and related molecules (180); and lastly, (j) tie receptor family predominantly expressed in endothelial cells and involved with angiogenesis. They contain three EGF-like domains, two immunoglobulin-like domains, and three fibronectin type III–like domains in their extracellular compartment (174,181).

In addition, many other receptors exhibiting intrinsic tyrosine kinase activity as well as these tyrosine kinases associated with cell surface receptors contain tyrosine residues that, upon phosphorylation, interact with other cytosolic proteins of the signaling cascade (182). These other proteins often contain domains of amino acid sequences homologous to a domain first identified in the c-Src proto-oncogene. These domains are termed SH2 domains (*Src homology domain 2*) (183). Significantly, interactions of SH2 domain–containing proteins with tyrosine kinase receptors or receptor-associated tyrosine kinases commonly promote tyrosine phosphorylation of the SH2-containing proteins. Phosphorylation of SH2 protein domains results in alteration (either positively or negatively) in their intrinsic signaling activity. Several SH2-containing proteins with intrinsic enzymatic activity include phospholipase C – γ(PLCγ), the proto-oncogene c-Ras-associated GTPase-activating protein (184), phosphatidy-linositol 3-kinase (185), protein phosphatase 1C, as well as members of the Src family of protein tyrosine kinases (186). Several of these are known to be activated by cell–surface interactions (see below), occupying an important part in the outside-in signal transduction process.

X. NONRECEPTOR PROTEIN TYROSINE KINASES

Most proteins of the nonreceptor protein tyrosine kinase family are cytoplasmic phosphorylating enzymes that couple to cellular receptors lacking their own endogenous enzymatic signaling activity. Subfamilies of the nonreceptor protein tyrosine kinase family include one related to the Src (short for sarcoma) protein, a tyrosine kinase first identified as the transforming protein (or proto-oncogene) in Rous sarcoma virus (186–188). Subsequently, a cellular homologue was identified as c-Src (189).

Other members of the nonreceptor tyrosine kinases are the *Ja*nus *k*inase or "*J*ust *a*nother *k*inase" (Jak), involved in the Jak/STAT (*s*ignal *t*ransducers and *a*ctivators of *t*ranscription) pathway initiated by cytokines such as interleukin-2 (IL-2) and interferon (190). Jak1 and Jak3 have a critical role in IL-2-mediated proliferative signaling (191). The STAT transcription factors are downstream targets of Jaks. STATs are located in the cytoplasm and are translocated to the nucleus following activation by Jak kinases via phosphorylation on specific tyrosine residues. The nuclear proto-oncogene, *sis*, is known to be the critical target of the Jak/STAT signaling pathway (192). Clinically, it has been shown that a specific inhibitor of Jak3 is effective in the treatment of amyotrophic lateral sclerosis (ALS), or Lou Gehrig's disease, a progressive, fatal neurodegenerative disorder (193). Additional nonreceptor protein tyrosine kinases involved with IL-2 signaling include Syk/Zap-70 family known to also be coupled to T- and B-cell antigen receptors and induce cell growth via the *c-myc* proto-oncogene (194,195); and the Src family which are linked to at least three signaling pathways: the *c-fos/c-jun*, the *c-myc*, and the *bcl-2* induction pathways (196).

XI. RECEPTOR SERINE/THREONINE KINASES

The transmembrane serine/threonine receptor kinases identified to date act as receptors for pleotropic bone morphogenetic proteins [BMPs, part of the transforming growth factor β (TGF-β) superfamily] (197); the activins (homodimers) and inhibins (heterodimers), involved in regulation of mammary epithelial cell differentiation through mesenchymal–epithelial cell interactions (198); and various TGF-βs (also members of the TGF-β superfamily) (199). Although these families of proteins can induce and/or inhibit cellular proliferation or differentiation, the signaling receptors and pathways utilized are different from those for cell receptors with intrinsic tyrosine kinase activity or those that associate with intracellular tyrosine kinases, mentioned in the previous section. Mechanisms of cellular responses to the receptor serine/threonine kinases are not as clearly understood as those of receptor tyrosine kinases. One nuclear protein involved in the responses of cells to the TGF-β family is the proto-oncogene transcriptional regulator, c-myc, which directly affects the expression of genes harboring myc-binding elements in response to serine/threonine kinase receptor activation. Because of the involvement of serine/threonine kinases with TGF-β superfamily pleotropic factors, implications for this receptor family with targeted growth factor delivery systems or immobilized growth factor surfaces are significant. Combinations of controlled growth factor delivery with degradable tissue scaffolds hold promise to facilitate some limited manipulation of cell behavior that is only now in early stages of study (200).

XII. NONRECEPTOR SERINE/THREONINE KINASES

Several nonreceptor serine/threonine kinases function in signal transduction pathways. Two more commonly known examples are cAMP-dependent protein kinase A (PKA) and PKC. Additional nonreceptor serine/threonine kinases important for signal transduction are the MAPK family noted below.

XIII. PROTEIN KINASE C

PKC (structure of its conserved regions is shown in Fig. 3) was originally identified as a serine/threonine kinase activated within the cell by DAG, a well-known membrane lipid product of the phosphatidylinositol cycle and also identified as an intracellular receptor for tumor-promoting phorbol esters (201,202). At least 10 proteins are known to compose the PKC enzyme family. Each of these enzymes exhibits specific patterns of tissue expression and calcium-dependent activation by lipids (203). PKCs are involved in the signal transduction pathways initiated by certain hormones, growth factors, and neurotransmitters. Phosphorylation of various proteins by PKC leads to either increased or decreased protein activity. Of particular importance is the phosphorylation of the EGF receptor by PKC, which down-regulates the tyrosine kinase activity of this important receptor. This effectively limits the length of the cellular responses initiated through the EGF receptor (204). Recently, EGF has been patterned onto biomaterials surfaces in order to control cellular function, primarily through this EGF–PKC ligand–receptor cell signaling cascade (205,206).

XIV. MAP KINASES

Mitogen-activated protein kinase (MAPK) cascades initiate when a protein kinase (an MAPK) is regulated by dual phosphorylation on both threonine and tyrosine residues—a type of switch mechanism that transmits information of increased intracellular tyrosine phosphorylation to that of serine/threonine phosphorylation. MAPKs were identified by virtue of their activation in response to growth factor stimulation of cells in culture; hence the name *m*itogen-*a*ctivated *p*rotein *k*inases. Mammalian members of the MAPK family include ERK1 and ERK2, p45 and p54 Jun kinase, and p38/CSBP (181). Not all of the substrates of each MAPK have been defined, but it is clear that transcription factors are important targets for MAPK cascades (207,208). Each MAPK is activated by a phosphorylation event by MAPK kinase (MAPKK), considered a dual-specificity kinase because it in turn is activated by a serine/threonine kinase, MAPKK kinase (MAPKKK). Small GTPases (see below) link transmembrane signaling to activation of the MAPK cascade by direct interaction with MAPKKK or with an upstream kinase. In the ERK pathway, p21Ras (see below) interacts with Raf during the initial signaling cascade (209,210). GTPases of the Rho family appear to be involved in the activation of the Jun kinases and p38

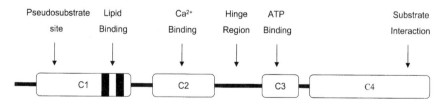

Figure 3 Schematic of the conserved regions of the protein kinase C (PKC) isoenzymes, an important cytoplasmic regulatory component in cell signaling. The DNA sequence for this part of the protein structure has been used as a probe to find more enzymes that belong to the PKC family. (Adapted from Ref. 168, p. 225.)

pathways (211). Furthermore, mechanical stress, as opposed to soluble or insoluble extracellular signaling molecules, can trigger the MAPK intracellular signaling cascade (see below) (212,213).

XV. PHOSPHOLIPASES AND PHOSPHOLIPIDS IN CELLULAR SIGNAL TRANSDUCTION

Phospholipases are soluble, ubiquitous, membrane-active lipid hydrolases that interact with membrane phospholipids to assist with transmission of ligand receptor–induced signals from the plasma membrane to intracellular proteins. The enzyme target affected by phospholipase activation is PKC (discussed above). As shown in Figs 1 and 4, PLC hydrolyzes the membrane phospholipid phosphatidylinositol 4,5-biphosphate (PIP$_2$), producing two secondary messengers: inositol 1,4,5-triphosphate (IP$_3$) and DAG (214,215). Three mammalian families of PLC are known: PLCβ, γ, and δ (216). The principal intracellular mediators of PKC activity are receptors coupled to activation of PLCγ. PLCγ contains SH2 domains that facilitate interaction with tyrosine-phosphorylated receptor tyrosine kinases (217). This allows PLCγ to be intimately associated with the signal transduction complexes of the membrane as well as membrane phospholipids that are its substrates. IP$_3$, one of the signaling molecules produced by PLCγ, interacts with intracellular membrane receptors leading to an increased release of stored calcium ions (transients) from intracellular vesicles. Together, the increased DAG and intracellular free calcium ion concentrations lead to increased PKC activity (214,218). This pathway then cascades to activation of MAPK, then to c-fos, c-myc, and other transcriptional regulators in the nucleus.

Recent evidence indicates that phospholipases D and A$_2$ (PLD and PLA$_2$) are also involved in the sustained activation of PKC through their hydrolysis of membrane phosphatidylcholine (PC) (219). PLD action on PC leads to the release of phosphatidic acid, which in turn is converted to DAG by a specific phosphatidic acid phosphomonoesterase (220). PLA$_2$ hydrolyzes PC to yield free fatty acids and lysoPC, both of which have been shown to potentiate the DAG-mediated activation of PKC (221). Of medical significance is the ability of phorbol ester tumor promoters to activate PKC directly. This leads to elevated and unregulated activation of PKC and the consequent disruption in normal cellular growth and proliferation control leading ultimately to neoplasia (202,222). Such an analogous mechanism possibly is involved in tumor-associated biomaterial implants through uncontrolled biomaterial surface activation of PKC.

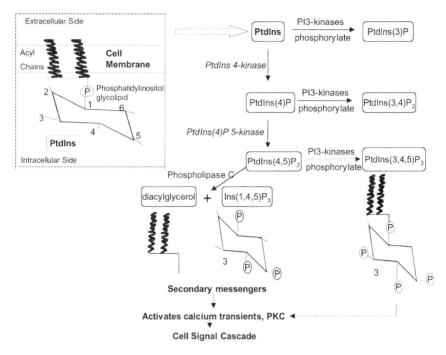

Figure 4 Phosphoinositide signaling pathways. The glycolipid phosphatidylinositol resides largely on the cytoplasmic leaflet (interior) of the cell membrane. Enzymatic manipulation of this lipid through directed mono- and multiphosphorylation events via PI kinases produces various second-messenger molecules with varieties of functions within the cell. Ins(1,4,5)P$_3$ is involved in the protein kinase C (PKC) signaling pathway, and diacylglycerol (DAG) binds to PKC. Both of these molecules are secondary messengers. PtdIns(3,4,5)P$_3$ is involved in regulating cell migration and motility through influences on cytoskeletal movement (see Fig. 1). (Adapted from Ref. 168, p. 251.)

XVI. PHOSPHATIDYLINOSITIDE 3-KINASE (PI$_3$ KINASES)

The soluble receptor-associated, nonreceptor tyrosine kinase, PI$_3$ kinase, was first identified in bovine brain after the realization that 3-phosphorylated inositol lipids are important signal transducers (223–225). PI$_3$ kinase is tyrosine phosphorylated and subsequently activated by various receptor tyrosine kinases and receptor-associated protein tyrosine kinases. PI$_3$ kinase, schematically depicted in Fig. 5 (its enzymatic activity is shown in Fig. 4), is a heterodimeric protein containing 85-kDa (or p85) and 110-kDa (p110) subunits. The p85 subunit contains SH2 domains that interact with

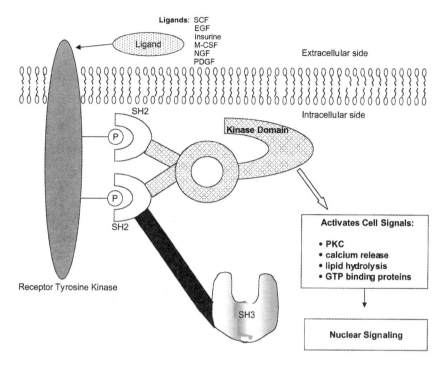

Figure 5 Generic structure of membrane receptor–associated receptor-activated heterodimeric phosphoinositide 3-kinase (PI_3 kinase). Src homology 2 (SH2) domains bind phosphotyrosines and Src homology 3 (SH3) domains bind polyproline sequences. Signals transduced by extracellular tyrosine kinase receptor binding produces kinase activity intracellularly. Extracellular receptors include the platelet-derived growth factor (PDGF), epidermal growth factor (EGF), insulin, insulin-like growth factor type I (IGF-I), hepatocyte growth factor (HGF), and nerve growth factor (NGF) receptor families. Interactions of PI_3 kinase, SH2, with these tyrosine kinase receptors or receptor-associated tyrosine kinases promote tyrosine phosphorylation of it and all related SH2-containing proteins. Phosphorylation of the SH2 protein domains results in changes in enzymatic activity. Besides PI_3 kinase, SH2-containing proteins with intrinsic enzymatic activity include phospholipase $C\gamma(PLC\gamma)$, the proto-oncogene c-Ras-associated GTPase activating protein, protein phosphatase-1C, as well as members of the Src family of protein tyrosine kinases. Several of these are known to be activated by cell–surface interactions (see text). (Adapted from Ref. 168, p. 254.)

activated receptors or other receptor-associated protein tyrosine kinases and is itself subsequently tyrosine phosphorylated and activated (226). The 85-kDa subunit is noncatalytic. However, it contains a domain homologous to

GTPase-activating (GAP) proteins (see below) (227). The 110-kDa subunit is enzymatically active, containing the lipid kinase domain (228). PI_3 kinase associates with and is activated by PDGF, EGF, insulin, IGF-I1, HGF, and NGF receptors (229–235) (schematically demonstrated in Fig. 5). Active PI_3 kinase then phosphorylates various membrane phosphatidylinositol lipids at the 3 position of the inositol ring as shown in Fig. 4 (236,237). This activity generates additional substrates for $PLC\gamma$, allowing a cascade of DAG and IP_3 to be generated by a single activated receptor tyrosine kinase or other protein tyrosine kinase (201,214). Some of the cellular responses resulting from PI_3 kinase activity include DNA synthesis (238), actin rearrangement (239), neutrophil oxidative burst and superoxide production (240), membrane ruffling (241), and activation of glucose transport (242). Physiologically, these cellular events are demonstrated by cell survival (243), oocyte maturation (244), differentiation (245), chemotaxis (246), and neurite outgrowth (247,248)—events clearly important to tissue engineering.

XVII. G-PROTEIN-COUPLED RECEPTORS

The family of cell membrane receptors ("R_7G" receptors) coupled to GTP-binding regulatory proteins (G proteins) is one of the largest to be characterized in mammalian cells. Initially, these receptors were discovered to be similar to the seven transmembrane-spanning bacteriophage rhodopsin proteins (249,250), but continuing new discoveries within this G-protein-coupled receptor family have served to underscore the broad, general importance of this conserved receptor signaling mechanism. These receptors provide the link between an extracellular ligand (hormone) and an intracellular amplifier (adenylate cyclase) via a soluble intracellular transducing enzyme, the guanine nucleotide–binding or G protein (251–254).

Several different classifications of cell receptors couple signal transduction to soluble intracellular G proteins. Three different classes are discussed: (a) G-protein-coupled receptors that modulate adenylate cyclase activity, activating associated G proteins and leading to the production of cAMP as the second messenger. Receptors of this class include the β-adrenergic, glucagon, calcitonin, parathyroid hormone, and odorant molecule receptors (255). Increases in the production of cAMP lead to increases in the activity of cAMP-dependent PKA in the case of β-adrenergic and glucagon receptors. In the case of odorant molecule receptors found only in olfactory sensory neurons mediated by the G protein, G_{olf}, one member of the large family of G proteins (discussed below) increases in cAMP lead to activation of cell transmembrane ion channels. In contrast to increased adenylate cyclase activity, the α-adrenergic receptors are coupled to inhibitory G proteins that repress adenylate cyclase activity upon receptor activation (256); (b) G-protein-coupled receptors that activate PLCγ leading to hydrolysis of polyphosphoinositides (e.g., PIP$_2$) generating the second messengers, DAG and IP$_3$, as shown in Fig. 4 (257). This class of receptors includes the angiotensin, bradykinin, somatostatin, and vasopressin receptors; (c) novel G-protein-coupled photoreceptors. This class is coupled to the G protein transducin, which activates a phosphodiesterase leading to a decrease in the level of cyclic guanosine monophosphate (cGMP) (258). The drop in cGMP then results in the closing of a Na^+/Ca^{2+} channel leading to hyperpolarization of the cell and resulting photoactivated signaling pathways. G-protein cascade mechanisms are outlined below.

XVIII. G PROTEINS AND THEIR REGULATORS

G-protein-coupled receptors, as implicit in their name, exert their transduction functions by coupling to G proteins. G proteins consume GTP in the course of their activity, prompting their GTPase label. They cycle reversibly between active GTP-bound and inactive GDP-bound states, serving as molecular switches in the cytosol, controlled by extracellular stimuli via receptors, to mediate cell attachment, spreading, and growth functions. The heterotrimeric family of G proteins are considered the large class of G proteins as opposed to monomeric small G proteins (e.g., Ras, Rho, Ran1, Rab, Sar1, Cdc42). Heterotrimeric G proteins comprise an α subunit that binds and hydrolyzes GTP, and β and γ subunits, which are regarded as a functional entity associated with the GDP-loaded α subunit when the G protein is in an inactivated state (259). Binding of G$\alpha \cdot$ GDP $\cdot$ G$_\beta$G$_\gamma$ to a cell hormone–receptor complex induces the Gα subunit to exchange its bound GDP for GTP, and, in doing so, to dissociate from G$_\beta$G$_\gamma$. Binding of GTP to Gα also increases its affinity for adenylate cyclase, which in turn activates adenylate cyclase to convert ATP to cAMP and activate further cell cascades (Fig. 1) (260).

Some G-protein-coupled hormone receptors inhibit rather than stimulate adenylate cyclase via activation of an inhibitory, or "i," class of heterotrimeric G proteins. These include the α_2-adrenoreceptors, as well as receptors for thrombin, opoids, thyrotropin, and somatostatin (181). The inhibitory protein, termed G$_i$, most likely has the same β and γ subunits as the stimulatory G protein, G$_s$, but has a different α subunit, G$_{i\alpha}$. G$_i$ acts similarly to G$_s$ in binding to its corresponding hormone–receptor complex:

its $G_{i\alpha}$ subunit exchanges bound GDP to GTP and dissociates from $G_\beta G_\gamma$ to inhibit further signals. Interaction of $G_{i\alpha}$ with adenylate cyclase then inhibits its activity by direct interaction and possibly because the unbound $G_\beta G_\gamma$ sequesters $G_{s\alpha}$ (260).

The Ras GTPase or G-protein superfamily make up the small molecular weight (about 21,000 Da, hence "p21") G-protein monomeric class (261). The proto-oncogenic protein Ras (name derived from discovery of viral oncogenes in *Ha*rvey and *Ki*rsten rat sarcoma viruses, hence the prefixes, Ha-ras and Ki-ras, as opposed to wild-type or *n*ormal ras, N-ras) is involved in the genesis of numerous forms of cancer (184,210), which are capable of transforming mammalian cells when activated by point mutations. Of particular clinical significance is the fact that oncogenic activation of Ras occurs with higher frequency than that of any other gene in the development of colorectal cancers (262,263). Normal p21^{ras} binds GTP and hydrolyzes it to GDP via its enzymatic action. The p21^{ras} plays a central role in many cell signal transduction pathways stimulated by both environmental input, as well as mitogens and cytokines. The activation of p21^{ras} in turn triggers other protein kinases, including Raf-1 and MEKK/ MAPKK, that through the increasingly important extracellular signal–regulated kinases (ERKs) (264,265), proceeds through c-jun N-terminal kinase (JNK) or through p62^{TCF} (protein of molecular weight 62 Da called *t*ernary *c*omplex *f*actor) to activate c-fos, both gene transcriptional regulators of transcription factor, AP-1 transcriptional response element (TRE) (jun-fos heterodimer), and gene expression. These signal pathways can be activated chemically (phorbol ester), biochemically (cytokines, growth factors), by insoluble matrix cues (ECM), and by fluid shear and mechanics, producing signal cascades leading to differential gene expression (266). Biomaterials, therefore, are passively (i.e., their compliance mismatch equates with mechanics, discontinuity or resultant fluid shearing from device conduits) or actively (growth factor delivery or inflammatory mediation) producing signaling via these routes, whether intended or not, but certainly not in a well-controlled or understood manner.

The activity of G proteins with respect to GTP hydrolytic turnover is regulated by a family of proteins termed GTPase-activating proteins (GAPs) (267). As shown in Fig. 6, GAPs act as a negative regulator on normal Ras proteins (see below), but are ineffective on activated mutants of p21^{ras} (268,269); hence, the cancerous phenotype mentioned above. Several other GAP proteins besides p120^{GAP} are important in cell signal transduction, and these include p190^{GAP} (Rac/Rho pathway) and NF1 (Ras pathway). Interestingly, the NF1 GAP catalytic fragment has a much higher affinity for p21^{ras} than does p120^{GAP}, but has a slower turnover number. The neurofibromatosis type 1 (NF1) protein (270) is therefore expected to

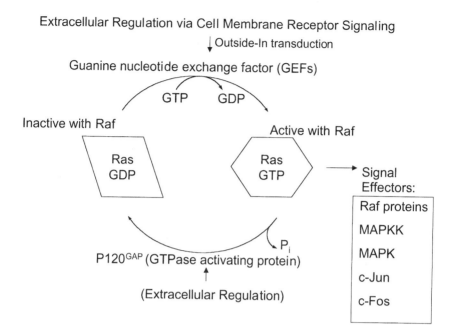

Figure 6 G-protein regulation. The ras superfamily of G proteins (small GTPases rho, rac, ras, cdc42) are coupled to membrane receptor activation. The activity of G proteins with respect to GTP hydrolysis is regulated by a respective family of proteins termed GTPase-activating proteins, (GAPs; see Fig. 1). Guanine nucleotide exchange factors (GEFs) facilitate the exchange of GDP to GTP to control G-protein activity. Integrin receptor binding of ECM has been shown to trigger various G-protein responses, including cascades involving both rho and rac, which include regulation of focal adhesion assembly via focal adhesion kinase (FAK), cytoskeleton formation through rho-associated serine/threonine kinase 1 (ROCK-1) and LIM-kinase (a kinase containing the LIM domain, named from the Lin-11, Isl-1, and Mec-3 genes), and transcriptional regulation through the MAPK cascade to c-fos and c-jun. This has important implications for influences of biomaterial-adsorbed ECM on integrin pathways under G-protein control.

inactivate p21^{ras} more efficiently than p120^{GAP} at low but not high concentrations (271).

Proteins that act as activating control factors for G proteins in general and p21^{ras} in particular are the exchange factors, or guanine nucleotide exchange factors (GEFs) (272), also shown in Figs 6 and 7. Cellular factors that stimulate exchange of GDP to GTP prompt G proteins or p21^{ras} to bind more GTP, since this is the predominant guanine nucleotide found in

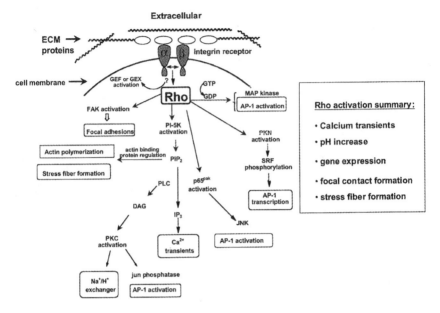

Figure 7 Outside-in ECM-integrin modulation of G-protein Rho. Integrin recognition of ECM motifs producing transmembrane activation of Rho family proteins intracellularly leading to many signaling pathway activations. This pathway has been interrogated in the context of biomaterial surfaces and mechanotransduction. *Abbreviations*: ECM, extracellular matrix; GEF/GEX, guanine nucleotide exchange factor; GTP, guanine triphosphate; GDP, guanine diphosphate; FAK, focal adhesion kinase; PI-5K, phosphatidylinositol 5-kinase; PIP_2, phosphatidylinositol 4,5-biphosphate; IP_3, inositol 1,4,5-triphosphate; PLC, phospholipase C; DAG, diacylglycerol; PKC, protein kinase C; PKN, protein kinase N (also known as PRK-1, PKC-related kinase 1); SRF, serum response factor; p65^{pak}, p21-activated kinase 1; JNK, c-Jun NH$_2$-terminal kinase; AP-1, activating protein 1.

the cytosol (271). For example, in the Rho family of GTPases, members of the Dbl/Cdc24 proteins have interacting GEFs that are known to be oncogenic (273–275). The GTPase Rho is a member of the Ras superfamily, and has an essential role in controlling the assembly of actin cytoskeleton and of integrin-dependent adhesion processes. Figure 7 depicts outside-in signal transduction through integrin receptors for RhoA, a member of the Rho GTPase family. Cdc24 is a GEF that activates the exchange of GDP to GTP in Cdc 42 (monomeric G protein that is a member of the Rho GTPase family); and Dbl is an oncogene found in mammals that also interacts with Cdc42. Both Cdc24 and Dbl are members of the same family of GEFs based on sequence similarities (267). Dbl proteins (products of the *Dbl* oncogene) are potent inducers of cell focus formation (reflecting a loss of contact inhibition, characteristic of tumor phenotype) in fibroblast transfection assays (276,277). Because of their ubiquitous receptor association, and their involvement in many cell behaviors of interest to cell–surface activation, inflammation, and cancer phenotypes, G proteins are an increasing focus for tissue engineering and biomaterials-associated studies (31,32,278).

XIX. INTRACELLULAR HORMONE RECEPTORS

The steroid/thyroid hormone receptor superfamily (e.g., glucocorticoid, vitamin D, retinoic acid, and thyroid hormone receptors) is a class of proteins that reside in the cytoplasm and bind the lipophilic steroid/thyroid hormones. These hormones have low, intrinsic solubilities (low abundance) but are capable of freely penetrating the hydrophobic plasma membrane. Upon binding ligand, the hormone–receptor complex translocates to the nucleus and binds to specific DNA sequences, termed hormone response elements (HREs). Binding of the complex to this element results in altered transcription rates of the associated gene. Thus, most lipophilic hormone receptors are proteins that effectively bypass all of the signal transduction pathways previously described by residing intracellularly, within the cytoplasm, as opposed to on or near the cell membrane. In addition, all of the hormone receptors are bifunctional in that they are capable of binding steroid hormones of the thyroxine and retinoic acid classes, as well as directly activating gene transcription (279). A local delivery system releases testosterone using a zinc-based, self-setting, ceramic bone substitute and tricalcium phosphate-lysine (280,281). Steriod hormones have also been delivered from biomaterials to adult castrated rams (282), and dexamethasone has been shown to be released from biomaterials to reduce inflammation and fibrosis at implant cites (283,284). Hence, these pathways are currently being manipulated by biomaterials strategies, although with as-yet-unknown signal influences.

XX. PHOSPHATASES IN SIGNAL TRANSDUCTION

As described above, evidence links both tyrosine and serine/threonine phosphorylation with increased cellular growth, proliferation, and differentiation. Removal of the incorporated phosphates must be a necessary event in order to reversibly turn on/off these proliferative signals. Work on reversible protein phosphorylation was highlighted by the 1992 Nobel Prize awards in physiology and medicine to Edmond Fischer and Edwin Krebs (285,286). Reversible protein phosphorylation mediates the regulation of cell growth, cell division, and differentiation as well as responses to kinase activity within the cell. Thus, phosphatases are just as important as kinases in signal transduction cascades for their ability to participate in the on off switching mechanisms of phosphorylated signaling molecules within cells.

The first transmembrane protein tyrosine phosphatase characterized was the leukocyte cell surface glycoprotein, CD45 (287–289). This protein was shown to have homology to the intracellular protein tyrosine phosphatase, PTP1B (290). CD45 is involved in regulation of T-cell activation, and is known to dephosphorylate a Tyr residue in Lck, which is associated with T-cell antigens, CD4, and CD8 (291–294). Two broad classes of protein tyrosine phosphatases are now known. One class is the receptor-type enzymes which contain the phosphatase activity domain in the intracellular portion of the protein, contain a transmembrane region, and have an extracellular portion that often contains domains homologous to immunoglobulin G and fibronectin type III repeats (295–298). The other class comprises the soluble nonreceptor type of enzymes localized intracellularly (299–302).

The C-terminal residues of many intracellular protein tyrosine phosphatases are very hydrophobic, suggesting that these sites are membrane localization domains (303). One role of intracellular protein tyrosine phosphatases is in the maturation of *Xenopus* oocytes in response to hormones (304). Overexpression of protein tyrosine phosphatase 1B (PTP1B) in oocytes resulted in a marked retardation in the rate of insulin- and progesterone-induced maturation (305,306). These results suggest a role for PTP1B in countering the signals leading to cellular activation. Other members of these protein tyrosine phosphatases include subclass members: cdc25, VH1, MEG1, MEG2, PEST, LMWP, and others (307).

Other phosphatases that recognize serine- and/or threonine-phos- phorylated proteins also exist in cells (308–310). At least 15 distinct phosphatases of this category have been identified (311,312). The type 2A protein serine phosphatases exhibit selective substrate specificity toward PKC-phosphorylated proteins, in particular serine- and threonine-phos- phorylated receptors (313,314). The type 2A protein serine phosphatases have two subunits (a regulatory and a catalytic) both of which can associate with one of the tumor antigens of the DNA tumor virus, polyoma (315). Transformation by DNA tumor viruses such as polyoma appears to be mediated by formation of a signal transduction unit consisting of a virally encoded T antigen and several host-encoded proteins. Several host proteins are tyrosine kinases of the src family. Polyoma middle T antigen also can bind to PI-3K (316). The association of type 2A protein serine phosphatases

in these complexes may lead to dephosphorylation of regulatory serine/
threonine-phosphorylated sites, resulting in increased signal transduction
and subsequent cellular proliferation.

XXI. CELL ADHESION–DEPENDENT SIGNALING

Focal adhesions found in attachment-dependent cells are known to result
from integrin recognition of ECM via Ras small GTPase superfamily (Rac,
Ras, Rho, cdc42) convergent signaling pathways. Focal adhesion assembly
is known to be regulated by combinations of the nonreceptor tyrosine
kinase, Src-focal adhesion kinase (FAK), signal paths (317–319), regulated
by the Ras superfamily in as-yet-unelucidated ways. Src is activated through
autophosphorylation induced by paracrine growth factors, including EGF
and PDGF, and by proximity to receptor tyrosine kinases (320).
Additionally, ECM-integrin recognition activates Src to phosphorylate
FAK. This then cascades to phosphorylate several focal adhesion proteins
(321). As represented in Fig. 1 for this pathway, focal adhesions on the
cytosolic membrane surface comprise FAK, integrin domains, paxcillin,
vinculin, and possibly other nonreceptor protein kinases (e.g., Src),
providing direct physical connections through integrin transmembrane
domains between ECM and internal cell signaling pathways. Overexpression
of c-Src promotes cell adhesion and migration in culture systems (322).
Actin–myosin II interactions in part responsible for cell migration are cued
by MLCK signaling pathway (323). Cell traction—a primary cell motility
mechanism—proceeds once the membrane is anchored via focal adhesions,
likely generated through these actin–myosin II interactions and coordinated
integrin release from focal adhesions at cells' trailing edges on surfaces.
Myosin light chain phosphorylation by calcium-dependent/calmodulin-
dependent serine/threonine kinase (MLCK) initiates interactions between
actin and myosin II (324): fasudil, a known MLCK inhibitor, has been
shown to suppress cell migration (325). Other work has shown that MLCK
is activated by Rho kinase (326–328) and phosphorylated by MAPK p44
and p42 that are activated as in typical MAPK pathways by pleotropic
factors, FGF, VEGF, EGF, and PDGF (329). MLCK is inhibited by p21-
activated kinases (330). These growth factors are responsible for several
gene products important to cell adhesion and motility (331). One recent
study supports the involvement of the receptor tyrosine kinase-MAPK
signaling pathway in up-regulation of these gene products in response to
growth factors (323). This work showed that activation of p44 and p42
MAPKs proceeds through autophosphorylation of receptor tyrosine kinases
activated by cognate receptors. This MAPK activation step involves Raf

and MAPK extracellular signal–regulated kinase kinase and leads to direct phosphorylation of MLCK and then to phosphorylation of myosin light chains (323,324) to promote actin interactions.

Other cell migratory activities, including actin polymerization, calcium transients, activation of membrane antiporters, and focal adhesions, while linked to focal assembly and actin–myosin interaction, are also likely to be regulated by similar kinase pathways. Evidence points to common receptor-activated (integrin) pathways involving Rho, Rac, cdc42, and Ras GTPases. Transfected forms of constitutively active GTPases in cells support distinct roles for each Ras family GTPase in these activities (332–334). Analogous receptor activation of GTPases in connection with surface chemistry has been shown for attachment-dependent cells (31,32). Other work has shown that Rho activates Rho kinase which cascades to LIM kinase to produce actin polymerization (335). Additionally, pleotropic factors, including FGF, VEGF, PDGF, and possibly EGF, activate both Rho and Rac through receptor tyrosine kinases and PI$_3$ kinase (318,336).

XXII. MECHANICAL STRESS, FLUID SHEAR, AND CELL SIGNALING

One disadvantage of decades of cell–materials work has been the predominant historical focus on static culture conditions, often considered irrelevant to physiological conditions. An additional presumption, now known to be false, is that anchored cells on materials experience no adverse stress or strain influences. More recent work has shown that, in addition to long-known, well-studied effects of culture or substrate chemistry on cell attachment mechanisms and the implications for receptor-mediated pathways, mechanical effects, including static and oscillatory shear stresses, also activate important signaling pathways that influence many cell functions. Conditions more relevant to physiological environments under continuous or pulsatile flow, tension, or flexure (e.g., vascular entholelium, lung tissue, bone tissues) are shown in vitro to influence in significant ways the behavior and phenotypic properties of cells. More significantly, these changes are increasingly linked to specific stress-activated signaling pathways involving several protein kinases, as shown in Fig. 8. Cells experience stress stimuli from several sources, including dynamic fluid and mechanical stresses, prompting mechanotransduction of signals and cascade initiation ending at the genetic level. Many signal pathways are identical to these observed in static cells stimulated with soluble mitogens or cytokines in standard assays (266,337).

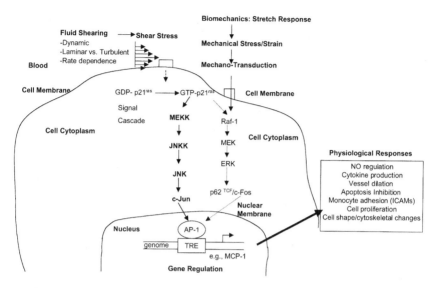

Figure 8 The hemodynamic stress–initiated and mechanical stress signal transduction pathways activated in endothelium by mechanical-to-biochemical coupling transduced by the endothelial cell membrane via receptors such as integrins. Membrane-associated $p21^{ras}$ furthermore activates a number of pathways. Shown here are the MEKK-JNKK-JNK pathway (shown bold-faced in the figure), which is preferential in the fluid shear stress model over the Raf-MEK-ERK pathway in activation of AP-1 ternary complex transcription factor formation upon binding and activation of TRE promoters. Expression of chemokine MCP-1 from endothelium due to this shear stress can attract monocytes, T cells, and natural killer cells to the target endothelial cell, which has potential cancer treatment capabilities by increasing monocyte (anti-tumoral) activity (370). *Abbreviations*: MEKK, an MAPKKK (mitogen-activated protein kinase kinase kinase) or extracellular signal–regulated kinase kinase; JNKK, c-Jun NH_2-terminal kinase kinase; JNK, c-Jun NH_2-terminal kinase; AP-1, activating protein-1; TRE, thyroid hormone response element; MEK, an MAPKK (mitogen-activated protein kinase kinase) or extracellular signal–regulated kinase; ERK, extracellular signal–regulated kinase, an MAPK; $p62^{TCF}$, also known as Elk-1, a 62-kDa ternary complex factor that mediates growth factor stimulation by binding to the c-Fos promoter in part with SRF (serum response factor). (Adapted from Ref. 266.)

Fluid shear stress is known to influence or even control the behavior of cells in vascular tissues (338–340). Vascular shear stress, the fluid dynamic force acting tangentially to cell surfaces in vasculature, has been shown to change cell cytoskeletal morphology (341), alter growth factor expression (342,343), regulate cell proliferation (344,345), and apoptosis (344,346) (Fig.

8). Recent work has implicated a connection between shear stress effects on vascular endothelial cell signaling migration behavior of smooth muscle cells (347,348), and cyclic strain on tissue-engineered smooth muscle (278). While this shear stress could be a mechanically transduced effect onto both cell populations located in adjacent radial layers in the vascular tissue, protein kinase–mediated signaling from endothelial cells directly exposed to blood fluid shear (or alterations in natural shear due to device placement) to smooth muscle cells peripheral and adjacent to them is also possible. Shear strain rate dependence on cell signals is not well studied to date but seems likely to be important since oscillatory effects on signaling are notable. Mechanotransduction influences should also be studied in the context of implant-associated healing where mechanical and oxidative stresses are coupled (278,349,350).

XXIII. BIOLOGICAL AND BIOCHEMICAL TECHNIQUES FOR THE DETECTION AND ANALYSIS OF SIGNALING MOLECULES

While many signal pathways in cells have been and continue to be elucidated, knowledge of their synergy, redundancy, overlap, feedback, and more intimate mechanistic details are lacking for most pathways. Nonetheless, many of these transduction mechanisms are operative in normal attachment-dependent cells and are likely perturbed in complex ways by the presence of any biomaterial. Differentiation of signal mechanisms, nuclear and genetic targets, transcriptional influence, phenotypic regulation and control over cell behavioral traits would be valuable to assess for cells proliferating on tissue engineering matrices and biomaterials where local and global chemical and mechanical stimuli are altered. Little is known about cell signaling mechanisms or control in the surgical implant environment, or simply in cell culture systems with biomaterials;—this is an enormous opportunity to gain insight. This relatively unexplored research area requires refinement of experimental protocols in order to progress along these lines. The following experimental methods provide an ensemble of state-of-the-art methods to begin addressing these challenges. Yet, molecular cell biology methods continue to advance at such a rapid pace that this list will quickly be obsolete.

A. ^{3}H-Thymidine Incorporation (Mitogen Assay)

This experiment is relatively straightforward if radioactivity capabilities are available. A mitogenic assay is one way of measuring cell proliferation upon cellular stimulation by a mitogenic factor, such as a growth factor, an antigen, a synthetic (drug) molecule, or a culture substrate. Cell activation is determined by the incorporation of a soluble, added radiolabeled nucleotide into cellular DNA. In this assay, metabolic genomic uptake of ^{3}H-thymidine can be monitored by scintillation counting of cell lysate after this radiolabeled base is added to cellular growth medium under the test conditions desired, followed by an incubation period of 48–72 h at 37°C. Actively proliferating cells incorporate more ^{3}H-thymidine into their DNA than slowly proliferating or nonproliferating cells, as exemplified in Ref. 191.

B. SDS-PAGE and Western Blotting

Sodium dodecyl sulfate–polyacrylamide gel electrophoresis [SDS-PAGE] (351) and the subsequent development of Western blotting are now routine methods of detecting cell proteins and carbohydrates. The former method separates a mixture of soluble biological molecules by mass to charge ratio, whereas the latter method allows for the transfer of proteins/carbohydrates onto a membrane that is probed with a chosen antibody specific to that antigen. Application of an appropriate secondary sandwich-tagging antibody (e.g., if the first antibody has been sourced from rabbit sera, then the second antibody should be antirabbit) conjugated with an enzyme such as horseradish peroxidase (HRP) or alkaline phosphatase (AP), is used to detect the molecule of interest upon addition of a substrate for the enzyme that produces a colorimetric, fluorescent, or chemiluminescent signal at the separated protein band on the membrane.

C. Polymerase Chain Reaction and Reverse Transcriptase

Polymerase chain reaction (PCR) and reverse-transcriptase PCR (RT-PCR) are excellent methods to identify the expression of a particular gene or transcribed gene product, especially since these methods amplify the amount of cellular genetic material originally isolated from cells grown under desired test conditions. Minimal detection is about 1 μg of RNA (352) and 1 ng of DNA. This means that approximately 10^3 cells from identical environments must be collected for genetic analysis, or that genetic amplification methods must be employed on smaller cell extract samples to produce sufficient copies of DNA or RNA for analysis. Detection limits for DNA or RNA can be reduced if the number of PCR thermocycles is 30–40. These methods rely on the ability of a thermally stable enzyme (*Taq* polymerase), operating under cyclically applied temperatures that denature the oligonucleotides primer strands from the genes of interest, to promote continual synthesis of complementary DNA (cDNA) in the presence of the appropriate primers, buffering conditions, and free dNTPs (commercial sources provide kits complete with all necessary instructions and reagents). This often requires knowledge of the DNA sequences for the gene of interest and construction of complementary 5' and 3' primers along specific 20- to 30-bp subsequences on this gene to enable amplification. The final amplified nucleotide products can be analyzed and visualized on agarose gel in the presence of an optically active DNA intercalator (e.g., ethidium bromide). Also, commercially available molecular weight markers allow for base pair size comparison within the same gel (final products are double-stranded cDNAs).

One problem with RT-PCR is that RNA is thermodynamically more unstable than DNA and very susceptible to ubiquitous RNase degradation. Although RNA isolation kits (Ambion, PCG Scientific, Qiagen) can help prevent degradation of sample RNA, it is always a question of whether or not the absence of bands in a gel is due to this degradation. Also, mRNA expression may vary from cell/tissue type, both in amount and isoform. Thus, RT-PCR primers should be designed toward a conserved mRNA sequence, or else careful design of primers should be undertaken in order to target a rarer or unique form of mRNA that may be specific to a particular cell/tissue type or to expression within the cell cycle. Finally, because so many manipulations of the original amount of DNA/RNA take place, the quantitation of actual starting material is difficult. Many researchers use "housekeeping genes," such as GAPDH, as an internal control (when using a thermocycler), or else use newly developed instruments, such as the LightCycler (Roche Diagnostics), which claims quantitative PCR and RT-PCR methods. Other companies that currently sell PCR and RT-PCR thermocyclers include Biometra, Bio-Rad, Eppendorf, Hybaid, MJ Research, Perkin–Elmer, and Techne; the machines offered by these companies offer various improvements in older-style equipment, including real-time/quantitative PCR and multiple amplification software associated with multiple machines (Biometra) allowing for simultaneous data analyses. New developments in this important and rapidly developing method will continue to improve its bioanalytical capabilities and potentially to rapid single-cell analysis.

D. Southern (DNA) and Northern (mRNA) Blotting

Both of these protocols (353) involve the blotting of single-stranded sample nucleic acids from cells of interest onto a charged membrane and then probing with a complementary strand labeled with $^{32}PO_4$ nucleotides (most sensitive but also most hazardous, and laboratory conditions must be approved for radioactive work), deoxyginin (Roche Diagnostics Labeling

Kit), biotin (354), chemiluminesence (355,356) or other possible probes. The blotted DNA or RNA cell sample fragments complementary to the applied specific probe hybridize with it, and their location on the filter can be revealed by autoradiography. The advantage of this technique is that it is quantitative (when compared with PCR and RT-PCR): one DNA sequence or gene (1 part in 10^6) from 5 μg of DNA (amount of DNA in about 10^6 cells) can usually be detected (279). The Western blots (see above) for proteins were also developed from this original idea, and the protein of interest is probed using a labeled antibody instead of labeled cDNA. Problems with Southerns and Northerns are sensitivity limitations, and protecting the mRNA from degrading RNAses, as discussed under PCR and RT-PCR. Nevertheless, the payoff can be quantitative information on genetic regulation in contact with biomaterials and other relevant conditions.

E. Enzyme-Linked Immunosorbent Assay

Enzyme-linked immunosorbent assay (ELISA) is a useful method to assay just about any molecule of interest as long as there is an antibody available against it. These experiments are useful because ELISA plates have many sample wells (96, 384, and even 1536) in which scaled-down, small-volume molecular assays are performed and instruments rapidly measure each well. Many types of experiments using ELISA can be designed. For example, an adsorbed protein can be probed with a monoclonal antibody against a particular domain of that protein (e.g., adsorption of Fn to a biomaterial and then probing with an anti-RGD antibody) to determine the conformation of the adsorbed protein in the plate wells. Serially diluted inhibitors can provide an IC_{50} value, a number roughly related to the K_d binding coefficient. Pierce and Bio-Rad both have commercially available reagents which allow for protein quantitation assays using a microplate design. An advantage of this technique is that there typically are enough wells to run the appropriate controls—both positive and negative—against the actual experiment and, if necessary, against other components used in the test (i.e., one may want to try various surface blocking conditions, like albumin or nonfat milk; different batches of secondary antibodies; or varying concentrations of components to permit optimal signal over noise readout). Some caveats with ELISAs are that they require a plate-reading assay instrument (many companies manufacture these: Molecular Devices, Phenix, Bio-Tek, Packard, etc.) for detection of the generated substrate (optical density, fluorescence, or chemiluminescence), and although the absorbance values typically tend to be not as wildly fluctuating as fluorescence or chemiluminescence, they are also not as sensitive. Also, data from these experiments are relative because conditions usually vary from plate to plate; hence the need for running controls or internal standards per plate.

F. Immunofluorescence—Molecular Tagging

Cytoskeletal reorganization occurs within cells attached to surfaces (357). Immunofluorescence microscopy utilizes fluorescently tagged antibodies to mark specific, accessible intracellular cytoskeletal components or organelles, thus demonstrating where a particular protein of interest is located within the cell by distinct microscopic observation of the cell. Formation of focal adhesions, for example, can be studied by immunofluorescence by staining components such as paxillin, actinin, or vinculin with probe-tagged antibodies to these cytoskeletal proteins (31,32).

G. Ribonuclease Protection Assays

The ribonuclease (RNase) protection assay is an extremely sensitive technique for the quantitation of specific RNAs in solution (359–361). This assay can be performed on total cellular RNA or poly(A)-selected mRNA as a target for analysis. RNase protection assays are highly sensitive due to the use of a complementary high-specific-activity ^{32}P-labeled antisense probe. The probe and target RNA are hybridized in solution, after which the mixture is diluted and treated with RNase to degrade all remaining RNA. The hybridized portion of the probe will be protected from digestion and can be visualized via electrophoresis of the mixture on a denaturing polyacrylamide gel (as opposed to agarose gels, which are typically used for nucleotide analysis) followed by autoradiography. The resulting signal will be directly proportional to the amount of complementary RNA in the sample.

The ribonuclease protection assay provides advantages over Northern blots for the detection and quantitation of low abundance RNAs. With Northern blots, RNA transfer and binding to the membrane may be inefficient because some RNA molecules may not be accessible for hybridization (after binding to the membrane). Finally, sample integrity influences the degree to which the signal is localized in a single band (362). Also, improvements in the RNase protection assay system have overcome the shortcomings of the original S1 nuclease protection assay because with S1 mapping procedures, lower temperatures are used to favor single-stranded cleavage and AU-rich regions are attacked nonspecifically, creating artifacts (360,363).

Both PharMingen and Promega have helped to revolutionize the RNase protection assay system by developing kits useful for these experiments (364,365). Promega's RNase Protection Assay System utilizes RNase ONE (366), one of the few known ribonucleases that cleaves the phosphodiester bond between any two ribonucleotides and degrading single-stranded RNA to a mixture of monomers and oligomers (367,371). In addition, RNase ONE is inactivated by 0.1% SDS (368), thus eliminating the need for time-consuming phenol/chloroform extractions to remove the RNase before gel analysis, which helps to improve the accuracy and reproducibility of this system (358).

PharMingen's ribonuclease protection assay kits also have beneficial features, such as utilizing template mRNA sequences that are capable of analyzing up to 13 RNA species in a single sample of RNA (369). Another advantage of using PharMingen's RiboQuant Multi-Probe RNase Protection Assay System is that the company currently offers up to 91 Multi-Probe Template sets, including cytokines, cytokine receptors, apoptosis-related molecules, cell cycle regulators, tumor suppressor genes, DNA damage and repair molecules, angiogenesis molecules, developmental genes, signal transduction pathway molecules, and more. The advantage of the multi-probe system is comparative analyses of different mRNAs within samples and among separate experiments since the mRNAs of "housekeeping" genes are included in the kits. Finally, this assay system is very specific and quantitative due to the sensitivity of the ribonuclease for mismatched base pairs and the use of Le Chatelier's principle, where excess probe induces completion of solution-based hybridization (369).

XXIV. SUMMARY

Biomaterial designs can currently elicit very limited cell responses using limited controlled growth factor release and homogeneous adhesion peptide immobilization (1,2). These strategies can only prompt cell–surface communication and integrating cell signaling responses in very primitive ways, producing numerous clinical performance deficiencies from these materials because phenotypic traits are not well preserved in the long term.

Progress in molecular and cell biology assays of cell signals, receptor-mediated stimuli, and intracellular pathways leading to transcriptional regulation should prove immensely useful to addressing long-standing challenges surrounding the interface between living cells and tissues and biomaterials. Interrogation of modes of communication both intra- and intercellularly in the context of cell surface, mechanical, and dynamic fluid shearing stimuli is now increasingly valuable and relevant. Many new opportunities are available to exploit new knowledge of cell signal transduction mechanisms in the design of high-performance biomaterials for implants and tissue engineering. Ultimately, a more complete sorting of signal pathways must be achieved. This should be accompanied by a fuller understanding of autoregulation in the host by soluble (e.g., cytokine) and insoluble (ECM matrix) cues, and predictable disruption or alteration of normal regulation by biomaterial interfaces (both chemically and mechanically). Progress in these areas will naturally elucidate control strategies by which biomaterials designs might effectively tailor implant device properties to manipulate or integrate into cell signaling pathways so as to enhance clinical performance and even promote cell differentiation into tissue-like constructs. Using such an approach, tissue-engineered biomaterials might someday be capable of combining cell-sourced signals, scaffold-encapsulated or immobilized cues, and versatile, dynamic menus of signal prompts in both temporal and spatial domains to grow tissue sources comprising multiple cell types in complex organizational and functional designs.

ACKNOWLEDGMENTS

The authors thank Jordan Nestlerode for preparation of the figures; Colleen McKiernan, PhD, for technical discussions regarding G-protein-coupled receptors, G proteins, and G protein regulators sections; Jimmy McColery for EndNote technical support. The authors also acknowledge support from NIH Grant R01 GM56751-01.

REFERENCES

1. AL Koenig, DW Grainger. Cell-synthetic surface interactions: targeted cell adhesion. In: Atala A, Lanza R, eds. Methods of Tissue Engineering. San Diego: Academic Press, 2001, pp. 751–770.
2. RG LeBaron, KA Athanasiou. Extracellular matrix cell adhesion peptides: functional applications in orthopedic materials. Tissue Eng 6:85–103, 2000.
3. F Grinnell. Fibronectin adsorption on material surfaces. Ann N Y Acad Sci 516:280–290, 1987.
4. F Grinnell, PA Shere. Inhibition of cellular adhesiveness by sulfhydryl blocking agents. J Cell Physiol 78:153–158, 1971.
5. F Grinnell, M Milam, PA Shere. Studies on cell adhesion. II. Adhesion of cells to surfaces of diverse chemical composition and inhibition of adhesion by sulfhydryl binding reagents. Arch Biochem Biophys 153:193–198, 1972.
6. F Grinnell, M Milam, PA Srere. Studies on cell adhesion. 3. Adhesion of baby hamster kidney cells. J Cell Biol 56:659–665, 1973.

7. F Grinnell, M Milam, PA Srere. Attachment of normal and transformed hamster kidney cells to substrata varying in chemical composition. Biochem Med 7:87–90, 1973.

8. AL Koenig, V Gambillara, DW Grainger. Correlating fibronectin adsorption with endothelial cell adhesion and signaling on polymer substrates. J Biomed Mater Res, accepted, 2002.

9. F Grinnell, JL Marshall. Coating bacteriological dishes with fibronectin permits spreading and growth of human diploid fibroblasts. Cell Biol Int Rep 6:1013–1018, 1982.

10. S Downes, DJ Wood, AJ Malcolm, SY Ali. Growth hormone in polymethylmethacrylate cement. Clin Orthop 294–298, 1990.

11. S Downes. Methods for improving drug release from poly(methyl)methacrylate bone cement. Clin Mater 7:227–231, 1991.

12. S Downes, M Patel, L Di Silvio, H Swai, K Davy, M Braden: Modifications of the hydrophilicity of heterocyclic methacrylate copolymers for protein release. Biomaterials, 16:1417–1421, 1995.

13. CJ Goodwin, M Braden, S Downes, NJ Marshall: Investigation into the release of bioactive recombinant human growth hormone from normal and low-viscosity poly(methylmethacrylate) bone cements. J Biomed Mater Res 34:47–55, 1997.

14. RC Straw, BE Powers, SJ Withrow, MF Cooper, AS Turner: Effect of intramedullary polymethylmethacrylate on healing of intercalary cortical allografts in a canine model. J Orthop Res 10:434–439, 1992.

15. MC Trindade, M Lind, SB Goodman, WJ Maloney, DJ Schurman, RL Smith: Interferon-gamma exacerbates polymethylmethacrylate particle-induced interleukin-6 release by human monocyte/macrophages in vitro. J Biomed Mater Res 47:1–7, 1999.

16. MC Trindade, DJ Schurman, WJ Maloney, SB Goodman, RL Smith. G-protein activity requirement for polymethylmethacrylate and titanium particle-induced fibroblast interleukin-6 and monocyte chemoattractant protein-1 release in vitro. J Biomed Mater Res 51:360–368, 2000.

17. A Gopferich, SJ Peter, A Lucke, L Lu, AG Mikos. Modulation of marrow stromal cell function using poly(D,L-lactic acid)- block-poly(ethylene glycol)–monomethyl ether surfaces. J Biomed Mater Res 46:390–398, 1999.

18. MA Tracy, KL Ward, L Firouzabadian, Y Wang, N Dong, R Qian, Y Zhang: Factors affecting the degradation rate of poly(lactide-co-glycolide) microspheres in vivo and in vitro. Biomaterials 20:1057–1062, 1999.

19. BD Boyan, CH Lohmann, A Somers, GG Niederauer, JM Wozney, DD Dean, DL Carnes, Jr., Z Schwartz: Potential of porous poly-D,L-lactide-co-glycolide particles as a carrier for recombinant human bone morphogenetic protein-2 during osteoinduction in vivo. J Biomed Mater Res 46:51–59, 1999.

20. JWM Vehof, PHM Spauwen, JA Jansen: Bone formation in calcium-phosphate-coated titanium mesh. Biomaterials 21:2003–2009, 2000.

21. S Vercaigne, JGC Wolke, I Naert, JA Jansen: Effect of titanium plasma-sprayed implants on trabecular bone healing in the goat. Biomaterials 19:1093–1099, 1998.

22. AA Comu, S Shortkroff, X Zhang, M Spector. Association of fibroblast orientation around titanium in vitro with expression of a muscle actin. Biomaterials 21:1887–1896, 2000.

23. KE Healy, P Ducheyne. Hydration and preferential molecular adsorption on titanium in vitro. Biomaterials 13:553–561, 1992.

24. KE Healy, P Ducheyne. A physical model for the titanium–tissue interface. ASAIO Trans 37:M150–151, 1991.

25. CH Thomas, JB Lhoest, DG Castner, CD McFarland, KE Healy. Surfaces designed to control the projected area and shape of individual cells. J Biomech Eng 121:40–48, 1999.

26. R Suzuki, JA Frangos. Inhibition of inflammatory species by titanium surfaces. Clin Orthop 280–289, 2000.

27. DM Brunette, P Tengvall, M Textor, P Thomsen. Titanium in Medicine: Material and Surface Science and Engineering, Biological Performance, Medical Applications. Heidelberg: Springer-Verlag, 2001, p 1019.

28. M Textor S-JX, G Kenausis. Biochemical surface treatment of titanium. In: Titanium in Medicine: Material and Surface Science and Engineering, Biological Performance, Medical Applications. Heidelberg: Springer-Verlag, 2001, pp 417–456.

29. GM Whitesides, KL Prime. Self-assembled organic monolayers: model systems for studying the adsorption of proteins at surfaces. Science 252:1164–1167, 1991.

30. CA Scotchford, E Cooper, GJ Leggett, S Downes. Growth of human osteoblast-like cells on alkanethiol on gold self-assembled monolayers: the effect of surface chemistry. J Biomed Mater Res 41:431–442, 1998.

31. KB McClary, T Ugarova, DW Grainger. Modulating fibroblast adhesion, spreading, and proliferation using self-assembled monolayer films of alkylthiolates on gold. J Biomed Mater Res 50:428–439, 2000.

32. KB McClary, DW Grainger. RhoA-induced changes in fibroblasts cultured on organic monolayers. Biomaterials 20:2435–2446, 1999.

33. BT Houseman, M Mrksich. The microenvironment of immobilized Arg-Gly-Asp peptides is an important determinant of cell adhesion. Biomaterials 22:943–955, 2001.

34. S Downes, CJ Clifford, C Scotchford, CP Klein. Comparison of the release of growth hormone from hydroxyapatite, heat-treated hydroxyapatite, and fluoroapatite coatings on titanium. J Biomed Mater Res 29:1053–1060, 1995.

35. RG Courteney-Harris, MV Kayser, S Downes. Comparison of the early production of extracellular matrix on dense hydroxyapatite and hydro-xyapatite-coated titanium in cell and organ culture. Biomaterials 16:489–495, 1995.

36. MD Ball, S Downes, CA Scotchford, EN Antonov, VN Bagratashvili, VK Popov, WJ Lo, DM Grant, SM Howdle. Osteoblast growth on titanium foils

coated with hydroxyapatite by pulsed laser ablation. Biomaterials 22:337–347, 2001.

37. Y Sugimura, M Spector. Interfacial fracture toughness of a plasma sprayed hydroxyapatite coating used for orthopedic implants. Mater Res Soc Symp Proc 550:367–371, 1998.

38. AJ Garcia, P Ducheyne, D Boettiger. Effect of surface reaction stage on fibronectin-mediated adhesion of osteoblast-like cells to bioactive glass. J Biomed Mater Res 40:48–56, 1998.

39. JA Neff, PA Tresco, KD Caldwell. Surface modification for controlled studies of cell-ligand interactions. Biomaterials 20:2377–2393, 1999.

40. K Webb, V Hlady, PA Tresco. Relative importance of surface wettability and charged functional groups on NIH 3T3 fibroblast attachment, spreading, and cytoskeletal organization. J Biomed Mater Res 41:422–430, 1998.

41. K Webb, K Caldwell, PA Tresco. Fibronectin immobilized by a novel surface treatment regulates fibroblast attachment and spreading. Crit Rev Biomed Eng 28:203–208, 2000.

42. JA Neff, KD Caldwell, PA Tresco. Novel method for surface modification to promote cell attachment to hydrophobic substrates. J Biomed Mater Res 40:511–519, 1998.

43. K Kim, C Kim, Y Byun. Preparation of a PEG-grafted phospholipid Langmuir-Blodgett monolayer for blood-compatible material. J Biomed Mater Res 52:836–840, 2000.

44. JH Kim, MJ Song, HW Roh, YC Shin, SC Kim. The in vitro blood compatibility of poly(ethylene oxide)-grafted polyurethane/polystyrene inter-penetrating polymer networks. J Biomater Sci Polym Ed 11:197–216, 2000.

45. JH Lee, KO Kim, YM Ju. Polyethylene oxide additive-entrapped polyvinyl chloride as a new blood bag material. J Biomed Mater Res 48:328–334, 1999.

46. Y Byun, HA Jacobs, SW Kim. Heparin surface immobilization through hydrophilic spacers: thrombin and antithrombin III binding kinetics. J Biomater Sci Polym Ed 6:1–13, 1994.

47. LJ Suggs, RS Krishnan, CA Garcia, SJ Peter, JM Anderson, AG Mikos. In vitro and in vivo degradation of poly(propylene fumarate-co-ethylene glycol) hydrogels. J Biomed Mater Res 42:312–320, 1998.

48. LJ Suggs, EY Kao, LL Palombo, RS Krishnan, MS Widmer, AG Mikos. Preparation and characterization of poly(propylene fumarate-co-ethylene glycol) hydrogels. J Biomater Sci Polym Ed 9:653–666, 1998.

49. LJ Suggs, AG Mikos. Development of poly(propylene fumarate-co-ethylene glycol) as an injectable carrier for endothelial cells. Cell Transplant 8:345–350, 1999.

50. LJ Suggs, MS Shive, CA Garcia, JM Anderson, AG Mikos. In vitro cytotoxicity and in vivo biocompatibility of poly(propylene fumarate-co-ethylene glycol) hydrogels. J Biomed Mater Res 46:22–32, 1999.

51. LJ Suggs, JL West, AG Mikos. Platelet adhesion on a bioresorbable poly(propylene fumarate-co-ethylene glycol) copolymer. Biomaterials 20:683–690, 1999.

52. S He, MJ Yaszemski, AW Yasko, PS Engel, AG Mikos. Injectable biodegradable polymer composites based on poly(propylene fumarate) cross-linked with poly(ethylene glycol)-dimethacrylate. Biomaterials 21:2389–2394, 2000.
53. NA Peppas, KB Keys, M Torres-Lugo, AM Lowman. Poly(ethylene glycol)-containing hydrogels in drug delivery. J Controlled Release 62:81–87, 1999.
54. RA Scott, NA Peppas. Highly crosslinked, PEG-containing copolymers for sustained solute delivery. Biomaterials 20:1371–1380, 1999.
55. V Tangpasuthadol, SM Pendharkar, RC Peterson, J Kohn. Hydrolytic degradation of tyrosine-derived polycarbonates, a class of new biomaterials. Part II: 3-yr study of polymeric devices. Biomaterials 21:2379–2387, 2000.
56. V Tangpasuthadol, SM Pendharkar, J Kohn. Hydrolytic degradation of tyrosine-derived polycarbonates, a class of new biomaterials. Part I: Study of model compounds. Biomaterials 21:2371–2378, 2000.
57. P Vermette, GB Wang, JP Santerre, J Thibault, G Laroche. Commercial polyurethanes: the potential influence of auxiliary chemicals on the biodegradation process. J Biomater Sci Polym Ed 10:729–749, 1999.
58. RS Labow, E Meek, JP Santerre. The biodegradation of poly(urethane)s by the esterolytic activity of serine proteases and oxidative enzyme systems. J Biomater Sci Polym Ed 10:699–713, 1999.
59. JP Santerre, P ten Hove, JL Brash. Polyurethanes bearing pendant amino acids: fibrinogen adsorption and coagulant properties. J Biomed Mater Res 26:1003–1018, 1992.
60. JP Santerre, P ten Hove, NH VanderKamp, JL Brash. Effect of sulfonation of segmented polyurethanes on the transient adsorption of fibrinogen from plasma: possible correlation with anticoagulant behavior. J Biomed Mater Res 26:39–57, 1992.
61. DJ Wheatley, L Raco, GM Bernacca, I Sim, PR Belcher, JS Boyd. Polyurethane: material for the next generation of heart valve prostheses? Eur J Cardiothorac Surg 17:440–448, 2000.
62. GM Bernacca, DJ Wheatley. Surface modification of polyurethane heart valves: effects on fatigue life and calcification. Int J Artif Organs 21:814–819, 1998.
63. GM Bernacca, MJ Gulbransen, R Wilkinson, DJ Wheatley. In vitro blood compatibility of surface-modified polyurethanes. Biomaterials 19:1151–1165, 1998.
64. DB Holt, RC Eberhart, MD Prager. Endothelial cell binding to Dacron modified with polyethylene oxide and peptide. ASAIO J 40:M858–863, 1994.
65. YC Paquay, JE de Ruijter, JP van der Waerden, JA Jansen. Tissue reaction to Dacron velour and titanium fibre mesh used for anchorage of percutaneous devices. Biomaterials 17:1251–1256, 1996.
66. YW Tong, MS Shoichet. Enhancing the interaction of central nervous system neurons with poly(tetrafluoroethylene-co-hexafluoropropylene) via a novel surface amine-functionalization reaction followed by peptide modification. J Biomater Sci Polym Ed 9:713–729, 1998.

67. YW Tong, MS Shoichet. Peptide surface modification of poly(tetrafluoro-ethylene-co-hexafluoropropylene) enhances its interaction with central nervous system neurons. J Biomed Mater Res 42:85–95, 1998.

68. A Guo, LL Rife, NA Rao, RE Smith. Anterior segment prosthesis development: evaluation of expanded polytetrafluoroethylene as a sclera-attached prosthetic material. Cornea 15:210–214, 1996.

69. M Deng, RA Latour, AA Ogale, SW Shalaby. Study of creep behavior of ultra-high-molecular-weight polyethylene systems. J Biomed Mater Res 40:214–223, 1998.

70. FJ Buchanan, B Sim, S Downes. Influence of packaging conditions on the properties of gamma-irradiated UHMWPE following accelerated ageing and shelf ageing. Biomaterials 20:823–837, 1999.

71. OK Muratoglu, CR Bragdon, DO O'Connor, M Jasty, WH Harris, R Gul, F McGarry. Unified wear model for highly crosslinked ultra-high molecular weight polyethylenes (UHMWPE). Biomaterials 20:1463–1470, 1999.

72. SP James, S Blazka, EW Merrill, M Jasty, KR Lee, CR Bragdon, WH Harris. Challenge to the concept that UHMWPE acetabular components oxidize in vivo. Biomaterials 14:643–647, 1993.

73. JE Babensee, MV Sefton. Viability of HEMA-MMA microencapsulated model hepatoma cells in rats and the host response. Tissue Eng 6:165–182, 2000.

74. JE Babensee, RM Cornelius, JL Brash, MV Sefton. Immunoblot analysis of proteins associated with HEMA-MMA microcapsules: human serum proteins in vitro and rat proteins following implantation. Biomaterials 19:839–849, 1998.

75. NK Mongia, KS Anseth, NA Peppas. Mucoadhesive poly(vinyl alcohol) hydrogels produced by freezing/thawing processes: applications in the development of wound healing systems. J Biomater Sci Polym Ed 7:1055–1064, 1996.

76. CS Brazel, NA Peppas. Modeling of drug release from swellable polymers. Eur J Pharm Biopharm 49:47–58, 2000.

77. JV Cauich-Rodriguez, S Deb, R Smith. Effect of cross-linking agents on the dynamic mechanical properties of hydrogel blends of poly(acrylic acid)–poly(vinyl alcohol-vinyl acetate). Biomaterials 17:2259–2264, 1996.

78. I Strzinar, MV Sefton. Preparation and thrombogenicity of alkylated polyvinyl alcohol coated tubing. J Biomed Mater Res 26:577–592, 1992.

79. GR Llanos, MV Sefton. Heparin-poly(ethylene glycol)-poly(vinyl alcohol) hydrogel: preparation and assessment of thrombogenicity. Biomaterials 13:421–424, 1992.

80. JL West, SM Chowdhury, AS Sawhney, CP Pathak, RC Dunn, JA Hubbell. Efficacy of adhesion barriers. Resorbable hydrogel, oxidized regenerated cellulose and hyaluronic acid. J Reprod Med 41:149–154, 1996.

81. KP Vercruysse, GD Prestwich. Hyaluronate derivatives in drug delivery. Crit Rev Ther Drug Carrier Syst 15:513–555, 1998.

82. Y Luo, KR Kirker, GD Prestwich. Cross-linked hyaluronic acid hydrogel films: new biomaterials for drug delivery. J Controlled Release. 69:169–184, 2000.

83. M Mason, KP Vercruysse, KR Kirker, R Frisch, DM Marecak, GD Prestwich, WG Pitt. Attachment of hyaluronic acid to polypropylene, polystyrene, and polytetrafluoroethylene. Biomaterials 21:31–36, 2000.

84. LA Solchaga, JE Dennis, VM Goldberg, AI Caplan. Hyaluronic acid-based polymers as cell carriers for tissue-engineered repair of bone and cartilage. J Orthop Res 17:205–213, 1999.

85. LA Solchaga, JU Yoo, M Lundberg, JE Dennis, BA Huibregtse, VM Goldberg, AI Caplan. Hyaluronan-based polymers in the treatment of osteochondral defects. J Orthop Res 18:773–780, 2000.

86. MJ Kujawa, AI Caplan. Hyaluronic acid bonded to cell-culture surfaces stimulates chondrogenesis in stage 24 limb mesenchyme cell cultures. Dev Biol 114:504–518, 1986.

87. S Nehrer, HA Breinan, A Ramappa, S Shortkroff, G Young, T Minas, CB Sledge, IV Yannas, M Spector. Canine chondrocytes seeded in type I and type II collagen implants investigated in vitro. J Biomed Mater Res 38:95–104, 1997.

88. LJ Chamberlain, IV Yannas, A Arrizabalaga, HP Hsu, TV Norregaard, M Spector. Early peripheral nerve healing in collagen and silicone tube implants: myofibroblasts and the cellular response. Biomaterials 19:1393–1403, 1998.

89. CS Chen, IV Yannas, M Spector. Pore strain behaviour of collagen-glycosaminoglycan analogues of extracellular matrix. Biomaterials 16:777–783, 1995.

90. N Dubey, PC Letourneau, RT Tranquillo. Guided neurite elongation and schwann cell invasion into magnetically aligned collagen in simulated peripheral nerve regeneration. Exp Neurol 158:338–350, 1999.

91. D Ceballos, X Navarro, N Dubey, G Wendelschafer-Crabb, WR Kennedy, RT Tranquillo. Magnetically aligned collagen gel filling a collagen nerve guide improves peripheral nerve regeneration. Exp Neurol 158:290–300, 1999.

92. MJ Yaszemski, RG Payne, WC Hayes, R Langer, AG Mikos. In vitro degradation of a poly(propylene fumarate)-based composite material. Biomaterials 17:2127–2130, 1996.

93. T Katsumura, T Koshino, T Saito. Viscous property and osteogenesis induction of hydroxyapatite thermal decomposition product mixed with gelatin implanted into rabbit femurs. Biomaterials 19:1839–1844, 1998.

94. JE Hulshoff, K van Dijk, JP van der Waerden, JG Wolke, LA Ginsel, JA Jansen. Biological evaluation of the effect of magnetron sputtered Ca/P coatings on osteoblast-like cells in vitro. J Biomed Mater Res 29:967–975, 1995.

95. JE Hulshoff, K van Dijk, JP van der Waerden, W Kalk, JA Jansen. Histological and histomorphometrical evaluation of screw-type calciumphosphate (Ca-P) coated implants; an in vivo experiment in maxillary cancellous bone of goats. J Mater Sci Mater Med 7:603–609, 1996.

96. H Caulier, S Vercaigne, I Naert, JP van der Waerden, JG Wolke, W Kalk, JA Jansen. The effect of Ca-P plasma-sprayed coatings on the initial bone healing of oral implants: an experimental study in the goat. J Biomed Mater Res. 34:121–128, 1997.

97. K Webb, V Hlady, PA Tresco. Relationships among cell attachment, spreading, cytoskeletal organization, and migration rate for anchorage-dependent cells on model surfaces. J Biomed Mater Res 49:362–368, 2000.

98. L Orienti, M Fini, M Rocca, G Giavaresi, M Guzzardella, A Moroni, R Giardino. Measurement of insertion torque of tapered external fixation pins: a comparison between two experimental models. J Biomed Mater Res 48:216–219, 1999.

99. W Heidemann, KL Gerlach, KH Grobel, HG Kollner. Influence of different pilot hole sizes on torque measurements and pullout analysis of osteosynthesis screws. J Craniomaxillofac Surg 26:50–55, 1998.

100. IM Kung, FF Wang, YC Chang, YJ Wang. Surface modifications of alginate/poly(L-lysine) microcapsular membranes with poly(ethylene glycol) and poly(vinyl alcohol). Biomaterials 16:649–655, 1995.

101. FY Hsu, SW Tsai, FF Wang, YJ Wang. The collagen-containing alginate/poly(L-lysine)/alginate microcapsules. Artif Cells Blood Substit Immobil Biotechnol 28:147–154, 2000.

102. JK West, R Latour, Jr., LL Hench. Molecular modeling study of adsorption of poly-L-lysine onto silica glass. J Biomed Mater Res 37:585–591, 1997.

103. Y Tabata, Y Ikada. Vascularization effect of basic fibroblast growth factor released from gelatin hydrogels with different biodegradabilities. Biomaterials 20:2169–2175, 1999.

104. OA Trentz, A Platz, N Helmy, O Trentz. Response of osteoblast cultures to titanium, steel and hydroxyapatite implants. Swiss Surg 4:203–209, 1998.

105. G Braun, D Kohavi, D Amir, M Luna, R Caloss, J Sela, DD Dean, BD Boyan, Z Schwartz. Markers of primary mineralization are correlated with bone-bonding ability of titanium or stainless steel in vivo. Clin Oral Implants Res 6:1–13, 1995.

106. PJ Sell, R Prakash, CW Hastings. Torsional moment to failure for carbon fibre polysulphone expandable rivets as compared with stainless steel screws for carbon fibre-reinforced epoxy fracture plate fixation. Biomaterials 10:182–184, 1989.

107. T Albrektsson, HA Hansson. An ultrastructural characterization of the interface between bone and sputtered titanium or stainless steel surfaces. Biomaterials 7:201–205, 1986.

108. E Rouslahti. Fibronectin and its receptors. Annu Rev Biochem 57:375–413, 1988.

109. MD Pierschbacher, E Rouslahti, J Sundelin, P Lind, PA Peterson. The cell attachment domain of fibronectin. Determination of the primary structure. J Biol Chem 257:9593–9597, 1982.

110. SK Akiyama, KM Yamada. Fibronectin. Adv Enzymol Relat Areas Mol Biol 59:1–57, 1987.

111. EG Hayman, MD Pierschbacher, S Suzuki, E Rouslahti. Vitronectin—a major cell attachment-promoting protein in fetal bovine serum. Exp Cell Res 160:245–258, 1985.

112. JL Myles, BT Burgess, RB Dickenson. Modification of the adhesive properties of collagen by covalent grafting with RGD peptides. J Biomater Sci Polym Ed 11:69–86, 2000.

113. GB Fields, JL Lauer, Y Dori, P Forns, YC Yu, M Tirrell. Protein-like molecular architecture: biomaterial applications for inducing cellular receptor binding and signal transduction. Biopolymers 47:143–151, 2998.

114. YC Yu, V Roontga, VA Daragan, KH Mayo, M Tirrell, GB Fields. Structure and dynamics of peptide-amphiphiles incorporating triple-helical protein-like molecular architecture. Biochemistry 38:1659–1668, 1999.

115. CM Kielty, I Hopkinson, ME Grant. Collagen: the collagen family— structure, assembly and organization in the extracellular matrix. In: Royce PM, Steinmann B, eds. Connective Tissue and Its Heritable Disorders: Molecular, Genetic, and Medical Aspects. New York: John Wiley and Sons, 1992, pp 103–147.

116. AL Boskey. Noncollagenous matrix proteins and their role in mineralization. Bone Miner 6:111–123, 1989.

117. C Stanford, J Keller. The concept of osseointegration and bone matrix expression. Crit Rev Oral Biol Med 2:83–101, 1991.

118. B Savage, ZM Ruggeri. Selective recognition of adhesive sites in surface-bound fibrinogen by glycoprotein IIb–IIIa on nonactivated platelets. J Biol Chem 266:11227–11233, 1991.

119. PC Johnson, RA Shepeck, SR Hribar, ML Bentz, J Janosky, CS Dickson. Inhibition of platelet retention on artificial microvascular grafts with monoclonal antibodies and a high-affinity peptide directed against platelet membrane glycoproteins. Arteriosc Thromb 11:552–560, 1991.

120. SP Massia, SS Rao, JA Hubbell. Covalently immobilized laminin peptide Tyr-Ile-Gly-Ser-Arg (YIGSR) supports cell spreading and co-localization of the 67-kilodalton laminin receptor with alpha-actinin and vinculin. J Biol Chem 268:8053–8059, 1993.

121. A Dekker, AA Poot, JA van Mourik, MP Workel, T Beugeling, A Bantijes, J Feijen, WG van Aken. Improved adhesion and proliferation of human endothelial cells on polyethylene precoated with monoclonal antibodies directed against cell membrane antigens and extracellular matrix proteins. Thromb Haemost 66:715–724, 1991.

122. DW Staatz, KF Fok, MM Zutter, SP Adams, BA Rodriguez, SA Santoro. Identification of a tetrapeptide recognition sequence for the $\alpha2\beta1$ integrin in collagen. J Biol Chem 266:7363, 1991.

123. F Ruggiero, H Chanut, A Fichard. Production of recombinant collagen for biomedical devices. BioPharm 32–37, 2000.

124. E Ruoslahti. RGD and other recognition sequences for integrins. Annu Rev Cell Dev Biol 12:697–715, 1996.

125. AI Caplan. Tissue engineering designs for the future: new logics, old molecules. Tissue Eng 6:1–8, 2000.
126. WS Craig, S Cheng, DG Mullen, J Blevitt, MD Pierschbacher. Concept and progress in the development of RGD-containing peptide pharmaceuticals. Biopolymers 37:157–175, 1995.
127. Y Cadroy, RA Houghten, SR Hanson. RGDV peptide selectively inhibits platelet-derived thrombus formation in vivo. Studies using a baboon model. J Clin Invest 84:939–944, 1987.
128. JP Bearinger, DG Castner, SL Gollege, A Rezania, S Hubchak, KE Healy. P(Amm-co-EG) interpenetrating polymer networks grafted to oxide surfaces: surface characterization, protein adsorption, and cell attachment studies. Langmuir 13:5175–5183, 1997.
129. DM Ferris, GD Moodie, PM Dimond, CWD Gioranni, MG Ehrlich, RF Valentini. RGD-coated titanium implants stimulate increased bone formation in vivo. Biomaterials 2323–2331, 1999.
130. GD Moodie, DM Ferris, BA Hertzog, N Wimmer, H Morgan, CY Chen, F Mathiowitz, RF Valentini. Early osteoblast attachment, spreading, and focal adhesions on RGD coated surfaces. Proc Mater Res Soc Symp 550:207–214, 1998.
131. KC Dee, TT Andersen, R Bizios. Cell function on substrates containing immobilized bioactive peptides. Mater Res Soc Symp Proc 331:115–119, 1993.
132. PD Drumheller, JA Hubbell. Polymer networks with grafted cell adhesion peptides for highly biospecific cell adhesive substrates. Anal Biochem 222:380–388, 1994.
133. CD McFarland, S Mayer, C Scotchford, BA Dalton, JG Steele, S Downes. Attachment of cultured human bone cells to novel polymers. J Biomed Mater Res 44:1–11, 1999.
134. J Aigner, J Tegeler, P Hutzler, D Campoccia, A Pavesio, C Hammer, E Kastenbauer, A Naumann. Cartilage tissue engineering with novel nonwoven structural biomaterial based on hyaluronic acid benzyl ester. J Biomed Mater Res 42:172–181, 1998.
135. A Tona, RF Valentini. Derivatized hyaluronic acid films support mesenchymal stem cell attachment and proliferation. Soc Biomater 849, 1996.
136. CD McFarland, CH Thomas, C DeFilippis, JG Steele, KE Healy. Protein adsorption and cell attachment to patterned surfaces. J Biomed Mater Res 49:200–210, 2000.
137. JJ Grzesiak, MD Pierschbacher, MF Amodeo, TI Malaney, JR Glass. Enhancement of cell interactions with collagen/glycosaminoglycan matrices by RGD derivatization. Biomaterials 18:1625–1632, 1997.
138. T Yoneyama, M Ito, K Sugihara, K Ishihara, N Nakabayashi. Small diameter vascular prosthesis with a nonthrombogenic phospholipid polymer surface: preliminary study of a new concept for functioning in the absence of pseudo- or neointima formation. Artif Organs 24:23–28, 2000.
139. AE Aplin, A Howe, SK Alahari, RL Juliano. Signal transduction and signal modulation by cell adhesion receptors: the role of integrins, cadherins,

immunoglobulin-cell adhesion molecules, and selectins. Pharmacol Rev 50:197–263, 1998.

140. A Howe, AE Aplin, SK Alahari, RL Juliano. Integrin signaling and cell growth control. Curr Opin Cell Biol 10:220–231, 1998.

141. J Folkman, A Moscona. Role of cell shape in growth control. Nature 273:345–349, 1978.

142. M Stoker, C O'Neill, S Berryman, V Waxman. Anchorage and growth regulation in normal and virus-transformed cells. Int J Cancer 3:683–693, 1968.

143. GA van Seventer, Y Shimizu, KJ Horgan, S Shaw. The LFA-1 ligand ICAM-1 provides an important co-stimulatory signal for T cell receptor–mediated activation of resting T cells. J Immunol 144:4579–4586, 1990.

144. LC Burkly, A Jakubowski, BM Newman, MD Rosa, G Chirosso, RR Lobb. Signaling by vascular adhesion molecule-1 (VCAM-1) through VLA-4 promotes CD3-dependent T cell proliferation. Eur J Immunol 21:2871–2875, 1991.

145. JE Meredith, B Fazeli, MA Schwartz. The extracellular matrix as a cell survival factor. Mol Biol Cell 4:953–961, 1993.

146. H Frisch SMF. Disruption of epithelial cell–matrix interactions induces apoptosis. J Cell Biol 12:619–626, 1994.

147. PC Brooks, AMP Montgomery, M Rosenfeld, RA Reisfeld, T Hu, et al. Integrin alphaVbeta3 anagonists promote tumor regression byb inducing apoptosis of angiogenic blood vessels. Cell 79:1157–1164, 1994.

148. CH Streuli, N Bailey, MJ Bissell. Control of mammary epithelial differentiation: basement membrane induces tissue-specific gene expression in the absence of cell–cell interaction and morphological polarity. J Cell Biol 115:1383–1395, 1991.

149. T Volk, LI Fessler, JH Fessler. A role for integrin in the formation of sarcomeric cytoarchitecture. Cell 63:525–536, 1990.

150. DE Ingber, J Folkman. How does extracellular matrix control capillary morphogenesis? Cell 58:803–805, 1989.

151. DE Ingber. Integrins as mechanochemical transducers. Curr Opin Cell Biol 3:841–848, 1991.

152. KC Chang, DF Tees, DA Hammer. The state diagram for cell adhesion under flow: leukocyte rolling and firm adhesion. Proc Natl Acad Sci USA 97:11262–11267, 2000.

153. CE Orsello, DA Lauffenburger, DA Hammer. Molecular properties in cell adhesion: a physical and engineering perspective. Trends Biotechnol 19:310–316, 2001.

154. J-S Chun, BS Jacobson. Spreading of Hela cells on a collagen substratum requires a second messenger formed by the lipoxygenase metabolism of arachidonic acid released by collagen receptor clustering. Mol Biol Cell 3:271–281, 1992.

155. E Vuori KaR. Activation of protein kinase C precedes alpha5beta1 integrin-mediated cell spreading on fibronectin. J Biol Chem 268:21459–21462, 1993.

156. DE McNamee HMI, MA Schwartz. Adhesion to fibronectin stimulates inositol lipid synthesis and enhances PDGF-induced inositol lipid breakdown. J Cell Biol 121:673–678, 1992.
157. RO Hynes. Integrins: Versatility, modulation, and signaling in cell adhesion. Cell 69:11–25, 1992.
158. JJ Grzesiak, MD Pierschbacher, MF Amodeo, TI Malaney, JR Glass. Enhancement of cell interactions with collagen/glycosaminoglycan matrices by RGD derivatization. Biomaterials 18:1625–1632, 1997.
159. WJ Kao, JA Hubbell, JM Anderson. Protein-mediated macrophage adhesion and activation on biomaterials: a model for modulating cell behavior. J Mater Sci Mater Med 10:601–605, 1999.
160. KY Lee, DJ Mooney. Hydrogels for tissue engineering. Chem Rev 101:1869–1879, 2001.
161. KH Bouhadir, KY Lee, E Alsberg, KL Damm, KW Anderson, DJ Mooney. Degradation of partially oxidized alginate and its potential application for tissue engineering. Biotechnol Prog 17:945–950, 2001.
162. JA Rowley, G Madlambayan, DJ Mooney. Alginate hydrogels as synthetic extracellular matrix materials. Biomaterials 20:45–53, 1999.
163. SP Massia, J Stark, DS Letbetter. Surface-immobilized dextran limits cell adhesion and spreading. Biomaterials 21:2253–2261, 2000.
164. SP Massia, J Stark. Immobilized RGD peptides on surface-grafted dextran promote biospecific cell attachment. J Biomed Mater Res 56:390–399, 2001.
165. GM Cruise, OD Hegre, FV Lamberti, SR Hager, R Hill, DS Scharp, JA Hubbell. In vitro and in vivo performance of porcine islets encapsulated in interfacially photopolymerized poly(ethylene glycol) diacrylate membranes. Cell Transplant 8:293–306, 1999.
166. JA Hubbell. Bioactive biomaterials. Curr Opin Biotechnol 10:123–129, 1999.
167. WJ Kao, JA Hubbell. Murine macrophage behavior on peptide-grafted polyethyleneglycol-containing networks. Biotechnol Bioeng 59:2–9, 1998.
168. DK Han, KD Park, JA Hubbell, YH Kim. Surface characteristics and biocompatibility of lactide-based poly(ethylene glycol) scaffolds for tissue engineering. J Biomater Sci Polym Ed 9:667–680, 1998.
169. LC Groenen, EC Nice, AW Burgess. Structure–function relationships for the EGF/TGF-alpha family of mitogens. Growth Factors 11:235–256, 1994.
170. DE James, M Strube, M Mueckler. Molecular cloning and characterization of an insulin-regulatable glucose transporter. Nature 338:83–87, 1989.
171. MF White, CR Kahn. The insulin signaling system. J Biol Chem 269:1–4, 1994.
172. WJ Fantl, DE Johnson, LT Williams. Signalling by receptor tyrosine kinases. Annu Rev Biochem 62:453–481, 1993.
173. G Crumley, F Bellot, JM Kaplow, J Schlessinger, M Jaye, CA Dionne. High-affinity binding and activation of a truncated FGF receptor by both aFGF and bFGF. Oncogene 6:2255–2262, 1991.
174. T Mustonen, K Alitalo. Endothelial receptor tyrosine kinases involved in angiogenesis. J Cell Biol 129:895–898, 1995.

175. E Gherardi, J Gray, M Stoker, M Perryman, R Furlong. Purification of scatter factor, a fibroblast-derived basic protein that modulates epithelial interactions and movement. Proc Natl Acad Sci USA 86:5844–5848, 1989.

176. G Gaudino, A Follenzi, L Naldini, et al. RON is a heterodimeric tyrosine kinase receptor activated by the HGF homologue MSP. EMBO J 13:3524–3532, 1994.

177. CA Smith, T Farrah, RG Goodwin. The TNF receptor superfamily of cellular and viral proteins: activation, costimulation, and death. Cell 76:959–962, 1994.

178. M Tessier-Lavigne. Eph receptor tyrosine kinases, axon repulsion, and the development of topographic maps. Cell 82:345–348, 1995.

179. BC Varnum, C Young, G Elliot, et al. Axl receptor tyrosine kinase stimulated by the vitamin K-dependent protein encoded by growth-arrest-specific gene 6. Nature 373:623–626, 1995.

180. TN Stitt, G Conn, M Gore, et al. The anticoagulation factor protein S and its relative, Gas6, are ligands for the Tyro 3/Axl family of receptor tyrosine kinases. Cell 80:661–670, 1995.

181. PJ Parker, T Pawson. Cancer Surveys. Cold Spring Harbor, NY: Cold Spring Harbor Laboratory Press, 1996, p 386.

182. T Hunter. A thousand and one protein kinases. Cell 50:823, 1987.

183. T Hunter, BM Sefton. Transforming gene product of Rous sarcoma virus phosphorylates tyrosine. Proc Natl Acad Sci USA 77:1311–1315, 1980.

184. M Barbacid. ras Genes. Annu Rev of Biochem 56:779–827, 1987.

185. SR Coughlin, JA Escobedo, LT Williams. Role of phosphatidylinositol kinase in PDGF receptor signal transduction. Science 243:1191–1194, 1989.

186. SA Courtneidge. Activation of the pp60c-src kinase by middle T antigen and dephosphorylation. EMBO 4:1471–1477, 1985.

187. MS Collett, RL Erikson. Protein kinase activity associated with the avian sarcoma virus src gene product. Proc Natl Acad Sci USA 75:2021–2024, 1978.

188. RF Doolittle, MW Hunkapiller, LE Hood, SG Devare, KC Robbins, SA Aaronson, HN Antioniades. Simian sarcoma virus onc gene, v-sis, is derived from the gene (or genes) encoding a platelet-derived growth factor. Science 221:275–276, 1983.

189. D Stehelin, HE Varmus, JM Bishop, PK Vogt. DNA related to the transforming gene(s) of avian sarcoma viruses is present in normal avian DNA. Nature 260:170–173, 1976.

190. JE Darnell, IM Kerr, GR Stark. Jak-STAT pathways and transcriptional activation in response to IFNs and other extracellular signaling proteins. Science 264:1415–1421, 1994.

191. T Miyazaki, A Kawahara, H Fujii, Y Nakagawa, Y Minami, ZJ Liu, I Oishi, O Silvennoinen, BA Witthuhn, JN Ihle et al. Functional activation of Jak1 and Jak3 by selective association with IL-2 receptor subunits. Science 266:1045–1047, 1994.

192. A Kawahara, Y Minami, T Miyazaki, JN Ihle, T Taniguchi. Critical role of the interleukin 2 (IL-2) receptor gamma-chain-associated Jak3 in the IL-2-

induced c-fos and c-myc, but not bcl-2, gene induction. Proc Natl Acad Sci USA 92:8724–8728, 1995.

193. VN Trieu, FM Uckun. Genistein is neuroprotective in murine models of familial amyotrophic lateral sclerosis and stroke. Biochem Biophys Res Commun 258:685–688, 1999.

194. JE Hutchcroft, ML Harrison, RL Geahlen. Association of the 72-kD protein-tyrosine kinase PTK72 with the B cell antigen receptor. J Biol Chem 267:8613–8619, 1992.

195. DB Straus, A Weiss. The CD3 chains of the T cell antigen receptor associate with the ZAP-70 tyrosine kinase and are tyrosine phosphorylated after receptor stimulation. J Exp Med 178:1523–1530, 1993.

196. T Miyazaki, ZJ Liu, A Kawahara, Y Minami, K Yamada, Y Tsujimoto, EL Barsoumian, RM Permutter, T Taniguchi. Three distinct IL-2 signaling pathways mediated by bcl-2, c-myc, and lck cooperate in hematopoietic cell proliferation. Cell 81:223–231, 1995.

197. K Arora, H Dai, SG Kazuko, et al. The Drosophila schnurri gene acts in the Dpp/TGF-beta signaling pathway and encodes a transcription factor homologous to the human MBP family. Cell 81:781–790, 1995.

198. L Attisano, JL Wrana, S Cheifetz, J Massague. Novel activin receptors: distinct genes and alternative mRNA splicing generate a repertoire of serine/threonine kinase receptors. Cell 68:97–108, 1992.

199. L Attisano, J Carcamo, F Ventura, et al. Identification of human activin and TGF-beta type I receptors that form heteromeric kinase complexes with type II receptors. Cell 75:671–680, 1993.

200. SR Winn, JM Schmitt, D Buck, Y Hu, D Grainger, JO Hollinger. Tissue-engineered bone biomimetic to regenerate calvarial critical-sized defects in athymic rats. J Biomed Mater Res 45:414–421, 1999.

201. Y Nishizuka. Intracellular signaling by hydrolysis of phospholipids and activation of protein kinase C. Science 258:607–614, 1992.

202. M Castagna, Y Takai, K Kaibuchi, K Sano, U Kikkawa, Y Nishizuka. Direct activation of calcium-activated, phospholipid-dependent protein kinase by tumor-promoting phorbol esters. J Biol Chem 257:7847–7851, 1982.

203. G Kochs, R Hummel, B Feibich, TF Sarre, D Marme, H Hug. Activation of purified human protein kinase C alpha and beta I isoenzymes in vitro by Ca^{2+}, phosphatidylinositol and phosphatidylinositol 4,5-bisphosphate. Biochem J 291:627–633, 1993.

204. M Ido, K Sekiguchi, U Kikkawa, Y Nishizuka. Phosphorylation of the EGF receptor from A431 epidermoid carcinoma cells by three distinct types of protein kinase C. FEBS Lett 219:215–219, 1987.

205. Y Ito, G Chen, Y Imanishi. Micropatterned immobilization of epidermal growth factor to regulate cell function. Bioconjug Chem 9:277–282, 1998.

206. PR Kuhl, LG Griffith-Cima. Tethered epidermal growth factor as a paradigm for growth factor–induced stimulation from the solid phase. Nat Med 2:1022–1027, 1996.

207. R Marias, J Wynne, R Treismann. The SRF accessory protein Elk-1 contains a growth factor–related transcriptional activation domain. Cell 73:381–393, 1993.

208. I Sanchez, RT Hughes, BJ Mayer, et al. Role of SAPK/ERK kinase-1 in the stress-activated pathway regulating transcription factor c-Jun. Nature 372:794–798, 1994.

209. L van Aelst, M Barr, S Marcus, A Polverino, M Wigler. Complex formation between RAS and RAF and other protein kinases. Proc Natl Acad Sci USA 90:6213–6217, 1993.

210. M Malumbres, A Pellicer. RAS pathways to cell cycle control and cell transformation. Front Biosci 3:d887–912, 1998.

211. MF Olson, A Ashworth, A Hall. An essential role for Rho, Rac, and Cdc42 GTPases in cell cycle progression through G1. Science 269:1270–1272, 1995.

212. Y Zou, Y Hu, B Metzler, Q Xu. Signal transduction in arteriosclerosis: mechanical stress–activated MAP kinases in vascular smooth muscle cells (review). Int J Mol Med 1:827–834, 1998.

213. S Lehoux, A Tedgui. Signal transduction of mechanical stresses in the vascular wall. Hypertension 32:338–345, 1998.

214. SB Lee, SG Rhee. Significance of PIP_2 hydrolysis and regulation of phospholipase C isoenzymes. Curr Opin Cell Biol 7:183–189, 1995.

215. Y Nishizuka. Protein kinase C and lipid signaling for sustained cellular responses. FASEB J 9:484–496, 1995.

216. AL Drayer, PJM van Haastert. Molecular cloning and expression of a phosphoinositide-specific phospholipase C of dictyostelium discoideum. J Biol Chem 267:18387–18392, 1992.

217. M Mohammadi, AM Honegger, D Rotin, R Fischer, F Bellot, W Li, CA Dionne, M Jaye, M Rubinstein, J Schlessinger. A tyrosine-phosphorylated carboxy-terminal peptide of the fibroblast growth factor receptor (Flg) is a binding site for the SH2 domain of phospholipase C-gamma 1. Mol Cell Biol 11:5068–5078, 1991.

218. T Pawson, J Schlessinger. Growth factor receptors. Curr Biol 3:434–442, 1993.

219. R Graber, C Sumida, EA Nunez. Fatty acids and cell signal transduction. J Lipid Mediat Cell Signal 9:91–116, 1994.

220. MR Boarder. A role for phospholipase D in control of mitogenesis. Trends Pharmacol Sci 15:57–62, 1994.

221. WA Khan, GC Blobe, YA Hannun. Arachidonic acid and free fatty acids as second messengers and the role of protein kinase C. Cell Signal 7:171–184, 1995.

222. YA Hannun, RM Bell. Phorbol ester binding and activation of protein kinase C on Triton X-100 mixed micelles containing phosphatidylserine. J Biol Chem 261:9341–9347, 1986.

223. SJ Morgan, AD Smith, PJ Parker. Purification and characterization of bovine brain type I phosphatidylinositol kinase. Eur J Biochem 191:761–767, 1990.

224. M Otsu, ID Hiles, I Gout, et al. Characterization of two 85 kD proteins that associate with receptor tyrosine kinases, middle T/pp60c-src complexes, and PI3-kinase. Cell 65:91–104, 1991.

225. ID Hiles, M Otsu, S Volinia, et al. Phosphatidylinositol 3-kinase: structure and expression of the 110 kd catalytic subunit. Cell 70:419–429, 1992.

226. GB Cohen, R Ren, D Baltimore. Modular binding domains in signal transduction proteins. Cell 80:237–248, 1995.

227. M Reedijk, XQ Liu, T Pawson. Interactions of phosphatidylinositol 3-kinase, GTPase-activating protein (GAP), and GAP-associated proteins with the colony stimulating factor 1 receptor. Mol Cell Biol 10:5601–5608, 1990.

228. R Dhand, I Hiles, G Panayotou, et al. PI 3-kinase is a dual specificity enzyme: autoregulation by an intrinsic protein-serine kinase activity. EMBO J 13:522–533, 1994.

229. M Alimandi, A Romano, MC Curia, et al. Cooperative signalling of ErbB3 and ErbB2 in neoplastic transformation and human mammary carcinomas. Oncogene 10:1813–1821, 1995.

230. H-H Kim, SL Sierke, JG Koland. Epidermal growth factor receptor–dependent association of phosphatidylinositol 3-kinase with the erbB3 gene product. J Biol Chem 269:24747–24755, 1994.

231. A Obermeier, R Bradshaw, K Seedorf, A Choidas, J Schlessinger, A Ullrich. Neuronal differentiation signals are controlled by nerve growth factor receptor/Trk binding sites for SHC and PLC-gamma. EMBO J 13, 1994.

232. S Roche, M Koegl, SA Courteneidge. The phosphatidylinositol 3-kinase is required for DNA synthesis induced by some, but not all, growth factors. Proc Natl Acad Sci USA 91:9185–9189, 1994.

233. SP Soltoff, SL Rabin, SC Cantley, DR Kaplan. Nerve growth factor promotes the activation of phosphatidylinositol 3-kinase and its association with the trk tyrosine kinase. J Biol Chem 267, 1992.

234. FS Vassbotn, OK Havnen, CH Heldin, H Holmsen. Negative feedback regulation of human platelets via autocrine activation of the platelet-derived growth factor alpha-receptor. J Biol Chem 269:13874–13879, 1994.

235. FS Vassbotn, A Ostman, N Langeland, H Holmsen, B Westermark, CH Heldin, M Nister. Activated platelet-derived growth factor autocrine pathway drives the transformed phenotype of a human glioblastoma cell line. J Cell Physiol 158:381–389, 1994.

236. M Whitman, DR Kaplan, B Schaffhausen, L Cantley, TM Roberts. Association of phosphatidylinositol kinase activity with polyoma middle-T component for transformation. Nature 315:239–242, 1985.

237. M Whitman, CP Downes, M Keeler, T Keller, L Cantley. Type I phosphatidylinositol kinase makes a novel inositol phospholipid, phosphatidylinositol-3-phosphate. Nature 332:644–646, 1988.

238. WJ Fantl, JA Escobedo, GA Martin, CW Turck, M del Rosario, F McCormick, LT Williams. Distinct phosphotyrosines on a growth factor receptor bind to specific molecules that mediate different signaling pathways. Cell 69:413–423, 1992.

239. M Wymann, A Arcaro. Platelet-derived growth factor–induced phosphatidylinositol 3-kinase activation mediates actin rearrangements in fibroblasts. Biochem J 298 Pt 3:517–520, 1994.

240. L Stephens, FT Cooke, R Walters, T Jackson, S Volinia, I Gout, MD Waterfield, PT Hawkins. Characterization of a phosphatidylinositol-specific phosphoinositide 3-kinase from mammalian cells. Curr Biol 4:203–214, 1994.

241. S Wennstrom, P Hawkins, F Cooke, K Hara, K Yonezawa, M Kasuga, T Jackson, L Claesson-Welsh, L Stephens. Activation of phosphoinositide 3-kinase is required for PDGF-stimulated membrane ruffling. Curr Biol 4:385–393, 1994.

242. K Hara, K Yonezawa, H Sakaue, A Ando, K Kotani, T Kitamura, Y Kitamura, H Ueda, L Stephens, TR Jackson, et al. 1-Phosphatidylinositol 3-kinase activity is required for insulin-stimulated glucose transport but not for RAS activation in CHO cells. Proc Natl Acad Sci USA 91:7415–7419, 1994.

243. S Roche, M Koegl, SA Courtneidge. The phosphatidylinositol 3-kinase alpha is required for DNA synthesis induced by some, but not all, growth factors. Proc Natl Acad Sci USA 91:9185–9189, 1994.

244. R Yao, GM Cooper. Requirement for phosphatidylinositol-3 kinase in the prevention of apoptosis by nerve growth factor. Science 267:2003–2006, 1995.

245. Q Hu, A Klippel, AJ Muslin, WJ Fantl, LT Williams. Ras-dependent induction of cellular responses by constitutively active phosphatidylinositol-3 kinase. Science 268:100–102, 1995.

246. SP Soltoff, SL Rabin, LC Cantley, DR Kaplan. Nerve growth factor promotes the activation of phosphatidylinositol 3-kinase and its association with the trk tyrosine kinase. J Biol Chem 267:17472–17477, 1992.

247. V Kundra, JA Escobedo, A Kazlauskas, HK Kim, SG Rhee, LT Williams, BR Zetter. Regulation of chemotaxis by the platelet-derived growth factor receptor-beta. Nature 367:474–476, 1994.

248. S Wennstrom, A Siegbahn, K Yokote, AK Arvidsson, CH Heldin, S Mori, L Claesson-Welsh. Membrane ruffling and chemotaxis transduced by the PDGF beta-receptor require the binding site for phosphatidylinositol 3′ kinase. Oncogene 9:651–660, 1994.

249. RAF Dixon, BK Kobilka, DJ Strader, et al. Cloning of the gene and cDNA for mammalian beta-adrenergic receptor and its homology with rhodopsin. Nature 321:75–79, 1986.

250. Y Yarden, H Rodriguez, SKF Wong, et al. The avian beta-adrenergic receptor: primary structure and membrane topology. Proc Natl Acad Sci USA 83:6795–6799, 1986.

251. M Rodbell. Nobel Lecture. Signal transduction: evolution of an idea. Biosci Rep 15:117–133, 1995.

252. M Rodbell. G proteins: out of the cytoskeletal closet. Mt Sinai J Med 63:381–386, 1996.

253. M Rodbell. The complex regulation of receptor-coupled G-proteins. Adv Enzyme Regul 37:427–435, 1997.

254. JK Northup, PC Sternweis, MD Smigel, LS Schleifer, EM Ross, AG Gilman. Purification of the regulatory component of adenylate cyclase. Proc Natl Acad Sci USA 77:6516–6520, 1980.

255. AB Schreiber, PO Couraud, C Andre, B Vray, AD Strosberg. Anti-alprenolol anti-idiotypic antibodies bind to beta-adrenoreceptors and modulate catecholamine sensitive adenylate cyclase. Proc Natl Acad Sci USA 77:7385–7389, 1980.

256. TM Savarese, CM Fraser. In vitro mutagenesis and the search for structure–function relationships among G protein–coupled receptors. Biochem J 283:1–19, 1992.

257. L Birnbaumer. Receptor-to-effector signaling through G proteins: roles for beta gamma dimers as well as alpha subunits. Cell 71:1069–1072, 1992.

258. R Henderson, JM Baldwin, TAK Cesca, F Zemlin, E Beckmann, KH Downing. Model for the structure of bacteriorhodopsin based on high-resolution electron cryomicroscopy. J Mol Biol 213:899–929, 1990.

259. S Offermanns, MI Simon. Organization of transmembrane signalling by heterotrimeric G proteins. In: Parker PJ, Pawson T, eds. Cell Signalling. Cold Spring Harbor, NY: Cold Spring Harbor Laboratory Press, 1996, vol. 27, pp 177–198.

260. D Voet, JG Voet. Biochemistry: Biochemistry. New York: John Wiley and Sons, 1995, pp 1276–1278.

261. IG Macara, KM Lounsbury, SA Richards, C McKiernan, D Bar-Sagi. The Ras superfamily of GTPases. FASEB J 10:625–630, 1996.

262. S Srivastava, M Verma, DE Henson. Biomarkers for early detection of colon cancer. Clin Cancer Res 7:1118–1126, 2001.

263. M Esteller, S Gonzalez, RA Risques, E Marcuello, R Mangues, JR Germa, JG Herman, G Capella, MA Peinado. K-ras and p16 aberrations confer poor prognosis in human colorectal cancer. J Clin Oncol 19:299–304, 2001.

264. AM de Vries-Smits, BM Burgering, SJ Leevers, CJ Marshall, JL Bos. Involvement of p21ras in activation of extracellular signal–regulated kinase 2. Nature 357:602–604, 1992.

265. A Minden, A Lin, M McMahon, C Lange-Carter, B Derijard, RJ Davis, GL Johnson, M Karin. Differential activation of ERK and JNK mitogen-activated protein kinases by Raf-1 and MEKK. Science 266:1719–1723, 1994.

266. YS Li, JY Shyy, S Li, J Lee, B Su, M Karin, S Chien. The Ras-JNK pathway is involved in shear-induced gene expression. Mol Cell Biol 16:5947–5954, 1996.

267. MS Boguski, F McCormick. Proteins regulating Ras and its relatives. Nature 366:643–654, 1993.

268. H Adari, DR Lowy, BM Willumsen, CJ Der, F McCormick. Guanine nucleosine triphosphatase activating protein (GAP) interacts with p21 ras effector binding domain. Science 240:518–521, 1988.

269. C Cales, JF Hancock, CJ Marshall, A Hall. The cytoplasmic protein GAP is implicated as the target for regulation by the ras gene product. Nature 332:548–551, 1988.

270. V Riccardi, J Eichner. Neurofibromatosis: Phenotype, Natural History and Pathogenesis. Baltimore: Johns Hopkins University Press, 1986.

271. J Downward. Control of Ras activation. In: Parker PJ, Pawson T, eds. Cell Signalling. Cold Spring Harbor, NY: Cold Spring Harbor Laboratory Press, 1996, vol. 27, pp 87–100.

272. AG Gilman. G proteins: transducers of receptor-generated signals. Annu Rev Biochem 56:615–649, 1987.

273. A Eva, SA Aaronson. Isolation of a new human oncogene from a diffuse B-cell lymphoma. Nature, 316:273–275, 1985.

274. D Ron, M Zannini, M Lewis, RB Wickner, LT Hunt, G Graziani, SR Tronick, SA Aaronson, A Eva. A region of proto-dbl essential for its transforming activity shows sequence similarity to a yeast cell cycle gene, CDC24, and the human breakpoint cluster gene, bcr. New Biol 3:372–379, 1991.

275. T Miki, CL Smith, JE Long, A Eva, TP Fleming. Oncogene ect2 is related to regulators of small GTP-binding proteins. Nature 362:462–465, 1993.

276. MJ Hart, A Eva, D Zangrilli, SA Aaronson, T Evans, RA Cerione, Y Zheng. Cellular transformation and guanine nucleotide exchange activity are catalyzed by a common domain on the dbl oncogene product. J Biol Chem 269:62–65, 1994.

277. R Khosravi-Far, M Chrzanowska-Wodnicka, PA Solski, A Eva, K Burridge, CJ Der. Dbl and Vav mediate transformation via mitogen-activated protein kinase pathways that are distinct from those activated by oncogenic Ras. Mol Cell Biol 14:6848–6857, 1994.

278. BS Kim, J Nikolovski, J Bonadio, DJ Mooney. Cyclic mechanical strain regulates the development of engineered smooth muscle tissue. Nat Biotechnol 17:979–983, 1999.

279. J Darnell, H Lodish, D Baltimore. Molecular Cell Biology. New York: WH Freeman, 1990.

280. E Gordon, A Lasserre, P Stull, PK Bajpai, B England. A zinc based self setting ceramic bone substitute for local delivery of testosterone. Biomed Sci Instrum 33:131–136, 1997.

281. M Varnado, M Tucci, Z Cason, A Mohamed, H Benghuzzi. Germinal cell alterations associated with sustained delivery of testosterone enanthate in adult male rats. Biomed Sci Instrum 33:161–165, 1997.

282. H Benghuzzi, B England. Biocompatibility of steroid-HA delivery system using adult castrated rams as a model. Biomed Sci Instrum 37:275–280, 2001.

283. N Wisniewski, F Moussy, WM Reichert. Characterization of implantable biosensor membrane biofouling. Fresenius J Anal Chem 366:611–621, 2000.

284. F Pavanetto, I Genta, P Giunchedi, B Conti, U Conte. Spray-dried albumin microspheres for the intra-articular delivery of dexamethasone. J Microencapsul 11:445–454, 1994.

285. EH Fischer, NK Tonks, H Charbonneau, MF Cicirelli, DE Cool, CD Diltz, EG Krebs, KA Walsh. Protein tyrosine phosphatases: a novel family of

enzymes involved in transmembrane signalling. Adv Second Messenger Phosphoprotein Res 24:273–279, 1990.

286. EH Fischer, H Charbonneau, NK Tonks. Protein tyrosine phosphatases: a diverse family of intracellular and transmembrane enzymes. Science 253:401–406, 1991.

287. ML Thomas. The leukocyte common antigen family. Annu Rev Immunol 7:339–369, 1989.

288. IS Trowbridge. CD45. A prototype for transmembrane protein tyrosine phosphatases. J Biol Chem 266:23517–23520, 1991.

289. NK Tonks, H Charbonneau, CD Diltz, EH Fischer, KA Walsh. Demonstration that the leukocyte common antigen CD45 is a protein tyrosine phosphatase. Biochemistry 27:8695–8701, 1988.

290. H Charbonneau, NK Tonks, S Kumar, CD Diltz, M Harrylock, DE Cool, EG Krebs, EH Fischer, KA Walsh. Human placenta protein-tyrosine-phosphatase: amino acid sequence and relationship to a family of receptor-like proteins. Proc Natl Acad Sci USA 86:5252–5256, 1989.

291. HL Ostergaard, IS Trowbridge. Coclustering CD45 with CD4 or CD8 alters the phosphorylation and kinase activity of p56lck. J Exp Med 172:347–350, 1990.

292. T Mustelin, A Altman. Dephosphorylation and activation of the T cell tyrosine kinase pp56lck by the leukocyte common antigen (CD45). Oncogene 5:809–813, 1990.

293. M Guttinger, M Gassmann, KE Amrein, P Burn. CD45 phosphotyrosine phosphatase and p56lck protein tyrosine kinase: a functional complex crucial in T cell signal transduction. Int Immunol 4:1325–1330, 1992.

294. JA Ledbetter, JP Deans, A Aruffo, LS Grosmaire, SB Kanner, JB Bolen, GL Schieven. CD4, CD8 and the role of CD45 in T-cell activation. Curr Opin Immunol 5:334–340, 1993.

295. BA Cunningham, JJ Hemperly, BA Murray, EA Prediger, R Brackenbury, GM Edelman. Neural cell adhesion molecule: structure, immunoglobulin-like domains, cell surface modulation, and alternative RNA splicing. Science 236:799–806, 1987.

296. L Patthy. Homology of a domain of the growth hormone/prolactin receptor family with type III modules of fibronectin. Cell 61:13–14, 1990.

297. K Umezawa, AR Kornblihtt, FE Baralle. Isolation and characterization of cDNA clones for human liver fibronectin. FEBS Lett 186:31–34, 1985.

298. SM Brady-Kalnay, NK Tonks. Protein tyrosine phosphatases as adhesion receptors. Curr Opin Cell Biol 7:650–657, 1995.

299. KH Lau, JR Farley, DJ Baylink. Phosphotyrosyl protein phosphatases. Biochem J 257:23–36, 1989.

300. NK Tonks, CD Diltz, EH Fischer. Characterization of the major protein-tyrosine-phosphatases of human placenta. J Biol Chem 263:6731–6737, 1988.

301. NK Tonks, CD Diltz, EH Fischer. Purification of the major protein-tyrosine-phosphatases of human placenta. J Biol Chem 263:6722–6730, 1988.

302. SW Jones, RL Erikson, VM Ingebritsen, TS Ingebritsen. Phosphotyrosyl-protein phosphatases. I. Separation of multiple forms from bovine brain and purification of the major form to near homogeneity. J Biol Chem 264:7747–7753, 1989.

303. S Brown-Shimer, KA Johnson, JB Lawrence, C Johnson, A Bruskin, NR Green, DE Hill. Molecular cloning and chromosome mapping of the human gene encoding protein phosphotyrosyl phosphatase 1B. Proc Natl Acad Sci USA. 87:5148–5152, 1990.

304. D Huchon, R Ozon, JG Demaille. Protein phosphatase-1 is involved in Xenopus oocyte maturation. Nature 294:358–359, 1981.

305. C Le Goascogne, N Sananes, M Gouezou, EE Baulieu. Alkaline phospha-tase activity in the membrane of Xenopus laevis oocytes: effects of steroids, insulin, and inhibitors during meiosis reinitiation. Dev Biol 119:511–519, 1987.

306. P Cormier, O Mulner-Lorillon, R Belle. In vivo progesterone regulation of protein phosphatase activity in Xenopus oocytes. Dev Biol 139:427–431, 1990.

307. BJ Goldstein. Tyrosine Phosphoprotein Phosphatases. Oxford: Oxford University Press, 1998, p 260.

308. P Cohen. Protein phosphorylation and hormone action. Proc R Soc Lond B Biol Sci 234:115–144, 1988.

309. P Cohen. The role of protein phosphorylation in neural and hormonal control of cellular activity. Nature 296:613–620, 1982.

310. PT Cohen, ND Brewis, V Hughes, DJ Mann. Protein serine/threonine phosphatases; an expanding family. FEBS Lett 268:355–359, 1990.

311. P Cohen, S Alemany, BA Hemmings, TJ Resink, P Stralfors, HY Tung. Protein phosphatase-1 and protein phosphatase-2A from rabbit skeletal muscle. Meth Enzymol 159:390–408, 1988.

312. P Cohen, PT Cohen. Protein phosphatases come of age. J Biol Chem 264:21435–21438, 1989.

313. AT Sim, JD Scott. Targeting of PKA, PKC and protein phosphatases to cellular microdomains. Cell Calcium 26:209–217, 1999.

314. R Ricciarelli, A Azzi. Regulation of recombinant PKC alpha activity by protein phosphatase 1 and protein phosphatase 2A. Arch Biochem Biophys 355:197–200, 1998.

315. A Garcia, X Cayla, E Sontag. Protein phosphatase 2A: a definite player in viral and parasitic regulation. Microbes Infect 2:401–407, 2000.

316. A Garcia, S Cereghini, E Sontag. Protein phosphatase 2A and phosphatidy-linositol 3-kinase regulate the activity of Sp1-responsive promoters. J Biol Chem 275:9385–9389, 2000.

317. MB Calalb, TR Polte, SK Hanks. Tyrosine phosphorylation of focal adhesion kinase at sites in the catalytic domain regulates kinase activity: a role for Src family kinases. Mol Cell Biol 15:954–963, 1995.

318. JT Parsons, SJ Parsons. Src family protein tyrosine kinases: cooperating with growth factor and adhesion signaling pathways. Curr Opin Cell Biol 9:187–192, 1997.

319. CR Hauck, CK Klingbeil, DD Schlaefer. Focal adhesion kinase functions as a receptor-proximal signaling component required for directed cell migration. Immunol Res 21:293–303, 2000.

320. J Schlessinger. New roles for Src kinases in control of cell survival and angiogenesis. Cell 100:293–296, 2000.

321. A Richardson, RK Malik, JD Hildebrand, JT Parsons. Inhibition of cell spreading by expression of the C-terminal domain of focal adhesion kinase (FAK) is rescued by coexpression of Src or catalytically inactive FAK: a role for paxillin tyrosine phosphorylation. Mol Cell Biol 17:6906–6914, 1997.

322. BS Verbeek, TM Vroom, G Rijksen. Overexpression of c-Src enhances cell–matrix adhesion and cell migration in PDGF-stimulated NIH3T3 fibroblasts. Exp Cell Res 248:531–537, 1999.

323. RL Klemke, S Cai, AL Giannini, PJ Gallagher, P de Lanerolle, DA Cheresh. Regulation of cell motility by mitogen-activated protein kinase. J Cell Biol 137:481–492, 1997.

324. KA Giuliano, J Kolega, RL DeBiasio, DL Taylor. Myosin II phosphorylation and the dynamics of stress fibers in serum-deprived and stimulated fibroblasts. Mol Biol Cell 3:1037–1048, 1992.

325. N Negoro, M Hoshiga, M Seto, E Kohbayashi, M Ii, R Fukui, N Shibata, T Nakakoji, F Nishiguchi, Y Sasaki, T Ishihara, N Ohsawa. The kinase inhibitor fasudil (HA-1077) reduces intimal hyperplasia through inhibiting migration and enhancing cell loss of vascular smooth muscle cells. Biochem Biophys Res Commun 262:211–215, 1999.

326. M Amano, M Ito, K Kimura, Y Fukata, K Chihara, T Nakano, Y Matsuura, K Kaibuchi. Phosphorylation and activation of myosin by Rho-associated kinase (Rho-kinase). J Biol Chem 271:20246–20249, 1996.

327. K Kimura, M Ito, M Amano, K Chihara, Y Fukata, M Nakafuku, B Yamamori, J Feng, T Nakano, K Okawa, A Iwamatsu, K Kaibuchi. Regulation of myosin phosphatase by Rho and Rho-associated kinase (Rho-kinase). Science 273:245–248, 1996.

328. T Matsui, M Amano, T Yamamoto, K Chihara, M Nakafuku, M Ito, T Nakano, K Okawa, A Iwamatsu, K Kaibuchi. Rho-associated kinase, a novel serine/threonine kinase, as a putative target for small GTP binding protein Rho. Embo J 15:2208–2216, 1996.

329. MJ Robinson, MH Cobb. Mitogen-activated protein kinase pathways. Curr Opin Cell Biol 9:180–186, 1997.

330. LC Sanders, F Matsumura, GM Bokoch, P Lanerolle. Inhibition of myosin light chain kinase by p21-activated kinase. Science 283:2083–2085, 1999.

331. Y Imai, DR Clemmons. Roles of phosphatidylinositol 3-kinase and mitogen-activated protein kinase pathways in stimulation of vascular smooth muscle cell migration and deoxyriboncleic acid synthesis by insulin-like growth factor-I. Endocrinology 140:4228–4235, 1999.

332. A Hall. Rho GTPases and the actin cytoskeleton. Science 279:509–514, 1998.

333. L Kjoller, A Hall. Signaling to Rho GTPases. Exp Cell Res 253:166–179, 1999.

334. A Hall. Signal transduction pathways regulated by the Rho family of small GTPases. Br J Cancer 80 Suppl 1:25–27, 1999.

335. M Maekawa, T Ishizaki, S Boku, N Watanabe, A Fujita, A Iwamatsu, T Obinata, K Ohashi, K Mizuno, S Narumiya. Signaling from Rho to the actin cytoskeleton through protein kinases ROCK and LIM-kinase. Science 285:895–898, 1999.

336. JT Parsons. Integrin-mediated signalling: regulation by protein tyrosine kinases and small GTP-binding proteins. Curr Opin Cell Biol 8:146–152, 1996.

337. N Wang, JP Butler, DE Ingber. Mechanotransduction across the cell surface and through the cytoskeleton. Science 260:1124–1127, 1993.

338. LV McIntire, JE Wagner, M Papadaki, PA Whitson, SG Eskin. Effect of flow on gene regulation in smooth muscle cells and macromolecular transport across endothelial cell monolayers. Biol Bull 194:394–399, 1998.

339. RM Nerem, RW Alexander, DC Chappell, RM Medford, SE Varner, WR Taylor. The study of the influence of flow on vascular endothelial biology. Am J Med Sci 316:169–175, 1998.

340. PF Davies. Flow-mediated endothelial mechanotransduction. Physiol Rev 75:519–560, 1995.

341. PR Girard, RM Nerem. Shear stress modulates endothelial cell morphology and F-actin organization through the regulation of focal adhesion–associated proteins. J Cell Physiol 163:179–193, 1995.

342. JA Frangos, SG Eskin, LV McIntire, CL Ives. Flow effect on prostacyclin production by cultured human endothelial cells. Science 227:1477–1479, 1985.

343. SQ Liu. Focal expression of angiotensin II type 1 receptor and smooth muscle cell proliferation in the neointima of experimental vein grafts: relation to eddy blood flow. Arterioscler Thromb Vasc Biol 19:2630–2639, 1999.

344. JA Frangos, V Gahtan, B Sumpio. Localization of atherosclerosis: role of hemodynamics. Arch Surg 134:1142–1149, 1999.

345. SQ Liu. Influence of tensile strain on smooth muscle cell orientation in rat blood vessels. J Biomech Eng 120:313–320, 1998.

346. S Dimmeler, AM Zeiher. Nitric oxide—an endothelial cell survival factor. Cell Death Differ 6:964–968, 1999.

347. SQ Liu. Regulation of neointimal morphogenesis by blood shear stress. Adv Bioeng 48:61–62, 2000.

348. SQ Liu, J Goldman. Regulation of vascular smooth muscle cell migration by blood shear stress. IEEE Trans Biomed Eng 48:474–483, 2001.

349. ME Goldschmidt, KJ McLeod, WR Taylor. Integrin-mediated mechano-transduction in vascular smooth muscle cells: frequency and force response characteristics. Circ Res 88:674–680, 2001.

350. AB Howard, RW Alexander, RM Nerem, KK Griendling, WR Taylor. Cyclic strain induces an oxidative stress in endothelial cells. Am J Physiol 272:C421–427, 1997.

351. UK Laemmli. Cleavage of structural proteins during the assembly of the head of bacteriophage T4. Nature 227:680–685, 1970.

352. F Bonino, J Milanini, J Pouyssegur, G Pages. RT-PCR method to quantify vascular endothelial growth factor expression. BioTechniques 30:1254–1260, 2001.

353. EM Southern. Detection of specific sequences among DNA fragments separated by gel electrophoresis. J Mol Biol 98:503–517, 1975.

354. JM Foster, IH Kamal, J Daub, MC Swan, JR Ingram, M Ganatra, J Ware, D Guiliano, A Abookaker, L Moran, M Blaxter, BE Slatko. Hybridization to high-density filter arrays of a Brugia malayi BAC library with biotinylated oligonucleotides and PCR products. Biotechniques 30:1216–1224, 2001.

355. D Guiliano, M Ganatra, J Ware, J Parrot, J Daub, L Moran, H Brennecke, JM Foster, T Supali, M Blaxter, AL Scott, SA Williams, BE Slatko. Chemiluminescent detection of sequential DNA hybridizations to high-density, filter-assayed cDNA libraries: a subtraction method for novel gene discovery. Biotechniques 27:146–152, 1999.

356. WH Benjamin Jr, LS McDaniel, JS Sheffield. Detection of DNA in Southern blots by chemiluminescence. Biotechniques 12:836–839, 1992.

357. DE Ingber. The architecture of life. Sci Am 278:48–57, 1998.

358. P Chomczynski, N Sacchi. Single-step method of RNA isolation by acid guanidinium thiocyanate- phenol-chloroform extraction. Anal Biochem 162:156–159, 1987.

359. DA Melton, PA Krieg, MR Rebagliati, T Maniatis, K Zinn, MR Green. Efficient in vitro synthesis of biologically active RNA and RNA hybridization probes from plasmids containing a bacteriophage SP6 promoter. Nuc Acids Res 12:7035–7056, 1984.

360. J Sambrook, EF Fritsch, T Maniatis. Synthesis of RNA Probes by In Vitro Transcription of Double-Stranded DNA Templates by Bacteriophage DNA-Dependent RNA Polymerases. Cold Spring Harbor, NY: Cold Spring Harbor Laboratory Press, 1989, pp 10.27–10.37.

361. M Gilman. Ribonuclease Protection Assay. New York: John Wiley and Sons, 1993, pp 4.7.1–4.7.8.

362. J Stone, T de Lange, G Ramsay, E Jakobovits, JM Bishop, H Varmus, W Lee. Definition of regions in human c-myc that are involved in transformation and nuclear localization. Mol Cell Biol 7:1697–1709, 1987.

363. R Lehman. The Enzymes XV, Part A. New York: Academic Press, 1982.

364. M Bordonaro, JS Chen, JL Nordstrom, CF Saccomanno. A faster ribonuclease protection assay. Biotechniques 13:846–850, 1992.

365. Y Hod. A simplified ribonuclease protection assay. Biotechniques 13:852–854, 1992.

366. J Meador III, D Kennell. Cloning and sequencing the gene encoding Escherichia coli ribonuclease I: exact physical mapping using the genome library. Gene 95:1–7, 1990.

367. J Meador, 3rd, B Cannon, VJ Cannistraro, D Kennell. Purification and characterization of Escherichia coli RNase I. Comparisons with RNase M. Eur J Biochem 187:549–553, 1990.

368. G Brewer, E Murray, M Staeben. Promega Notes 38:1, 1992.

369. Pharmingen. Multi-Probe RNAse Protection Assay (RPA) System. San Diego, 1999.

370. Y Manome, PY Wen, A Hershowitz, T Tanaka, BJ Rollins, DW Kufe, HA Fine. Monocyte chemoattractant protein-1 (MCP-1) gene transduction: an effective tumor vaccine strategy for non-intracranial tumors. Cancer Immunol Immunother 41:227–235, 1995.

371. V Shen, D Schlessinger. In: Boyer PD, ed. The Enzymes. Vol. XV. San Diego: Academic Press, 1982.

372. NB Holland, RE Marchant. Individual plasma proteins detected on rough biomaterials by phase imaging AFM. J Biomed Mater Res 51:307–315, 2000.

373. CJ Doillon, K Cameron. New approaches for biocompatibility testing using cell culture. Int J Artif Organs 13:517–520, 1990.

374. KJ Zehr, PC Lee, RS Poston, AM Gillinov, RH Hruban, DE Cameron. Protection of the internal mammary artery pedicle with polytetrafluoroethylene membrane. J Card Surg 8:650–655, 1993.

375. SP Massia, JA Hubbell. Human endothelial cell interactions with surface-coupled adhesion peptides on a nonadhesive glass substrate and two polymeric biomaterials. J Biomed Mater Res 25:223–242, 1991.

376. DW Grainger, G Pavon-Djavid, V Migonney, M Josefowicz. Assessment of fibronectin conformation adsorbed to polytetrafluoroethylene surfaces from serum protein mixtures and correlation to support of cell attachment in culture. J Biomat Sci Polym Ed, accepted, 2002.

8

Biomaterials
Synthetic and Engineering Strategies

Scott M. Cannizzaro and Robert Langer
Massachusetts Institute of Technology, Cambridge, Massachusetts

I. INTRODUCTION AND DEFINITIONS

A. Biomaterials and Biopolymers

This chapter focuses on biomaterials and synthetic strategies used to improve their performance in vivo. The last 20 years witnessed a synergy among chemists, biologists, medical doctors, and engineers in developing biomedical materials. Today we commonly deploy materials in the body that provide significant therapeutic improvements to pharmaceuticals and to healing of diseased or damaged tissue. As a result, patient outcomes have been vastly improved in such diverse areas as cancer and burns.

In our laboratory the collaborative effort of multidisciplinary teams has become essential for continuing innovation in drug delivery and tissue engineering applications (1). The emphasis for this chapter will be on the chemical compositions, structure, and characterization of materials from research in our laboratory. We will also highlight some promising work that is leading to precise synthetic refinements of polymer materials for next-generation materials.

Some definitions may help to define the scope of work being pursued in this area. Biomaterials, the focus of this chapter, include synthetic materials that are born of man-made monomers. Polyurethane and polyethylene glycol are common synthetic materials of great medical importance. Biomaterials can also be composed of naturally occurring polymers, such as silk and cellulose.

Biomaterials can contain naturally occurring monomers. In the case of polylysine, which is frequently used in condensing genetic material for drug delivery (2,3), its monomer constituent is a naturally occurring amino acid. However, the homopolymer is synthetic, not corresponding to any natural protein sequence. This is further impacted by the noted immunogenicity of polylysine (4).

Collagen is also a frequently used, naturally occurring *biopolymer*. The synthetic manipulation of biopolymers is pursued to either better understand the properties or to improve on the functionality of these already biocompatible materials (5). The research by Jelinski et al. on incorporation of deuterium-labeled alanine into the diets of golden orb-weaver spiders to produce deuterium-labeled silk protein for nuclear magnetic resonance (NMR) analysis is a sophisticated example of how scientists are defining the form and function of biopolymers (6). Again, this manipulation of a natural protein sequence was undertaken to elucidate how a synthetic approach might lead to biomaterials with comparable or improved performance.

It is important to note that biomaterials research has grown from two major drivers. First, the ability to produce and manufacture synthetic materials can offer a significant advantage over harvesting of natural products. This is analogous to the efforts to work out synthetic protocols for natural products in medicinal chemistry. Second, the ability to tailor properties from the ground up can lead to more precise control of performance. In this chapter we generally focus on synthetic as opposed to naturally occurring biomaterials.

B. Smart and Biomimetic Polymers

The terms *smart* and *biomimetic* polymer are also increasingly used to describe materials. As a distinction, a "smart" material refers to the property of shape memory materials that conform, expand, or constrict in response to environmental stimuli like pH, light, or pressure (7,8). "Biomimetic" refers to the inherent ability of a material to reproduce or elicit a biological function.

C. Site-Specific and Targeted Delivery

Placement of a biomaterial construct, such as a wafer or microspheres, at a physiological site of concern, such as diseased tissue, is referred to as *site-specific delivery*. In many applications a localized approach to treatment is more efficient than a systemic approach.

However, the pinnacle of therapeutic treatment is to simply have a patient swallow a pill and design a therapeutic drug that targets a desired location or disease path. The effort to create targeted delivery has as one of its major goals the identification of specific ligand–receptor pairs that direct therapeutic uptake or dictate cell behavior.

D. Polymer Functionality

Functionality in biomaterials also needs clarification as the idea of functionality has two levels of meaning. To the polymer chemist, functionality is viewed from the perspective of chemical functionality, namely, hydroxyl, ether, amide, ester, carboxylic acid, anhydride, and so on. To the engineer it means: What can this material do? Does the performance of the polymer impart cell adhesion or site-specific drug delivery? In this chapter we will look at both, as they are inextricably related. The ability of chemists to add chemical functionality to biomaterials is leading the way for biomedical engineers to explore specific applications of these materials in vivo.

The terms *tissue engineering* and *drug delivery* are often written in the same sentence because of their intimate ties to biomaterials. The use of biomaterials in these applications is a common denominator. With a great degree of correlation, the rudimentary materials that have proven useful in drug delivery have also proven useful in tissue engineering. However, as our ability to impart functionality to biomaterials grows, we are seeing a departure from scientists using off-the-shelf or readily available materials to bioengineers who put a great deal of effort into tailoring material properties for very specific applications in medical products.

We will elucidate some of the history behind the evolution of biomaterials in use today and highlight some of the interesting work that will lead to development of the advanced biomimetic materials of tomorrow. In addition, a number of comprehensive reviews give an excellent background to some of the recent synthetic materials derived for medical applications of controlled release and tissue engineering (9–11).

II. SYNTHETIC DESIGN OF BIOCOMPATIBLE POLYMERS

A. Biodegradable Polymers: First Principal—Do No Harm

Medical doctors and biomaterials alike start from the same proposition: "Do no harm." This philosophy has given rise to the vast use of biodegradable and resorbable biomaterials. This is the simplest form of biomimicry. In particular, polymer systems that degrade or are absorbed into the physiological environment in which they are placed and that produce little or no response to their deployment are of great potential advantage in clinical use.

The common theme in degradable polymer systems is the presence of cleavable bonds along the polymer backbone. The most widely studied degradable materials are the polyesters. Polylactic acid (PLA), polygylcolic acid (PGA), and their copolymers (PLGA) have been intensively studied. They have even been used to carry out research in space (12). Their extensive use in drug delivery and tissue engineering applications is based on their biocompatibility and safety record in humans. PLA is typical of the commonly used polyester systems in its synthesis and degradation schemes. Degradation of these systems is characterized by bulk erosion from random hydrolytic cleavage of the ester bonds along the polymer backbone (Fig. 1).

The biocompatibility of the degradation product(s) often defines the biocompatibility for the polymer. The hydrolysis of PLA leads to degradation of the polymer back to the lactic acid repeat unit. As a natural metabolite of the body, lactic acid is a nontoxic degradation product. However, this is not always the case. In polylysine while the repeat unit is an amino acid, the polymer has a well-documented immunogenicity (4). Cationic polymers like polylysine are of great interest for their ability to condense and deliver DNA in drug delivery systems (13).

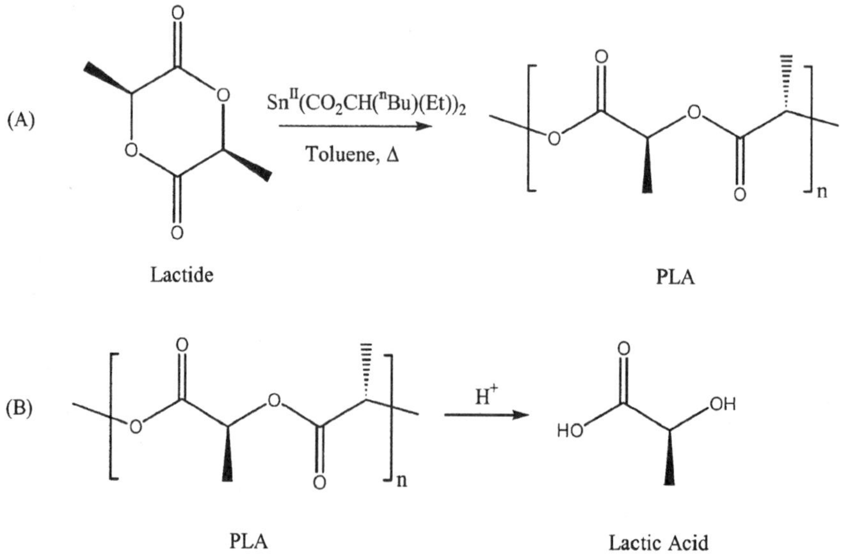

Figure 1   Synthesis and degradation of polylactic acid (PLA). (A) Polymer synthesis: ring-opening polymerization of lactide via stannous octoate to give PLA. (B) Polymer degradation: acid hydrolysis of PLA to give lactic acid.

However, polyester systems based on PLGA have been successfully used in DNA delivery systems for tissue engineering (14,15). For example, the authors found that an in vivo physiological response was only achieved through sustained release of plasmid DNA from PLGA matrices. In comparison, the direct subcutaneous injection of plasmid into the tissue did not produce a response (14).

DNA encoding for the protein platelet-derived growth factor (PDGF) was fabricated into three-dimensional DNA-polymer sponges utilizing a high-pressure gas foaming process followed by salt leaching to provide a highly porous, open-pore matrix. Release of the incorporated plasmid was demonstrated over time periods ranging from days to months depending on the PLGA copolymer composition. This example offers an interesting tact on how essentially a drug delivery system can affect a desired tissue engineering outcome. This offers an alternative to more traditional tissue engineering approaches of seeding cells onto polymer scaffolds for implantation. Furthermore, protein formulation in drug delivery systems is often difficult owing to concerns of maintaining protein stability and activity over time (16–18). The potential stability of plasmid DNA may offer an advantage over the use of proteins to gain a therapeutic response.

In an analogous example, Levy and coworkers used PLGA-coated stents to deliver plasmid DNA as a potential treatment for restenosis (obstruction) of arteries (19). Restenosis is a common failure of post–balloon angioplasty and stenting surgical procedures to clear occluded arteries. Using green fluorescent protein plasmid DNA as a model agent, these results also indicate that sustained release of plasmids from biomaterials may provide beneficial drug delivery and tissue engineering outcomes.

In an example of the synergy between polymers and biology, Niklason et al. demonstrated the growth of functional arterial grafts in vitro on tubular PGA scaffolds (20). The fabricated scaffolds were treated to a mild base hydrolysis to render the immediate surface hydrophilic for greater serum protein and, consequently, cell coverage. The basic physical properties and biocompatibility of PGA were enough to provide a suitable support environment for successful cell growth. However, it was the use of biomimetic culture conditions that lead to confluent endothelial cell and to differentiated smooth muscle cell growth that mimicked autologous arterial grafts. Scaffold cell constructs were cultured under pulsed-medium conditions in an engineered bioreactor. In animal studies, these arterial grafts remained open for up to 4 weeks (the duration of the experiment) following implantation (Fig. 2).

Recently, two groups examined engineering of degradable polyester systems with supercritical carbon dioxide (scCO$_2$). Howdle and colleagues

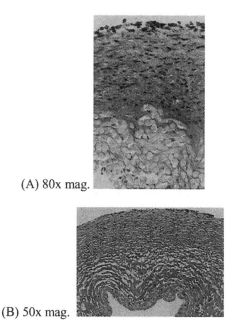

(A) 80x mag.

(B) 50x mag.

Figure 2 Bovine engineered vessels that have been cultured under (A) nonpulsatile or (B) pulsatile conditions for 8 weeks. Nonpulsed vessel has polymer fragments scattered about on the inside surface of the vessel, while the pulsed vessel has incorporated the polymer fragments and is more organized in structure. (Masson's trichrome stain. Polymer fragments are nonstaining and white in both images. Top side is the outer edge of the vessel wall; bottom is the inner vessel surface.)

demonstrated the ability to process PLGA in $scCO_2$ (21). They showed that efficient loading of bioactive enzymes could be achieved in a PLGA matrix and retain bioactivity after sustained release. Residual solvent is often problematic when encapsulating sensitive proteins in polymer constructs. Such processing conditions could alleviate the need for organic solvent–based processing techniques. Furthermore, it was established that by varying the rate of $scCO_2$ depressurization, the porosity of the final polymer constructs could be controlled.

Dillow et al. demonstrated that sterilization of PLGA microparticles could be achieved through use of $scCO_2$ (22). Typical sterilization techniques, such as steam treatment, would be detrimental to biodegradable polyesters. In challenge assays against clinically relevant bacteria, PLGA microspheres were left undamaged by $scCO_2$ exposure.

1. Increased Chemical Functionality to Biodegradable Systems

Understanding the biocompatibility of the monomers and the degradation products can serve as a strategic advantage in the design of new synthesis for biomaterials. The polyesters above that are functional from a biocompatible point of view typically lack the chemical functionality to have additional in vivo functionality added. Barrera et al. demonstrated the use of a novel monomer for the incorporation of amine functional groups into a PLA polymer system (23). Poly(lactic acid-*co*-lysine) (PLAL) was produce from the copolymerization of cyclic lactide and an analogous cyclic monomer containing the amino acid lysine. Inclusion of the amino acid lysine provides a free amine to conduct further chemical reactions and will not likely impact the overall biocompatibility of the polymer (Fig. 3).

Microspheres formulated from PLAL exhibited deep-lung delivery (24). Particles prepared from a double-emulsion technique were highly

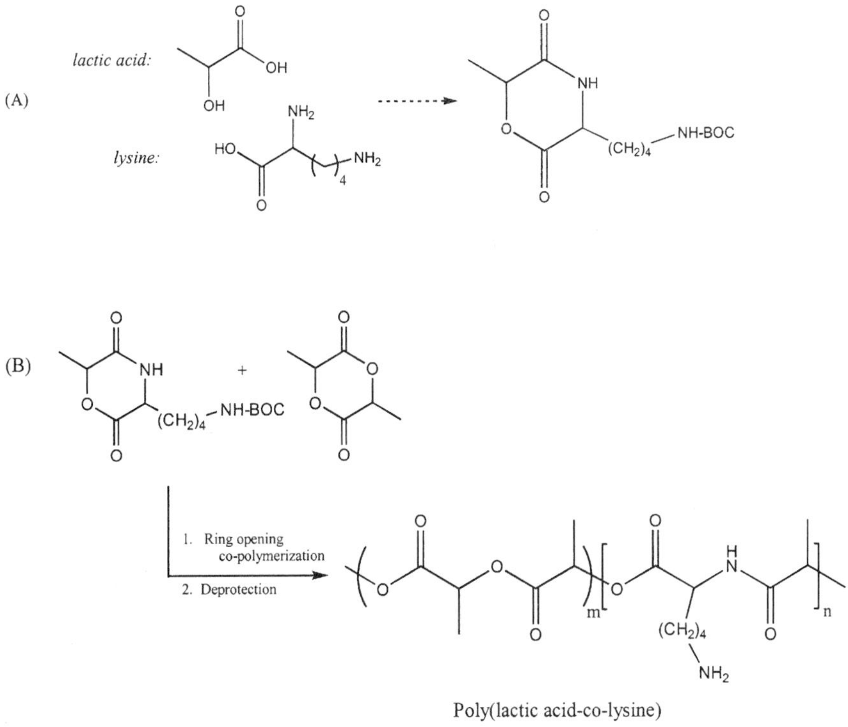

Figure 3   (A) Cyclic monomer incorporating lysine (analogous to lactide; see Fig. 1). (B) Poly(lactic acid-*co*-lysine) (PLAL) copolymer system.

porous and demonstrated superior performance in vitro using a cascade impactor system. These particles delivered close to a 60% respirable fraction as compared with only 20% for nonporous particles. These microspheres were relatively large having a mean diameter of 20 μm. In comparison, conventional particles for pulmonary use are on the order of 2 μm. These larger systems are likened to whiffle balls in that they have better in-(air)stream flight performance than smaller nonporous particles (Fig. 4).

2. Poly(Anhydride)

The mechanism of polymer degradation in the polyester systems is predominantly a *bulk* erosion process. However, we have also utilized *surface*-eroding polymers to control release profiles in drug delivery systems. Surface-eroding systems are differentiated from bulk-eroding systems in that they maintain their geometrical shape as they degrade. This is akin to a bar of soap as it slowly dissolves over time. A detailed discussion of polymer degradation and erosion can be found in review of controlled drug release by Uhrich et al. (9). Again, from the viewpoint of synthesizing biomaterials, the goal is to create new performance characteristics for polymers in vivo.

Some of the best known polyanhydrides are based on sebacic acid (SA) and *p*-carboxyphenoxypropane (CPP). By controlling the hydrophilic/ hydrophobic monomer content in polymers, the rate of surface erosion can be controlled for these polymer systems. Homopolymers based in SA degrade within days, whereas polymers based on CPH can degrade over

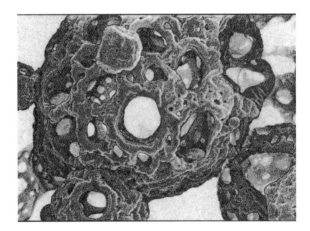

Figure 4   Porous particles made from biocompatible polymers.

(A)

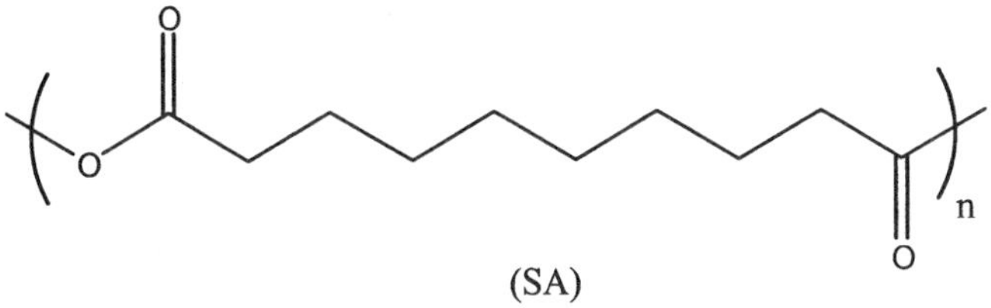

(SA)

(B)

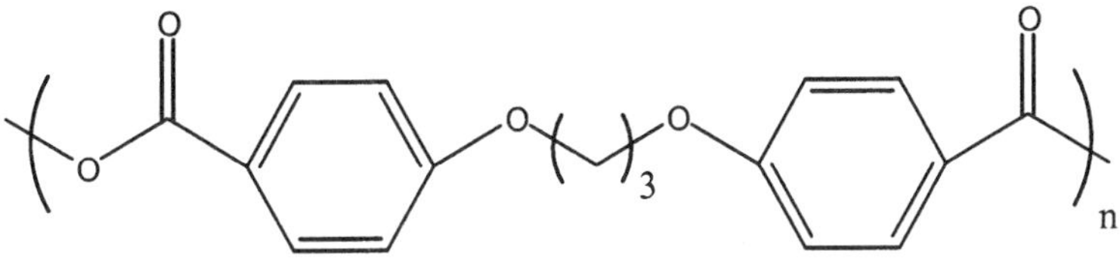

(CPP)

Figure 5 Polyanhydrides: (A) polysebacic acid (SA) and (B) poly-*p*-carboxyphe-noxypropane, (CPP).

months to years (25) (Fig. 5). The biocompatibility of these copolymer systems has been established (26), and the in vivo performance of these biomaterials makes them excellent candidates for use in medical applications.

Polyanhydride wafers containing chemotherapeutic agents are approved in treatment of brain cancer (27). This example of site-specific placement of a drug delivery system has proven to be a common theme in use of polymers in controlled release applications. Similar site-specific placement therapies are also being pursued, e.g., in lung, eye, and coronary arteries. Again, this is differentiated from targeted delivery where a systemic dose is preferentially taken up at a remote site.

Recently, Anseth et al. developed a novel class of photopolymerizable anhydrides (28,29). By synthesizing additional chemical functionality into anhydride monomers and oligomers, greater engineering functionality for the polymer was obtained. The goal was to expand on the biocompatibility of polyanhydrides and create a polymer system that could be cured in vivo. This will provide surgeons, for example, with greater flexibility in use and handling of implantable devices (Fig. 6).

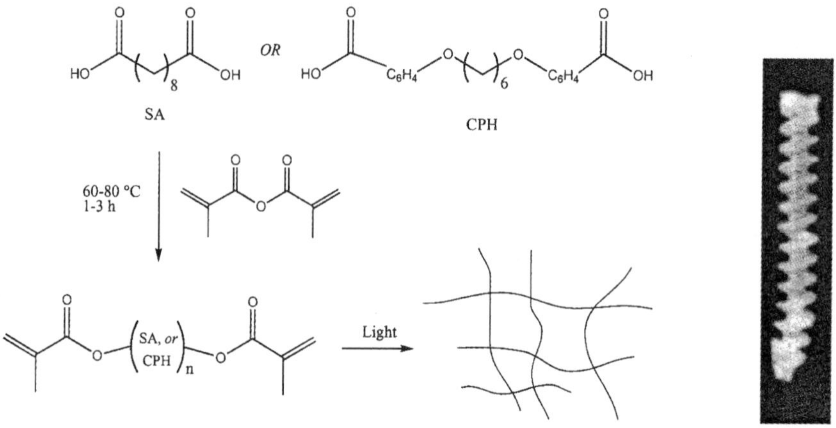

Figure 6   Synthesis of methacrylated anhydride oligomers for use in a photo-polymerizable polyanhydride system. (right) A degradable bone screw (length = 4 cm) produced in a mold from illuminating at the screw head only.

3. Polyaspirin: Polymer Therapeutics

Polymer therapeutics are a relatively new class of biomaterials in which the polymer itself acts as the active agent in promoting a therapeutic outcome. In one of the first examples of a degradable polymer therapeutic, Uhrich and coworkers have developed "PolyAspirin," a polyanhydride ester that incorporates the active component of aspirin, salicylic acid, within a degradable polymer backbone (30). These materials are a new class of *prodrugs*. Typically, prodrugs are a polymer or any adjuvant added to increase the therapeutic efficacy of an active agent or drug. In this example, hydrolytic degradation of the polymer leads to the production of salicylic acid (Fig. 7). The polymers have the potential to more effectively deliver aspirin to the intestines and avoid stomach irritation often associated with aspirin tablets. In animal studies related to bone restoration, the SA-derived polymers stimulated new-bone formation (31). Potentially this material could be applied as a coating to orthopedic and other medical devices.

B. Polyethylene Glycol: PEG and Related Systems

Polyethylene glycol (PEG), also referred to as polyethylene oxide (PEO) at high molecular weights, represents another widely used biomaterial that differs from the above polyester and polyanhydride systems insofar as PEG

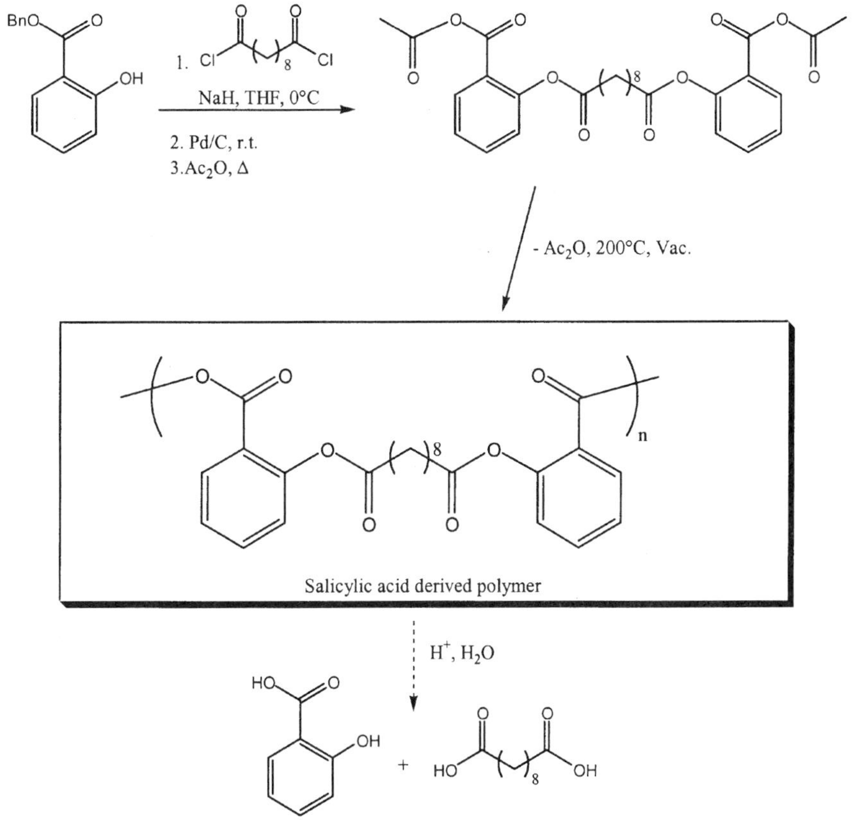

Figure 7 Synthesis of polyanhydride ester: PolyAspirin.

is resorbable but not degraded. Typically, PEG with molecular weights of 4000 amu is 98% excreted in man (32).

PEG is ubiquitous in biomaterial applications. It has been extensively researched in controlled-release systems and as a coating for medical devices. The hydrophilic nature of PEG leads to its ability to resist protein deposition (33). Much of the recent work on self-assembled monolayers (SAMs) has been invaluable in defining the behavior of molecules presented at surfaces. While SAMs offer an exacting surface environment in which to study ligands, these surfaces are difficult to replicate in vivo and are not readily adaptable for use in biomaterials. However, the application of PEG as a protein-inert background in SAMs has allowed for the study of ligand–

receptor binding and may lead to the elucidation of new motifs for biomimetic applications (34,35).

Many research groups are investigating PEG in block copolymer systems with degradable materials like the polyesters and polyanhydrides. PEG can be made with a range of terminal functional groups, which can lead to the formation of useful copolymer systems. PEG is typically terminated with hydroxyl groups, which can serve as a point of synthetic modification. The free hydroxyl groups of PEG are ring-opening initiators for lactide or glycolide. The synthesis and characterization of diblock and triblock systems have been reviewed (9) (Fig. 8).

One of the emerging drivers for inclusion of PEG in biomaterial applications arises from its protein resistivity. The hydrophilic nature of PEG is such that water hydrogen-bonds tightly with the polymer chain and thus excludes, or inhibits, protein adsorption. The inclusion of PEG in copolymer systems imparts extremely beneficial surface properties in the body because of the ability to repel proteins in aqueous environments. This repulsion inhibits the adsorption of proteins to the polymer surface and therefore prevents many polymer–cell interactions.

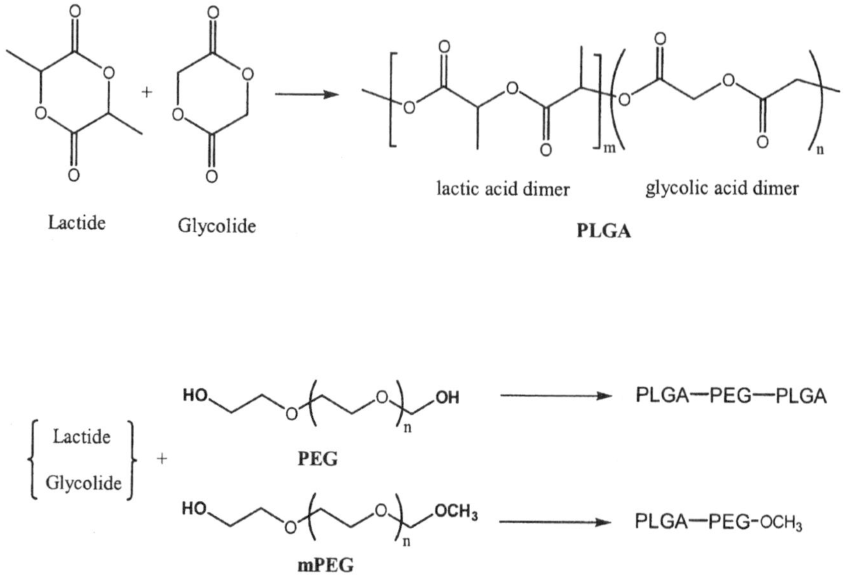

Figure 8 Synthesis of polyester-polyether block copolymers. Ring opening polymerization of lactide and glycolide from hydroxyl end group of PEG gives PLGA-PEG block polymers.

PLGA-PEG diblock copolymer systems possess surfactant properties because the PEG block is very hydrophilic and the PLGA block is hydrophobic. Therefore, when PLGA-PEG is employed in a fabrication process that uses an aqueous external phase, e.g., particle fabrication emulsion techniques, PEG enriches the surface. An important aspect of biomimetic materials is stealth. The body has an amazing capacity for recognizing foreign bodies and eliminating them. PEG-enriched surfaces allow for longer viability of biomaterials in the body by prolonging biological events, such as endocytosis, phagocytosis, liver uptake and clearance, and other adsorptive processes.

For example, particles of 90–150 nm were made from diblock PLGA-PEG copolymers. Importantly, the ester bond between the PEG and PLGA blocks showed less than 5% degradation after 24 h in buffered saline, confirming the stability of the particles' surface properties. In model studies with mice, the liver had cleared only 30% of optimized PLGA-PEG particles after 5 h. In comparison, 66% of nanospheres made of PLGA were cleared in only 5 min (36,37).

The synthetic versatility of end-group chemistry was further exploited in PLA-PEG-PLA triblock systems. Acrylate end groups were introduced to produce light-curable systems. These systems were described by Sawhney and have been reviewed by Anseth (38,39) (Fig. 9). When photoinitiated, a cross-linked, biodegradable hydrogel system is formed. Diacrylate end groups have also been introduced via anhydride bonds to produce polyether-anhydride networks (40). Light-curable systems represent a strategic approach in biomaterials synthesis and application. Intuitively, internal locations in the body are dark, and the development of light-curable biomaterials will allow for the delivery of prepolymer systems to remote locations (via minimally invasive surgery) where complex shapes or implantation of preformed polymers may be difficult. Tissue engineering applications in reconstructive and augmentation surgery are potential benefactors from these systems (41).

In work by West and Hubbell, PEG is synthesized with short peptide sequences that have specific activity with enzymes important to wound healing (42). In one example, the tetramer peptide sequence Ala-Pro-Gly-Leu was chosen as a mimic to type 1 collagen for specific cleavage by collagenase. These PEG systems were also functionalized with terminal acrylate groups and form cross-linked hydrogels (Fig. 10). The PEG-peptide polymers showed significant degradation in the presence of their targeted enzyme, collagenase, but proved to be stable in the presence of other proteases. This represents a departure from relying on hydrolysis for degradation of biomaterials and instead tailoring degradation to specific enzymatic activity.

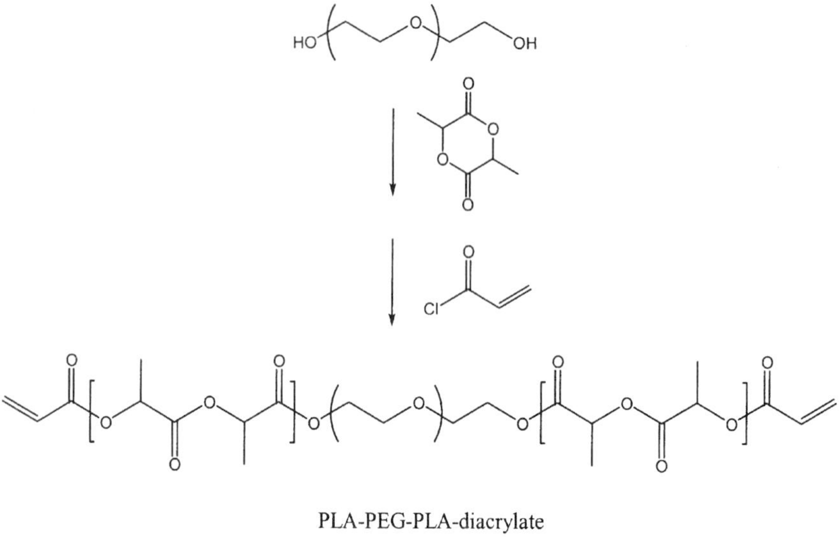

PLA-PEG-PLA-diacrylate

Figure 9   End-group modification of a polyester-polyether triblock copolymer with acrylate functionality.

Russell et al. have produced hydrogel systems based on cross-linking PEG via a 2 + 2 cycloaddition of pendant cinnamylidene acetyl groups (43). The cycloaddition forms cyclobutane cross-links between "four-armed" PEG derivatives. These hydrogels are reversible through photoscission of the cinnamylidene dimer back to cinnamylidene acetyl groups. Such light-responsive systems may allow for the controlled release of agents from hydrogels (Fig. 11).

A clever approach to biomimetic, reversible hydrogel systems was achieved through creation of an antigen-responsive hydrogel (44). Corresponding antigen–antibody pairs were utilized to form reversible non-covalent cross-links in a polyacrylamide system. In the presence of excess free antigen the hydrolgels can swell and in the absence of free antigen collapse back to a cross-linked network (Fig. 12). Swelling did not occur upon the addition of foreign antigens (to the antibody), proving this system to have an antigen-specific response. Pulsatile release of the model protein hemoglobulin was demonstrated for this system.

Thermosensitive hydrogel materials based on PLA-PEG have also been developed (45). In this example the authors synthesized PEG-PLA-PEG systems through use of a urethane linkage. These materials exhibited a gel-sol transition. Above physiological temperatures ($> 37°C$) the polymer

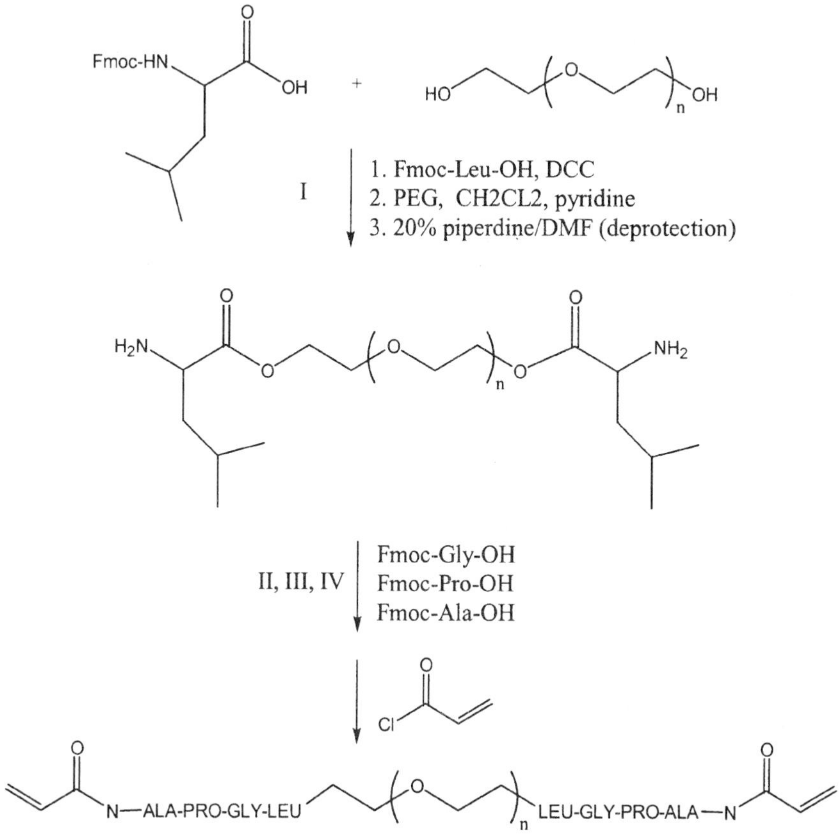

Figure 10 PEG derivatives containing short peptide sequences.

systems are free flowing and can be admixed with a desired therapeutic. Upon injection into the body, these polymers "cool" and gel to provide sustained release.

C. Summary: Biocompatible Systems

Biodegradable and resorbable biomaterials serve as supports and delivery vehicles for therapeutic applications in medicine and medical devices. The in vivo tolerance of these materials makes them an advantageous starting point in development of more complex biomimetic systems. Improving the performance of these polymers has focused on engineering of bulk material

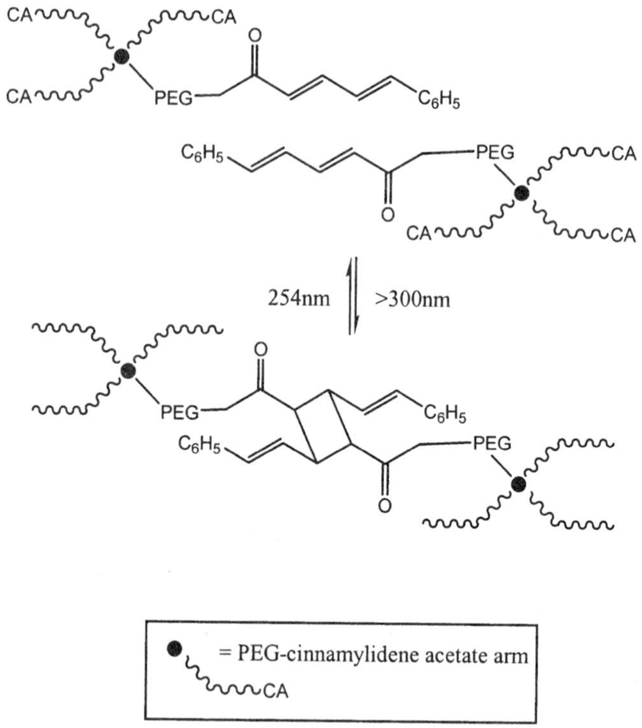

Figure 11   Reversible PEG hydrogel.

and creating additional chemical and biological functionality. Biodegradable polymers have even been incorporated into materials with shape memory properties (46).

When engineering these materials for in vivo use, one must bear in mind that the material will interact with physiological environment in which it is placed. Degradation products must be predictable. For in situ polymerizations one must be mindful of exothermic heat given off from polymerization that might be damaging to surrounding tissue, but need to cure in a timely fashion useful to surgeons.

Continued development of synthetic schemes (47) and process engineering (48) for degradable systems will lead to the development of highly functional materials for in vivo use. While we have highlighted the synthesis and engineering of biodegradable systems, biomimetic materials will be important. As an example, carbohydrates offer excellent synthetic versatility (49) and are commonly implicated in biological functions. It is

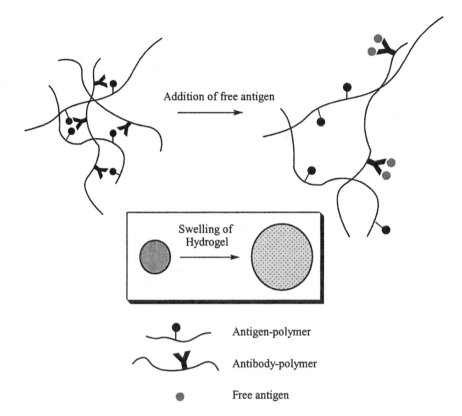

Figure 12 Hydrogel formed via antigen–antibody cross-links. Competition of free antigen for bound antibody causes swelling in the polymer matrix. (Reproduced with permission from *Nature*.)

clear that materials will continue to evolve in sophistication as we increase our understanding of biology and the interactions of these materials with their physiological environment.

III. ADDING BIOMIMETIC FUNCTIONALITY

A. Cell-Adhesive Biological Tags

As our knowledge of ligand molecules that elicit a biological response grows, it is inevitable that they will play a crucial role in the next generation of biomaterials. Attempts to add biomimetic functionality to polymer

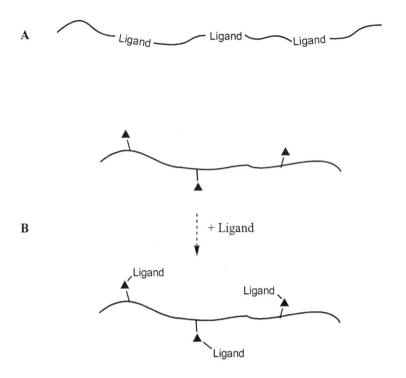

Figure 13 General depiction of synthetic bulk modification of polymers. Biomimetic ligand incorporated (A) directly into polymer backbone and (B) at side chain functionalities along the polymer backbone.

systems has predominantly come from the addition of such ligands to the bulk polymer (50) (Fig. 13). While the synthesis of peptide sequence into bulk polymers has been explored, it is often the case that the peptide or ligand need only be present at the surface of a construct. For example, patterning cell growth on polymers requires that a cell-adhesive ligand be present in discrete areas, not throughout the polymer matrix. Such design criteria may be important in promoting cocultures and cell in-growth on polymeric scaffolds. In drug delivery applications of microspheres, the ability to attach ligands for targeting or to promote cellular uptake would necessarily need to be present only at the surface. Bulk modification of materials can suffer from underutilization of a precious ligand by masking its function in the bulk while only a small percentage is exposed at the surface. This concern can be particularly exasperated if hydrophilic/ hydrophobic process conditions of a construct preferentially bury the ligand in the bulk. Generally, bulk modification suffers from the fact that if the desired ligand is optimized or altered, it requires a completely new polymer synthesis to incorporate it, making it difficult to evaluate new ligands in a facile manner.

One approach to solving some of these challenges has been to introduce chemical functionality into the bulk polymer and attach the ligand in a postfabrication event. Again, introduction of chemical functionality into the bulk polymer is subject to the drawbacks mentioned above. Furthermore, it can adversely affect the polymerization reaction and resulting polymer. Covalent attachment of ligands after, say, microsphere formation may be limited if the reaction conditions are too harsh to preserve the microsphere architecture.

Recently, we expanded on the PLA-PEG copolymer system to produce a PLA-PEG-biotin biomaterial that could be readily adapted with ligands that impart biomimetic function (51,52). The goal was to maintain the beneficial bulk properties of PLA-PEG copolymers and provide a method of facile surface modification with biological ligands. PLA-PEG systems offer a unique advantage in that the hydrophilic nature of the PEG chains causes them to behave with surfactant-like qualities. In aqueous emulsion techniques to create microspheres or solvent casting techniques to produce films, the surface of PLA-PEG copolymers is enriched with the hydrophilic PEG chains. Therefore, these constructs require only the derivatization of the PEG chain for surface engineering. By functionalizing the PEG block with biotin, a surface engineering strategy was developed using avidin as a bridge between the biotinylated polymer and a biotinylated ligand. Avidin's tetrameric structure contains four biotin binding sites; as such, avidin immobilized on the material surface retains the ability to further bind biotin. The goal of surface engineering is then reduced to established synthetic protocols for biotinylation of ligands (53). More-over, the surface modification is a postfabrication event under mild conditions allowing for any architecture to be rapidly modified with a ligand, without damage to either (Fig. 14). Surface analysis of PLA-PEG-biotin systems by x-ray photoelectron spectroscopy (XPS) reveals that the surface density of PEG chains (and subsequently biotin) can be tailored by varying the PLA molecular weight (54) (Fig. 15). Deconvolution of the carbon signals in XPS corresponding to PLA and PEG, respectively, shows that as the PLA block molecular weight is decreased, the amount of PEG at the surface is increased.

PLA-PEG-biotin polymers have been fabricated into microspheres and thin films for drug delivery and tissue engineering systems, respectively. Fluorescence confocal microscopy confirmed that the biotin-avidin-biotin binding scheme could be used to render surfaces with ligands. Micro-

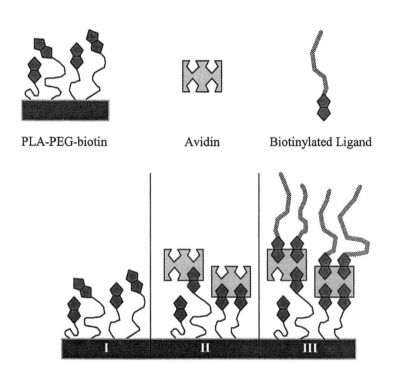

PLA-PEG-biotin

PLA-PEG-biotin   Avidin   Biotinylated Ligand

Figure 14 PLA-PEG-biotin as a general, facile method for coupling biomimetic ligands to a biomaterial constructs.

particles made from these materials were first incubated with avidin fluorescently labeled with Texas red (Fig. 16A). Subsequent incubation with biotin labeled with fluorescein isothrocyanate revealed an nearly exact distribution to the surface-bound avidin (Fig. 16B). In contrast, PLA-PEG

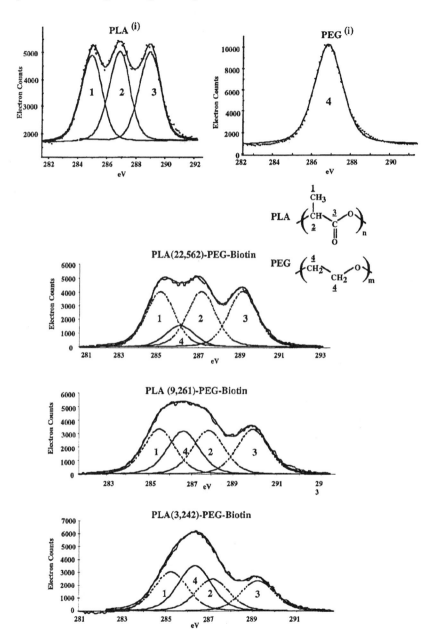

Figure 15 XPS characterization of PLA-PEG-biotin films shows increasing PEG surface content with decreasing PLA molecular weight. C(1s) region data for PLA, PEG, and the PLA-PEG-biotin copolymers.

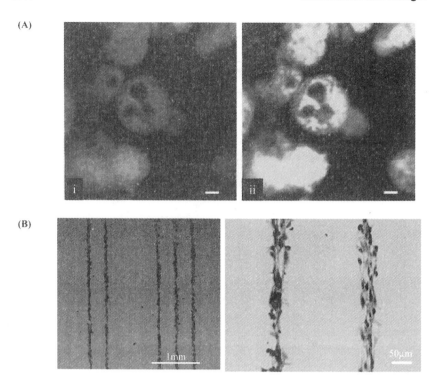

Figure 16 PLA-PEG-biotin constructs with ligand-modified surfaces. (A) Microspheres for drug delivery (i) incubated with fluorescently labeled avidin and (ii) fluorescently labeled biotin; same field viewed by a dual-channel confocal microscope. Bar is 50 μm. (B) Tissue engineering polymer films patterned for directed cell adhesion (shown: bovine aortic endothelial cells on patterned RGD surfaces).

(no biotin) microparticles showed no surface fluorescence when incubated with labeled avidin or biotin (51).

PLA-PEG-biotin films facilitated surface patterning of aortic endothelial cells and PC12 nerve cells using biotinylated RGD and IKVAV peptide sequences, respectively. Again, the use of PEG in these experiments allowed for surfaces that were protein and cell resistant unless modified with a biomimetic ligand.

Shakesheff et al. demonstrated an alternative to PLA surface modification through surface entrapment of ligand motifs. In this work, PLA was swelled in a solvent to nonsolvent system causing gelation of the polymer surface. When ligands are dissolved in this solvent system they become entangled at the polymer surface. Subsequent collapse of the polymer surface by addition of an excess of nonsolvent causes the ligands to become entrapped. They demonstrated that one could obtain 75% surface coverage of PLA when PEG is used as a model ligand (55).

B. Cell Transport Ligands

PEG-based systems have a demonstrated ability to carry drugs through the body and reduce clearance. This is one facet of designing biomaterials that achieve a desired biomimetic function. In drug delivery, cellular uptake is another function that is required. As differentiated from a cellular response as invoked by the use of RGD peptide sequences, cellular uptake is vital for effective drug candidates.

The ability to directly access sites like the lung and the eye make it easy to appreciate the advantage of site-specific application of biomaterials. Diseases that affect these areas offer the potential to design systems that can be treated by direct placement of biomaterials at the site of the affected area. In the case of the Gliadel wafer, this idea is taken further by placing a degradable wafer carrying a therapeutic dose to a site that is being accessed during surgery. After closing, the benefit of a drug regime is localized to an otherwise inaccessible location (Fig. 17).

However, it is not always desirable (or possible) to access all locations of the body. One goal of medicine is to reduce the need for surgical intervention. The pinnacle of drug delivery is to obtain the maximum therapeutic dose at the site of concern while minimizing systemic levels that might be toxic and cause adverse side effects. The recent advancements in defining receptor-mediated response in cells are being incorporated into "smarter" drug delivery systems. A major hurdle to increasing the therapeutic benefit of drugs is providing for efficient cellular uptake.

One of the main drivers of biomimetic materials is the delivery of a therapeutic benefit at a specific site in the body. While many of the bulk polymer systems described here can serve as scaffolds to support cell growth or carry therapeutic payloads, they are increasingly being equipped with specific ligands such as peptide and carbohydrate, which can enable greater biological specificity to the materials.

One of the greatest barriers to increasing efficiency and bioavailability of therapeutics is not only getting them where they are needed most but also ensuring that cellular uptake of the drugs occurs when they are there. Several groups have demonstrated the ability to trigger endocytosis as a means of targeting intracellular space.

Wender and colleagues synthesized mimics to a Tat protein segment known to permeate cell membranes. An arginine-rich domain found within

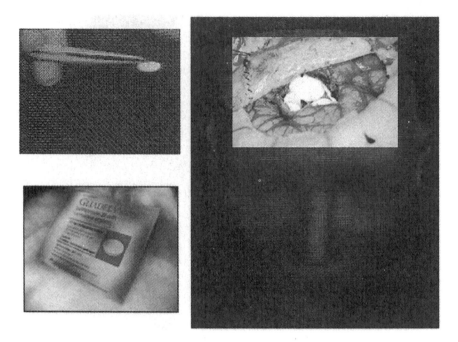

Figure 17 Gliadel wafers for the treatment of brain tumors placed at the site of a tumor resection following surgery.

a nine-residue sequence encoded by HIV-1, Tat_{49-57} has been successfully coupled to proteins for delivery into cells. (56–60). Wender's group set out to improve on the function of the Tat_{49-57} peptide fragment and increase transport efficiencies (61). They showed that improvements could be achieved through synthetic modification of the original Tat_{49-57} sequence. A peptide consisting of nine repeating units of the amino acid L-arginine (Arg9), showed a 20-fold increase in cellular response compared with the native Tat sequence. Moreover, the unnatural D-arginine isomer sequence showed more than a 100-fold improvement likely owing to its ability to avoid protease degradation. This work elucidated the importance of the guanidinium side chain group. From these findings "peptoid" analogues were synthesized that feature side chain guanidinium groups along a polyamide backbone analogous to Arg9. These materials, called "peptoids," are more readily prepared and proved to have even greater kinetic transport than the peptide derivatives (Fig. 18).

Recently, an arginine heptomer (Arg7) was coupled to cyclosporin A (CsA) (62). Oral administration of CsA is a well-known treatment for skin

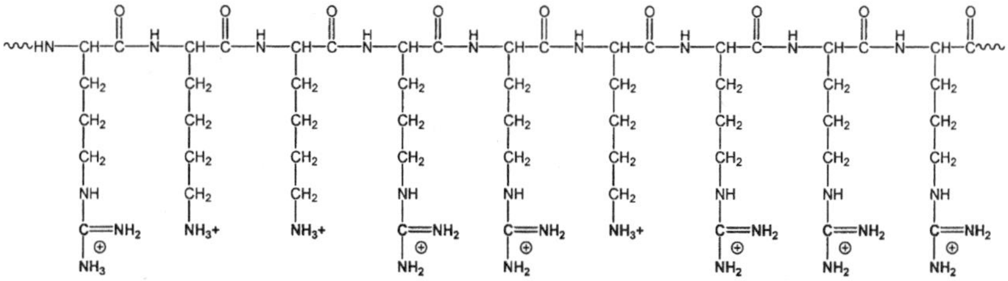

Tat$_{49\text{-}57}$

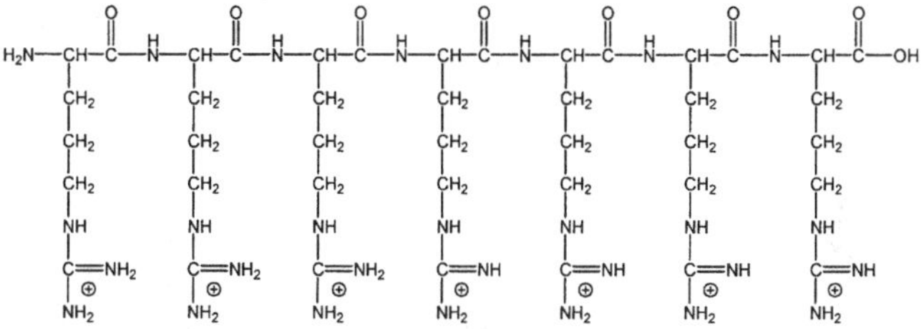

Arg7

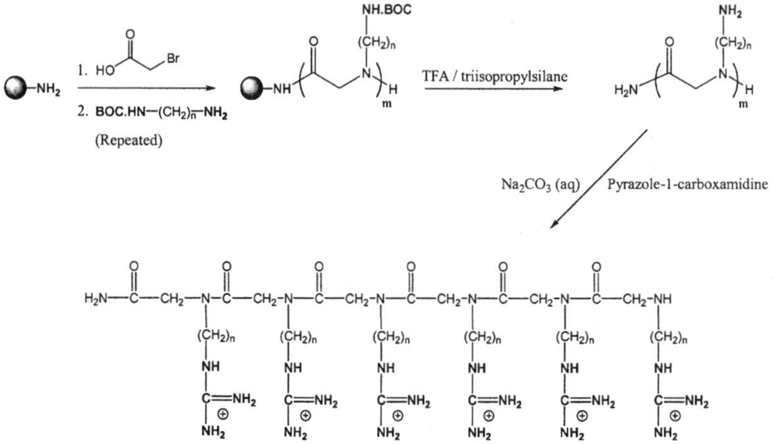

Synthesis of Peptoid Mimic to Arg7

Figure 18 (top) HIV-1 Tat$_{49\text{–}57}$ peptide sequence shown to facilitate transport across cell membranes. (middle) Arginine heptomer; Arg7. (bottom) Synthesis of peptoid mimic to Arg7.

ailments but, as is common with many systemic treatments, efficacy is limited by deleterious side effects and topical administration of CsA has been limited by poor bioavailability. Topically applied CsA-Arg7 conjugates demonstrated 74% reduction in ear inflammation (mice) while the other ear (control: untreated) showed no improvement, proving the treatment to be a local effect with release of the drug in the target cells and with no systemic uptake occurring.

C. Targeting Ligands

Many groups have demonstrated the use of amino acid sequences and other molecules for obtaining improved biological function of materials and therapeutics. One of the main goals for this research is to target active agents to proteins, cells, and organs specifically, so that systemic applications can have local effects.

The discovery of a cyclic decapeptide by Pasqualini that inhibits matrix metalloproteinases (MMP-2 and MMP-9 specifically), inhibits tumor cell migration, and targets angiogenic vessels is an example of how protein–target interactions are defining new motifs to be included in biomimetic architectures (63,64). The peptidomimetic CysThrThrHisTrpGlyPheThrLeuCys owes it cyclic structure to a disulfide bond. When the sulfide side chains contained in the cysteine residues are replaced with serine, the resulting linear analogue has a markedly lower activity. Maintaining the structure–activity relationships of biomimetic peptide fragments is important if they are to be successfully included in synthetic schemes.

Bertozzi has advanced a recent strategy in cell targeting (65–67). This work demonstrated the ability to express chemical functionality at cell surfaces that could serve as homing agents for targeting cells. A cell surface presents numerous motifs that regulate cellular function. These motifs consist of a diverse array of functionalities, lipids, peptides, and carbohydrates. However, ketones were seen as a unique chemical functionality, atypical to the chemistry presented at a cell surface. It was reasoned that if modified precursors to cell surface ligands were fed into the cell biosynthetic machinery, this modification would become expressed in the cell surface ligands. Sialic acid, a common terminal component of cell surface ligands, are derived from N-Acetylmannosamine. N-acetylmannosamine can then be modified to carry a ketone group and the ketone chemical functionality preserved in the expressed cell surface ligand. Hydrazide chemistry, for example, can then be used to target the ketone in a selective ligation event (Fig. 19).

Several research groups are actively pursuing novel motifs for targeting tumors (68–70), and reviews on drug targeting offer insight into

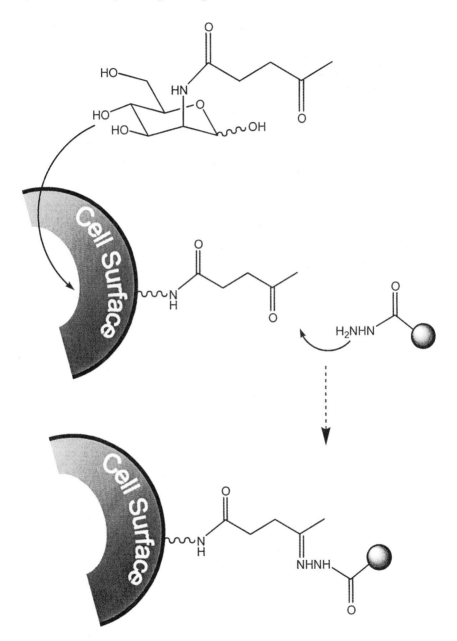

Figure 19 Cell surface engineering is achieved by modification of cell surface ligand precursor. Cell expression of a chemospecific site allows for targeted delivery.

biomimetic transport (71–74). The RGD sequence, noted as a cell-adhesive ligand, has demonstrated potential as a targeting vector for tumor vasculature (75).

D. Summary: Ligands for Biomimetic Function

Synthesis and engineering will combine the components of polymers and biomolecules to bring us to a new generation of biomaterials with exacting performance characteristics. The research surrounding polymers for medical applications is advancing from simple biocompatible systems to multicomponent systems that can service specific biological functions.

The ability to add specific biological function to polymeric systems is inevitable in their evolution. Identification and synthetic refinement of protein sequences like the RGD peptide sequence and the Tat-peptoid analogues will be crucial in developing novel biomaterials. One can envision the creation of tissue scaffolds that can promote and direct growth of cells and biomaterial systems with greater therapeutic payload efficiencies. The discovery of ligands with exquisite specificity for targets will ultimately become part of the synthetic repertoire for biomaterials.

REFERENCES

1. R Langer. Biomaterials in drug delivery and tissue engineering: one laboratory's experience. Acc Chem Res 33(2):94–101, 2000.
2. CB Matthews, et al. Gene Ther 6(9):1558–1564, 1999.
3. P Mulders, et al. Cancer Res 58(5):956–961, 1998.
4. H Vermeersch, JP Remon. Immunogenicity of poly(D-lysine), a potential polymeric drug carrier. J Controlled Release 32(3):225–229, 1994.
5. IV Yannas. Natural materials. In: BD Ratner et al., eds. Biomaterials Science. San Diego: Academic Press, 1996, pp. 84–94.
6. AH Simmons, CA Michal, LW Jelinski. Molecular orientation of two-component nature of the crystalline fraction of spider dragline silk. Science 271(5245):84–87, 1996.
7. IY Galaev, B Mattiasson. "Smart" polymers and what they could do in biotechnology and medicine. Trends Biotechnol 17:335–340, 1999.
8. J Kost, R Langer. Responsive polymer systems for controlled delivery of therapeutics. Trends Biotechnol 10(4):127–131, 1992.
9. KE Uhrich, et al. Polymeric systems for controlled drug release. Chem Rev 99(11):3181–3198, 1999.
10. BD Ratner, et al. (eds). Biomaterials Science. San Diego: Academic Press, 1996.
11. NA Peppas, R Langer. New challenges in biomaterials. Science 263:1715–1720, 1994.

12. LE Freed, et al. Tissue engineering of cartilage in space. Proc Natl Acad Sci USA 94:13885–13890, 1997.
13. D Putnam, et al. Polymer-based gene delivery with low cytotoxicity by a unique balance of side-chain termini. Proc Natl Acad Sci USA 98(3):1200–1205, 2001.
14. LD Shea, et al. DNA delivery from polymer matrices for tissue engineering. Nature Biotechnol 17:551–554, 1999.
15. WM Saltzman. Delivering tissue regeneration. Nature Biotechnol 17:534–535, 1999.
16. K Fu, et al. Visual evidence of acidic environment within degrading poly(lactic-co-glycolic acid) (PLGA) microspheres. Pharm Res 17(1):100–106, 2000.
17. K Fu, et al. FTIR characterization of the secondary structure of proteins encapsulated within PLGA microspheres. J Controlled Release 58(3):357–366, 1999.
18. SP Schwendeman, et al. Stabilization of tetanus and diphtheria toxoids against moisture-induced aggregation. Proc Natl Acad Sci USA 92:11234–11238, 1995.
19. BD Klugherz, et al. Gene delivery from a DNA controlled-release stent in porcine coronary arteries. Nature Biotechnol 18:1181–1184, 2000.
20. LE Niklason, et al. Functional arteries grown in vitro. Science 284:489–493, 1999.
21. SM Howdle, et al. Supercritical fluid mixing: preparation of thermally sensitive polymer composites containing bioactive materials. Chem Commun 109–110, 2001.
22. AK Dillow, et al. Bacterial inactivation by using near- and supercritical carbon dioxide. Proc Natl Acad Sci USA 96:10344–10348, 1999.
23. D Barrera, et al. J Am Chem Soc 115(11010), 1993.
24. D Edwards, et al. Large porous particles for pulmunary delivery. Science 276:1868–1871, 1997.
25. K Leong, B Brott, R Langer. J Biomed Mater Res 19:941, 1985.
26. C Laurencin, et al. J Biomed Mater Res 24:1463, 1990.
27. H Brem, R Langer. Sci Med 3:52, 1996.
28. KS Anseth, VR Shastri, R Langer. Photopolymerizable degradable polyanhydrides with osteocompatibility. Nature Biotechnol 17:156–159, 1999.
29. AK Burkoth, KS Anseth. A review of photocrosslinked polyanhydrides: in situ forming degradable networks. Biomaterials 21:2395–2404, 2000.
30. L Erdmann, KE Uhrich. Synthesis and degradation characteristics of salicylic acid–derived poly(anhydride-esters). Biomaterials 21:1941–1946, 2000.
31. L Erdmann, B Macedo, KE Uhrich. Degradable poly(anhydride-ester) implants: effects of localized salicylic acid release on bone. Biomaterials 21:2507–2512, 2000.
32. R Shields, J Harris, M Davis. Gastroenterology 54, 1968.
33. P Kingshott, HJ Griesser. Surfaces that resist bioadhesion. Curr Opin Solid State Mater Sci 4:403–412, 1999.
34. RG Chapman, et al. Polymeric thin films that resist the adsorption of proteins and the adhesion of bacteria. Langmuir 17(4):1225–1233, 2001.

35. CS Chen, et al. Geometric control of cell life and death. Science 276:1425–1428, 1997.
36. R Gref, et al. Biodegradable long-circulating polymeric nanospheres. Science 263:1600–1603, 1994.
37. R Gref, et al. The controlled intravenous delivery of drugs using PEG-coated sterically stabilized nanospheres. Adv Drug Del Rev 16:215–233, 1995.
38. AS Sawhney, PP Chandrashekhar, JA Hubbell. Macromolecules 26(4):581–587, 1993.
39. AT Metters, KS Anseth, CN Bowman. Fundamental studies of a novel, biodegrable PEG-b-PLA hydrogel. Polymer 41:3993–4004, 2000.
40. BSH Kim, S Jeffrey, R Langer. Synthesis and characterization of novel degradable photocrosslinked poly(ether-anhydride) networks. J Polym Sci A Polym Chem 38(8):1277–1282, 2000.
41. J Elisseeff, et al. Transdermal photopolymerization for minimally invasive implantation. Proc Natl Acad Sci USA 96:3104–3107, 1999.
42. JL West, JA Hubbell. Polymeric biomaterials with degradation sites for proteases involved in cell migration. Macromolecules 32:241–244, 1999.
43. FM Andreopoulos, et al. Photoscissable hydrogel synthesis via rapid photopolymerization of novel PEG-based polymers in the absence of photoinitiators. J Am Chem Soc 118(26):6235–6240, 1996.
44. T Miyata, N Asami, T Uragami. A reversibly antigen-responsive hydrogel. Nature 399:766–768, 1999.
45. B Jeong, et al. Biodegradable block copolymers as injectable drug-delivery systems. Nature 388(6645):860–862, 1997.
46. A Lendlein, AM Schmidt, R Langer. AB-polymer networks based in oligo(ε-caprolactone) segments showing shape-memory properties. Proc Natl Acad Sci USA 98(3):842–847, 2001.
47. DM Lynn, R Langer. Degradable poly(beta-amino esters): synthesis, characterization, and self-assembly with plasmid DNA. J Am Chem Soc 122(44):10761–10768, 2000.
48. VP Shastri, I Martin, R Langer. Macroporous polymer foams by hydrocarbon templating. Proc Natl Acad Sci USA 97(5):1970–1975, 2000.
49. GS Hird, TJ McIntosh, MW Grinstaff. Supramolecular structures of novel carbohydrate-based phospholipids. J Am Chem Soc 122(33):8097–8098, 2000.
50. KM Shakesheff, SM Cannizzaro, R Langer. Creating biomimetic microenvironments with synthetic polymer-peptide hybrid molecules. J Biomater Sci Polym Edn 9(5):507–518, 1998.
51. SM Cannizzaro, et al. A novel biotinylated degradable polymer for cell-interactive applications. Biotech Bioeng 58(5):529–535, 1998.
52. N Patel, et al. Spatially controlled cell engineering on biodegradable polymer surfaces. FASEB J 12:1447–1454, 1998.
53. JP Diamandis, TK Christopoulos. Clin Chem 37:625–636, 1991.
54. FE Black, et al. Surface engineering and surface analysis of a biodegradable polymer with biotinylated end groups. Langmuir 15(9):3157–3161, 1999.

55. RA Quirk, et al. Surface engineering of poly(lactic acid) by entrapment of modifying species. Macromolecules 33(2):258–260, 2000.

56. AM Vocero-Akbani, et al. Nat Med 5:29–33, 1999.

57. DR Gius, et al. Cancer Res 59:2577–2580, 1999.

58. H Nagahara, et al. Nat Med 4:1449–1452, 1998.

59. DT Kim, et al. J Immunol 159:1666–1668, 1997.

60. RB Pepinsky, et al. DNA Cell Biol 13:1011–1019, 1994.

61. PA Wender, et al. The design, synthesis and evaluation of molecules that enable or enhance cellular uptake: peptoid molecular transporters. Proc Natl Acad Sci USA 97(24):13003–13008, 2000.

62. JB Rothbard, et al. Conjugation of arginine oligomers to cyclosporin A facilitates topical delivery and inhibition of inflammation. Nat Med 6(11):1253–1257, 2000.

63. E Koivunen, et al. Tumor targeting with a selective gelatinase inhibitor. Nature 17:768–774, 1999.

64. J Folkman. Angiogenic zip codes. Nature 17:749, 1999.

65. LK Mahal, KJ Yarema, CR Bertozzi. Engineering chemical reactivity on cell surfaces through oligosaccharide biosynthesis. Science 276:1125–1128, 1997.

66. E Saxon, CR Bertozzi. Cell surface engineering by a modified staudinger reaction. Science 287:2007–2010, 2000.

67. HC Hang, CR Bertozzi. Ketone Isosteres of 2-*N*-acetamidosugars as substrates for metabolic cell surface engineering. J Am Chem Soc 123(6):1242–1243, 2001.

68. FD Hong, GL Clayman. Isolation of a peptide for targeted drug delivery into human head and neck solid tumors. Cancer Res 60(23):6551–6556, 2000.

69. J Sudimack, RJ Lee. Targeted drug delivery via the folate receptor. Adv Drug Del Rev 41(2):147–162, 2000.

70. Z-R Lu, P Kopeckova, J Kopecek. Polymerizable Fab' antibody fragments for targeting of anticancer drugs. Nat Biotechnol 17(11):1101–1104, 1999.

71. DF Ranney. Biomimetic transport and rational drug delivery. Biochem Pharmacol 59(2):105–114, 2000.

72. VP Torchilin. Drug targeting. Eur J Pharm Sci 11, 2000.

73. WM Pardridge. Vector-mediated drug delivery to the brain. Adv Drug Del Rev 36:299–321, 1999.

74. AS Kearney. Prodrugs and targeted drug delivery. Adv Drug Del Rev 19:225–239, 1996.

75. W Arap, R Pasqualini, E Ruoslahti. Cancer treatment by targetted drug delivery to tumor vasculature in a mouse model. Science 279:377–380, 1998.

9
Scaffolds for Directing Cellular Responses and Tissue Formation

Pamela K. Kreeger and Lonnie D. Shea
Northwestern University, Evanston, Illinois

I. INTRODUCTION

Tissue loss and organ failure are two of the most substantial health problems in the United States. Approximately 50% of the total health care costs in the United States annually, in excess of $400 billion, is spent on patients suffering from these conditions (1). Numerous therapies are available to combat these health problems, including organ or tissue transplantation and the use of synthetic prosthetic devices. However, the transplantation approach is limited by a shortage of suitable donor tissue and synthetic prostheses typically do not replace all functions of a lost tissue or organ. The limitations inherent in these approaches have motivated the development of a new strategy for tissue and organ replacement, termed tissue engineering (2).

Tissue engineering has been formally defined as a "combination of the principles and methods of the life sciences with those of engineering to elucidate fundamental understanding of structure–function relationships in normal and diseased tissues, to develop materials and methods to repair damaged or diseased tissue, and to create entire tissue replacements" (1). This field integrates tissue/organ transplantation with synthetic prostheses by combining cells with synthetic extracellular matrices to develop natural biological substitutes that restore or replace tissue structure and function. Three general strategies have emerged for the engineering of tissues— conductive, inductive, and cell transplantation (3)—all of which employ a scaffold to influence tissue structure and function. In the conductive approach, a scaffold is provided that supports tissue formation and functions to provoke infiltration of desired cell types (4,5). Inductive approaches combine synthetic scaffolds with bioactive factors to enhance cell infiltration and induce the formation of a specific tissue. In the cell transplantation approach, cells are seeded onto scaffolds and cultured in vitro for subsequent implantation to the desired anatomical location.

Scaffolds designed to engineer tissues must have several basic requirements, which include being biodegradable and biocompatible, having a high surface area/volume ratio with sufficient mechanical integrity, and having the ability to provide a suitable environment for new-tissue formation that can integrate with the surrounding tissue (3). A scaffold that degrades at a rate comparable to that of new-tissue formation can direct tissue formation but will ultimately leave a completely natural tissue composed only of the cells and their products. Importantly, the degradation products should be easily cleared or resorbed by the body to minimize any inflammatory response in the host tissue. Another critical feature is a high surface area/volume ratio, which enables sufficient surface area to support cell adhesion. A high surface area/volume ratio can be achieved using a highly porous scaffold, which initially can support nutrient transport by diffusion from the surrounding tissue; however, the material must have sufficient mechanical properties to create and maintain a space and to resist collapse of the porous structure. An interconnected pore structure also provides for cell infiltration from the surrounding tissue, which is important not only for integration of the engineered tissue with the host but for development of a vascular network throughout the tissue to supply the necessary metabolites once the tissue has developed.

Perhaps the most complex aspect of scaffold design is the presentation of the appropriate signals or stimuli to guide the development of a tissue that fulfills the required structure and function. A fundamental premise of the conductive, inductive, and transplantation approaches is that the cells occupying the scaffold have the potential to regenerate the desired tissue and restore its function. However, to realize this potential the scaffold must provide the appropriate environment to support and stimulate the cellular processes involved in tissue development, such as proliferation, migration, matrix deposition, and differentiation. The delivery of the appropriate signals within this environment may be capable of directing cellular gene expression and subsequent cellular processes. These signals can be presented to the cells from their multiple interactions with the microenvironment, which include interactions with the scaffold surface, other cells, soluble factors, and responses to mechanical stimuli within the system. Each of these stimuli presents unique opportunities for directing cellular functions, and the scaffold must provide the appropriate combination of these signals to initiate a specific program of gene expression that ultimately leads to tissues with the desired properties. The objective of this chapter is to review the mechanisms by which tissue engineering scaffolds can direct cellular processes through regulation of cell–substrate interactions, the mechanical environment, and the delivery of bioactive factors.

II. CELL–SUBSTRATE INTERACTIONS

The natural extracellular matrix (ECM) is a complex chemically and physically cross-linked network of proteins and glycosaminoglycans. The matrix performs numerous functions, such as the organization of cells and the presentation of environmental signals to direct site-specific cellular recognition. The interaction between cells and the ECM is bidirectional and dynamic: cells are constantly accepting information about their environment from cues in the ECM, and cells are frequently remodeling this ECM. Tissue engineering scaffolds are being developed to mimic these functions of the ECM by regulating the surface or material with which cells interact.

A. Cell Adhesion

Naturally occurring materials, such as collagen or hyaluronan, are advantageous for use as tissue engineering scaffolds because they provide for specific cellular interactions. One of the most widely used materials for fabricating tissue engineering scaffolds is collagen (6,7), the major component of mammalian connective tissue. Collagen provides a structure to the tissue and is involved in numerous developmental and physiological functions, such as cell attachment, differentiation, and chemotaxis. Cellular interactions with the ECM occur primarily through a class of receptors termed integrins, which can lead to morphological changes that include cell spreading, formation of focal contacts that extend toward the ECM surface, clustering of integrin receptors at the sites of focal contact, and assembly of accessory proteins to the cytoplasmic face of clustered integrins to form connections with the cytoskeleton (8). Integrin occupancy triggers cell-signaling mechanisms, including tyrosine kinase activation, growth factor responsiveness, and alterations in gene expression. Another natural material that provides fundamentally different properties from collagen is hyaluronan, a heteropolysaccharide that has been implicated in biological processes such as tissue hydration, cell differentiation, movement, proliferation, and angiogenesis (9). Hyaluronan is found in high concentrations in the ECM surrounding migrating and proliferating cells during regeneration and wound healing, but is reduced upon differentiation (10). Cells interact with hyaluronan through two receptors: CD44 and receptor for hyaluronic acid–mediated mobility (RHAMM) (11). Tissue engineering scaffolds are being formed by chemical modification or cross-linking of hyaluronan for a variety of applications, such as bone and cartilage (12–15).

Synthetic polymers have been utilized to provide greater versatility than natural materials for designing tissue engineering scaffolds with controlled properties. Synthetic materials can be manufactured reproducibly on a large scale and can be processed into exogenous ECM in which the macrostructure, mechanical properties, and degradation time can be readily controlled and manipulated. Perhaps the most widely used synthetic material for the creation of tissue engineering scaffolds are poly-L-lactic acid (PLLA), polyglycolic acid (PGA), and copolymers of these materials (PLG). Scaffolds can be formed as a mesh of fibers wound together or the polymer can be processed into a highly porous structure (16–19). These scaffolds contain an interconnected open-pore structure (Fig. 1) that allows for cells to be seeded throughout the scaffold in vitro or allows for cells to invade into the entire scaffold in vivo. This material is not intrinsically recognized by cell surface receptors; however, cell–substrate interactions are supported through proteins that adsorb to the surface. This adsorption is a result of an entropic gain as water is released from the hydrophobic material

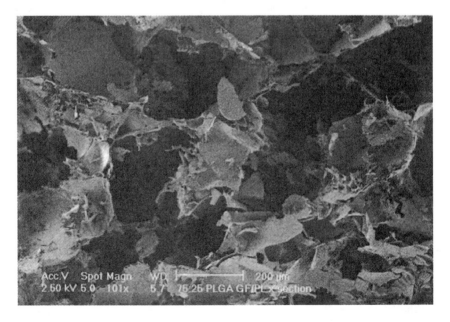

Figure 1 Scanning electron micrograph of the cross-section of a 75:25 PLG scaffold fabricated by a gas foaming/particulate leaching process. (From Ref. 96.)

surface (20). The complexity inherent in protein–surface interaction complicates the ability to precisely control the concentration, conformation, and bioactivity of adsorbed proteins (20–22); thus, techniques are being developed to more specifically regulate the surface of these polymers, such as processing to regulate adsorption (23) or the development of materials that self-assemble on surfaces (24). The typical procedure for protein adsorption involves the immersion of PLG scaffolds in serum-containing media, which results in the adsorption of the serum proteins to the surface. Vitronectin appears to be the major component of serum that adsorbs to the PLG surface (25). Alternatively, the material can be coated with specific ECM molecules, such as laminin, fibronectin, and collagen, to provide specific interactions with the cells.

The chemistry of the scaffold can direct cellular interactions that subsequently affects such processes as proliferation, migration, and matrix deposition. Scaffolds of PGA, 85:15 PLG, and collagen seeded with smooth muscle cells have shown differences in proliferation rates and in ECM deposition (25). The PGA scaffold had the highest proliferation rate and the highest rate of elastin production, whereas the collagen scaffold had the lowest proliferation rate with the highest rate of collagen production. Similarly, chondrocytes cultured on PGA scaffolds had enhanced proteoglycan synthesis relative to collagen scaffolds (26). These differences are hypothesized to result from the different receptor interactions with the material surface, which is consistent with studies performed with the adsorption of specific ECM proteins onto the polymer surface. For example, dorsal root ganglia were able to extend neurites on a PLG copolymer coated with laminin but not on a polylysine-coated polymer (27). Keratinocytes exhibited rapid migration across PLG surfaces coated with type I collagen but not those coated with fibronectin (22).

Hydrogels, which typically exhibit little protein adsorption relative to PLG, can be modified with peptides or proteins to selectively interact with specific receptors and direct cellular responses such as proliferation or differentiation. Commonly used hydrogels include alginate, a polysaccharide found naturally in algae, polyethylene glycol (PEG), polyacrylamide, and polyvinyl alcohol (PVA) (28). Hydrogels frequently exhibit minimal interactions with cells prior to modification but have chemical groups along their backbone that can be functionalized. Thus, oligopeptides that mimic natural adhesion proteins of the ECM can be chemically incorporated into the polymer surface to allow interactions between the material and cellular receptors. The RGD sequence, which is found in several ECM molecules, represents the minimal sequence necessary to interact with integrin receptors in order to induce adhesion to the substrate. The attachment of these adhesion ligands can cause cells to adhere to an otherwise noninteractive

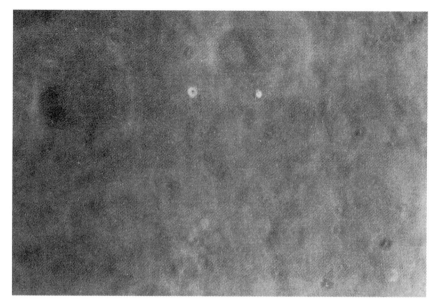

(a)

Figure 2 Photomicrograph of myoblasts on alginate surfaces that are either (a) unmodified or (b) modified with the adhesion peptide GRGDY. GRGDY-modified alginate surface showed spreading and adherence after 1 day of culture. (From Ref. 29, with permission from Elsevier Science.)

surface. For example, unmodified alginate does not provide for cell adhesion (Fig. 2a), whereas GRGDY ligands covalently linked to calcium alginate enables mouse skeletal myoblasts to attach and spread, eventually showing a differentiated phenotype (Fig. 2b) (29). In vivo implantation of RGD-modified alginate supports stromal invasion, which is not observed without the modifications (30). The ability of the tethered peptide to support cellular interactions is dependent on its design. For example, the inclusion of a spacer arm between the substrate surface and the adhesion sequence RGD enhances cell spreading and improves specificity relative to no spacer (31).

The sequence of the attached peptide can dictate the receptors that interact with the surface and thereby direct the cellular responses. The sequence RGD has been identified in numerous ECM proteins, such as collagen type I, fibronectin, and vitronectin. Modification of the flanking residues can modulate the receptor specificity. For example, RGDV from vitronectin has preferences for the $\alpha_v\beta_3$ integrin and the RGDS sequence

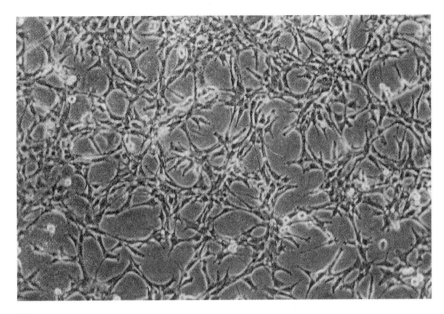

(b)

Figure 2

from fibronectin for the $\alpha_5\beta_1$ integrin (32). Alternatively, peptide sequences exist that regulate adhesion to nonintegrin receptors, such as the sequence YIGSR from laminin which is specific for the 67-kDa monomeric laminin receptor that is involved in the adhesion of many cell types. Some peptide sequences may be recognized by specific cell types, which can be used to separate cell types. KRSR is a peptide specific for the heparin sulfate–modified osteoblast adhesion mechanism; it enhances the adhesion of osteoblasts to surfaces but not endothelial cells or fibroblasts (33). The sequence REDV is specific for endothelial cells, with interactions seen at concentrations of less than $20\,fmol/cm^2$, resulting in morphologically and functionally normal monolayers (34). Combinations of adhesion peptides may also be used to produce the desired proliferation and differentiation. Surfaces modified with concentrations of 25:75, 50:50, and 75:25 RGD and FHRRIKA (a heparin binding domain) were prepared and cultured with osteoblast-like cells (35). The 25:75 and 50:50 surfaces supported a greater degree of cell spreading and greater mineralization than homogeneous RGD or FHRRIKA surfaces.

The density of covalently immobilized peptides or adsorbed proteins regulates cell adhesion, spreading, and morphology and the subsequent cellular processes, such as ECM deposition and migration. A surface density of $0.1\,fmol/cm^2$ of covalently attached RGD enabled fibroblast cell adhesion, but spreading was observed only at densities higher than $1\,fmol/cm^2$ (36). However, focal contacts and stress fibers were not observed until densities of $10\,fmol/cm^2$ and higher were used. Interestingly, these concentrations are significantly lower than the minimal surface concentrations needed for adhesion on surfaces with adsorbed RGD-containing proteins. The concentration of adsorbed protein or immobilized peptide has been shown to have a biphasic effect on cell migration, likely due to increases in cell adhesion. At low densities of adsorbed fibronectin, increases in protein adsorption led to increases in migration speed of smooth muscle cells (37). However, at high densities of adsorbed protein, additional increases in protein adsorption decrease the migration speed. In three-dimensional RGD-modified type I collagen gels, a similar biphasic relationship was observed between the distance traveled in a particular direction and the ligand density (38). The peptide and protein density also has an affect on ECM deposition. Smooth muscle cells and endothelial cells cultured on surfaces with varying peptide density were observed to decrease their ECM production with increasing density (39). An issue that is related to ligand density is the clustering of ligands, which may allow for receptor aggregation upon adhesion and spreading (40). YGRGD presented singly and in clusters of five or nine ligands using star polyethylene oxide (PEO) tethers on an inert PEO hydrogel led to different morphologies and migration rates (41). Individual peptides promoted adhesion and migration; however, the presence of the clustered ligands allowed full spreading and cell migration at lower average ligand densities.

The patterning of surfaces with one or more adhesion molecules can control the arrangement of cells and provide spatial guidance over tissue formation. Surfaces patterned with RGD molecules spatially controlled the adhesion and spreading of bovine aortic endothelial cells on lines 50- to 70-µm-wide stripes (42). Using the same method, neuronal cells cultured on a surface patterned with IKVAV selectively adhered to the peptide-coated surface and neurite extension was stimulated by the patterned ligands. In these cells, extended neurites were observed to approach but not cross the boundary between the patterned and nonpatterned surface. A 20-µm-wide YIGSR pattern was followed by the NG108-15 cells for 3 days and a 300-µm-wide IKVAV pattern selectively adhered PC12 cells for 3 days (43).

Carbohydrate-based cell recognition has also been investigated for the ability to affect cellular responses and tissue formation from substrate surfaces. Oligosaccharides are known to stimulate signal transduction processes for many cellular functions, particularly in hepatocytes. PEO surfaces prepared with varied galactose concentrations, which bind to the asialoglycoprotein receptor on hepatocytes, specifically affected hepatocyte spreading, in a manner similar to that of immobilized RGD peptides (44). Degradable polyesters patterned by a three-dimensional printing process with PEO–PPO (polypropylene oxide)–PEO copolymers are not adhesive for either hepatocytes or fibroblasts (45). By modifying the PEO chain end with carbohydrate ligands specific for the hepatocyte receptors, hepatocytes selectively adhere, which may prove useful in controlling spatial organization of varied cell types.

B. Immobilized Cytokines

In vivo, the ECM serves as a reservoir for growth factors and cytokines that protects against degradation, presents these factors more efficiently to their receptors, or affects their synthesis (46). Thus, the ECM can locally regulate the concentration and biological activity of these factors. The linkage of proteins, hormones, and other bioactive molecules to tissue engineering scaffolds is aimed at recapitulating the functions of the natural ECM and controlling the timing and location of growth factor presentation. In addition to the normal challenges associated with tethering peptides to surface, the tethering of cytokines and hormones is complicated by the need to retain the native three-dimensional structure of the molecule to maintain its activity.

The covalent immobilization of cytokines and growth factors to surfaces can maintain the bioactivity of the protein while stimulating cellular responses in a way different from soluble delivery of the same factors. Transforming growth factor $\beta2$ (TGF-$\beta2$) has been immobilized to fibrillar collagen to increase its stability and bioactivity (47). After 1 week in vivo, the immobilized TGF-$\beta2$ had similar responses to unbound TGF; however, the immobilized TGF-$\beta2$ retained activity for up to 4 weeks as compared to 1 week for unbound TGF. Similarly, the immobilization of insulin on polymethyl methacrylate surfaces demonstrated increased growth rates relative to controls with free insulin (48). The coimmobilization of insulin and fibronectin was found to act synergistically to further accelerate growth and enhance adhesion and spreading. Furthermore, hepatocytes cultured on surfaces with epidermal growth factor (EGF) tethered through the only primary amine (the N-terminal amine) initiated responses similar to those of soluble EGF, including DNA synthesis and morphological changes, and cell motility (49). Adsorbed EGF had no effect, illustrating the importance of developing an immobilization method that retains protein bioactivity.

III. MECHANICAL PROPERTIES

Mechanical stimuli have been implicated in the development of various tissues and the gene expression of many cell types in culture. Mechanical signals are conveyed to cells via their adhesion to the ECM. Integrin receptors are the major structural components of adhesion complexes at the cell membrane and serve both signaling and mechanical functions. They physically link the ECM to the cytoskeleton, and hence are responsible for establishing a mechanical continuum by which forces are transmitted between the outside and the inside of cells in both directions. Upon mechanical stimulation via the ECM, signals that lead to adaptive cellular responses are initiated either by integrins, proteins in the focal contacts, or cytoskeletal proteins (50). A more comprehensive discussion of mechanical stress effects on cell and tissue function can be found in several review articles (51,52). In order to engineer functional structural tissues, the correct mechanical stimuli may have to be provided during the process of tissue development via an appropriate synthetic ECM. For example, cartilage engineered without mechanical stimuli has mechanical strength less than that of native tissue, although they appear similar histologically (53).

The stiffness and compliance of the matrix are critical to the transmission of external forces to resident cells in that matrix. Upon seeding into a tissue engineering scaffold, cells exhibit a tractional force. The scaffold should have sufficient stiffness to resist these tractional forces and maintain its original size and shape, which is important for regenerating tissues of predefined sizes. The mechanical support provided by the scaffold should be maintained until the engineered tissue has sufficient mechanical integrity to support itself. If the stiffness of the matrix is insufficient to counter the tractional forces, the matrix will contract and collapse the three-dimensional structure during tissue growth. This behavior has been observed for fibroblasts cultured on collagen gels (54) and smooth muscle cells cultured on PGA scaffolds (55). The mechanical properties of the scaffold may be directly sensed by cells, thus affecting their behavior. Alginate hydrogels modified with adhesion peptide have been fabricated with varying mechanical strengths through variations in cross-linking (56). Cell proliferation and myoblast fusion were observed to differ on the substrates with varying mechanical properties. Similarly, the effects of matrix compliance on the cellular response have been observed for fibroblasts cultured on collagen gels (54).

Alternatively, the cell/scaffold construct can be mechanically manipulated to affect the organization of cells and deposited ECM, which can enhance the mechanical properties of the engineered tissue. Mechanical stimulation has been applied to three-dimensional tissues in multiple ways, such as a pulsatile flow through the lumen of tubular constructs (57) or a cyclic strain of polymer scaffolds (58). One application of mechanical strain involves smooth muscle cells, which are critical components of cardiovascular, gastrointestinal, and urological tissues and reside in mechanically dynamic environments. The pulsatile stimulation of the tubular constructs increased the collagen content and burst strengths over that of nonpulsed constructs (57). Interestingly, the burst strengths of the pulsed tubular constructs were greater than that of native human saphenous veins. Alternatively, mechanical stimulation of a cell-seeded scaffold with a cyclic strain applied at a frequency of 1 Hz and an amplitude of 7% resulted in alignment of cells in the direction of the applied strain (Fig. 3) and an increase in the mechanical properties of the engineered tissue (58). Mechanical stimulation led to increased elastin and type I collagen mRNA levels, and the resulting tissue contained a greater elastin content than control tissues.

IV. DELIVERY OF BIOACTIVE FACTORS

Soluble factors, such as growth factors and hormones, are critical regulators of cellular responses and phenotype; however, these factors may not be present in sufficient quantities in an engineered or regenerating tissue. The combination of drug delivery technology with the fabrication of polymer scaffolds has led to the fabrication of tissue engineering scaffolds capable of controlled release of proteins, DNA, or other bioactive factors. This technology has potential to locally control cellular process for prolonged times through a sustained release of the appropriate factors directly into the cell microenvironment.

Controlled-release systems provide a number of potential advantages for the therapeutic delivery of drugs (59). Drug encapsulation within the polymer can protect against degradation and loss in bioactivity until release. Injection or implantation of the polymer into the body can be used to target a particular cell type or tissue. Drug release from the polymer and into the tissue can be designed to occur rapidly, as in a bolus delivery, or to occur over an extended period; thus, a delivery system can be tailored to a particular application. For bolus delivery, drug levels quickly rise and decline as the drug is cleared or degraded. For sustained delivery, the drug concentration is maintained within a therapeutic window by adjusting the release rate (e.g., through the polymer choice). Drug release from polymeric systems occurs primarily through three mechanisms (60): diffusion of the drug from the system, degradation of the polymer to release the encapsulated protein, or countercurrent diffusion of aqueous medium into

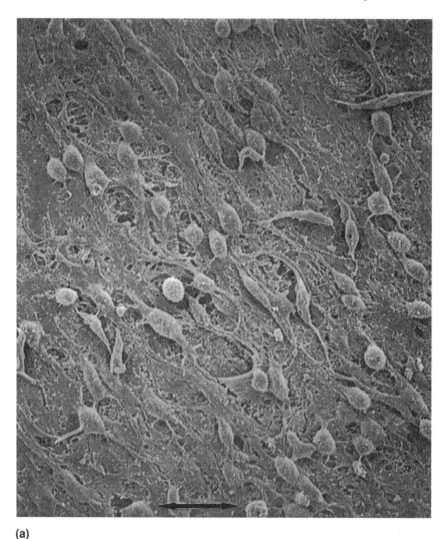

(a)

Figure 3 Scanning electron micrograph of cells on the surface of smooth muscle tissues engineered with type I collagen scaffolds subjected to cyclic strain after 10 weeks (a) and 20 weeks (b). Arrow indicates direction of applied strain. (From Ref. 25.)

the polymer. In the first mode, the pore size in the polymer and the size of the drug interact to control the diffusion rate. The second mode is controlled by the degradation mechanism of the polymer, which can be modified to give varied release rates. In the final mechanism, osmosis or swelling as a

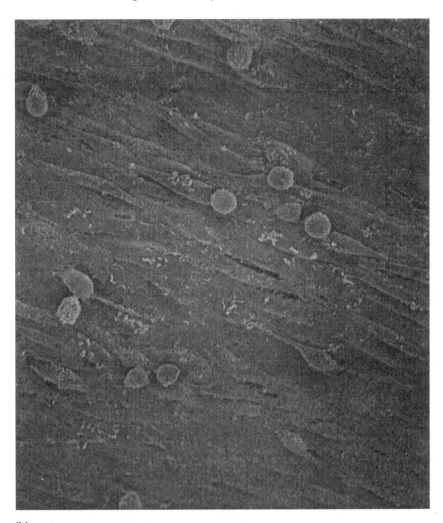

(b)

Figure 3

result of fluid entering the polymer helps control the release of the drug from the matrix.

A. Protein Delivery

Growth factors regulate many facets of cell activity by binding to specific cellular receptors, which then inhibit or promote cellular processes. The delivery of proteins either in vitro or in vivo can locally stimulate cellular processes to facilitate the inductive and cell transplantation approaches to tissue engineering. However, the in vivo delivery of proteins is complicated by the short biological half-lives of many growth factors as well as unfavorable pharmacokinetics (61,62). To overcome these barriers, proteins are being incorporated directly into the tissue engineering scaffold during fabrication for localized delivery.

Scaffolds composed of natural polymers and hydrogels have been used to deliver growth factors, often with improved preservation of bioactivity compared to growth factor in solution. Alginate has been used to encapsulate and release various proteins, such as EGF, fibroblast growth factor (FGF), insulin, nerve growth factor (NGF), and TGF (63). Small molecules diffuse through the alginate pores independent of the alginate structure, while larger molecules (e.g., proteins) show diffusion that depends on molecular weight, giving controlled release. For example, vascular endothelial growth factor (VEGF), a growth factor specific for endothelial cells and capable of stimulating angiogenesis, encapsulated in alginate beads showed a small initial burst of 8% and a constant release of 5% per day for 2 weeks in vitro (64). The released VEGF activity was determined to be three to five times greater than the same mass of VEGF directly applied to endothelial cells in culture. It was hypothesized that an interaction exists between VEGF and alginate that preserves VEGF's bioactivity and slows its release from the gel. When used to encapsulate endothelial cell growth factor (ECGF), 64% was released during the first 2 weeks, followed by decreasing release rates for the following 6 weeks (65). The ECGF maintained bioactivity throughout this time, and in vivo assays showed angiogenesis in rats when compared to unmodified alginate implants. Similar results with protein delivery have been obtained for hydrogels of hyaluronan, collagen, and fibrin. Incorporation and release of FGF and platelet-derived growth factor (PDGF) enhanced proliferation and sustained the biological activity (66). An alternative approach involves developing scaffolds that restrict the passive diffusion of proteins from the material and maintains an elevated concentration within the scaffold. Fibrin matrices modified with peptides containing a heparin-binding domain can immobilize heparin-binding growth factors electrostatically rather than covalently (67). It is hypothesized that the electrostatic interaction of the fibrin matrix limits passive diffusion of basic fibroblast growth factor (bFGF), thus enabling release following enzymatic degradation of the fibrin matrix by infiltrating cells. In vitro studies of heparin-bFGF scaffolds enhanced neurite extension nearly 100% in comparison with unmodified fibrin.

Controlled drug release in the cellular environment can alternatively be achieved through incorporation of drug-loaded microspheres into the tissue engineering scaffold. Numerous techniques can be employed to fabricate microspheres loaded with tissue-inductive proteins that are capable of controlled and sustained release (68). Microspheres can be incorporated into the scaffolds during fabrication or can be mixed with cells that are subsequently seeded onto the scaffold. PLG microspheres have been fabricated that release EGF for up to a month in vitro, and have demonstrated the ability to stimulate DNA synthesis and cell division and to improve the survival of isolated hepatocytes (69). Mixing of the microspheres with hepatocytes and subsequent seeding onto a PLA scaffold and in vivo implantation increased hepatocyte engraftment. Similarly, TGF-$\beta1$ was encapsulated in microspheres and incorporated into a polypropylene fumarate substrate (70). Marrow stromal cells cultured on the scaffold showed an enhanced proliferation and osteoblastic differentiation. Lipid microcylinders have been developed that encapsulate and release physiologically significant levels of nerve growth factor for at least 7 days in vitro (71). Embedding of these cylinders into laminin-modified hydrogels of agarose has stimulated the directional neurite extension from dorsal root ganglia.

Recently, synthetic tissue engineering scaffolds have been fabricated into which proteins are incorporated directly into the polymer. The processing techniques create a highly porous structure with an interconnected open-pore structure and retain the activity of the incorporated growth factor. Supercritical CO_2 has been used to fabricate scaffolds from PLG with encapsulated bFGF (72). The release kinetics showed no large initial burst with nearly constant release for 3 weeks. However, there was a reduction in the activity of the protein. High-pressure CO_2 was similarly used in a gas foaming/particulate leach process has been used to fabricate PLG scaffolds with incorporated VEGF (73,74). An initial release of 20% of the incorporated protein was observed to occur in the 2 days followed by a sustained release for up to 40 days. The release kinetics of protein could be regulated by using different copolymer ratios. Importantly, protein collected during the first 14 days of release retained more than 90% of its bioactivity. Release of VEGF from the tissue engineering scaffolds may stimulate angiogenesis by endothelial cells in the surrounding tissue that is necessary to supply the developing tissue with the necessary nutrients. PLLA scaffolds loaded with sulfohodamine B and alkaline phosphatase show an initial burst followed by slow release of protein, with a loss of only 25% of bioactivity (75).

Nerve guidance channels capable of sustained release of neurotrophic factors have been developed to stimulate the regeneration of damaged nerves. A dip molding technique was used to fabricate tubular devices of ethylene vinyl acetate (EVA) with entrapped bFGF and bovine serum albumin (BSA) (76). Ethylene vinyl acetate is a nondegradable polymer in which drug is released through interconnected pores created by the incorporated proteins. The exterior of the tubular device was coated with EVA (without protein) to ensure that the protein release was directed to the lumen. More recently, the purine analogue inosine has been incorporated and released from cylindrical polymer foams of PLG that were formed by an injection molding process (77). The incorporated drug was released over a period of at least 9 weeks in vitro, and in vivo studies have demonstrated an increase in the mean fiber diameter of a regenerating nerve.

B. Gene Delivery

The delivery of genes encoding for therapeutic or tissue inductive proteins—an approach termed gene therapy—represents a powerful alternative to direct delivery of the protein. The aim of gene therapy is to treat disease by delivering DNA, RNA, or antisense sequences that alter gene expression within a specific cell population, thereby manipulating cellular processes and responses. The delivery of genes encoding for therapeutic proteins that increases their expression is the traditional view of somatic gene therapy; however, we include in our definition antisense and antigene approaches, aimed at blocking expression at the level of transcription or translation (78,79). Though gene therapy was originally devised for the treatment of inherited genetic disorders, such as cystic fibrosis, recent work has expanded the applications of gene therapy to include wound healing and tissue engineering (80,81).

Cellular gene expression can be manipulated either ex vivo or in vivo. The ex vivo approach involves genetically modifying cells, isolated either from the patient or from a donor, that are subsequently implanted into the patient (82). Ex vivo gene delivery provides a relatively high gene transfer efficiency. Once modified, the cells can be seeded onto tissue engineering scaffolds and implanted. The genetically modified cells are typically designed to act as bioreactors for the localized secretion of tissue inductive or wound healing growth factors. This approach has been utilized for numerous applications (reviewed in Refs. 83–85) such as the modification of keratinocytes to enhance dermal repair or Schwann cells to enhance nerve regeneration (86). The duration and amount of protein production by these transplanted cells, which must be sufficient to stimulate physiological responses, may be affected by the supporting scaffold (87).

In vivo delivery of DNA can avoid the need for cell transplantation but is limited by the ability to deliver DNA safely and efficiently to the desired cell population (88). Viral vectors generally provide the most efficient gene transfer, which is a result of viruses having evolved efficient methods to introduce DNA into host cells. The limited space to insert genes in the viral genome combined with issues associated with virus production and safety have inspired the development of systems to deliver nonviral DNA. Nonviral approaches typically involve plasmid DNA (i.e., circular loops of DNA), which are generally considered safe; however, the gene transfer efficiency is significantly less than that of viral vectors and must be improved for many therapeutic applications. Effective in vivo delivery requires that the plasmid be delivered to the desired cell population, be efficiently internalized by the cell, and be transported to the appropriate cellular compartment. Many barriers are present that limit the efficiency of delivery, including degradation (89), clearance from the tissue (90,91), and the inability to cross biological membranes due to its size and charge density (92). The polymeric systems developed to deliver biologically active proteins have been adapted to deliver nonviral DNA in order to overcome some of these limitations. Encapsulation of DNA in the polymer can protect against its degradation. Sustained-delivery systems can overcome difficulties associated with clearance from the tissue and can increase gene transfer (93). Finally, many of the polymeric materials used for encapsulation also support cell adhesion (e.g., collagen, PLG); thus, the cells are adhered to the material from which the DNA is being released, which may create a high concentration at the cell surface that can enhance gene transfer (94). This association of DNA with the ECM to obtain localized gene delivery is an approach used by viruses to enhance uptake (95).

DNA release from tissue engineering scaffolds has led to expression of the transgene in sufficient quantities to stimulate physiological responses and new-tissue formation in vivo (96,97). These scaffolds were implanted at a specific anatomical location to create and maintain a space for tissue formation. Cells from the adjacent tissue subsequently infiltrated the scaffold, where they encountered DNA that had been encapsulated. Thus far, genes encoding for secreted hormones or growth factors have been utilized to increase their production locally. Collagen-based systems for plasmid delivery have been used for applications in bone regeneration (97,98). In these applications, collagen functions to entrap the nonviral DNA and also provides a scaffold that supports cell attachment and cell migration. The nonviral DNA is incapable of diffusing through the collagen carrier. Thus, the matrix serves to hold DNA in situ until endogenous repair fibroblasts infiltrate the scaffold, internalize the DNA, and express the encoded protein. The delivery of 100 mg of PTH plasmid from collagen matrices resulted in bone regeneration across a 1.6-cm defect over a 6-month period. Alternatively, PLG scaffolds with entrapped DNA were fabricated using the gas foaming/particulate leaching process (96) with an incorporation efficiency of 50%. Release studies demonstrated a sustained release of

DNA for more than 30 days. Implantation of these matrices into a subcutaneous pocket led to transfected cells throughout the polymer (Fig. 4). Release of a plasmid encoding for PDGF resulted in sufficient protein production to induce physiological responses at 4 weeks in vivo that were significantly greater than that obtained by delivery of a control plasmid (Fig. 5).

Antisense oligonucleotides (ONs)—short single-stranded pieces of DNA that bind to messenger RNA and block translation—have similarly been delivered from polymer systems to direct responses both in vitro and in vivo. Bolus delivery of ONs can typically alter gene expression for only 24 to 48 hours (78,99); thus, sustained delivery may be particularly effective for the delivery of antisense ONs (100). Antisense ONs targeted to genes involved in cell proliferation have been delivered from polymeric systems to inhibit proliferation of smooth muscle cells both in vitro and in vivo (101–103). Although this approach has potential to manipulate cellular responses, delivery from within tissue engineering scaffolds has yet to be examined.

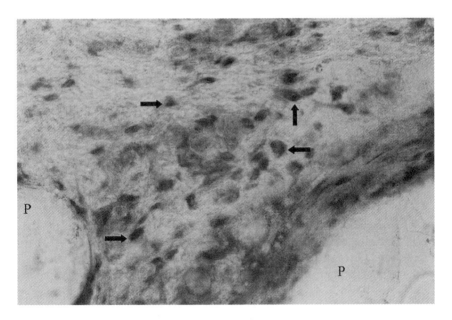

Figure 4 Photomicrograph of cross-section of tissue containing polymer matrix loaded with nuclear targeted β-galactosidase (400×) 4 weeks after implantation. Samples were cryosectioned and stained with X-gal. Polymer is labeled with P and arrows indicate stained nuclei. (From Ref. 96.)

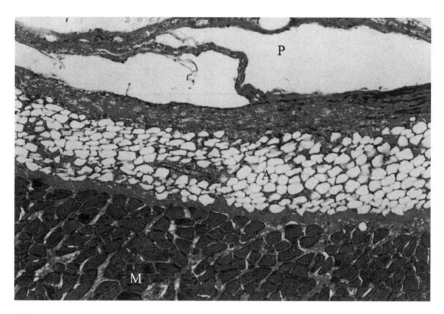

(a)

Figure 5 Photomicrographs of tissue cross-section after 4 weeks of implantation for matrix releasing (a) a control plasmid and (b) a plasmid encoding PDGF. Photomicrographs (100×) are labeled for polymer (P), granulation tissue (G), muscle layer (M), and adipose tissue (A). (From Ref. 96.)

V. CONCLUSIONS AND FUTURE DIRECTIONS

The development of scaffolds with controlled surfaces, mechanical properties, and controlled drug delivery have considerable promise for the three approaches to tissue engineering: conductive, inductive, and cell transplantation. The scaffold functions as a controlled environment into which specific signals can be delivered to direct cellular responses. The ultimate goal in the development of these scaffolds is to obtain temporal and spatial control over the presentation or delivery of specific signals in order to precisely direct the complex series of events that normally occur during tissue formation. Though the signals were presented individually in this chapter, there exists a synergy between them, e.g., (104), which can be incorporated into the design. For example, a system was recently developed in which mechanical stimulation of the implant enhanced the release rate of encapsulated drug (105). These tissue engineering scaffolds can be used as model systems to investigate the signals necessary to stimulate tissue

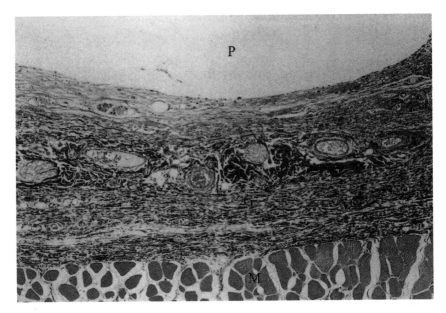

(b)

Figure 5 Continued

formation and the preferred mechanism by which to deliver those signals (e.g., protein vs. gene). These fundamental studies combined with the development of novel systems for the controlled presentation of these signals will eventually lead to novel therapeutic strategies for patients suffering from tissue loss or organ failure.

REFERENCES

1. R Langer, JP Vacanti. Tissue engineering. Science 260:920–926, 1993.
2. AJ Putnam, DJ Mooney. Tissue engineering using synthetic extracellular matrices. Nat Med 2:824–826, 1996.
3. WL Murphy, DJ Mooney. Controlled delivery of inductive proteins, plasmid DNA and cells from tissue engineering matrices. J Periodontal Res 34:413–419, 1999.
4. R O'Neal, HL Wang, RL MacNeil, MJ Somerman. Cells and materials involved in guided tissue regeneration. Curr Opin Periodontol 141–156, 1994.
5. RC Williams, JD Beck, SN Offenbacher. The impact of new technologies to diagnose and treat periodontal disease. A look to the future. J Clin Periodontol 23:299–305, 1996.

6. KP Rao. Recent developments of collagen-based materials for medical applications and drug delivery systems. J Biomater Sci Polym Ed 7:623–645, 1995.
7. JM Pachence. Collagen-based devices for soft tissue repair. J Biomed Mater Res 33:35–40, 1996.
8. FG Giancotti, E Ruoslahti. Integrin signaling. Science 285:1028–1032, 1999.
9. JR Fraser, TC Laurent, UB Laurent. Hyaluronan: its nature, distribution, functions and turnover. J Intern Med 242:27–33, 1997.
10. BP Toole. Hyaluronan in morphogenesis. J Intern Med 242:35–40, 1997.
11. J Entwistle, CL Hall, EA Turley. HA receptors: regulators of signalling to the cytoskeleton. J Cell Biochem 61:569–577, 1996.
12. K Tomihata, Y Ikada. Crosslinking of hyaluronic acid with water-soluble carbodiimide. J Biomed Mater Res 37:243–251, 1997.
13. GD Prestwich, DM Marecak, JF Marecek, KP Vercruysse, MR Ziebell. Controlled chemical modification of hyaluronic acid: synthesis, applications, and biodegradation of hydrazide derivatives. J Controlled Release 53:93–103, 1998.
14. P Bulpitt, D Aeschlimann. New strategy for chemical modification of hyaluronic acid: preparation of functionalized derivatives and their use in the formation of novel biocompatible hydrogels. J Biomed Mater Res 47:152–169, 1999.
15. LA Solchaga, JU Yoo, M Lundberg, JE Dennis, BA Huibregtse, VM Goldberg, AI Caplan. Hyaluronan-based polymers in the treatment of osteochondral defects. J Orthop Res 18:773–780, 2000.
16. AG Mikos, AJ Thorsen, LA Czerwonka, Y Bao, R Langer. Peparation and characterization of poly(L-lactic acid) foams. Polymer 35:1068–1077, 1994.
17. DJ Mooney, CL Mazzoni, C Breuer, K McNamara, D Hern, JP Vacanti, R Langer. Stabilized polyglycolic acid fibre-based tubes for tissue engineering. Biomaterials 17:115–124, 1996.
18. YS Nam, TG Park. Biodegradable polymeric microcellular foams by modified thermally induced phase separation method. Biomaterials 20:1783–1790, 1999.
19. LD Harris, BS Kim, DJ Mooney. Open pore biodegradable matrices formed with gas foaming. J Biomed Mater Res 42:396–402, 1998.
20. JA Hubbell. Biomaterials in tissue engineering. Biotechnology (N Y) 13:565–576, 1995.
21. JA Chin. Biomaterials: protein–surface interactions. In: JD Bronzino, ed. The biomedical engineering handbook. Boca Raton: CRC Press, 1995, pp 1597–1608.
22. JS Tjia, BJ Aneskievich, PV Moghe. Substrate-adsorbed collagen and cell secreted fibronectin concertedly induce cell migration on poly(lactide-glycolide) substrates. Biomaterials 20:2223–2233, 1999.
23. J Gao, L Niklason, R Langer. Surface hydrolysis of poly(glycolic acid) meshes increases the seeding density of vascular smooth muscle cells. J Biomed Mater Res 42:417–424, 1998.

24. JJ Hwang, DA Harrington, SI Stupp. Self-assembling biomaterials on tissue engineering scaffolds. In: A Atala, R Lanza, ed. Methods of Tissue Engineering. San Diego: Academic Press, 2001, pp 741–750.

25. BS Kim, J Nikolovski, J Bonadio, E Smiley, DJ Mooney. Engineered smooth muscle tissues: regulating cell phenotype with the scaffold. Exp Cell Res 251:318–328, 1999.

26. DA Grande, C Halberstadt, G Naughton, R Schwartz, R Manji. Evaluation of matrix scaffolds for tissue engineering of articular cartilage grafts. J Biomed Mater Res 34:211–220, 1997.

27. N Rangappa, A Romero, KD Nelson, RC Eberhart, GM Smith. Laminin-coated poly(L-lactide) filaments induce robust neurite growth while providing directional orientation. J Biomed Mater Res 51:625–634, 2000.

28. WH Wong, DJ Mooney. Synthesis and properties of biodegradable polymers used as synthetic matrices for tissue engineering. In: A Atala, DJ Mooney, eds. Synthetic Biodegradable Polymer Scaffolds. Boston: Birkhauser, 1997, pp 49–80.

29. JA Rowley, G Madlambayan, DJ Mooney. Alginate hydrogels as synthetic extracellular matrix materials. Biomaterials 20:45–53, 1999.

30. JJ Marler, A Guha, J Rowley, R Koka, D Mooney, J Upton, JP Vacanti. Soft-tissue augmentation with injectable alginate and syngeneic fibroblasts. Plast Reconstr Surg 105:2049–2058, 2000.

31. DL Hern, JA Hubbell. Incorporation of adhesion peptides into nonadhesive hydrogels useful for tissue resurfacing. J Biomed Mater Res 39:266–276, 1998.

32. JA Hubbell. Matrix effects. In: RP Lanza, R Langer, WL Chick, eds. Principles of Tissue Engineering. Austin: R. G. Landes, 1997, pp 247–262.

33. KC Dee, TT Andersen, R Bizios. Design and function of novel osteoblast-adhesive peptides for chemical modification of biomaterials. J Biomed Mater Res 40:371–377, 1998.

34. JA Hubbell, SP Massia, NP Desai, PD Drumheller. Endothelial cell-selective materials for tissue engineering in the vascular graft via a new receptor. Biotechnology (N Y) 9:568–572, 1991.

35. A Rezania, KE Healy. Biomimetic peptide surfaces that regulate adhesion, spreading, cytoskeletal organization, and mineralization of the matrix deposited by osteoblast-like cells. Biotechnol Prog 15:19–32, 1999.

36. SP Massia, JA Hubbell. An RGD spacing of 440 nm is sufficient for integrin alpha V beta 3-mediated fibroblast spreading and 140 nm for focal contact and stress fiber formation. J Cell Biol 114:1089–1100, 1991.

37. PA DiMilla, JA Stone, JA Quinn, SM Albelda, DA Lauffenburger. Maximal migration of human smooth muscle cells on fibronectin and type IV collagen occurs at an intermediate attachment strength. J Cell Biol 122:729–737, 1993.

38. BT Burgess, JL Myles, RB Dickinson. Quantitative analysis of adhesion-mediated cell migration in three-dimensional gels of RGD-grafted collagen. Ann Biomed Eng 28:110–118, 2000.

39. BK Mann, AT Tsai, T Scott-Burden, JL West. Modification of surfaces with cell adhesion peptides alters extracellular matrix deposition. Biomaterials 20:2281–2286, 1999.

40. LG Griffith. Polymeric biomaterials. Acta. Mater. 48:263–277, 2000.

41. G Maheshwari, G Brown, DA Lauffenburger, A Wells, LG Griffith. Cell adhesion and motility depend on nanoscale RGD clustering. J Cell Sci 113:1677–1686, 2000.

42. N Patel, R Padera, GH Sanders, SM Cannizzaro, MC Davies, R Langer, CJ Roberts, SJ Tendler, PM Williams, KM Shakesheff. Spatially controlled cell engineering on biodegradable polymer surfaces. FASEB J 12:1447–1454, 1998.

43. JP Ranieri, R Bellamkonda, EJ Bekos, JA Gardella, Jr., HJ Mathieu, L Ruiz, P Aebischer. Spatial control of neuronal cell attachment and differentiation on covalently patterned laminin oligopeptide substrates. Int J Dev Neurosci 12:725–735, 1994.

44. LG Griffith, S Lopina. Microdistribution of substratum-bound ligands affects cell function: hepatocyte spreading on PEO-tethered galactose. Biomaterials 19:979–986, 1998.

45. A Park, B Wu, LG Griffith. Integration of surface modification and 3D fabrication techniques to prepare patterned poly(L-lactide) substrates allowing regionally selective cell adhesion. J Biomater Sci Polym Ed 9:89–110, 1998.

46. M Martins-Green. The dynamics of cell–ECM interactions with implications for tissue engineering. In: RP Lanza, R Langer, WL Chick, eds. Principles of Tissue Engineering. Austin: R. G. Landes, 1997, pp 23–46.

47. H Bentz, JA Schroeder, TD Estridge. Improved local delivery of TGF-beta2 by binding to injectable fibrillar collagen via difunctional polyethylene glycol. J Biomed Mater Res 39:539–548, 1998.

48. Y Ito, M Inoue, SQ Liu, Y Imanishi. Cell growth on immobilized cell growth factor. 6. Enhancement of fibroblast cell growth by immobilized insulin and/or fibronectin. J Biomed Mater Res 27:901–907, 1993.

49. PR Kuhl, LG Griffith-Cima. Tethered epidermal growth factor as a paradigm for growth factor-induced stimulation from the solid phase. Nat Med 2:1022–1027, 1996.

50. AJ Putnam, JJ Cunningham, RG Dennis, JJ Linderman, DJ Mooney. Microtubule assembly is regulated by externally applied strain in cultured smooth muscle cells. J Cell Sci 111:3379–3387, 1998.

51. DE Ingber, L Dike, L Hansen, S Karp, H Liley, A Maniotis, H McNamee, D Mooney, G Plopper, J Sims, et al. Cellular tensegrity: exploring how mechanical changes in the cytoskeleton regulate cell growth, migration, and tissue pattern during morphogenesis. Int Rev Cytol 150:173–224, 1994.

52. CG Galbraith, MP Sheetz. Forces on adhesive contacts affect cell function. Curr Opin Cell Biol 10:566–571, 1998.

53. PX Ma, R Langer. Morphology and mechanical function of long-term in vitro engineered cartilage. J Biomed Mater Res 44:217–221, 1999.

54. RT Prajapati, B Chavally-Mis, D Herbage, M Eastwood, RA Brown. Mechanical loading regulates protease production by fibroblasts in three-dimensional collagen substrates. Wound Repair Regen 8:226–237, 2000.

55. BS Kim, DJ Mooney. Engineering smooth muscle tissue with a predefined structure. J Biomed Mater Res 41:322–332, 1998.

56. JA Rowley, DJ Mooney. New Approach for Biomaterial Design: Controlling Cell Function through Mechanics. J Biomed Mater Res (in press).

57. LE Niklason, J Gao, WM Abbott, KK Hirschi, S Houser, R Marini, R Langer. Functional arteries grown in vitro. Science 284:489–493, 1999.

58. BS Kim, J Nikolovski, J Bonadio, DJ Mooney. Cyclic mechanical strain regulates the development of engineered smooth muscle tissue. Nat Biotechnol 17:979–983, 1999.

59. R Langer. Drug delivery and targeting. Nature 392:5–10, 1998.

60. WR Gombotz, DK Pettit. Biodegradable polymers for protein and peptide drug delivery. Bioconjug Chem 6:332–351, 1995.

61. ME Nimni. Polypeptide growth factors: targeted delivery systems. Biomaterials 18:1201–1225, 1997.

62. JE Babensee, LV McIntire, AG Mikos. Growth factor delivery for tissue engineering. Pharm Res 17:497–504, 2000.

63. S Wee, WR Gombotz. Protein release from alginate matrices. Adv Drug Deliv Rev 31:267–285, 1998.

64. MC Peters, BC Isenberg, JA Rowley, DJ Mooney. Release from alginate enhances the biological activity of vascular endothelial growth factor. J Biomater Sci Polym Ed 9:1267–1278, 1998.

65. CY Ko, V Dixit, WW Shaw, G Gitnick. Extensive in vivo angiogenesis from the controlled release of endothelial cell growth factor: implications for cell transplantation and wound healing. J Controlled Release 44:209–214, 1997.

66. F Roy, C DeBlois, CJ Doillon. Extracellular matrix analogs as carriers for growth factors: in vitro fibroblast behavior. J Biomed Mater Res 27:389–397, 1993.

67. SE Sakiyama-Elbert, JA Hubbell. Development of fibrin derivatives for controlled release of heparin-binding growth factors. J Controlled Release 65:389–402, 2000.

68. H Okada, H Toguchi. Biodegradable microspheres in drug delivery. Crit Rev Ther Drug Carrier Syst 12:1–99, 1995.

69. DJ Mooney, PM Kaufmann, K Sano, SP Schwendeman, K Majahod, B Schloo, JP Vacanti, R Langer. Localized delivery of epidermal growth factor improves the survival of transplanted hepatocytes. Biotechnol Bioeng 50:422–429, 1996.

70. SJ Peter, L Lu, DJ Kim, GN Stamatas, MJ Miller, MJ Yaszemski, AG Mikos. Effects of transforming growth factor beta1 released from biodegradable polymer microparticles on marrow stromal osteoblasts cultured on poly (propylene fumarate) substrates. J Biomed Mater Res 50:452–462, 2000.

71. X Yu, GP Dillon, RB Bellamkonda. A laminin and nerve growth factor-laden three-dimensional scaffold for enhanced neurite extension. Tissue Eng 5:291–304, 1999.

72. DD Hile, ML Amirpour, A Akgerman, MV Pishko. Active growth factor delivery from poly(D,L-lactide-*co*-glycolide) foams prepared in supercritical CO(2). J Controlled Release 66:177–185, 2000.

73. MH Sheridan, LD Shea, MC Peters, DJ Mooney. Bioabsorbable polymer scaffolds for tissue engineering capable of sustained growth factor delivery. J Controlled Release 64:91–102, 2000.

74. WL Murphy, MC Peters, DH Kohn, DJ Mooney. Sustained release of vascular endothelial growth factor from mineralized poly(lactide-*co*-glycolide) scaffolds for tissue engineering. Biomaterials 21:2521–2527, 2000.

75. H Lo, MS Ponticello, KW Leong. Fabrication of Controlled Release Biodegradable Foams by Phase Separation. Tissue Eng 1:15–28, 1995.

76. P Aebischer, AN Salessiotis, SR Winn. Basic fibroblast growth factor released from synthetic guidance channels facilitates peripheral nerve regeneration across long nerve gaps. J Neurosci Res 23:282–289, 1989.

77. T Hadlock, C Sundback, R Koka, D Hunter, M Cheney, J Vacanti. A novel, biodegradable polymer conduit delivers neurotrophins and promotes nerve regeneration. Laryngoscope 109:1412–1416, 1999.

78. CF Bennett. Antisense oligonucleotides: is the glass half full or half empty? Biochem Pharmacol 55:9–19, 1998.

79. PP Chan, PM Glazer. Triplex DNA: fundamentals, advances, and potential applications for gene therapy. J Mol Med 75:267–282, 1997.

80. C Andree, WF Swain, CP Page, MD Macklin, J Slama, D Hatzis, E Eriksson. In vivo transfer and expression of a human epidermal growth factor gene accelerates wound repair. Proc Natl Acad Sci USA 91:12188–12192, 1994.

81. J Bonadio, SA Goldstein, RJ Levy. Gene therapy for tissue repair and regeneration. Adv Drug Del Rev 33:53–69, 1998.

82. PL Chang, KM Bowie. Development of engineered cells for implantation in gene therapy. Adv Drug Del Rev 33:31–43, 1998.

83. SM Shenaq, ED Rabinovsky. Gene therapy for plastic and reconstructive surgery. Clin Plast Surg 23:157–171, 1996.

84. SA Eming, JR Morgan, A Berger. Gene therapy for tissue repair: approaches and prospects. Br J Plast Surg 50:491–500, 1997.

85. AN Salyapongse, TR Billiar, H Edington. Gene therapy and tissue engineering. Clin Plast Surg 26:663–676, 1999.

86. N Weidner, A Blesch, RJ Grill, MH Tuszynski. Nerve growth factor-hypersecreting Schwann cell grafts augment and guide spinal cord axonal growth and remyelinate central nervous system axons in a phenotypically appropriate manner that correlates with expression of L1. J Comp Neurol 413:495–506, 1999.

87. MJ Petersen, J Kaplan, CM Jorgensen, LA Schmidt, L Li, JR Morgan, MK Kwan, GG Krueger. Sustained production of human transferrin by

transduced fibroblasts implanted into athymic mice: a model for somatic gene therapy. J Invest Dermatol 104:171–176, 1995.

88. WF Anderson. Human gene therapy. Nature 392:25–30, 1998.
89. K Kawabata, Y Takakura, M Hashida. The fate of plasmid DNA after intravenous injection in mice: involvement of scavenger receptors in its hepatic uptake. Pharm Res 12:825–830, 1995.
90. KA Choate, PA Khavari. Direct cutaneous gene delivery in a human genetic skin disease. Hum Gene Ther 8:1659–1665, 1997.
91. MY Levy, LG Barron, KB Meyer, FC Szoka, Jr. Characterization of plasmid DNA transfer into mouse skeletal muscle: evaluation of uptake mechanism, expression and secretion of gene products into blood. Gene Ther 3:201–211, 1996.
92. FD Ledley. Pharmaceutical approach to somatic gene therapy. Pharm Res 13:1595–1614, 1996.
93. T Imaoka, I Date, T Ohmoto, T Yasuda, M Tsuda. In vivo gene transfer into the adult mammalian central nervous system by continuous injection of plasmid DNA–cationic liposome complex. Brain Res 780:119–128, 1998.
94. D Luo, WM Saltzman. Enhancement of transfection by physical concentration of DNA at the cell surface. Nat Biotechnol 18:893–895, 2000.
95. DA Williams. Retroviral-fibronectin interactions in transduction of mammalian cells. Ann N Y Acad Sci 872:109–113; discussion 113–104, 1999.
96. LD Shea, E Smiley, J Bonadio, DJ Mooney. DNA delivery from polymer matrices for tissue engineering. Nat Biotechnol 17:551–554, 1999.
97. J Bonadio, E Smiley, P Patil, S Goldstein. Localized, direct plasmid gene delivery in vivo: prolonged therapy results in reproducible tissue regeneration. Nat Med 5:753–759, 1999.
98. J Fang, YY Zhu, E Smiley, J Bonadio, JP Rouleau, SA Goldstein, LK McCauley, BL Davidson, BJ Roessler. Stimulation of new bone formation by direct transfer of osteogenic plasmid genes. Proc Natl Acad Sci USA 93:5753–5758, 1996.
99. SW Ebbinghaus, N Vigneswaran, CR Miller, RA Chee-Awai, CA Mayfield, DT Curiel, DM Miller. Efficient delivery of triplex forming oligonucleotides to tumor cells by adenovirus-polylysine complexes. Gene Ther 3:287–297, 1996.
100. E Wickstrom. Antisense c-myc inhibition of lymphoma growth. Antisense Nucleic Acid Drug Dev 7:225–228, 1997.
101. ER Edelman, M Simons, MG Sirois, RD Rosenberg. c-myc in vasculoproliferative disease. Circ Res 76:176–182, 1995.
102. AE Villa, LA Guzman, EJ Poptic, V Labhasetwar, S D'Souza, CL Farrell, EF Plow, RJ Levy, PE DiCorleto, EJ Topol. Effects of antisense c-myb oligonucleotides on vascular smooth muscle cell proliferation and response to vessel wall injury. Circ Res 76:505–513, 1995.
103. RL Cleek, AA Rege, LA Denner, SG Eskin, AG Mikos. Inhibition of smooth muscle cell growth in vitro by an antisense oligodeoxynucleotide released from

poly(DL-lactic-co-glycolic acid) microparticles. J Biomed Mater Res 35:525–530, 1997.

104. G Maheshwari, A Wells, LG Griffith, DA Lauffenburger. Biophysical integration of effects of epidermal growth factor and fibronectin on fibroblast migration. Biophys J 76:2814–2823, 1999.

105. KY Lee, MC Peters, KW Anderson, DJ Mooney. Controlled growth factor release from synthetic extracellular matrices. Nature 408:998–1000, 2000.

10
Chitosan as a Molecular Scaffold for Biomimetic Design of Glycopolymer Biomaterials

Howard W. T. Matthew
Wayne State University, Detroit, Michigan

I. INTRODUCTION

Polysaccharides have long been recognized as a unique family of polymeric materials with an array of properties that have made them indispensable for applications ranging from adhesives to viscosity modifiers. The characteristics have included such features as high swelling ratios in aqueous media, environmentally controlled gellation properties, high-viscosity solutions at low concentrations, and so forth. As a result, they have found wide acceptance as food and drug additives designed to enhance rehydration, texture, and various other physical properties. Over the past 20 years, the biological properties of a variety of oligosaccharides and polysaccharides have been explored and a growing body of work has served to raise their profile as mediators and modulators of receptor-based phenomena such as cell signaling and direct cell–cell and cell–pathogen interactions. Yet despite their recognized strengths and intriguing properties, these materials have remained underutilized as components of implantable material structures. However, in recent years the explosion of research in tissue engineering and regenerative medicine has created a growing demand for biologically active materials whose properties may be harnessed to facilitate tissue assembly and organization. As a result, more attention is being paid to saccharide-based materials for implant applications.

While many polysaccharides possess potentially useful biological activities, relatively few also exhibit material properties that would allow their use as structural materials or tissue scaffolds within the tissue engineering paradigm. For example, the tissue polysaccharides termed glycosaminoglycans exhibit a very broad array of biologically useful interactions with enzymes, matrix proteins, and cell surface receptors. But their direct water solubility limits applications to cases where they can be covalently attached to more structurally suitable materials. Chitosan [β(1–3)poly-D-glucosamine] is one glycopolymer that exhibits both structural potential and useful biological activity. As such it is an excellent starting template for the design of a wide variety of modified glycopolymers that may exhibit superior performance in several areas, including the tunability of physical and degradation properties, and modulation of cell and tissue responses. A generic biomimetic approach to generating such materials may involve adding relatively simple functional groups that introduce molecular features that essentially encode the biological activity of other saccharide moieties while retaining the capability to perform as a structural polymer. Alternatively, simple architectural modifications can be used to tune the physical or biological properties of the polymer by creating new intra- or intermolecular interactions. In this chapter, various approaches to controlling and adjusting chitosan's physical, mechanical, and biological properties will be discussed.

II. STRUCTURE AND MOLECULAR FEATURES

The chitosan family of materials are derivatives of chitin, the primary structural polymer in arthropod exoskeletons. Chitin is a high molecular weight glycopolymer composed of N-acetyl-D-glucosamine units linked via β(1→4) glycosidic bonds. Chitosans are prepared by deacetylating chitin to varying degrees. The primary source for chitin/chitosan is shells from crustaceans such as crab or shrimp. Shells are ground, demineralized with HCl, deproteinized with a protease or dilute NaOH, and then deacetylated with concentrated NaOH. Structurally, chitosans are very similar to cellulose. The polymer is linear, consisting of β(1→4)-linked D-glucosamine residues with a variable number of randomly located N-acetylglucosamine groups (Fig. 1). In essence, chitosan is cellulose with the 2-hydroxyl group replaced by an amino or acetylated amino group. Depending on the source and preparation procedure, molecular weights may range from 50 kDa to 1000 kDa. Preparations with degrees of deacetylation ranging from 70% to 90% are commercially available. Higher degrees of deacetylation are not usually prepared because the reaction time required results in excessive depolymerization and a low molecular weight product.

Chitosan is a semicrystalline polysaccharide with the degree of crystallinity being a function of the degree of deacetylation. Crystallinity

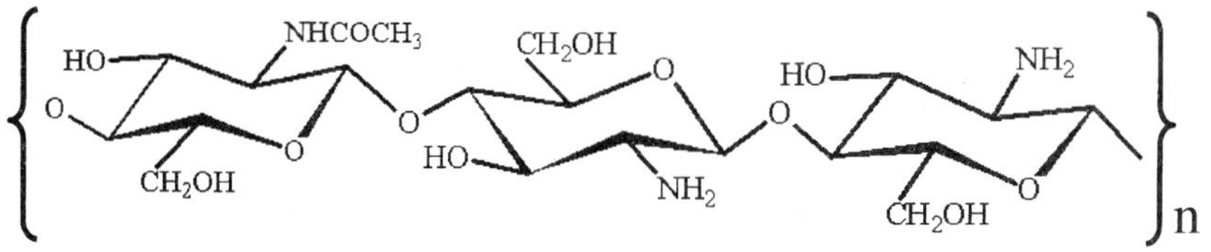

Figure 1 Repeating structure of chitosan. An acetylated residue is shown linked to two deacetylated residues.

exhibits maxima for both native chitin (i.e., 0% deacetylated) and fully (i.e., 100%) deacetylated chitosan. Minimal crystallinity is achieved at intermediate degrees of deacetylation. The crystalline structure results in the polymer being insoluble in neutral or basic aqueous solutions. However, in dilute acids (pH < 6) the protonation of free amino groups produces crystallite disruption, swelling, and dissolution. Charge repulsion in solution causes the polymer chain to extend into a flexible rod conformation. Upon raising the pH, amino groups are increasingly deprotonated and become available for hydrogen bonding. At some critical pH, which is dependent on the degree of deacetylation and molecular weight, the molecules in solution develop enough hydrogen bonds to establish a gel network. As the pH is raised further, deprotonation continues and the molecules establish additional hydrogen bonds, ultimately rearranging to establish miniature crystalline domains. This effect results in an increase in gel stiffness and is associated with increased light scattering (i.e., opacity of the gel) and some gel contraction.

Unlike its analogue cellulose, chitosan is clearly hydrolyzed enzymatically in vivo. The primary agent is lysozyme, which appears to target acetylated residues (1). However, there is evidence that a number of proteolytic enzymes show significant hydrolytic activity with chitosan. The most active proteases include pepsin, papain, and pancreatin (2,3). The lysozyme-mediated degradation products are chitosan oligosaccharides of variable length. The degradation kinetics appear to be inversely related to the degree of crystallinity. In fact, the low degradation rate of highly deacetylated chitosan implants is believed to be due to the inability of hydrolytic enzymes to penetrate the crystalline microstructure. Highly deacetylated forms (e.g., > 85%) exhibit the lowest degradation rates and may last several months in vivo, whereas samples with lower levels of deacetylation degrade more rapidly. This issue has been addressed by derivatizing the molecule with side chains of various types (4–7). Such treatments alter molecular chain packing and increase the amorphous fraction, allowing more rapid degradation. They also inherently affect both the mechanical and solubility properties.

As a gel-forming polymer, chitosan has been widely studied for applications in systems for the controlled release of various drugs and therapeutic agents. These applications have been extensively reviewed (8–10).

III. INTRINSIC BIOLOGICAL PROPERTIES

The chitosan repeat structure contains motifs specifically glucosamine and N-acetylglucosamine which are found in a number of glycosaminoglycans (GAGs). As such the molecule possesses features that may be recognized as innocuous components of the extracellular matrix (ECM). Alternatively, the GAG-like structure may encode some of the biological activity associated with GAGs or other cell surface saccharide structures. However, the positive charge imparted by the free amino group is not found among the GAGs, which are invariably anionic. This feature may allow chitosan to interact with cellular receptors and matrix proteins in unique ways based on a combination of stereospecific glycan binding and nonspecific charge interactions. In fact, chitosan oligosaccharides have been shown to have stimulatory activity on macrophages, and the effect has been linked to the acetylated residues (11). It has also been shown that chitosan oligosaccharides synergize with interferon-γ to enhance nitric oxide release and the tumor killing capabilities of macrophages (12,13). This effect was apparently mediated by chitosan's enhancement of the level of tumor necrosis factor-α (TNF-α) secretion. Furthermore, both chitosan and its parent molecule chitin have been shown to exert chemoattractive effects on neutrophils in vitro and in vivo (14–17).

A number of researchers have examined the tissue response to an assortment of chitosan-based implants (4,18–27). In general, these materials have been found to evoke a minimal foreign body reaction. In most cases, no significant fibrous encapsulation developed. Formation of normal granulation tissue, often with accelerated angiogenesis, appears to be the typical course of healing (28–30). In the short term (< 10 days), significant accumulation of neutrophils in the vicinity of the implants is often seen, but this dissipates rapidly and a chronic inflammatory response does not develop. The stimulatory effects of chitosan oligosaccharides on immune cells, mentioned above, probably plays a major role in these favorable tissue responses. Specifically, release of growth factors and cytokines by stimulated macrophages may induce local fibroblast and endothelial cell proliferation.

Ultimately, this leads to formation of a highly cellular and well-vascularized repair, followed by integration of the chitosan implant with the host tissue. Overall, the published results indicate that chitosan-based materials exhibit a very high degree of biocompatibility in a variety of subcutaneous and intraperitoneal implantation models. The precise mechanisms leading to broad biocompatibility and good tissue acceptance are still not well understood. However, a relatively benign interaction with plasma proteins leading to low or negligible rates of protein denaturation and fragmentation on the implant surface may be one factor contributing to the generally positive tissue responses.

In the area of blood interactions, chitosan has been shown to have a strong hemostatic capacity. Blood coagulation is achieved rapidly even under conditions of heparin anticoagulation (31,32). The process involves fibrin-independent aggregation of erythrocytes, possibly through direct chitosan interactions with erythrocyte membrane proteins (31–34). Platelets have been shown to adhere to and be activated by chitosan. However, it is not clear if this is mediated by a direct interaction mechanism or is merely the result of a platelet response to bound plasma protein components.

IV. MODIFICATIONS IN MOLECULAR ARCHITECTURE

From a chemical properties standpoint, the simplest modifications to native chitosan involve changes to the molecular architecture that can be accomplished without significantly altering the main chemical features of the molecule. As mentioned above, chitosan exhibits a linear, semirigid rod conformation in acidic solution. This conformation facilitates the formation of polymer crystallites during neutralization/gellation or casting operations. As with most semicrystalline polymers, the properties of chitosan materials are intimately affected by the level of crystallinity. As a result, molecular changes that affect the ability of the molecules to assemble into crystallites can be expected to affect a variety of material and possibly biological properties. The two simplest alterations to chitosan's molecular architecture involve (a) reducing the molecular weight and (b) introducing molecular branching. Both approaches can be used to tune the physicomechanical properties of chitosan materials.

Reduction of average molecular weight results in shorter chitosan molecules that exhibit greater molecular mobility and are thus more capable of assembling into crystallites. This change may be expected to increase the stiffness and reduce the elasticity of chitosan materials by increasing the overall level of crystallinity. Molecular weight reductions can be accomplished by enzymatic or chemical depolymerization. Both lysozyme and chitinases have been used to cleave chitosan to varying degrees. However, control of the enzymatic process is difficult given the uncertainty associated with enzymatic activity and the time and concentration dependence of the final product. Hence, the chemical depolymerization process is recommended. Chitosan can be stoichiometrically depolymerized in solution by reacting with nitrous acid (35,36). A reaction schematic is shown in Fig. 2. In practical terms, chitosan dissolved in a dilute acid reacts with nitrous acid generated by addition of a nitrite salt (typically $NaNO_2$) with evolution of nitrogen gas. The glucosamine residue on the reducing side of the cleavage point is deaminated and transformed into a 2,5-anhydro-D-mannose residue with a pendant aldehyde group. The stoichiometry of the reaction is such that each nitrite ion cleaves exactly one glycosidic bond. This 1:1 relationship dictates that the average molecular weight of the product is therefore dependent only on the molar ratio of nitrite ion to chitosan glucosamine and is independent of the chitosan molecular weight for preparations with a typical high starting molecular weight. In a well-mixed reaction solution, the average molecular weight of the product can be predicted with a fair degree of precision from the following simplified

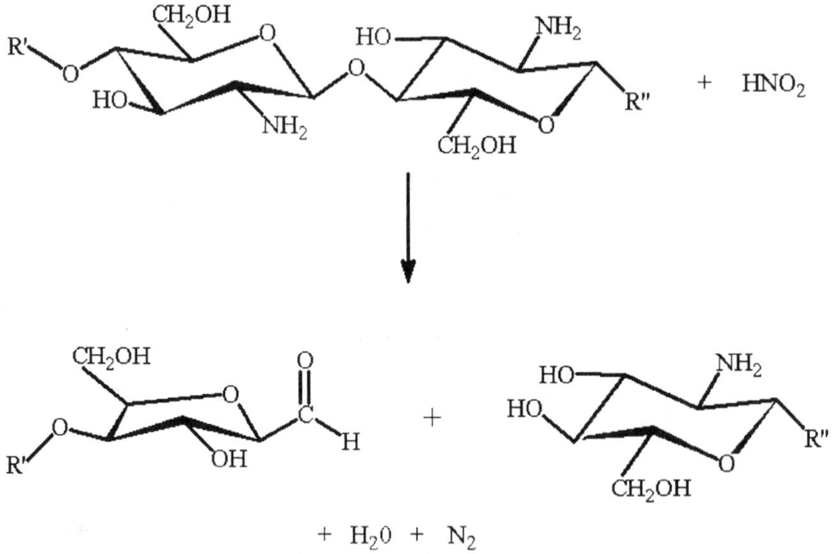

Figure 2   Reaction schematic for the nitrous acid cleavage of a chitosan chain. "R" groups represent extended sections of the chitosan polymer chain. The reaction produces an anhydro-D-mannose residue containing a pendant aldehyde group on the reducing side of the cleavage point.

relationship.

$$M_2 = \frac{m_1}{n(1 - f_d)}$$

where M_2 is the final number average molecular weight, m_1 is the mass of chitosan in solution, n is the number of moles of nitrite added, and f_d is the fraction of nitrous acid that vaporizes or decomposes without reacting. The value of f_d and hence errors in the prediction can be kept below 5% if the chitosan concentration is maintained above 1.5 wt %. The decomposed fraction can be reduced further by minimizing the area of free liquid surface available for HNO_2 evaporation in the reaction vessel (35,36).

Another method of controlling material properties through molecular architecture involves the addition of linear branches identical in structure to the main polymer chain. Branching in chitosan can be easily achieved by grafting low or intermediate molecular weight chitosan chains to amino groups on a high molecular weight chain. Adding branches or side chains increases the molecular weight. However, from a material properties standpoint, its major effect is to reduce the overall crystallinity of the material. Short side chains can interfere with the dense packing and associated hydrogen bonding of the main chains in polymer crystallites and thus reduce the overall material crystallinity. The actual effects of side chain addition on the physical properties of a chitosan hydrogel will be strongly dependent on both the average molecular weight of the side chains and the grafting density of side chains. At one end of the scale, grafting of high molecular weight branches to main chains with similar degrees of polymerization may generate a star polymer architecture. This type of arrangement should exhibit properties not far removed from those of the main chain since the mobility of the side chains would allow crystallite formation similar to that of the unbranched polymer. On the other hand, dense grafting of very low molecular weight side chains would effectively prevent extensive crystallite formation and may produce materials that exhibit very weak gelation or even complete water solubility over the entire pH range.

Chitosan molecules can be grafted to amino groups of other chitosan molecules by the process of reductive amination. In brief, the reducing or aldehyde end of the planned branch molecule is reacted with chitosan amino groups in alcoholic solution to form a Schiff base linkage. The unstable carbon–nitrogen double bond is then reduced to a stable single bond with an appropriate reducing agent (e.g., sodium cyanoborohydride). While every chitosan molecule has a reducing end capable of reacting with amino groups, the fraction of ends that are in the open and reactive (aldehyde) configuration at any instant is very small. As a result, the overall rate of reaction is very low. In contrast, the nitrous acid depolymerization described above generates an aldehyde group as part of the anhydro-D-mannose unit at the reducing end. This permanent aldehyde exhibits much higher reaction rates. Yalpani and coworkers have described the preparation of many oligosaccharide grafted chitosan derivatives with a number of interesting rheological and solubility properties (37–40). However, the biomaterials potential of these and related derivatives remain to be investigated.

The product yield and degree of substitution achievable with the reductive amination procedure may be limited by two phenomena. First, hydrolysis of the Schiff base formed by the initial reaction can regenerate the reactive species. Second, a significant percentage of the available reducing ends exist in the unreactive cyclic conformation. As an alternative scheme, reaction in supercritical fluids may provide a route to superior yield. Specifically, treatment of chitosan with reducing sugars or oligosaccharides in supercritical carbon dioxide has been shown to generate the corresponding branched derivatives with high levels of conversion (41).

V. MATERIAL PROCESSING APPROACHES

One of chitosan's most useful features is its ability to be processed under mild conditions into structures suitable for use as tissue scaffolds or drug carriers. Many tissue engineering approaches to repairing or regenerating damaged tissues make use of polymer scaffolds which serve to support and organize the regenerating tissue (42–45). Release of bioactive substances in order to influence the behavior of seeded or ingrowing cells may also be desirable. Furthermore, many application scenarios call for the use of biodegradable matrices that are amenable to integration with growing tissue. In order to achieve these goals, porous scaffold microstructures are usually employed. Porous chitosan structures can be easily formed by a phase separation method involving freezing and lyophilization of chitosan solutions in suitable molds (46). During the freezing process, ice crystals nucleate from solution and grow along the lines of heat flux. Exclusion of the chitosan salt from the ice crystal phase and subsequent ice removal by lyophilization generates a porous material whose mean pore size can be controlled by varying the freezing conditions. Some control over pore orientation can also be obtained by manipulating the direction of thermal gradients during freezing. Figure 3 illustrates the morphology of typical porous chitosan slabs produced by freezing and lyophilization of a 1.5 wt % chitosan solution in 0.1 M acetic acid.

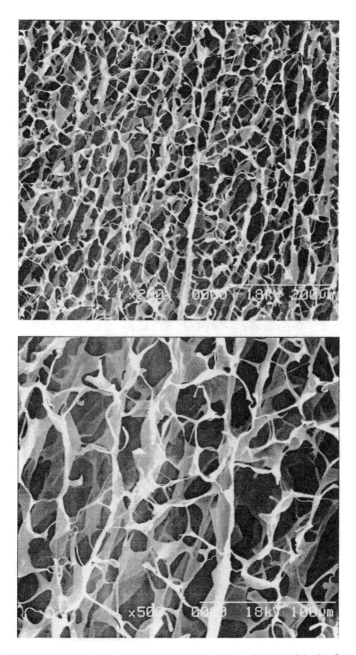

Figure 3   Scanning electron micrographs of porous chitosan blocks formed by freezing and lyophilizing a chitosan solution (1.5 wt % chitosan in 0.1 M acetic acid).

The mechanical properties of these chitosan scaffolds are mainly dependent on the pore sizes and pore orientations. Tensile testing of hydrated samples shows that porous membranes have greatly reduced elastic moduli (0.1–0.5 MPa) compared with nonporous chitosan membranes (5–7 MPa). The extensibility (maximal strain) of porous membranes varied from values similar to nonporous chitosan (~30%) to greater than 100% as a function of both pore size and orientation. The porous membranes also exhibit a stress–strain curve with two distinct regions typical of composite materials: a low-modulus region at low strains and a transition to a several-fold higher modulus at higher strains. For all pore orientations, membranes formed at lower freezing rates exhibited higher moduli in both curve regions. The differences were most notable for samples with a random pore orientation. This suggests that in addition to larger pores, the lower freezing rate produces a more crystalline (and hence stiffer) chitosan phase. The tensile strengths of these porous structures were in the range 30–60 kPa.

As an alternative to the phase separation method, porous tissue scaffolds can also be generated from polymer fibers using nonwoven (or felted) fabric technology. Chitosan materials can be prepared as fibers for this type of application. Chitosan solutions can be extruded through spinnarets of small-gauge needles and gelled in basic solutions (e.g., 5% ammonia) or baths containing nonsolvents (e.g., methanol) (47). These gel fibers can be subsequently drawn and dried to form dense fibers that exhibit much higher strength and stiffness even when hydrated. The polymer has been extensively studied for industrial applications based on film and fiber formation, and the preparation and mechanical properties of these forms have been reviewed previously (8,48). Woven and nonwoven fiber–based structures have potential for applications as implantable biomaterials but have been investigated to only a limited extent (47,49).

VI. ADDITION OF FUNCTIONAL GROUPS

Addition or grafting of functional groups into the chitosan backbone can be used to enhance or drastically alter most of chitosan's physical and biological properties. The effects of adding chitosan oligosaccharides and polymers have already been discussed. Addition of smaller functional groups can have profound effects on the behavior of the molecule, and the effects can be varied over a continuum defined by the degree of substitution and the molecular weight of the side group. The free amino groups are the most common derivatization targets, but there are methods available for targeting the C-3 and C-6 hydroxyl groups. In the sections below, the effects of adding various functional groups and small molecules are described.

A. Ionic Functional Groups

The character of chitosan as cationic, hemostatic, and insoluble at high pH can be completely reversed by the addition of anionic functional groups. Both carboxymethyl and sulfonate derivatives of chitosan have been synthesized. At high degrees of substitution, these molecules tend to be water soluble over a wide pH range. The introduction of these functional groups creates structural motifs that are found in the glycosaminoglycans and, as a result, can impart a number of interesting biological activities similar to those of the GAGs. Carboxymethylation of chitosan can be easily accomplished by reacting with chloroacetic acid (50). The C-6 and C-3 hydroxyl groups and the C-2 amino group are the potential derivatization sites using this scheme. A recent report describes a number of approaches for generating regioselective carboxymethyl and sulfated derives of chitosan and related polysaccharides (51). Thus, glyoxilic acid may be used to selectively carboxymethylate the amino groups. Carboxymethylchitosan has been shown to chelate calcium ions, forming cross-linked gels in a manner very similar to that of alginates. Lyophilized versions of these gels were implanted in vivo and found to promote healing of an experimental nonhealing bone defect in a sheep model (52). N-Carboxymethylchitosan was found to enhance the intestinal absorption of low molecular weight heparin for anticoagulation (53), possibly by a mechanism similar to chitosan's recognized ability to weaken epithelial cell tight junctions (54). A chitosan–polyacrylic acid graft copolymer has been prepared by graft polymerization of acrylic acid onto chitosan backbones (55). The resultant amphiphilic polymer exhibited unusual nonlinear solubility and swelling behavior as a result of the presence of free carboxyl and amino groups capable of pH-dependent ionic cross-linking. Introduction of carboxyl groups can also be accomplished by reacting chitosan with anhydrides of dicarboxylic acids such as succinic anhydride. Highly succinated chitosan is water soluble over a wide pH range and has been shown to circulate in the bloodstream with a half-life (in mice) of more than 100 hours (56,57).

Sulfated chitosan derivatives may be prepared by a number of reaction schemes, including reaction with trimethylamine–sulfur trioxide complexes (51) or concentrated sulfuric acid (oleum) (58). In blood, soluble sulfated chitosan derivatives formed complexes with antithrombin and effectively inhibited both thrombin and factor Xa–mediated coagulation (58,59). Sulfation of the C-6 position was determined to be essential for antic-oagulant activity. However, while sulfation at the C-2 (amino) or C-3 (hydroxyl) positions eliminated chitosan's usual hemostatic/procoagulant activity, these locations conferred negligible anticoagulation activity. In contrast, sulfation at C-2 and C-3 induced potent antiretroviral activity in vitro (60). Complexes of sulfated chitosan with collagen have also been found to support fibroblast attachment and matrix contraction to a much greater extent than collagen–chitosan complexes (61).

B. Nonionic Functional Groups

A number of small, uncharged molecules have been grafted onto chitosan to alter its properties. Grafting of chitosan oligosaccharide side chains has already been described above. Similarly, almost any mono-, di-, or oligosaccharide with a reducing end can be coupled to chitosan via reductive amination. As described for chitosan oligosaccharides, reliance on the native reducing end for reaction typically requires long reaction times. Yalpani and coworkers have described the preparation of many saccharide-modified chitosans using reductive amination methods and reaction times have ranged from several hours to several days (37–40,62,63). However, those studies generally were aimed at forming fully substituted, water-soluble derivatives. If chitosan's structural material potential is to be retained in the modified materials, lower degrees of substitution may be desired and correspondingly lower reaction times may be appropriate.

Other side chain structures that have been grafted include acyl chains and polyethylene glycol (PEG) chains of various molecular weights. Acyl chains have been attached to the amino groups by directly reacting chitosan with anhydrides of organic acids. This reaction produces an amide bond linking the amino and carboxyl groups of the two components. Use of acetic anhydride acetylates amino groups to generate chitosan with lower degrees of deacetylation. At high levels of substitution water insoluble chitin is formed. Chitosan has been derivatized with several carboxylic acid anhydrides, including propionic, n-butanoic, and n-hexanoic anhydrides. N-Acylation levels of 20–50% have been achieved without inducing gelation of the reaction solutions. Examination of the blood compatibility of these products demonstrated that blood compatibility increased with the length of the acyl chain. Thus, while N-acetylchitosan surfaces rapidly accumulated thrombus, no coagulation occurred on the N-hexanoyl derivative (6,34). Lysozyme hydrolysis studies also showed that the rate of degradation of N-acylchitosan films increased with the degree of derivatization. Sulfation of N-acylchitosans generated water-soluble derivatives that tended to aggregate in solution forming polymer micelles for acyl chain lengths greater than 10 carbons (64). These micellar preparations were able to solubilize hydrophobic compounds, and their solvation capacity increased with the length of the acyl chain. Interestingly, while these modified materials showed promising biological properties, no detailed examination of their biomaterials potential has been conducted.

Methoxy-polyethylene glycol (mPEG) side chains have been grafted to chitosan using reductive amination with mPEG aldehydes. This modification reduces the elastic modulus of cast chitosan membranes in direct proportion to the PEG content. Since PEG is a neutral, water-soluble, inert polymer with a large excluded volume, the grafted side chains serve to mask the chitosan surface under hydrated conditions. This masking effect has been shown to reduce the spreading and proliferation of endothelial and smooth muscle cells seeded onto PEG-chitosan membranes as compared with unmodified chitosan membranes (HWT Matthew, unpublished data). PEG dialdehydes have also been used to cross-link chitosan, producing insoluble, swellable hydrogels (3). Surprisingly, while the swollen hydrogels could be digested with papain, no degradation was observed with lysozyme.

VII. FORMATION OF IONIC COMPLEXES

Chitosan's cationic nature allows it to form insoluble polyelectrolyte complexes with a wide variety of water-soluble anionic polymers. Complex formation has been documented with anionic polysaccharides such as heparin and alginates, as well as synthetic polyanions like polyacrylic acid (65–68). Because the chitosan charge is pH dependent, transfer of these polyelectrolyte complexes to a higher pH may result in partial dissociation of the immobilized polyanion. This property can be used as a technique for local delivery of biologically active polyanions such as heparin or even DNA. Heparin release from ionic complexes may enhance the effectiveness of growth factors released by inflammatory cells in the vicinity of an implant (28,69). In the case of DNA, complexation with chitosan has been shown to protect plasmids from degradation by nucleases and also facilitates cellular transfection by poorly understood interactions with cell membranes (70–72). This section of the chapter will focus on chitosan complexes with glycosaminoglycans because of their potential for biomaterials applications.

A. Glycosaminoglycans

Glycosaminoglycans (GAGs) are polysaccharides that occur ubiquitously within the ECM (73). They are unbranched heteropolysaccharides, consisting of repeated disaccharide units, with the general structure: (uronic acid–amino sugar)$_n$. In their native form, several GAG chains are covalently linked to a central protein core, and the protein–polysaccharide complex is termed a *proteoglycan*. Proteoglycans have a major role in organizing and determining the properties and functionality of the ECM, and GAG chains are the major factor in determining proteoglycan properties.

There are six different types of GAGs: chondroitin sulfates, dermatan sulfate, keratan sulfate, heparan sulfate, heparin, and hyaluronic acid. Table 1 lists the component monosaccharides, primary source tissues and molecular features of the commonly occurring GAGs. The monosaccharides in GAGs are sulfated to varying degrees, with the exception of hyaluronic acid, which is not sulfated. Unlike the other GAGs, hyaluronate exists as a free, high molecular weight molecule with no covalently attached protein.

GAGs are usually obtained as salts of sodium, potassium, or ammonia, and in this form they are all water soluble. The presence of strongly ionizing sulfate groups means that the charge density of these molecules is much less pH dependent than in the case of chitosan, and as a result these molecules are soluble over a wide pH range. The disaccharide repeat structure and the resultant alternating glycosidic bond types prevent this family of materials from forming high-strength, crystalline structures in the solid state, and the dried or precipitated GAGs are essentially amorphous. The three-dimensional configurations that do form in solution tend to be flexible coil structures, extended as a result of the charge effects. For example, heparin is known to form single-chain helical structures in solution. The only GAG with significant gel-forming ability is hyaluronate. This high molecular weight molecule is the primary gelling agent in the vitreous humor of the eye and can form very-high-viscosity solutions at concentrations as low as 0.3 wt %.

The biomaterials potential of the GAGs stems not from their intrinsic physical properties but from their biological activity, which is a direct result of their numerous interactions with many important biomolecules. This biological activity can be exploited by binding, complexing, or covalently linking GAG moieties to other polymers with superior structural or mechanical characteristics. Formation of composites of this type can endow the structural polymer with desirable tissue interaction properties and drastically improve its overall biocompatibility. Thus, combining chitosan's structural properties with GAG biological activity in an ionic complex may produce biomaterials with superior potential for tissue repair and regeneration.

B. Glycosaminoglycan Biological Activity

Interactions with enzymes are the most extensively characterized of all GAG–protein interactions. In particular, the anticoagulant activity of heparin, via the activation of the protease inhibitor antithrombin III

Table 1 Glycosaminoglycan Sources and Molecular Properties

Glycosaminoglycan	Source tissues	Molecular weight (kDa)	Charges per disaccharide	Component monosaccharides
Hyaluronate	Vitreous humor, Cartilage	250–8000	1.0	N-Acetyl-D-glucosamine, D-Glucuronic acid
Chondroitin 4-sulfate	Cartilage, cornea, Skin, artery	5–50	1.1–2.0	N-Acetyl-D-galactosamine, D-Glucuronic acid
Chondroitin 6-sulfate	Cartilage, cornea, Skin, artery	5–50	1.2–2.3	N-Acetyl-D-galactosamine, D-Glucuronic acid
Dermatan sulfate	Skin, heart valve, Tendon, artery	15–40	2.0–2.2	N-Acetyl-D-galactosamine, L-Iduronic acid, D-Glucuronic acid
Keratan sulfate	Cartilage, cornea, Vertebral disks	2.5–20	0.9–1.8	N-Acetyl-D-glucosamine, D-Galactose
Heparan sulfate	Lung, artery, Cell surfaces	5–50	1.1–2.8	D-Glucosamine, N-Acetylglucosamine, L-Iduronic acid, D-Glucuronic acid
Heparin	Mast cells in: Lung, liver, skin, Intestinal mucosa	5–25	3–5	D-Glucosamine, L-Iduronic acid, D-Glucuronic acid

Source: Adapted from Ref. 73 with modifications.

(ATIII), has been thoroughly characterized (74,75). ATIII inactivates several proteases in the coagulation cascade, the most important of which is thrombin. Binding of heparin to ATIII increases the inactivation kinetics by as much as 2000-fold. ATIII binding and activation involves highly specific recognition of a pentasaccharide sequence found in both heparin and heparan sulfate. Heparin and heparan sulfate are also known to bind and activate the enzyme lipoprotein lipase (76–78). This property facilitates hydrolysis of triglycerides in lipoprotein particles in peripheral tissues. The fatty acids so formed are then available for uptake by adjacent cells. Lipoprotein lipase is normal found bound to endothelial cell surface heparan sulfate where it is active. The soluble enzyme is inactive in the absence of GAG. This property has been used to reduce the levels of circulating lipoprotein by activating inactive lipase via injections of soluble GAG.

A wide variety of polypeptide growth factors bind avidly to heparin and heparan sulfate. Lower affinity binding also occurs with the other sulfated GAGs. Members of the fibroblast growth factor (FGF) family have been most extensively studied, but heparin/GAG affinity has been demonstrated with epidermal growth factor (EGF), vascular endothelial growth factor (VEGF), a variety of interleukins (e.g., IL-3), as well as hematopoietic factors such as granulocyte colony-stimulating factor (G-CSF), granulocyte-macrophase colony-stimulating factor (GM-CSF) and stem cell factor (SCF). GAG binding can have a variety of effects on growth factors depending on the ratios of the two molecular species and the binding environment. Growth factors can be bound and sequestered in the ECM by GAGs. In the bound state, the polypeptides are often protected from proteolytic attack, and can be subsequently released from the ECM under the action of GAG lyases, matrix metalloproteinases, or changes in pH. Growth factor binding to GAGs can also induce conformational changes that enhance receptor–growth factor binding. GAGs may also enhance growth factor activity indirectly by mediating the clustering of growth factors or receptor–ligand complexes on the cell surface

Most ECM proteins have at least one GAG binding domain and many have several. These polypeptides bind heparin and heparan sulfate with the highest affinities, but binding of other GAGs is also known. The GAG–protein interaction may serve to facilitate the aggregation and organization of matrix proteins into ordered structures such as fibrils. Alternatively, the interaction may inhibit matrix protein organization. As an example, soluble GAG interactions can inhibit the assembly of type I collagen fibrils from solution at physiological pH, while ionic GAG–collagen complexes are precipitated under acidic conditions. Binding of heparan sulfate to fibronectin may affect the conformation of the protein and thereby regulate its function. Furthermore, the binding of fibronectin to collagen in vitro is stabilized by the presence of heparin. Similarly, the apparent affinity of fibronectin for its cell surface receptors on rat hepatocytes and peritoneal macrophages is increased in the presence of heparan sulfate (79).

C. The Tissue Response to Chitosan GAG Materials

Heparin has been most widely studied as the GAG of choice for tissue regeneration and wound healing applications primarily for two reasons. First, compared to other GAGs, it generally exhibits the highest level of biological activity with the broadest set of biological systems (80). Second, it is readily available at a fairly low cost, in contrast to its less sulfated counterpart, heparan sulfate. For wound healing and regeneration applications, heparin is generally complexed with or covalently linked to another polymer, which serves as the main structural component. Chitosan has been used for this purpose (26,69). Under these circumstances, the heparin can exert a number of influences dictated by the biological activities described above. Thus growth factors released in the vicinity of the implant by neutrophils and macrophages may be sequestered and stabilized within the implant structure by immobilized heparin and subsequently released and utilized by ingrowing tissue cells. The bound heparin may also facilitate the binding and organization of deposited ECM components to the implant and consequently enhance the integration of implant new tissue and existing tissue. Alternatively, heparin released from an implant may activate and protect growth factors from degradation in the vicinity of the implant, a phenomenon that may lead to accelerated healing and/or enhanced angiogenesis. The typical outcome of these implantation studies is formation of new tissue in and around the implant which is histologically and functionally intermediate between normal tissue and scar. Although heparin has garnered the most interest for tissue repair, the other sulfated GAGs have also been applied with similar goals (68).

VIII.   FUTURE TRENDS AND CONCLUDING REMARKS

Carbohydrates play a major role in almost all cellular contact interactions. Carbohydrates on the cell surface are involved in all cell–cell and cell–material interactions, ranging from specific cellular recognition, to signaling, to adhesion and migration. In addition, most soluble signaling proteins are glycosylated, and the oligosaccharide portions are heavily involved in determining receptor affinity. Polysaccharides on the cell surface and in the ECM bind and activate enzymes and growth factors. Likewise, polysaccharide binding can also down-regulate growth factor activity. In spite of this array of interactions, efforts to exploit carbohydrate chemistry and biology have traditionally lagged far behind those of proteins and peptides. The primary reason for this oversight has been the difficulty of synthesizing oligosaccharides and controlling the product structure to any significant degree.

Progress in tissue engineering research has intensified the need for new biologically active, biodegradable materials. There is a particular need for materials that either possess targeted biological activity or can be tuned to elicit desirable responses from specific cell types. Progress in the area of carbohydrate-based molecular recognition and signaling has resulted in greater understanding of the information content of polysaccharide sequences and their role in receptor-mediated cellular activity. This knowledge, together with recent developments in carbohydrate synthesis and modification, gives us the capability to conceptualize and synthesize materials with specific, sugar-based, cellular recognition features. Thus, recent advances in chemical and enzymatic oligosaccharide synthesis have opened the doors to many types of potentially interesting structural and functional modifications to existing glycomaterials (81–84). In particular, the recently reported one-step procedure for oligosaccharide synthesis is a quantum leap forward (84,85). The technique employs a defined series of monosaccharide derivatives with graded and stereospecific reactivity. Mixing the required monosaccharide components in a single reaction vessel and initiating reaction conditions produces the desired oligosaccharide at high yield. This advance can be expected to drastically reduce the time commitment and cost previously associated with any attempt to synthesize a defined oligosaccharide sequence. It also draws us closer to the commercial availability of an automated oligosaccharide synthesis device. Development of similar systems for proteins and nucleic acids were partly responsible for the revolution in molecular biology, and the field of polysaccharide biochemistry will soon undergo similar growth. In essence, we now have the tools to begin rational materials design with the goal of applying this underutilized class of materials within the tissue engineering/tissue regeneration paradigm.

Future work in the polysaccharide biomaterials area can now be based on the fundamental hypothesis that polysaccharide-based macromolecules can be designed to elicit specific cellular responses, while exhibiting mechanical and bioresorption properties suitable for many tissue applications. Such molecules may form the basis of superior scaffolding materials for tissue engineering applications. As more structure–function information becomes available, it should be possible to devise a set of rules or principles that will enable researchers to design carbohydrate moieties with targeted specificity.

REFERENCES

1. S Hirano, H Tsuchida, N Nagao. *N*-Acetylation in chitosan and the rate of its enzymic hydrolysis. Biomaterials 10:574–576, 1989.
2. M Yalpani, D Pantaleone. An examination of the unusual susceptibilities of aminoglycans to enzymatic-hydrolysis. Carbohydr Res 256:159–175, 1994.
3. A Dal Pezze, L Vanini, M Fagnoni, M Guerrini, A De Benedittis, RAA Muzzarelli. Preparation and characterization of poly(ethylene glycol)- cross-linked reacetylated chitosans. Carbohydr Polym 42:201–206, 2000.
4. RA Muzzarelli, C Zucchini, P Ilari, A Pugnaloni, M Mattioli Belmonte, G Biagini, C Castaldini. Osteoconductive properties of methylpyrrolidinone chitosan in an animal model. Biomaterials 14:925–929, 1993.
5. K Kamiyama, H Onishi, Y Machida, Biodisposition characteristics of *N*-succinyl-chitosan and glycol-chitosan in normal and tumor-bearing mice. Biol Pharm Bull 22:179–186, 1999.
6. KY Lee, WS Ha, WH Park. Blood compatibility and biodegradability of partially *N*-acylated chitosan derivatives. Biomaterials 16:1211–1216, 1995.
7. G Paradossi, E Chiessi, M Venanzi, B Pispisa, A Palleschi. Branched-chain analogues of linear polysaccharides: a spectroscopic and conformational investigation of chitosan derivatives. Int J Biol Macromol 14:73–80, 1992.
8. Y Qin, OC Agboh. Chitin and chitosan fibres. Med Device Technol 9:24–28, 1998.
9. WR Gombotz, DK Pettit. Biodegradable polymers for protein and peptide drug delivery. Bioconjug Chem 6:332–351, 1995.
10. O Felt, P Buri, R Gurny. Chitosan: a unique polysaccharide for drug delivery. Drug Dev Ind Pharm 24:979–993, 1998.
11. G Peluso, O Petillo, M Ranieri, M Santin, L Ambrosio, D Calabro, B Avallone, G Balsamo. Chitosan-mediated stimulation of macrophage function. Biomaterials 15:1215–1220, 1994.
12. W Seo, H Pae, N Kim, G Oh, I Park, Y Kim, Y Lee, C Jun, H Chung. Synergistic cooperation between water-soluble chitosan oligomers and interferon-gamma for induction of nitric oxide synthesis and tumoricidal activity in murine peritoneal macrophages. Cancer Lett 159:189–195, 2000.
13. H Jeong, H Koo, E Oh, H Chae, H Kim, S Suh, C Kim, K Cho, B Park, S Park, Y Lee. Nitric oxide production by high molecular weight water-soluble chitosan via nuclear factor-kappaB activation. Int J Immunopharmacol 22:923–933, 2000.
14. Y Usami, Y Okamoto, T Takayama, Y Shigemasa, S Minami. Chitin and chitosan stimulate canine polymorphonuclear cells to release leukotriene B4 and prostaglandin E2. J Biomed Mater Res 42:517–522, 1998.

15. Y Shibata, LA Foster, WJ Metzger, QN Myrvik. Alveolar macrophage priming by intravenous administration of chitin particles, polymers of N-acetyl-D-glucosamine, in mice. Infect Immun 65:1734–1741, 1997.

16. Y Usami, Y Okamoto, S Minami, A Matsuhashi, NH Kumazawa, S Tanioka, Y Shigemasa. Migration of canine neutrophils to chitin and chitosan. J Vet Med Sci 56:1215–1216, 1994.

17. Y Usami, Y Okamoto, S Minami, A Matsuhashi, NH Kumazawa, S Tanioka, Y Shigemasa. Chitin and chitosan induce migration of bovine polymorphonuclear cells. J Vet Med Sci 56:761–762, 1994.

18. H Onishi, Y Machida. Biodegradation and distribution of water-soluble chitosan in mice. Biomaterials 20:175–182, 1999.

19. RA Muzzarelli, M Mattioli-Belmonte, C Tietz, R Biagini, G Ferioli, MA Brunelli, M Fini, R Giardino, P Ilari, G Biagini. Stimulatory effect on bone formation exerted by a modified chitosan. Biomaterials 15:1075–1081, 1994.

20. RA Muzzarelli, G Biagini, M Bellardini, L Simonelli, C Castaldini, G Fratto. Osteoconduction exerted by methylpyrrolidinone chitosan used in dental surgery. Biomaterials 14:39–43, 1993.

21. RA Muzzarelli. Human enzymatic activities related to the therapeutic administration of chitin derivatives. Cell Mol Life Sci 53:131–140, 1997.

22. R Muzzarelli, G Biagini, A Pugnaloni, O Filippini, V Baldassarre, C Castaldini, C Rizzoli. Reconstruction of parodontal tissue with chitosan. Biomaterials 10:598–603, 1989.

23. R Muzzarelli, V Baldassarre, F Conti, P Ferrara, G Biagini, G Gazzanelli, V Vasi. Biological activity of chitosan: ultrastructural study. Biomaterials 9:247–252, 1988.

24. T Chandy, CP Sharma. Chitosan as a biomaterial. Biomater Artif Cells Artif Organs 18:1–24, 1990.

25. K Nishimura, S Nishimura, N Nishi, I Saiki, S Tokura, I Azuma. Immunological activity of chitin and its derivatives. Vaccine 2:93–99, 1984.

26. G Kratz, M Back, C Arnander, O Larm. Immobilised heparin accelerates the healing of human wounds in vivo. Scand J Plast Reconstr Surg Hand Surg 32:381–385, 1998.

27. T Hamano, A Teramoto, E Iizuka, K Abe. Effects of polyelectrolyte complex (PEC) on human periodontal ligament fibroblast (HPLF) function. II. Enhancement of HPLF differentiation and aggregation on PEC by L-ascorbic acid and dexamethasone. J Biomed Mater Res 41:270–277, 1998.

28. JM Chupa, AM Foster, SR Sumner, SV Madihally, HW Matthew. Vascular cell responses to polysaccharide materials: in vitro and in vivo evaluations. Biomaterials 21:2315–2322, 2000.

29. A Eser Elcin, YM Elcin, GD Pappas. Neural tissue engineering: adrenal chromaffin cell attachment and viability on chitosan scaffolds. Neurol Res 20:648–654, 1998.

30. YM Elcin, V Dixit, K Lewin, G Gitnick, Xenotransplantation of fetal porcine hepatocytes in rats using a tissue engineering approach. Artif Organs 23:146–152, 1999.

31. PR Klokkevold, DS Lew, DG Ellis, CN Bertolami. Effect of chitosan on lingual hemostasis in rabbits. J Oral Maxillofac Surg 49:858–863, 1991.

32. PR Klokkevold, H Fukayama, EC Sung, CN Bertolami. The effect of chitosan (poly-N-acetyl glucosamine) on lingual hemostasis in heparinized rabbits. J Oral Maxillofac Surg 57:49–52, 1999.

33. SB Rao, CP Sharma. Use of chitosan as a biomaterial: studies on its safety and hemostatic potential. J Biomed Mater Res 34:21–28, 1997.

34. S Hirano, Y Noishiki. The blood compatibility of chitosan and N-acylchitosans. J Biomed Mater Res 19:413–417, 1985.

35. GG Allan, M Peyron. Molecular weight manipulation of chitosan. I: Kinetics of depolymerization by nitrous acid. Carbohydr Res 277:257–272, 1995.

36. GG Allan, M Peyron. Molecular weight manipulation of chitosan. II: Prediction and control of extent of depolymerization by nitrous acid. Carbohydr Res 277:273–282, 1995.

37. LD Hall, M Yalpani. Formation of branched-chain, soluble polysaccharides from chitosan. J Chem Soc Chem Commun 1153–1154, 1980.

38. LD Hall, M Yalpani, N Yalpani. Ultrastructure of chitosan and some gel-forming, branched-chain chitosan derivatives. Biopolymers 20:1413–1419, 1981.

39. M Yalpani, LD Hall, MA Tung, DE Brooks. Unusual rheology of a branched, water-soluble chitosan derivative. Nature 302:812–814, 1983.

40. M Yalpani, LD Hall. Some chemical and analytical aspects of polysaccharide modifications. 3. Formation of branched-chain, soluble chitosan derivatives. Macromolecules 17:272–281, 1984.

41. M Yalpani. Supercritical fluids—Puissant media for the modification of polymers and biopolymers. Polymer 34:1102–1105, 1993.

42. R Langer, JP Vacanti. Tissue engineering. Science 260:920–926, 1993.

43. R Langer. Tissue engineering: a new field and its challenges. Pharm Res 14:840–841, 1997.

44. JA Hubbell. Biomaterials in tissue engineering. Biotechnology (N Y) 13:565–576, 1995.

45. SV Madihally, HW Matthew. Porous chitosan scaffolds for tissue engineering. Biomaterials 20:1133–1142, 1999.

46. SV Madihally, HW Matthew. Porous chitosan scaffolds for tissue engineering. Biomaterials 20:1133–1142, 1999.

47. S Hirano, M Zhang, M Nakagawa, T Miyata. Wet spun chitosan-collagen fibers, their chemical N-modifications, and blood compatibility. Biomaterials 21:997–1003, 2000.

48. TD Rathke, SM Hudson. Review of chitin and chitosan as fiber and film formers. Rev Macromol Chem Phys C34:375–437, 1994.

49. S Hirano, T Midorikawa. Novel method for the preparation of N-acylchitosan fiber and N-acylchitosan-cellulose fiber. Biomaterials 19:293–297, 1998.

50. GT Hermanson. Modification of hydroxyls with chloroacetic acid. In: Bioconjugate Techniques. San Diego: Academic Press, 1996, p 100.

51. H Baumann, V Faust. Concepts for improved regioselective placement of *O*-sulfo, *N*-sulfo, *N*-acetyl, and *N*-carboxymethyl groups in chitosan derivatives. Carbohydr Res 331:43–57, 2001.

52. RAA Muzzarelli, V Ramos, V Stanic, B Dubini, M Mattioli-Belmonte, G Tosi, R Giardino. Osteogenesis promoted by calcium phosphate *N,N*-dicarboxymethyl chitosan. Carbohydr Polym 36:267–276, 1998.

53. M Thanou, MT Nihot, M Jansen, JC Verhoef, HE Junginger. Mono-*N*-carboxymethyl chitosan (MCC), a polyampholytic chitosan derivative, enhances the intestinal absorption of low molecular weight heparin across intestinal epithelia in vitro and in vivo. J Pharm Sci 90:38–46, 2001.

54. NG Schipper, S Olsson, JA Hoogstraate, AG deBoer, KM Varum, P Artursson. Chitosans as absorption enhancers for poorly absorbable drugs. 2: Mechanism of absorption enhancement. Pharm Res 14:923–929, 1997.

55. M Yazdani-Pedram, J Retuert, R Quijada. Hydrogels based on modified chitosan. 1. Synthesis and swelling behavior of poly(acrylic acid) grafted chitosan. Macromol Chem Phy 201:923–930, 2000.

56. Y Kato, H Onishi, Y Machida. Biological fate of highly-succinylated *N*-succinyl-chitosan and antitumor characteristics of its water-soluble conjugate with mitomycin C at i.v. and i.p. administration into tumor-bearing mice. Biol Pharm Bull 23:1497–1503, 2000.

57. Y Kato, H Onishi, Y Machida. Evaluation of *N*-succinyl-chitosan as a systemic long-circulating polymer. Biomaterials 21:1579–1585, 2000.

58. RA Muzzarelli, F Tanfani, M Emanuelli, DP Pace, E Chiurazzi, M Piani. Sulfated *N*-(carboxymethyl)chitosans: novel blood anticoagulants. Carbohydr Res 126:225–231, 1984.

59. S Hirano, Y Tanaka, M Hasegawa, K Tobetto, A Nishioka. Effect of sulfated derivatives of chitosan on some blood coagulant factors. Carbohydr Res 137:205–215, 1985.

60. SI Nishimura, H Kai, K Shinada, T Yoshida, S Tokura, K Kurita, H Nakashima, N Yamamoto, T Uryu. Regioselective syntheses of sulfated polysaccharides: specific anti-HIV-1 activity of novel chitin sulfates. Carbohydr Res 306:427–433, 1998.

61. MR Mariappan, EA Alas, JG Williams, MD Prager. Chitosan and chitosan sulfate have opposing effects on collagen-fibroblast interactions. Wound Repair Regen 7:400–406, 1999.

62. LD Hall, M Yalpani. Enhancement of the metal-chelating properties of chitin and chitosan. Carbohydr Res 83:C5–C7, 1980.

63. M Yalpani, LD Hall. Some chemical and analytical aspects of polysaccharide modifications. 4. Electron-spin resonance studies of nitroxide-labelled chitin and chitosan derivatives. Can J Chem Rev Can Chim 62:975–980, 1984.

64. H Yoshioka, K Nonaka, K Fukuda, S Kazama. Chitosan-derived polymer-surfactants and their micellar properties. Biosci Biotechnol Biochem 59:1901–1904, 1995.

65. H Fukuda, Y Kikuchi. In vitro clot formation on the polyelectrolyte complexes of sodium dextran surface with chitosan. J Biomed Mater Res 12:531–539, 1978.

66. T Takahashi, K Takayama, Y Machida, T Nagai. Characteristics of polyion complexes of chitosan with sodium alginate and sodium polyacrylate. Int J Pharmaceut 61:35–41, 1990.

67. O Gaserod, O Smidsrod, G Skjak-Braek. Microcapsules of alginate-chitosan— I. A quantitative study of the interaction between alginate and chitosan. Biomaterials 19:1815–25, 1998.

68. A Denuziere, D Ferrier, O Damour, A Domard. Chitosan-chondroitin sulfate and chitosan-hyaluronate polyelectrolyte complexes: biological properties. Biomaterials 19:1275–1285, 1998.

69. G Kratz, C Arnander, J Swedenborg, M Back, CGI Falk, O Larm. Heparin-chitosan complexes stimulate wound healing in human skin. Scand J Plast Reconstr Surg Hand Surg 31:119–123, 1997.

70. KW Leong, HQ Mao, VL Truong-Le, K Roy, SM Walsh, JT August. DNA-polycation nanospheres as non-viral gene delivery vehicles. J Controlled Release 53:183–193, 1998.

71. FC MacLaughlin, RJ Mumper, J Wang, JM Tagliaferri, I Gill, M Hinchcliffe, AP Rolland, Chitosan and depolymerized chitosan oligomers as condensing carriers for in vivo plasmid delivery. J Controlled Release 56:259–272, 1998.

72. K Roy, HQ Mao, SK Huang, KW Leong. Oral gene delivery with chitosan— DNA nanoparticles generates immunologic protection in a murine model of peanut allergy [see comments]. Nat Med 5:387–391, 1999.

73. U Lindahl, M Hook. Glycosaminoglycans and their binding to biological macromolecules. Annu Rev Biochem 47:385–417, 1978.

74. I Bjork, U Lindahl. Mechanism of the anticoagulant action of heparin. Mol Cell Biochem 48:161–182, 1982.

75. B Bray, DA Lane, JM Freyssinet, G Pejler, U Lindahl. Anti-thrombin activities of heparin. Effect of saccharide chain length on thrombin inhibition by heparin cofactor II and by antithrombin. Biochem J 262:225–232, 1989.

76. T Olivecrona, G Bengtsson, SE Marklund, U Lindahl, M Hook. Heparin-lipoprotein lipase interactions. Fed Proc 36:60–65, 1977.

77. T Olivecrona, T Egelrud, PH Iverius, U Lindahl. Evidence for an ionic binding of lipoprotein lipase to heparin. Biochem Biophys Res Commun 43:524–529, 1971.

78. G Bengtsson, T Olivecrona, M Hook, J Riesenfeld, U Lindahl. Interaction of lipoprotein lipase with native and modified heparin-like polysaccharides. Biochem J 189:625–633, 1980.

79. E Ruoslahti, E Engvall. Complexing of fibronectin glycosaminoglycans and collagen. Biochim Biophys Acta 631:350–358, 1980.

80. DJ Tyrell, S Kilfeather, CP Page. Therapeutic uses of heparin beyond its traditional role as an anticoagulant. Trends Pharmacol Sci 16:198–204, 1995.

81. K Witte, P Sears, R Martin, CH Wong. Enzymatic glycoprotein synthesis: preparation of ribonuclease glycoforms via enzymatic glycopeptide condensation and glycosylation. J Am Chem Soc 119:2114–2118, 1997.
82. RL Halcomb, HM Huang, CH Wong. Solution-phase and solid-phase synthesis of inhibitors of Helicobacter-pylori attachment and E-selectin-mediated leukocyte adhesion. J Am Chem Soc 116:11315–11322, 1994.
83. KM Koeller, CH Wong. Complex carbohydrate synthesis tools for glycobiologists: enzyme-based approach and programmable one-pot strategies. Glycobiology 10:1157–1169, 2000.
84. P Sears, CH Wong. Toward automated synthesis of oligosaccharides and glycoproteins. Science 291:2344–2350, 2001.
85. ZY Zhang, IR Ollmann, XS Ye, R Wischnat, T Baasov, CH Wong. Programmable one-pot oligosaccharide synthesis. J Am Chem Soc 121:734–753, 1999.

11

"Cell-Internalizable" Ligand Microinterfaces on Biomaterials

Design of Regulatory Determinants of Cell Migration

Jane S. Tjia and Prabhas V. Moghe
Rutgers University, Piscataway, New Jersey

I. INTRODUCTION

The design of biomimetic materials can benefit from the systematic incorporation and presentation of specific ligand molecules that can selectively regulate cell functions, including cell proliferation, differentiation, adhesion, and migration (1,2). Various properties of ligands can affect cell signal transduction processes through interactions with surface receptors, e.g., ligand surface concentration, strength of ligand–receptor adhesion, degree of receptor occupancy by the ligand, and ligand affinity (3). Recently, the ligand microdistribution on biomaterial surfaces has also been shown to modulate the valency of receptor–ligand binding, with effects on cell spreading (4). The presence of three-dimensional microtopography can further alter ligand-elicited cell functional processes such as cell adhesive and motility responsiveness (5). Thus, the design of three-dimensionally clustered ligand interfaces may be warranted to mimic the regulatory control of cell function via native ligand presentation within the extracellular matrix (ECM) of a tissue. Ligand microinterfaces that exhibit more complex and dynamic cell interactions can also be envisioned, such as those that elicit receptor-mediated cell binding and adhesion but also activate cell signaling through active substrate internalization, through a process called phagocytosis (6). Such interfaces occur frequently in vivo, when cells contact a ligand-presenting surface and migrate on it through ligand internalization, a process called *phagokinetic migration* (7). For example, during wound healing, skin epidermal cells called keratinocytes have been shown to phagocytose ECM ligand debris that lies directly in their migratory path. Thus, the design of phagokinesis-promoting ligand interfaces may be of value to the development of tissue scaffold configurations that promote the kinetics of scaffold coverage or cell infiltration (8,9). This chapter presents key results of our study on the modulation of skin epidermal cell migratory behavior through the use of *ligand-associated microdepots* (LAMs) on synthetic polymers. The results focus on the short-term dynamic control of LAM regulation, as well as the longer term molecular control of the cell migratory response.

II. DESIGN OF CELL-INTERNALIZABLE LIGAND MICROINTERFACES AND ANALYSIS OF CELL RESPONSE

In order to simulate microinterfaces eliciting phagokinetic cell migration, a model system was developed in which ligand-adsorbed microdepots (LAMs) were incorporated onto substrates of ligand-adsorbed poly(lactide-glycolide) acid films such that the overall ligand density and the ligand loading per microcarrier were invariant (Fig. 1) (10). Glass coverslips (12-mm diameter) were cleaned using soap and sonication and stored in 100% ethanol until use. Thin polymer films were obtained by spin-coating a 1% w/ v solution of 50:50 poly-D,L-(lactide-*co*-glycolide) (PLGA) (Medisorb, Cincinnati, OH) in chloroform onto cleaned coverslips. We selected type I collagen (Collaborative, Bedford, MA) as our primary model ligand. PLGA films were then coated with type I rat tail tendon-extracted collagen (Collaborative, Bedford, MA) at a concentration of $5\,\mu g/cm^2$. As model microdepots, we used colloidal gold *microcarriers*, which have been previously shown to act as excellent depots for ligands, by forming monomolecular shells of proteins (11). Based on the protocol previously described (6), we prepared gold salts (diameter $\sim 400\,nm$) by combining 11 mL of distilled water with 6 mL of 36.5 mM Na_2CO_3 and 1.8 mL of 14.5 mL $AuCl_4H$ (J. T. Baker, Phillipsburg, NJ). The solution was heated just prior to boiling and 1.8 mL of 0.1% formaldehyde was added. In order to prevent any substrate denaturation, the solution was then cooled to below $70°C$. The cooled solution was layered over previously prepared collagen-PLGA substrates and incubated at room temperature for 45 min. The coverslips were then washed twice with PBS in preparation for cell plating. To obtain coverslips without microdepots, substrates were layered with a cooled solution that did not contain colloidal substrates. The

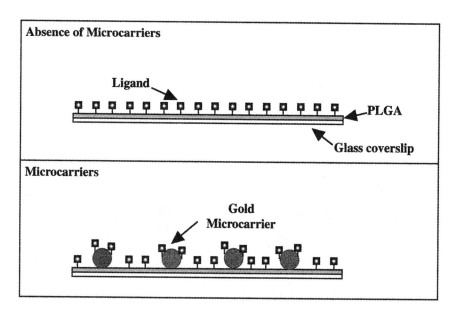

Figure 1 Schematic illustration of ligand-bound microinterface-coated substrates. Collagen ligands were adsorbed onto PLGA-coated coverslips in the presence or absence of ligand microinterfaces such that the overall surface concentration of the ligand was constant. The amount of bound collagen was quantified using trace amounts of ^{3}H-labeled collagen that were added to stock solutions and was found to be 612 ng/cm². Soluble fibronectin was added as an exogenous stimulus in selected conditions and is not diagrammed here.

coverslips were then washed twice with PBS in preparation for cell plating. Substrates prepared in this manner contain a final collagen concentration of 0.6 μg/cm² (17).

Primary human keratinocytes were isolated from neonatal foreskin and cultured in serum-free media (Clonetics, La Jolla, CA). For our experimental studies, keratinocytes were seeded with 30 ng/mL epidermal growth factor (Sigma, St. Louis, MO) stimulation and allowed to attach and migrate for varying periods of time. In selected studies, the cells were also stimulated with 10 μg/mL fibronectin (Sigma, St. Louis, MO), which was added to the media. As the keratinocytes migrated, they bound and phagocytosed the LAMs, leaving behind distinct, cleared tracks that were visible under transmitted light microscopy. The initial kinetics and short-term (5 h) regulation of keratinocyte migration due to the LAM microinterface were monitored using time-lapse microscopy and image analysis. The extent of cell migration on LAM surfaces was quantitated via the calculation of the cell random motility coefficient, μ, which relates the mean-squared displacement, $\langle d^2 \rangle$, of cells at various time intervals to the persistence time, P, via the following equation (12):

$$\langle d^2(t) \rangle = 4\mu \left[t - P \left(1 - e^{\frac{-t}{P}} \right) \right] \tag{1}$$

The average cell speed was also estimated in selected studies using the following equation:

$$\mu = \frac{1}{2} S^2 P \tag{2}$$

In addition, the area cleared by the cells as they migrated and phagocytosed the LAMs was determined directly via image analysis of experimental fields.

III. CELL MOTILITY RESPONSIVENESS TO LAM MICROINTERFACES: RESULTS AND DISCUSSION

In the absence of microcarriers, the extent of keratinocyte migration, as evaluated using time-lapse microscopy, was found to be minimal (Fig. 2). However, in the presence of collagen ligand–adsorbed microcarriers, the calculated random motility coefficient of migrating keratinocytes was found to increase significantly to a value of $49.69 \pm 12.25 \, \mu m^2/min$, suggesting that the presentation of ligand via the microcarriers leads to an enhanced activation of the signal transduction pathways necessary for migration (Figs 2 and 3). Furthermore, in the presence of ligand-deficient microcarriers, migration was not significantly improved (Fig. 3), indicating that the induction of migratory processes is dependent on the microcarrier-associated ligand, and not solely due to substrate-bound ligand.

Previous studies using substrate adsorbed cell adhesion proteins have shown that the rate of cell migration can be ultimately limited by the short-term adhesion strength of the cell to the substrate, which is governed by the number of ligand–receptor interactions (13,14). In contrast, using an enzymatic assay that measures the trypsin sensitivity of adhered cells (15,16), we found that the presence of the LAMs did not significantly alter the cell–substrate adhesion strength (Fig. 4). Thus, it appears in our system that the activation effects of the secondary, microcarrier-bound ligand may be rate limiting and the biophysical effects of the primary, substrate-immobilized ligand may play a secondary role. We expect that in our system with LAMs, the substrate–cell adhesion strength is primarily governed by

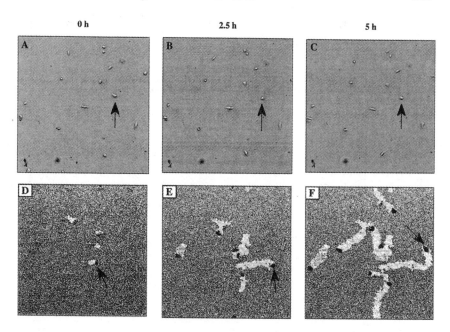

Figure 2 Enhanced keratinocyte migration on LAM microinterfaces. Keratinocytes were seeded onto prepared substrates with 30 ng/mL EGF stimulation, in the absence or presence of ligand microinterfaces, and tracked using time-lapse microscopy. Images were obtained every 3 min up to a total time of 5 h. Ligand microcarrier density in D–F is 1.21 LAMs/μm^2. Representative images are shown at 0 h (A, D), 2.5 h (B, E), and 5 h (C, F).

the number of ligand–receptor interactions at the substrate, not by the receptor–ligand interactions at the secondary LAM interface, which is relatively mobile in nature. Furthermore, since the overall collagen density used in our studies (0.6 $\mu g/cm^2$) (17) is significantly lower than that previously reported to be optimal for keratinocyte migration on collagen (3.7–4.4 $\mu g/cm^2$) (18,19), in all of our studies herein the cell–substrate adhesion is low. At low cell–substrate adhesion strengths, the weak traction forces on the underlying substrate due to a subcritical degree of cell–ligand interactions may likely limit keratinocyte motility. However, the presence of LAMs induces phagocytosis, due to which temporally coordinated forces within the cell cytostructure and cell spreading may result in the generation of a significant cell contractile force (20,21).

To verify that LAM internalization was necessary for enhanced migration, we performed experiments in which collagen LAMs were

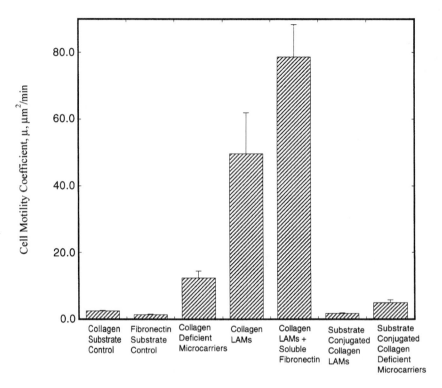

Figure 3 Effect of LAM internalization on the random motility coefficient. Estimates of the random motility coefficient for migrating cells were obtained in the absence or presence of collagen ligand on the microinterfaces and when internalization was inhibited by covalent attachment of the ligand-adsorbed microinterfaces to the substrate. In addition, experiments were also performed in the presence of stimulation with $10\,\mu g/mL$ fibronectin. Scanned images were processed using Image-Pro software (Media Cybernetics, Silver Spring, MD) to analyze the individual paths of migrating cells. Only cells whose paths did not intersect that of other cells over the migration periods were selected for analysis. All data were obtained at a carrier density of $1.21\,$microcarriers/μm^2. For each condition, 40–50 cells were analyzed. The error bars represent the standard error.

covalently attached to the underlying substrate, effectively blocking LAM internalization (22,23). Values of the random motility coefficient under these conditions were found to be significantly reduced in comparison with those observed on internalizable LAM substrates (Fig. 3). Thus, our studies show that keratinocyte binding to LAMs alone is not sufficient to activate significant migratory activity; LAM internalization appears to be an

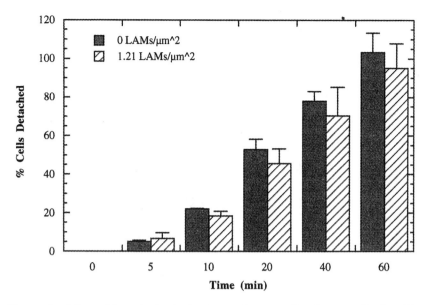

Figure 4 Effect of ligand-adsorbed microcarriers on cell–substrate adhesion. The relative adhesion strength of adhered keratinocytes was determined by enzymatic assay. Keratinocytes were seeded onto prepared substrates and allowed to adhere for 30 min. Adhered cells were then treated with 0.08% trypsin-EDTA (Clonetics, San Diego, CA) for 5 min to 1 h at 37°C with gentle shaking. Cells detached during treatment were counted using hemocytometers. Aliquots were taken at 5, 10, 20, 40, and 60 min, and initial volumes restored by addition of fresh trypsin-EDTA solution. The cumulative percentage of cells released after various times of enzymatic treatment was determined via hemocytometer cell counts.

essential coactivator for enhanced migration. Previous investigations have presented evidence suggesting that phagocytic internalization processes may contribute to cell migration by providing a means for membrane and integrin receptor recycling (24,25). Moreover, the phagocytic and migratory processes utilize similar cytoskeletal activation pathways, indicative of the possibility that phagocytosis may serve to enhance the cytoskeletally mediated events necessary for migration (26,27). It is possible, therefore, that the LAM internalization process contributes to cell migratory activation through temporally accumulated signaling intermediates that co-mediate migration as well as cytoskeletal processes and, like conventional phagocytic processes, effects faster receptor recyling.

Cell migration on ligands immobilized to substrates is induced via the activation of intracellular signal transduction pathways arising from receptor–ligand binding (28,29). By using ligand-presenting microcarriers or nanocarriers as secondary ligand depots in our system, we expect that the migratory activation may be promoted by altering the rate or degree of ligand exposure. The progressive increase in intracellular activation due to the presence of the LAMs is indicated by the differences observed in membrane spreading activity (30) (Fig. 5). In cells exposed to LAMs, a significant increase in the number of long filopodial extensions was

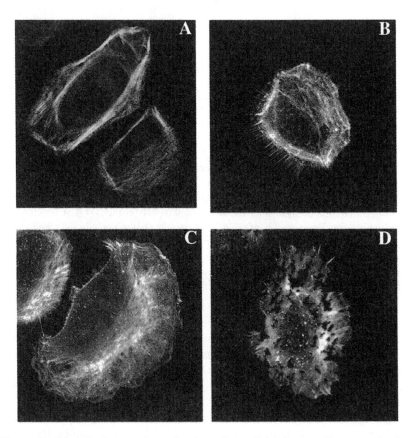

Figure 5   Ligand microcarrier activation of cytoskeletal stress fiber organization. Visualization of F-actin stress fibers (A) in the absence of microinterfaces, (B) in the presence of substrate-adsorbed ligand microinterfaces, (C) in the presence of ligand microinterfaces covalently attached to the substrate, and (D) in the presence of adsorbed microinterfaces without ligand. Cells were stained with fluorescein phalloidin (Molecular Probes, Eugene, OR) and visualized using a Zeiss Axiovert microscope (Carl Zeiss, Inc., Thornwood, NY).

observed; few filopodia were seen on purely ligand-immobilized substrates (no LAMs) or on uninternalizable LAM substrates. By exposing cells to collagen LAMs, we appear to be able to activate the signal transduction pathways necessary for migration beyond that which has previously been observed on substrate-bound ligand substrates.

Additional insights were gained from an examination of the cell speed and persistence times under various initial LAM substrate densities and stimulation conditions (10) (Figs 6 and 7). Regardless of the stimulatory conditions used, LAM density was observed to govern cell motility in a distinctly biphasic behavior (Fig. 6). It is notable that the accompanying changes in the cell persistence behavior were also distinctly biphasic (Table 1), particularly in the absence of exogenous fibronectin stimulation. We hypothesize that cell binding to LAMs accentuates the directional persistence behavior and that the local LAM density can intensify this further, within limits. Why 1.21 LAMs/μm^2 promotes persistence is unclear although it is likely that at this density, LAM clearance at the leading edge

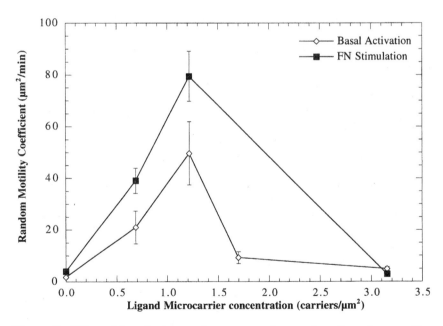

Figure 6 Effect of ligand microcarrier concentration on the cell random motility coefficient. Estimates of the random motility coefficient were obtained as previously described as a function of the initial ligand microinterface density. For each carrier concentration, 40–50 cells were analyzed. The error bars represent the standard error.

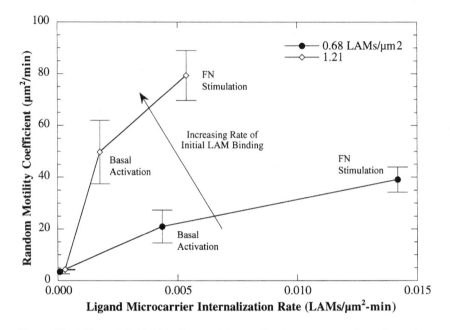

Figure 7 Effect of LAM binding and internalization rates on the cell random motility coefficient. The random motility coefficient was examined as a function of the initial LAM binding and initial LAM internalization rates. Initial LAM binding rates were determined by sparsely seeding cells onto substrates containing a known LAM density and incubating the samples for 1 h. The area cleared by singles cells was then determined using Image-Pro software and the number of LAMs effectively cleared from the surface was calculated. The cells were then trypsinized and stained with DiI, a membrane dye (Molecular Probes, Eugene, OR), and plated on glass slides for viewing under confocal microscopy. Under reflected light, ingested microinterfaces appeared white against a black background. The membrane dye was used to determine the cell boundaries under fluorescent light. Using the fluorescent and reflected confocal images together, the number of ingested microinterfaces was obtained. Subtracting the number of ingested microinterfaces from the total number of microcarriers cleared, the number of microcarriers was obtained.

of cells can be "spatially autocatalytic" for further LAM binding and clearance, thus eliciting tracks of a highly correlated nature. Cell motility has been similarly shown to correlate with persistence in systems where contact guidance due to ligand concentration predisposes persistence behavior (31). Interestingly, the presence of soluble fibronectin stimulation lowers persistence (indicating that cell binding has less regioselectivity), while enhancing cell speed [presumably via up-regulated activation path-

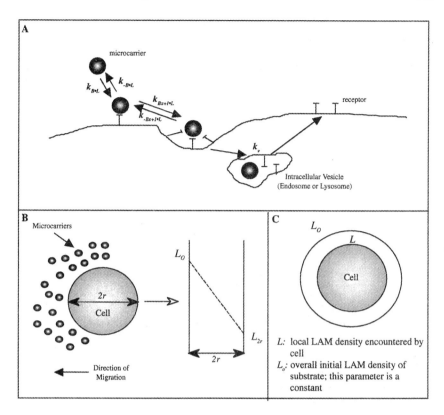

Figure 8 Schematic of proposed model. (A) Dynamics of cell–LAM interactions. Microinterfaces initially bind to one cell membrane/surface receptor. Before they can be internalized, additional membrane/receptors must be recruited in order to "activate" the interface for internalization. Once internalized, the interface dissociates from the membrane/receptor and the membrane/receptor gets recycled back to the cell surface. (B) Contribution of migration to model. Analogy to diffusion across a semi-infinite plane. (C) Cells encounter a local LAM density, L, as they migrate, which can differ from the initial overall LAM density of the system, L_0.

ways following LAM binding (17)], as well as enhancing the cell speed sensitivity to LAM density. The latter effect indicates that the time constant for binding and migration may be lowered in the presence of fibronectin. Overall, we believe that LAM density controls the initial rate of cell–LAM interactions and that there exists a threshold range of cell–LAM interactions at which migration is activated. Our data suggest that once migration is

Table 1 Effect of LAM Density on Cell Motility Parameters, Cell Speed, and Persistence Behavior, in the Presence and Absence of FN Stimulation[a]

LAM density	0 μg/mL FN stimulation		10 μg/mL FN stimulation	
	Cell speed (μm/min)	Persistence time (min)	Cell speed (μm/min)	Persistence time (min)
0	0.78 ± 0.12	22.52 ± 5.15	0.83 ± 0.09	20.55 ± 0.07
0.69	0.93 ± 0.23	37.70 ± 7.45	1.39 ± 0.23	40.38 ± 7.99
1.21	0.98 ± 0.10	104.23 ± 10.79	1.42 ± 0.34	54 ± 77 ± 7.90
3.15	0.60 ± 0.24	25.30 ± 1.64	0.69 ± 0.02	22.57 ± 3.12

[a]Estimates for root mean squared cell speed and directional persistence time were regressed from the mean squared displacement behavior versus time.

induced, the rate of cell–LAM interactions may be dependent on both the LAM density and the rate of cell migration. Therefore, there is an optimal LAM density that is able to stimulate migration at a rate that may be conducive to maintaining an optimal rate of cell–LAM interactions. At higher LAM densities, the rate of initial cell–LAM interactions is high, initially activating migration, but the rate of migration combined with the high LAM density may quickly lead to saturation of cell–LAM binding, resulting in reduced migration. At far lower LAM densities, the rate of cell–LAM interactions may not be rapid enough to activate migration.

Next, to gain further insight into the role of LAM dynamics on keratinocyte migration, we have examined the effects of LAM binding and internalization kinetics on migration through the development of a theoretical model.

IV. ROLE OF LAM DYNAMICS ON CELL MIGRATION: A MECHANISTIC UNDERSTANDING

The dynamic nature of the microdepots is evident given the rapid LAM binding and internalization by the cells. LAM dynamics can effect migratory signaling pathways via altered substrate ligand binding (through rapid ligand turnover) as well as through phagocytic activation. Because we have already established that LAM binding alone is insufficient for migration, it would be logical to assume that it is the internalization process that is critical for migratory activation. However, since binding must occur for internalization to take place, the roles of rates of LAM binding cannot be ignored. Thus, we have studied the possible relative contributions of LAM binding vs. internalization toward the induction of keratinocyte migration.

To rigorously analyze the effects of LAMs on cell migration, we attempted to decouple the binding and internalization aspects of the cell–LAM interactions. Quantitation of the initial LAM ingestion rate via fluorescence microscopy and image analysis established that (a) varying the initial substrate LAM density served to modulate the initial LAM binding rate; and (b) soluble stimulation with fibronectin significantly enhanced the initial internalization rate over the initial cell binding rate of LAMs. Thus, we were able to experimentally alter the relative LAM binding and internalization rates via modulation of the initial LAM density and soluble fibronectin stimulation. As expected, analysis of these results suggests that the effects of binding and internalization on the random motility coefficient are interdependent (Fig. 7). As the initial binding rate increases, the effects of increasing the initial internalization rate become greater, leading to enhanced motility. At lower initial binding rates, increases in the initial internalization rate lead to smaller increases in motility. Thus, an adequate rate of LAM binding is required, but not sufficient, for optimal migratory activation. While this analysis gives us some insight into the roles of binding vs. internalization in cell migration, it does not capture the possible temporal changes in LAM dynamics that may occur over the short term (hours) and critically affect migration. A theoretical mathematical formalism was therefore developed to further examine the possible temporal effects of cell–LAM dynamics on cell migration (32).

A. A Simple Theoretical Model for Cellular and LAM Interfacial Dynamics

1. LAM Internalization

The cell–LAM interactions were examined from a kinetic-mechanistic point of view (Fig. 8A) and were modeled using equations similar to those used in traditional Michaelis-Menton kinetics. The dominant mechanism by which phagocytosis is believed to occur is known as the "zipper" model (33). This model is based on previous studies showing that initial particle binding is not sufficient to induce ingestion; further sequential recruitment of cell surface receptors into interactions with the remainder of the particle surface is required (34–36). These receptor–ligand interactions control the advancement of the pseudopodial extension of that plasma membrane, which is engulfing the particle. If there are not sufficient receptors on the cell surface or ligands on the particle surface to allow engulfment of the particle, phagocytosis will not proceed. In keeping with the zipper model, we

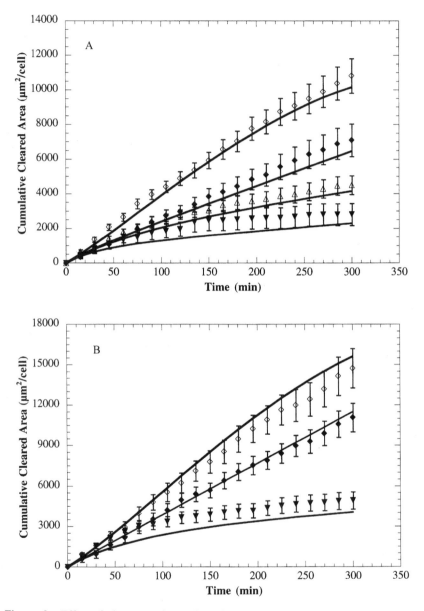

Figure 9 Effect of phagocytosis on cleared area. Using time-lapse microscopy and image analysis, the cumulative cleared area was experimentally determined at various carrier concentrations under conditions of (A) basal activation and (B) fibronectin stimulation. Theoretical simulation results are denoted by the solid lines and were obtained by simultaneously solving Eq. 3-11 using Matlab.

formulated the following set of ordinary differential equations describing the binding and release of a LAM, L, to cell–microcarrier binding site, B, to form either an initial cell–LAM complex, $B \bullet L$, or a partially "activated" cell–LAM complex, $B_{x+1} \bullet L$, where x represents the number of additional binding sites accumulated by the LAM. When $x = n$, the LAM has accumulated the additional number of binding sites necessary for phagocytosis and is consequently ingested to form an intracellular vesicle, V. The binding sites are then released and recycled back to the cell surface (Fig. 8A).

$$\frac{d[L]}{dt} = -k_{B \bullet L}[L][B] + k_{-B \bullet L}[B \bullet L] \tag{3}$$

$$\frac{d[B \bullet L]}{dt} = k_{B \bullet L}[L][B] - k_{-B \bullet L}[B \bullet L] - \sum_{x=1}^{n} k_{B_{x+1} \bullet L}[B \bullet L]$$

$$\times [B]^x + \sum_{x=1}^{n} k_{-B_{x+1} \bullet L}[B_{x+1} \bullet L] \tag{4}$$

$$\frac{d[B_{x+1} \bullet L]}{dt} = \sum_{x=1}^{n-1} k_{B_{x+1} \bullet L}[B \bullet L][B]^x - \sum_{x=1}^{n-1} k_{-B_{x+1} \bullet L}[B_{x+1} \bullet L];$$

$$x = 1 \ldots n - 1 \tag{5}$$

$$\frac{d[B_{n+1} \bullet L]}{dt} = k_{B_{n+1} \bullet L}[B \bullet L][B]^n - k_{-B_{n+1} \bullet L}[B_{n+1} \bullet L] - k_V$$

$$\times [B_{n+1} \bullet L] \tag{6}$$

$$\frac{d[V]}{dt} = k_V[B_{n+1} \bullet L] = k_V \frac{[B_T - B \bullet L][B \bullet L]}{K_m + s.[B \bullet L]} \tag{7}$$

where k_a and k_{-a} represent the binding and dissociation constant for species a, respectively; K_m determines the characteristic degree of bound complexes per unit area, and s, the equivalent cell membrane sites for LAM involution prior to internalization. For the time course of our experiments, the expression level of the cell or the total number of binding sites is assumed to remain constant and is given by the following expression.

$$B_T = B + \sum_{x=0}^{n} [(x+1)B_{x+1} \bullet L] \tag{8}$$

2. Cellular Migration Dynamics

Cell migration will affect the degree of exposure of LAMs to the cell, as migration would make new LAMs available for internalization. Previous studies have shown that in isotropic environments, migrating cells can be characterized as exhibiting a persistent random walk (37,38). This behavior indicates that they move along fairly linear paths over short periods of time, but show more randomly oriented paths over longer time intervals. A population of cells exhibiting this behavior can be characterized primarily in terms of μ, the random motility coefficient (39). In our system, as a first approximation, the overall density of LAMs, L_o, is assumed to be uniform and isotropic. Over relatively short times, the local binding and depletion of LAMs may bias the directionality of cell migration; however, over longer time periods, the mean-squared displacement of migrating cells as a function of time reaches linearity. Thus, we make use of the persistent random walk theory and use μ as the primary parameter characterizing migration in our system. Similar to molecular diffusion in a semi-infinite plane, we take a mass balance of LAMs encountered locally by the cell and make the assumption that the majority of the ingested LAMs are at the leading edge of the migrating cell (Fig. 8B, C). Thus, we obtain the following expression relating the rate of cell migration to the rate of change of the extracellular local LAM concentration:

$$\left.\frac{d[L]}{dt}\right|_{Migration} = \frac{\mu L_o}{\pi r^2} = \frac{\mu L_o}{A_{cell}} \tag{9}$$

Incorporating this equation into the phagocytic model, Eqn. (3) becomes:

$$\frac{d[L]}{dt} = -k_{B \bullet L}[L][B] + k_{-B \bullet L}[B \bullet L] + \frac{\mu L_o}{A_{cell}} \tag{10}$$

The net effects of cell migration were experimentally measured in terms of the rate at which cells effectively "clear" an area covered with ingestable LAMs. For a given initial surface particle concentration, the area of LAM clearance by a cell is given by the following expression:

$$\frac{d(cleared - area)}{dt} = \frac{1}{L_o}\left[\sum_{x=0}^{n}\frac{d[B_{x+1} \bullet L]}{dt} + \frac{d[V]}{dt}\right] \tag{11}$$

Values of parameters needed to solve the model were determined from experimental results described elsewhere (32). Selected model parameters are tabulated in Table 2. Analysis of the model equations was performed using an explicit Runga-Kutta method in Matlab (Mathworks, Inc., Natick, MA)

Table 2 Model Parameters[a]

	Parameter	Basal activation	Fibronectin stimulation
B_T	Total number of binding sites	12,708 particles	20,170 particles
n	Critical number of binding sites	1	2
k_{BP}	Kinetic constant of cell–LAM binding	$2.06\text{E-}3\ \mu m^2/$ particle-min	$1.52\text{E-}3\ \mu m^2/$ particle-min
k_v	Kinetic constant of LAM internalization	$1.28\text{E-}3\ min^{-1}$	$2.40\text{E-}3\ min^{-1}$
K_m	Kinetic constant of LAM activation (critical site equivalents, s)	0.7295 particles/ μm^2 $(s \sim 2)$	0.5012 particles/ μm^2 $(s \sim 3)$

[a]Model parameters were determined from experimental results (32). Values of the LAM binding capacity of the cell, B_T, were determined from the number of bound LAMs in the presence of excess LAM density. Knowing B_T and the average cell diameter, the critical number of binding sites, n, was then calculated. The kinetic constant of binding, k_{BP}, was determined from the slope of a plot of the initial number of bound LAMs as a function of the initial LAM density. The kinetic constant of internalization, k_v, was determined from a Lineweaver-Burk plot. K_m is a parameter that combines the kinetic constants found in eqs. (4)–(6) (32) and was also determined from a Lineweaver-Burk plot.

to provide clearance profiles under varying conditions of soluble stimulation and at varying initial LAM densities. Comparison of simulated clearance profiles with experimental results shows that the model can accurately capture the behavior of migratory activity observed at low to moderate LAM densities (Fig. 9).

B. Theoretical Studies of Cell Migration on LAM Microinterfaces: Results and Implications

Using the theoretical formalism model developed in this study, we have tested the premise that the internalizable nature of these ligand microcarriers can activate differential rates of cell migration. Analysis of the rates of LAM binding and internalization show that regardless of the initial LAM substrate density, (a) the rate of LAM binding is significantly greater than the rate of internalization; (b) the rate of LAM binding quickly reaches a steady state, the exact level of which depends on the initial LAM density (Fig. 10), and (c) depending on the initial LAM density, the rate of LAM internalization may steadily decrease (Fig. 10). Further analysis suggests that keratinocyte motility is differentially governed by the equilibrium net rate of carrier binding to the cell membrane (Fig. 11). Based on the fact that ligand concentration per carrier is invariant in our system (11), the net rate of carrier binding can be interpreted as the effective rate of accrued ligand on the cell surface or the net ligand sampling rate, indicating that migratory activity is an increasing function of the net rate of ligand binding. Our data also demonstrate that regardless of the conditions of activation (e.g., basal activation or secondary stimulation by soluble fibronectin), the relationship between the ligand binding rate and migratory activity remains qualitatively unchanged, suggesting that the LAMs activate receptors binding to different ligands (collagen vs. fibronectin) in qualitatively similar ways.

Previous studies on ligand-immobilized substrates have shown that ligand binding results in the activation of signal transduction pathways necessary for migration. On ligand-immobilized substrates, however, the extent of migratory signal pathway activation achieved through ligand binding processes is frequently limited by the substrate adhesion strength, which quickly becomes inhibitory as ligand binding increases. By presenting the ligand via a microinterface, we are able to significantly increase the degree of ligand binding without compromising the cell–substrate adhesion strength necessary for migration. The results of our model analysis can be used to explore the relative importance of LAM binding and internalization. Because the rate of LAM binding is an order of magnitude greater than the rate of LAM internalization, and since the rate of LAM internalization decreases over time at the LAM density that promotes the greatest migration ($1.21 \, LAMs/\mu m^2$), the internalization phenomena may be rate-wise, or signal-wise, limiting. Previous studies have shown that on ligand-adsorbed substrates a substantial fraction of integrin receptors are left behind on the substrate as the cell detaches and locomotes, while a smaller fraction are collected into vesicles and recycled (40). In order to sustain migration, cells must compensate for the loss of integrins with the synthesis of new integrins. We speculate that that internalizable and mobile nature of the LAMs may facilitate receptor recycling, resulting in a more efficient means of ligand removal, faster appearance of unbound receptors on the cell surface, and, thus, a faster rate of ligand binding.

The internalization process may also play a role in the cytoskeletal dynamics, which are required for the generation of a sufficient traction force needed for migration. Since the collagen ligand density used in our studies is lower than that previously reported to be optimal for keratinocytes, in all of

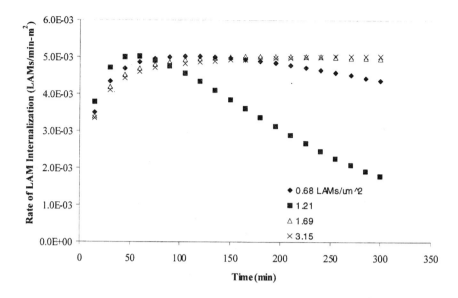

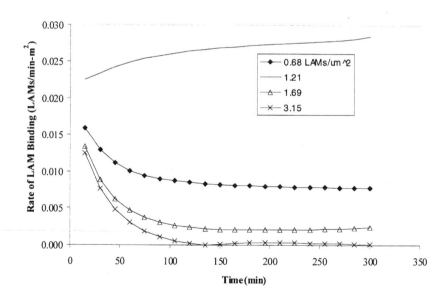

Figure 10 Theoretical temporal evolution of LAM binding and internalization rates. The model was used to generate average LAM binding and internalization rates as a function of time for various initial LAM densities.

our studies herein, cell–substrate adhesion strength is low and, in the absence of LAMs, weak traction forces on the underlying substrate limit keratinocyte motility. LAM internalization may allow increased activation of the signal transduction pathways initiated by ligand binding for the significant generation of a contractile force to overcome week adhesion to the substrates. In fact, previous investigations into the temporal coordination between the forces within the cell cytostructure and cell spreading during phagocytosis have shown that phagocytic ingestion results in the generation of a significant cell contractile force that is dependent on tyrosine phosphorylation (20,21). Pseudopod extension and binding, on the other hand, do not appear to necessarily require tyrosine kinase activity (21). Our own studies examining the tyrosine kinase activity of migrating keratinocytes show that, as the net LAM sampling rate increases, the proportion of cellular activity due to LAM internalization relative to that arising from LAM binding increases, suggesting that the increased migratory activity may be due to the increased activation of signaling pathways initiated by LAM internalization (Fig. 12). We propose that the efficiency of migratory

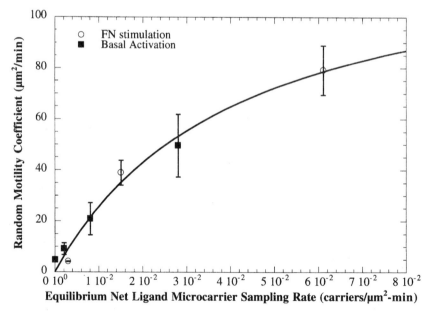

Figure 11   Theoretical relation between random motility coefficient and net ligand microcarrier sampling rate. Analysis of the model shows that the net rate of microinterfacial binding is directly proportional to the cell random motility coefficient (μ).

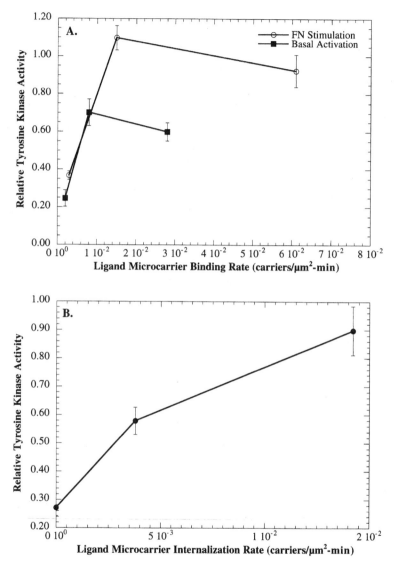

Figure 12   Effect of LAM sampling, binding, and internalization rates on cellular activation. (A) Effect of the relative tyrosine kinase activity on the LAM binding rate for both basal and fibronectin-stimulated activation states. (B) Effect of LAM internalization rates on the relative tyrosine kinase activity. Binding and internalization rates are theoretical values generated from model simulations. Tyrosine kinase activity values are the average of triplicate experiments samples from two experiments. Errors bars represent the standard error.

activation due to LAM internalization could be conceptualized in terms of the net tyrosine kinase (*ntk*) activity normalized to the underlying rate of LAM internalization, a parameter denoted by ε_i. A plot of ε_i vs. the LAM binding rate permits elucidation of the contributions of LAM binding and internalization to *ntk* activation (Fig. 13). When the LAM binding rate is relatively fast in comparison with the internalization rate, ε_i will be low and the extent of cell migration observed is minimal. Likewise, at relatively fast internalization rates and slow LAM binding rates, the amount of *ntk* activation due to internalization is high, but migration is still minimal. We believe that to achieve significant amounts of migration, cellular activation must be engendered via appropriate rates of both LAM binding and internalization, which we suggest, based on previous studies (21,41), in turn activate pathways leading to pseudopod extension and retraction, and the

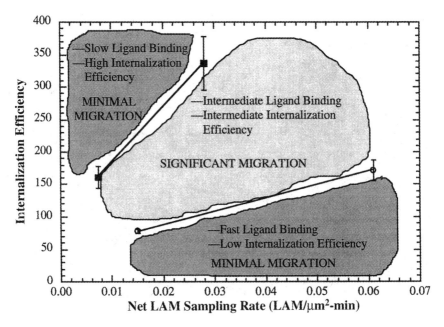

Figure 13 Map of internalization efficiency as a function of the rate of LAM binding. When the rate of LAM binding is relatively faster than the rate of internalization, activation efficiency of the internalization process is low and the extent of cell migration is minimal. Likewise, at relatively slow LAM binding rates compared with the internalization rate, where the majority of cellular activation is due to internalization, the efficiency of internalization is high but migration is still minimal. In order to achieve significant levels of migration, an intermediate rate of LAM binding and LAM internalization are necessary.

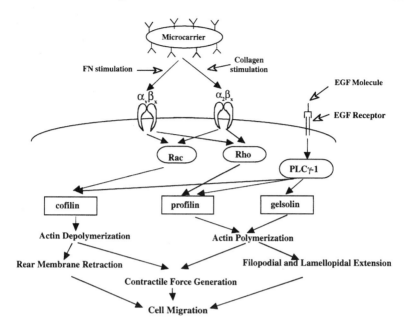

Figure 14 Intracellular signal activation pathways due to internalizable ligand-associated microdepots. We propose that exogenous ligand binding to LAMS followed by LAM internalization may activate cell migration by cooperative intensification of the native signaling pathways resulting from ligand–receptor binding and internalization mediated by phagocytic integrin receptors. For example, membrane ligation and internalization of integrin receptors leads to the activation of *rac* and *rho*, which ultimately leads to the polymerization and depolymerization of actin stress fibers. Stimulation with soluble fibronectin enables utilization of integrin receptors in addition to collagen-specific integrins, further stimulating the *rac* and *rho* pathways. While LAM binding primarily activates pathways used for the pseudopod extension and retraction, LAM internalization serves to activate pathways necessary for the generation of a contractile force. Notably, LAMs intensify migration in the presence of EGF, indicating overlap between EGF receptor-induced alterations in the actin cystoskeleton.

generation of a contractile force, respectively (Fig. 14). Our current understanding of LAM-induced activation pathways is limited: in future, the molecular details of the phosphorylation targets and their effects on migration will need to be resolved through studies of phosphoprotein dynamics.

V. MOLECULAR ACTIVATION OF CELL MIGRATION ON LAMS: LIGAND SPECIFICITY AND REMODELING

In this portion of our study, we have examined the molecular determinants underlying ligand regulation of LAM-based cell migration. Using two model ligands, collagen and fibronectin, we have evaluated the role of ligand specificity, growth factor stimulation, and ligand cooperativity, on LAM-elicited cell motility. Given their ability to enhance ligand responsiveness, LAM microinterfaces are a particularly attractive model system to examine ligand remodeling events that may occur over longer cell exposure to primary LAMs. The most comprehensive biomimetic signals designed for material interfaces are those that are derived or remodeled by cells themselves. Endogenous ligand synthesis and secretion may also be influenced by specific ligand–cell interactions, a concept known as dynamic reciprocity (42,43). In the present study, we have specifically tested ligand remodeling (collagen or fibronectin secretion) as a possible, secondary, biomimetic signal promoting cell motility responsiveness to the primary LAM-based ligand signal.

To that end, we have examined the longer term effects (48 h) of ligand-adsorbed microdepots on the matrix regulation and migration of keratinocytes (17). For these longer term studies, all experiments were performed at a constant LAM substrate density of 1.21 LAMs/μm^2 and quantitation of keratinocyte migration was done by exploiting the fact that migrating cells leave behind distinct, cleared tracks. Using image analysis, the extent of migration was quantified in terms of a "migration index," which was defined as the ratio of the area cleared by the cells to the area of the cells themselves. Two forms of regulatory mechanisms were investigated: the first, exogenously adsorbed ligands on LAM PLGA substrates, and the second, endogenously secreted ligands during cell secretion. As in our short-term studies, experiments were carried out under conditions of basal activation via epidermal growth factor in serum-free media.

A. Collagen-Lams Induce Keratinocyte Migration Whereas Fibronectin-Lams Do Not

In agreement with our short-term studies, we found that longer term keratinocyte migration on PLGA substrates containing ligand-deficient microdepots remained poor; but high levels of migration could be systematically induced through the use of ligand-adsorbed microdepots (Fig. 15). Unlike migration on collagen-adsorbed microdepots, however, keratinocyte migration on fibronectin-LAM PLGA substrates was found to be low, i.e., significantly lower than on fibronectin-LAM glass controls (data

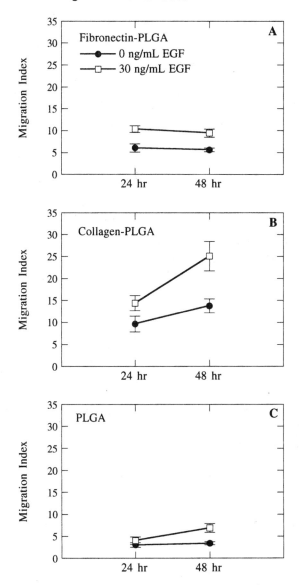

Figure 15 Quantitative analysis of keratinocyte migration on various substrates. Migration indices of keratinocytes showing effect of time and EGF stimulation on migration of keratinocytes on (A) fibronectin-LAM PLGA, (B) collagen-LAM PLGA, and (C) PLGA. Using image analysis, the total cleared area was quantitated and divided by the area of the cells to obtain a migration index. Results are the average of n analyzed images from four experiments. For PLGA, 0 ng/mL EGF samples, $n = 6$; for all other samples, $n \geq 10$.

not shown). These differences may be attributed, in part, to the lower biological activity of fibronectin adsorbed to the hydrophobic surface of the PLGA, even though greater amounts of fibronectin adsorb to the PLGA and the microcarriers. While we were unable to distinguish the conformation of fibronectin adsorbed to the microcarriers from that adsorbed directly to the PLGA, experiments using an antifibronectin antibody that binds to the cell binding region of fibronectin show that fewer cumulative fibronectin binding sites were available on fibronectin-LAM PLGA substrates than on fibronectin-LAM glass substrates. Thus, we conclude that the increase in the amount of adsorbed fibronectin is not enough to overcome the unfavorable conformation on PLGA, and is likely disallowing optimal cellular binding and leading to diminished basal levels of keratinocyte migration.

B. Ligand Remodeling Enhances Migration on Collagen-LAM Microinterfaces

We next examined possible roles of endogenously secreted collagen and fibronectin on keratinocyte migration. In order to examine the possible regulatory role of endogenously secreted collagen on LAM-mediated migration, experiments were performed in which the experimental media was supplemented with *cis*-4-hydroxy-L-proline (Sigma, St. Louis, MO), a proline analogue that inhibits the proper folding and secretion of triple-helical collagen (Fig. 16). The addition of this analogue to the media did not significantly alter the extent of migration on any of the LAM substrates studied, suggesting that *cis*-hydroxyproline-mediated collagen synthesis is not essential for elevated keratinocyte migration and that the cellular remodeling of collagen may not be a primary event during the activation of cell migration.

Addition of a polyclonal antifibronectin antibody to the media of keratinocytes migrating on collagen-adsorbed LAMs resulted in a significant decrease in migration that was not observed in the presence of fibronectin-adsorbed LAMs, indicating that fibronectin–collagen interactions may be a significant event in the activation of keratinocyte migration (Fig. 17). Fibronectin has previously been shown to be both haptotactic and chemotactic for keratinocytes, implicating the potential for a role of both substrate-bound and soluble forms of the protein in regulating migration. In addition, studies have reported migrating keratinocytes to deposit extracellular fibrillar fibronectin as well as secrete soluble fibronectin into the media (44–46). In our studies, keratinocytes were also found to secrete fibronectin (100–800 ng/mL/10^6 cells), although regulation of the amounts secreted and deposited were difficult to quantify, given the sparse cultures necessary to study migration. We attempted to discern the possible role of

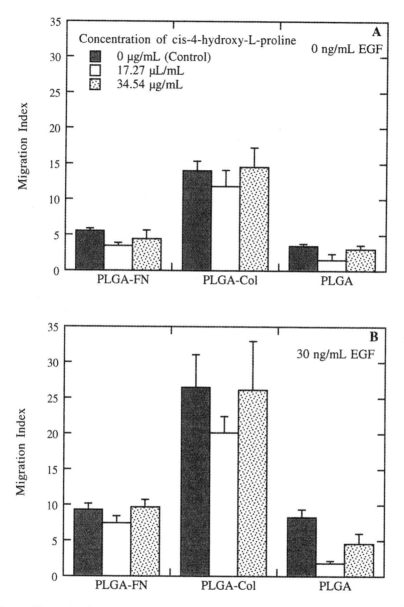

Figure 16 Role of collagen synthesis in keratinocyte migration. Quantitative levels of migration of keratinocytes cultured on various substrates using media supplemented with *cis*-4-hydroxy-L-proline. (A) 0 ng/mL EGF; (B) 30 ng/mL EGF. Results are the average of *n* analyzed images from three experiments. For PLGA samples, 17.27 μg/mL *cis*-proline, $n = 6$; for all other samples, $n \geq 9$.

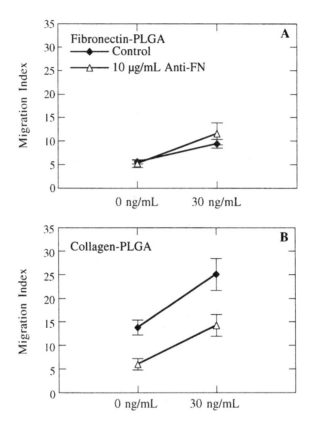

Figure 17   Role of fibronectin regulation during keratinocyte migration. Migration indices of keratinocytes showing effect of addition of rabbit antihuman fibronectin antibodies to cells cultured on (A) fibronectin-LAM PLGA, (B) collagen-LAM PLGA, and (C) PLGA. Results are the average of *n* analyzed images from three experiments. For PLGA samples, 10 µg/mL anti-FN, $n = 6$; for all other samples $n \geq 9$.

substrate deposited vs. soluble forms of fibronectin during the induction of cell motility. The exogenous addition of soluble fibronectin was found to augment migration on collagen-LAM PLGA substrates but not on fibronectin-LAM substrates of ligand-deficient substrates, indicating that while soluble fibronectin may be stimulating increased migration, its effects alone are not sufficient to achieve high levels of migration observed on collagen-LAM PLGA (Fig. 18a). A fairly high migration index ($\sim$15) observed even in the presence of antifibronectin antibodies or when

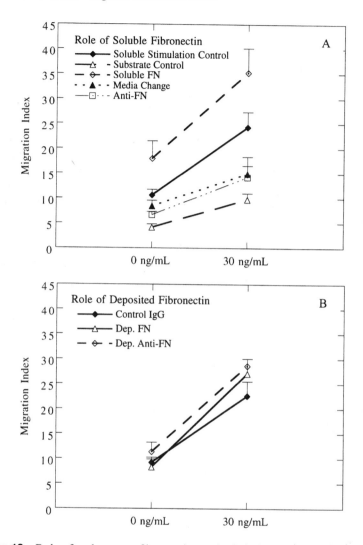

Figure 18 Role of endogenous fibronectin synthesis in keratinocyte migration on collagen-LAM PLGA substrates. Keratinocytes were seeded on collagen-LAM PLGA substrates and allowed to migrate for 48 h. (A) To determine the role of soluble fibronectin, 10 μg/mL soluble fibronectin was added simultaneously with the cells, or fresh media changes were done every 12 h. Soluble stimulation controls contained no soluble fibronectin in the media. Fibronectin-LAM PLGA served as substrate controls with 10 μg/mL soluble fibronectin added to the media. (B) To determine the effect of deposited fibronectin, fibronectin or anti-FN was preadsorbed onto substrates prior to seeding of cells. Results are the average of *n* analyzed images from three experiments. For all samples, $n \geq 9$.

fibronectin was depleted from the media, shows that the basal collagen-LAMs contributes significantly to the high levels of migration observed, even in the absence of fibronectin.

The role of deposited fibronectin was examined via two methods: either fibronectin or antifibronectin antibodies were deposited onto the collagen-LAMs prior to the addition of cells. Although both the fibronectin and the antifibronectin antibody were found to be functionally active, they failed to induce any inhibitory or stimulatory effects on cell migration (Fig. 18b). Thus, if deposited forms of fibronectin are important in the presence of collagen-LAMs, they may likely undergo cell-mediated postsecretory processing steps, such as fibrillogenesis, which we were unable to mimic in our experiments. Previous investigators have shown that secreted fibronectin undergoes fibrillogenesis to an insoluble, aggregated form that gets deposited directly onto the substrate in the pericellular space (45,46). Fibronectin fibrillogenesis is believed to be mediated in part by cell surface receptors specific for the 70-kDa amino-terminal matrix assembly domain of the fibronectin molecule. This matrix assembly domain is distinct from the cell adhesion RGD domain. In addition, since soluble fibronectin is reported to have at least a 10-fold greater affinity for the matrix assembly receptor than for the cell attachment receptor, cell-secreted fibronectin is believed to bind preferentially to fibronectin matrix assembly receptors rather than to cell adhesion receptors. Therefore, we hypothesize that cell-secreted fibronectin is first incorporated into pericellular fibronectin fibrils, which then bind to cell adhesion receptors and mediate migration. The progressive secretion and assembly of fibronectin and its adhesion to cell surface receptors may thus kinetically limit the process of migratory activation; this would be consistent with the temporal correlation we observed between the addition of soluble fibronectin to the culture media and the enhancement of migration, as well as that between the frequency of dilution of conditioned media and the inhibition of migration.

C. Cellular Effects of Ligand Remodeling on LAM Microinterfaces Are Receptor Mediated

A key step in the activation of cell migration by fibronectin is its binding to specific cell adhesion receptors. Experiments were therefore also carried out to determine the receptor-mediated mechanisms associated with the role of fibronectin in keratinocyte migration on collagen-LAM substrates. Indirect immunofluorescence experiments showed that integrin staining of α_5 and α_4 was diffuse, but levels of α_v were significantly elevated and were comparable to those observed in keratinocytes cultured on fibronectin-glass substrates (Fig. 19). Using media supplemented with function-blocking antibodies

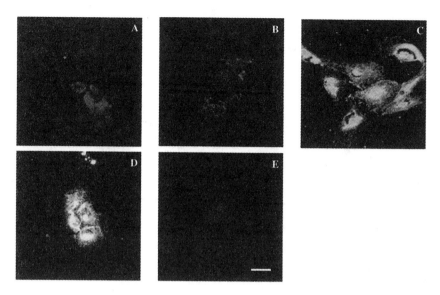

Figure 19 Keratinocyte expression of fibronectin-specific integrins. Keratinocytes were seeded on collagen-LAM PLGA substrates with EGF stimulation and allowed to migrate for 48 h. Cells were then stained for (A) α_5 integrins, (B) α_4 integrins, (C) α_v integrins, (D) α_v integrins on fibronectin-LAM glass substrates, and (E) negative control. Bar $= 25\mu$m.

against integrin receptors specific for fibronectin, we found that α_4 and α_5 integrin receptors do not appear to play a major role in the control of cell migration on collagen-LAM PLGA (Fig. 20). The $\alpha_5\beta_1$ receptor is known to be the primary integrin receptor regulating keratinocyte migration on fibronectin (49), and is believed to weakly regulate keratinocyte on native collagen (50). Moreover, the $\alpha_5\beta_1$ receptor is also believed to be involved in the assembly of fibronectin matrices (51,52). In the context of our findings, this suggests that $\alpha_5\beta_1$-mediated fibronectin fibrillogenesis may not play a key role in keratinocyte migration on collagen-LAM substrates. Furthermore, inhibition in cell migration due to anti-α_v antibodies was similar in magnitude to that observed in the presence of antifibronectin antibodies, suggesting that the migratory regulation exerted by cell-secreted fibronectin may be sensitively regulated by α_v integrins. However, our studies clearly indicate a role for α_v integrins in regulating keratinocyte migration on collagen-LAM PLGA substrates. Moreover, the inhibition of migration induced by the presence of anti-α_v antibodies was similar in magnitude to that elicited by antifibronectin antibodies, suggesting that the secreted

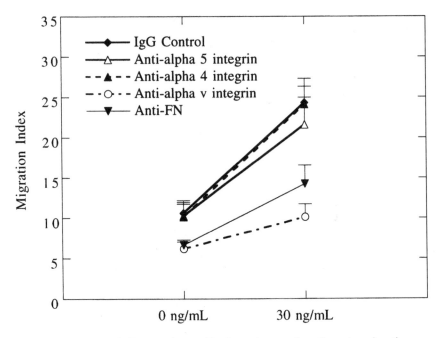

Figure 20 Role of fibronectin-specific integrins on keratinocyte migration on collagen-coated PLGA substrates. Keratinocytes were seeded on collagen-LAM PLGA substrates in the presence of $10\,\mu g/mL$ of either anti-α_5, anti-α_4 or anti-α_v integrin antibodies. Migration was evaluated after 48 h. Results are the average of n analyzed images from three experiments. For all samples, $n \geq 11$.

fibronectin may indeed be sensitively regulated by α_v integrins. During wound healing, keratinocytes have been shown to express the $\alpha_v\beta_6$ integrin, a fibronectin/tenascin receptor (53,54), as well as the $\alpha_v\beta_5$ integrin, which is specific for fibronectin and vitronectin (55). More recently, the $\alpha_v\beta_3$ integrin has been shown to play a role in the matrix assembly of fibronectin (56). Although it is unclear whether or not $\alpha_v\beta_3$ is present on human keratinocytes, if it is, it may suggest a role for α_v-mediated fibrillogenesis in the regulation of keratinocyte migration on collagen.

D. Ligand Dynamics Underlying Cell Matrix Reciprocity: A Model Biomimetic Interface

Because the effects of endogenously secreted fibronectin are unique to collagen-LAM PLGA substrates, there is most likely direct or indirect reciprocity between the roles of secreted fibronectin and adsorbed collagen. Based on bioactivity studies using an antibody specific for triple-helical collagen, in conjunction with transmission electron microscopy, we have confirmed that the collagen on the underlying PLGA substrate, as well as on the microcarriers, is rapidly denatured. These structural changes in collagen may effect the substrate sequestration of secreted or fibrillar forms of fibronectin, since the affinity of fibronectin for denatured collagen ($K_d = 2.5 \times 10^{-9}$M) is significantly greater than that for native collagen ($K_d = 7 \times 10^{-7}$M). We have calculated that for our experimental system, the bioactivity of soluble fibronectin bound to denatured collagen is at least threefold greater than that bound to native collagen adsorbed to glass. In Fig. 21 we present hypothetical pathways through which secreted fibronectin may be inducing cell migration. Several routes can be possible: (a) secreted fibronectin acts as chemoattractant, providing basal activation;

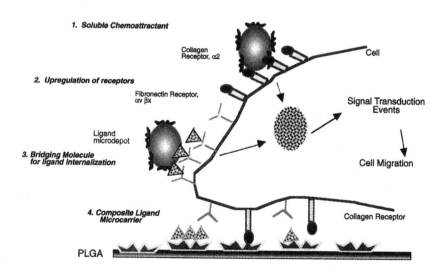

Figure 21 Hypothetical model of ligand dynamics governing the longer term induction of cell migration on LAM microinterfaces. The ligand dynamics possible include ligand remodeling (fibronectin secretion, assembly, substrate deposition) and cell–matrix reciprocity (collagen-fibronectin hybridization and cooperative cell activation). The remodeled ligand can activate cells in differential forms (soluble, assembled, substrate deposited) and promote migration rate, as well as enhance LAM internalization rate.

(b) secreted fibronectin binds to cell receptors that mediate pericellular fibrillogenesis and trigger further stimulation; and (c) secreted fibronectin is effectively sequestered on the denatured collagen on the underlying PLGA, facilitating adhesion as well as fibrillogenesis at the PLGA surface and, thereby, promoting migration. In addition to binding to cell adhesion receptors and mediating migration, fibronectin may also be contributing to migratory activation through the regulation of LAM internalization. The role of fibronectin and fibronectin-binding proteins in the phagocytosis of bacteria by neutrophils is well known. More recently, the importance of fibronectin in the epithelial phagocytosis has been deduced (47,48). These studies have shown that efficient binding to fibronectin via fibronectin-binding proteins is requisite for efficient internalization of bacteria. Thus, it is also possible that secreted fibronectin is binding to the collagen-adsorbed LAMs, thereby enhancing phagocytic internalization. Since the results of our previous mathematical analysis have shown that increasing internalization rates lead to an increase in the net LAM sampling rate, the increased phagocytic uptake of fibronectin-coated LAMs could result in increased migration. In fact, our short-term studies showed that soluble fibronectin stimulation did indeed result in increased LAM internalization (See Fig. 7). However, since predeposition of fibronectin onto collagen LAMs failed to significantly increase migration, it is unlikely that fibronectin interactions directly at the LAM–cell interface play an important role in the regulation of internalization in our system. Rather, it is more probable that secreted fibronectin is acting independently of the LAMs and activating cell signaling pathways that underlie increased internalization of the LAM-based primary ligand.

E. Growth Factor Activation of LAM-Induced Cell Migration Processes

Examination of the extent of keratinocyte migration in the presence and absence of EGF stimulation after 48 h shows that EGF caused a uniform, significant increase in migration on collagen-coated PLGA. In contrast, a significantly smaller increase was observed on plain PLGA and fibronectin-coated PLGA substrates. (Fig. 15). Since plain PLGA substrates do not contain any ECM ligands and the fibronectin adsorbed on fibronectin-coated PLGA substrates exhibits low bioavailability, it can be inferred that these substrates represent keratinocyte migration responses to EGF stimulation in the absence or at low levels of integrin-mediated interactions. The low migration indices observed on these substrates suggest that in the absence of significant integrin interactions, EGF stimulation alone cannot induce significant migratory activity. It should be noted that even in the absence of EGF, migration on collagen-coated PLGA substrates was greater than that observed on both fibronectin-PLGA and plain PLGA substrates, indicating that the basal contribution of ECM-mediated interactions was not insignificant. The presence of both EGF and substrate stimulation resulted in a migration index of about 25 on collagen-coated PLGA, a result greater than that expected from the additive combination of EGF and substrate effects alone (compare collagen-coated PLGA without EGF and plain PLGA with EGF). These results suggest that there are may be cooperative effects resulting from EGF stimulation and ligand-mediated migration.

The migration signaling pathways activated via EGF are known to involve gelsolin, phospholipase Cγ, and cofilin and profilin, among others (57). Gelsolin, cofilin, and profilin are also known to be involved in molecular pathways activated following integrin binding to ECM ligands (summarized in Fig. 14). In addition, previous studies have concluded that the extent of migration of EGF-stimulated keratinocytes reaches a plateau at an EGF concentration of 0.6 ng/mL (58). Thus, our studies represent responses under conditions of maximal (30 ng/mL) EGF stimulation. The cooperative responses observed in these studies suggest that ECM binding may stimulate an alternative molecular pathway leading to enhancement in migratory signals over those that have been maximally activated by EGF. Soluble stimulation via an appropriate cytokine may therefore be used in conjunction with ligand-induced activation to selectively enhance cell migratory signals.

VI. CONCLUDING REMARKS

In this work we have shown that on synthetic polymer substrates that poorly support cell migration, the controlled induction of phagocytic events through ligand-adsorbed microscale depots can be used to induce significant cell motility responsiveness. We hypothesize that the presentation of ligand on dynamic, mobile microcarrier substrates results in the enhanced activation of migratory signaling pathways and can sustain greatly increased migration due to the "decoupling" of the cell–substrate adhesion strength from the ligand–microcarrier activating effects. In addition, the internalization of the microcarriers may further enhance the intracellular activation process. Moreover, the selective use of a secondary, cell-secreted ligand can further increase migration via concerted interactions with the primary ligand that additionally modulate ligand dynamics. The results of these studies may provide new directions for the micromanipulation of cell motility process on artificial tissue analogue substrates, as well as to emerging fields of functional, noninvasive bioimaging and targeted drug delivery.

ACKNOWLEDGMENTS

The authors are grateful to Professor Brian Aneskievich, University of Connecticut, for his technical guidance. This study was supported by Johnson & Johnson Discovery Award, ConvaTec Young Professor Award, Hoechst Celanese Innovative Research Award, and a National Science Foundation Career Award to P. Moghe. The authors would like to thank Howard Salis, a NL Center for Biomaterials Summer Fellow, and Patrick Hossler for their help with image analysis. J. Tjia was partially supported by the Rutgers-UMDNJ National Institutes of Health Biotechnology Training Grant, and the Rutgers University Louis Bevier Fellowship.

REFERENCES

1. AS Hoffman. Molecular bioengineering of biomaterials in the 1990s and beyond: a growing liason of polymers with molecular biology. Artif Organs 16:43–49, 1992.
2. JA Hubbell. Biomaterials in tissue engineering Bio/Tech 13:565, 1995.
3. DA Hammer, M Tirrell. Biological adhesion at interfaces. Annu Rev Mater Sci 26:651–691, 1996.
4. LG Griffith, S Lopina. Microdistribution of substratum-bound ligands affects cell function: hepatocyte spreading on PEO-tethered galactose. Biomaterials 19:979–986, 1998.
5. CS Ranucci, PV Moghe. Substrate topography can enhance cell adhesive and migratory responsiveness to matrix ligand density. J Biomed Mater Res 54:140–161, 2001.
6. G Albrecht-Buehler. The phagokinetic tracks of 3T3 cells. Cell 11:395–404, 1977.
7. RAF Clark. The Molecular and Cellular Biology of Wound Repair, New York: Plenum Press, 1996.
8. GJ Beumer, CA Van Blitterswijk, D Bakker, M Ponec. Cell seeding and in vitro biocompatibility evaluation of polymeric matrices of PEO/PBT copolymers and PLLA. Biomaterials 14:598–604, 1993.
9. H Green. Cultured cells for the treatment of disease. Sci Am 96–102, Nov 1991.
10. JS Tjia, PV Moghe. Regulation of cell motility on polymer substrates via "dynamic," cell internalizable, ligand microinterfaces. Tissue Eng 8(2):247–261, 2002.
11. C De Roe, PJ Courtoy, P Baudhuin. A model for protein-colloidal gold interactions. J Histochem Cytochem 35:1191–1198, 1987.

12. PA DiMilla, JA Quinn, SM Albelda, DA Lauffenburger. Measurement of individual cell migration parameters for human tissue cells. AIChE J 38:1092–1104, 1992.

13. SP Palecek, JC Loftus, MH Ginsberg, DA Lauffenburger, AF Horwitz. Integrin-ligand binding properties govern cell migration speed through cell-substratum adhesiveness. Nature 385:537–540, 1997.

14. PA DiMilla, K Barbee, DA Lauffenburger. Mathematical model for the effects of adhesion and mechanics on cell migration speed. Biophy J 60:15–37, 1991.

15. M Lampin, R Warocquier-Clerout, C Legris, M Degrange, MF Sigot-Luizard. Correlation between substratum roughness and wettability, cell adhesion, and cell migration. J Biomed Mater Res 36:99–108, 1997.

16. JL Duval, M Letort, MF Sigot-Luizard. Comparative assessment of cell/substratum static adhesion using an in vitro organ culture method and computerized analysis system. Biomaterials 9:155–161, 1988.

17. JS Tjia, BJ Aneskievich, PV Moghe. Substrate-adsorbed collagen and cell-secreted fibronectin concertedly induce cell migration on poly(lactide-glycolide) substrates. Biomaterials 20:2223–2233, 1999.

18. DT Woodley, PM Bachmann, EJ O'Keefe. Laminin inhibits human keratinocyte migration. J Cell Physiol 136:140–146, 1988.

19. Y Sarret, DT Woodley, K Grigsby, K Wynn, EJ O'Keefe. Human keratinocyte locomotion: the effect of selected cytokines. J Invest Dermato 98:12–16, 1992.

20. E Evans, A Leung, D Zhelev. Synchrony of cell spreading and contraction force as phagocytes engulf large pathogens. J Cell Biol 122:1295–1300, 1993.

21. MB Lowry, A-M Duchemin, JM Robinson, CL Anderson. Functional separation of pseudopod extension and particle internalization during Fcγ receptor-mediated phagocytosis. J Exp Med 187:161–176, 1998.

22. S Saneinejad, MS Shoichet. Patterned glass surfaces direct cell adhesion and process outgrowth of primary neurons of the central nervous system. J Biomed Mater Res 42:13–19, 1998.

23. X Yi, J Huang-Xian, C Hong-Yuan. Direct electrochemistry of horseradish peroxidase immobilized on a colloid/cysteamine-modified gold electrode. Anal Biochem 278:22–28, 2000.

24. MS Bretscher. Circulating integrins: $\alpha_5\beta_1$, $\alpha_6\beta_4$ and Mac-1, but not $\alpha_3\beta_1, \alpha_4\beta_1$ or LFA-1. EMBO J 11:383–389, 1992.

25. MS Bretscher. Moving membrane up to the front of migrating cells. Cell 85:465–467, 1996.

26. KD Coutant, N Corvaia, NS Ryder. Bradykinin induces actin reorganization and enhances cell motility in HaCat keratinocytes. Biochem Biophys Res Commun 257–261, 1997.

27. T Ng, D Shima, A Squire, PIH Bastians, S Gschmeissner, MJ Humphries, PJ Parker. PKCa regulates b1 integrin-dependent cell motility through association and control of integrin traffic. EMBO J 18:3909–3923, 1999.

28. A Huttenlocker, MH Ginsberg, AF Horwitz. Modulation of cell migration by integrin-mediated cytoskeletal linkages and ligand-binding affinity. J Cell Biol 134:1551–1562, 1996.

29. S Miyamoto, H Teramoto, J Gutkind, KM Yamada. Integrins can collaborate with growth factors for phosphorylation of receptor tyrosine kinases and MAP kinases activation: roles of integrin aggregation and occupance of receptors. J Cell Biol 135:1633–1642, 1996.

30. E Kawahara, R Tokuda, I Nakanishi. Migratory phenotypes of HSC-3 squamous carcinoma cell line induced by EGF and PMA: relevance to migration of loosening of adhesion and vinculin-associated focal contacts with prominent filopodia. Cell Biol Inter 23:163–174, 1999.

31. BT Burgess, JL Myles, RB Dickinson. Quantitative analysis of adhesion-mediated cell migration in three-dimensional gels of RGD-grafted collagen. Ann Biomed Eng 28:110–118, 2000.

32. JS Tjia, PV Moghe. Activation of cell migration through cell-internalizable ligand microsubstrates: A phenomenological study. Ann Biomed Eng (submitted).

33. M Rabinovitch. Professional and non-professional phagocytes: an introduction. Trends Cell Biol 5:85–87, 1995.

34. FM Griffin, SC Silverstein. Sequential response of the macrophage plasma membrane to a phagocytic stimulus. J Exp Med 139:323–336, 1974.

35. FM Griffin, JA Griffin, JE Leider, SC Silverstein. Studies of the mechanism of phagocytosis: I. Requirements for circumferential attachement of particle-bound ligands to specific receptors on the macrophage plasma membrane. J Exp Med 142:1263–1282, 1975.

36. FM Griffin, JA Griffin, SC Silverstein. Studies on the mechanism of phagocytosis: II. The interactions of macrophages with anti-immunoglobulin IgG-coated bone marrow-derived lymphocytes. J Exp Med 144:788–809, 1976.

37. GA Dunn. Characterizing a kinesis response: time averaged measures of cell speed and directional persistence. Agents Actions (Suppl) 12:14–33, 1983.

38. HG Othmer, SR Dunbar, W Alt. Models of dispersal in biological systems. J Math Biol 26:263–298, 1988.

39. M Gail, C Boone. The locomotion of mouse fibroblasts in tissue culture. Biophys J 10:980–993, 1970.

40. SP Palecek, CE Schmidt, DA Lauffenburger, AF Horwitz. Integrin dynamics on the tail region of migrating fibroblasts. J Cell Sci 109:941–952, 1996.

41. P Defilippi, C Olivo, M Venturino, l Dolce, L Silengo, G Tarone. Actin cytoskeleton organization in response to integrin-mediated adhesion. Microsc Res Tech 47:67–78, 1999.

42. MJ Bissell, HG Hall, G Parry. How does the extracellular matrix direct gene expression? J Theor Biol 99:31–68, 1982.

43. CD Roskelley, MJ Bissell. Dynamic reciprocity revisited: a continuous, bidirectional flow of information between cells and the extracellular matrix regulates mammary epithelial cell function. Biochem Cell Biol 73:391–391, 1995.

44. M Kubo, M Kan, M Isenmura, I Yamane, H Tagami. Effects of extracellular matrices on human keratinocyte adhesion and growth and on its secretion and deposition of fibronectin in culture. J Invest Dermatol 88:594–601, 1987.

45. M Kubo, DA Norris, SE Howell, SR Ryan, RAF Clark. Human keratinocytes synthesize, secrete, and deposit fibronectin in the pericellular matrix. J Invest Dermatol 82:580–586, 1984.

46. EJ O'Keefe, D Woodley, G Castillo, N Russell, RE Payne. Production of soluble and cell-associated fibronectin by cultured keratinocytes. J Invest Dermatol 82:150–155, 1984.

47. K Dziewanowska, JM Patti, CF Deobald, KW Bayles, WR Trumble, GA Bohach. Fibronectin Binding Protein and host cell tyrosine kinase are required for internalization of Staphylococcus aureus by epithelial cells. Infect Immun 67:4673–4678, 1999.

48. M Zhao, M Jin, S He, C Spee, S Ryan, D Hinton. A distinct integrin-mediated phagocytic pathway for extracellular matrix remodeling by RPE cells. Invest Ophthalmol Vis Sci 40:2713–2723, 1999.

49. K Zhang, RH Kramer. Laminin 5 deposition promotes keratinocyte motility. Exp Cell Res 227:309–322, 1996.

50. JP Kim, K Zhang, RH Kramer, TJ Schall, DT Woodley. Integrin receptors and RGD sequences in human keratinocyte migration: unique anti-migratory function of $\alpha3\beta1$ epiligrin receptor. J Invest Dermatol 98:764–770, 1992.

51. FJ Fogerty, SK Akiyama, KM Yamada, DF Mosher. Inhibition of binding of fibronectin to matrix assembly sites by anti-integrin (alpha 5 beta 1) antibodies. J Cell Biol 111:699–708, 1990.

52. JA McDonald, BJ Quade, TJ Broekelmann, R LaChance, K Forsman, E Hasegawa, S Akiyama. Fibronectin's cell adhesive domain and an amino-terminal matrix assembly domain participate in its assembly in fibroblast pericellular matrix. J Biol Chem 262:2957–2967, 1987.

53. FM Watt, PH Jones. Expression and function of the keratinocyte integrins. Development (Suppl) 185–192, 1993.

54. K Haapasalmi, et al. Keratinocytes in human wounds express alpha v beta 6 integrin. J Invest Dermatol 106:42–48, 1996.

55. RAF Clark, GS Ashcroft, MJ Spencer, H Larjava, MWJ Ferguson. Re-epithelialization of normal excisional wounds is associated with a switch from $\alpha v\beta5$ to $\alpha v\beta6$ integrins. Br J Dermatol 135:46–51, 1996.

56. C Wu, PE Hughes, MH Ginsberg, JA McDonald. Identification of a new biological function for the integrin alpha v beta 3: initiation of fibronectin matrix assembly. Cell Adhes Commun 4:149–158, 1996.

57. A Wells. Tumor invasion: role of growth factor-induced cell motility. Adv Cancer Res 78:31–101, 2000.

58. D Cha, P O'Brien, EA O'Toole, DT Woodley, LG Hudson. Enhanced modulation of keratinocyte motility by transforming growth factor-α (TGF-α) relative to epidermal growth factor. J Invest Dermatol 106:590–597, 1996.

12
Biomimetic Strategies and Applications in the Nervous System

Jessica O. Winter and Christine E. Schmidt
University of Texas at Austin, Austin, Texas

I. INTRODUCTION

Biomimetic devices, which mimic the structure or function of biological systems, represent an area of intense research growth in the biotechnology industry. The nervous system provides several unique challenges. Although peripheral nerves regenerate after some injuries, current clinical treatment results in limited recovery. Central nerves, which contain different support cells than peripheral nerves, develop scar tissue that is inhibitory to regeneration. Many devices are being developed to imitate the structure of nerve and to promote regeneration in either the peripheral or central nervous system. These devices incorporate biological, mechanical, chemical, or electrical cues to recreate the native nerve environment. Although alteration of the local environment with individual cues has encouraged some regeneration, no single device has provided "the cure" to nervous system injury. Success in the peripheral nervous system has been confined to small injury gaps, while functional central nervous system repair is rarely evidenced. It is clear that future neural tissue analogues must integrate multiple cues to more closely imitate natural nerve structure. Due to the limited injury recovery in the nervous system, biomimetics are also being developed to replace neural function. Most technologies use microelectrodes to interact directly with nerve cells, with successful examples including cochlear and retinal implants. However, these digital approaches do not resemble nerve signaling, and future prosthetics will demand more faithful analogues, such as those available through neuromorphic engineering, an analogue computing approach. There is a clear need for biomimetic devices in the nervous system. Regeneration devices and prosthetics have already met some of this need. Combined approaches promise further improvements in compatibility and development of nerve–material interfaces never thought possible.

II. PHYSIOLOGY OF THE NERVOUS SYSTEM

A. Organization of the Nervous System

The nervous system is classified into two main subsystems: the peripheral nervous system (PNS) and the central nervous system (CNS). The PNS includes excitatory nerve extensions from the spinal cord, sensory nerve cell bodies (dorsal root ganglia), and their processes. Peripheral nerves innervate the muscular system, transmitting sensory and excitatory input to and from the spinal column. The CNS includes the brain and spinal cord, as well as optic, olfactory, and auditory systems. The CNS conducts and interprets signals, in addition to providing excitatory stimuli to the PNS (1).

B. Anatomy of the Peripheral and Central Nervous Systems

A nerve cell consists of a cell body (soma) and its extensions (axons and dendrites). Clusters of sensory nerve soma, known as ganglia, are located just outside the spinal column. Excitatory nerve soma are located inside the spinal cord or in the brain. Input signals to the soma are received through dendrites, which are short nerve extensions located close to the cell body. Output signals are carried in axons, processes that may extend for up to 1 m from the cell body. Nerves consist of a group of axons.

In the CNS, a primary organ is the spinal cord, a collection of dendrites, axons, and cell bodies. The center of the cord, a butterfly-shaped region known as gray matter, contains the cell bodies of excitatory neurons, as well as blood vessels and some support cells (glial cells) (Fig. 1). White matter surrounds the gray matter, insulating and protecting it from the immediate environment. White matter consists of axons and their associated glial cells, including oligodendrocytes, astrocytes, and microglia (immune cells) (2). Oligodendrocytes are the primary myelinating, or insulating, cells of the CNS, whereas astrocytes contribute to the formation of the blood–nerve barrier, separating the nervous system from blood proteins and cells. Axons project from the white matter in bundles, known as fascicles. These fascicles exit the encasing bone of the spinal column and enter the PNS.

In the peripheral system, fascicles join with projections from sensory neurons (ganglia) to produce a nerve. Nerves contain an outer covering, the epineurium, made of fibrocollagenous connective tissue. The epineurium

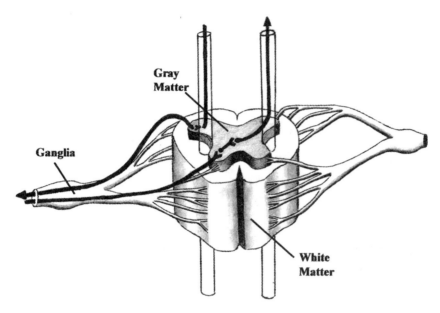

Figure 1 The spinal cord. Gray matter located in the center of the spinal cord contains the cell bodies of intermediate and excitatory neurons. The white matter surrounding the gray matter is comprised of axons emanating from gray matter cell bodies. Sensory nerve bodies are located outside the spinal cord in bulbous regions known as ganglia. (Adapted from JW McDonald. Sci Am Sep:67, 1999. Drawn by Timothy Liu, University of Texas, Austin, TX.)

binds the fascicles to neighboring components, including blood vessels (Fig. 2). Each fascicle is surrounded by a perineurium, made of flattened cells (i.e., fibroblasts) and collagen. Inside the fascicles, connective tissue, known as the endoneurium, unites individual axons. The endoneurium consists primarily of collagen fibers oriented parallel to axons. The basal lamina separates axons from the endoneurium and provides a site for axon attachment. The basal lamina is composed of laminin, collagen, and other extracellular matrix (ECM) components. Under the basal lamina, Schwann cells wrap around the axons, insulating them. The folds of the Schwann cell membrane surrounding the axon and the protein inside are collectively known as myelin (3).

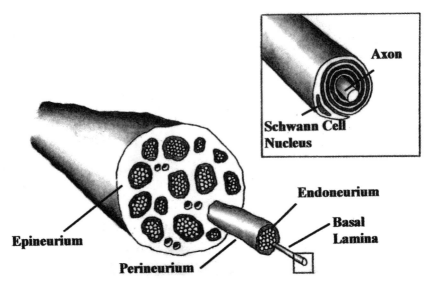

Figure 2 Anatomy of a peripheral nerve. The epineurium holds fascicles together. The perineurium covers the fascicles, while endoneurium binds the interior components of fascicles together. Each fascicle consists of several axons, each covered by the basal lamina and insulated by Schwann cell bodies. Proteins in the folds of the Schwann cell membrane are known as myelin. (Adapted from S. McKinnon, Surgery of the Peripheral Nerve, 1988. Drawn by Timothy Liu, University of Texas, Austin, TX.)

C. Response to Nervous System Injury

1. PNS Response

Injury and subsequent nerve regeneration are well-documented processes in the PNS. The earliest cellular changes begin moments after the axon is injured. The cytoskeleton begins to break down, followed shortly thereafter by a dissolution of the cell membrane. Degradation occurs primarily in the distal end of the nerve stump, the end farthest from the cell body. The proximal end of the nerve stump swells but experiences only minimal degradation (1). Originally, it was believed that the dissolution of the distal stump occurred because of isolation from nutrients provided by the cell body (4). However, axonal changes occur so rapidly that researchers now believe the disintegration results from direct proteolysis, induced by an influx of ions from the extracellular environment (5,6).

After the cytoskeleton and membrane degrade, Schwann cells surrounding the axons in the distal stump begin to shed their myelin lipids. Myelin protein is collected in ovoids, hollow football-shaped vacuoles, which flatten as the axon they enclose deteriorates. Eventually, the myelin lipids separate from the Schwann cells and are expelled. The response of myelin to neuronal injury indicates that signals from the axon are necessary to maintain both myelin protein production and Schwann cell insulation (5). The disruption of these signals leads to the loss of myelination. Phagocytotic cells, such as macrophages, clear myelin debris, though Schwann cells may also play a role (7). Debris clearance can take up to 7 months in humans (5), and is critical, as intact myelin protein has been shown to inhibit the elongation of new nerve fibers (8). In addition to clearing myelin, phagocytotic cells are also responsible for the production of cytokines, which encourage axon growth (5). Finally, the remaining Schwann cells in the proximal stump proliferate rapidly and form narrow tubes using their extensions, known as the bands of Bünger. The bands of Bünger provide a mechanical guide for axon migration.

Following breakdown of the axon and debris clearance, regeneration ensues. Regeneration begins from the proximal end and continues toward the distal stump. Sprouts usually emanate from the nodes of Ranvier, nonmyelinated areas of axons located between Schwann cells (9). In humans, axon regeneration occurs at a rate of 2–5 mm/day (10); thus, significant injury can take a while to heal.

In nerve guidance channels, conduits that span the injury gap (discussed further below), an additional step for regeneration has been evidenced. It is unclear as to whether this step also takes place in the absence of a conduit. After initial injury, a fibrin bridge extends across the site and through the conduit. The bridge includes macrophages and other leukocytes believed to be involved in debris clearance. The fibrin bridge retracts as Schwann cells and capillaries begin to grow across the gap, and regeneration proceeds as normal.

2. CNS Response

In the CNS, the initial cellular response to injury proceeds in much the same way as in the PNS. Injury allows an influx of ions that activate proteolysis. However, there are some marked differences in physiological response to axon degradation that appear to prevent regeneration in the CNS. For one, macrophages infiltrate the site of injury much more slowly in the CNS; therefore, inhibitory myelin removal is delayed (11,12). This is primarily due to the blood–spine barrier, which isolates blood components, such as monocytes/macrophages, from neurological tissue. Blood macrophages enter the nerve tissue primarily at the injury site, where barrier integrity is compromised. Native macrophages (microglia) are present in CNS nerve tissue, but their numbers are significantly lower than those seen in PNS injury response. In addition, cell adhesion molecules in the distal stump of the transected nerve do not up-regulate in a manner comparable to that of the PNS, discouraging macrophage recruitment. Another difference in the CNS is that oligodendrocytes, the myelinating cells of the CNS, do not eject their myelin in the same manner as Schwann cells. Oligodendrocytes have even been shown to inhibit regeneration, in a manner similar to myelin (8). Finally, astrocytes (CNS glial cells) proliferate in a manner similar to that of Schwann cells in the PNS. However, the proliferating cells do not produce bands of Bünger but instead become "reactive astrocytes," producing glial scars, that inhibit regeneration (13).

The progress of injury in the CNS also differs from that of the PNS. If injury is confined primarily to the gray matter, where the cell bodies are located, damage is limited to those cells involved in the injury. However, if the white matter is damaged, all nerve tracts below the injury site are affected due to the synaptic nature of axons. Furthermore, secondary injury results from swelling induced by the immune response. Swelling begins in the gray matter but proceeds in a lateral manner from the injury site into the white matter (2). If the nerve is pressed against bone fragments remaining from the initial trauma, additional damage may ensue. Ironically, the same blood–spine barrier that impedes macrophage infiltration may have evolved to protect the body from secondary injury resulting from swelling (14).

D. Current Clinical Approaches

Current clinical treatment is designed to speed regeneration, while minimizing harmful effects, such as inflammation, resulting from the injury. For peripheral nerve injury, treatment consists of end-to-end anastomosis or the autologous nerve graft (1). Short gaps can be managed by suturing the ends of the severed nerves together (end-to-end anastomosis); however, even this simple approach has drawbacks. Most notably, tension can be introduced into the nerve cable as it heals, and tension has been shown to inhibit nerve regeneration (26). For a larger nerve defect, the injury is spanned with an autologous nerve graft. A donor nerve from another site in the body is harvested and implanted between the two severed nerve ends of the injury site. The disadvantages of this technique include loss of function at the donor site and the need for multiple surgeries (1).

For CNS injury, and spinal cord injury in particular, clinical treatment is less promising. If bone fragments persist near the injury site, surgery may be attempted to reduce the risk of secondary injury. Anti-inflammatory drugs, such as methylprednisone, may also be administered to reduce swelling and secondary injury (2). However, there is no treatment available to restore function. After initial swelling has subsided, patients will begin a long period of rehabilitation, training remaining nerves to compensate for the injury.

E. Special Challenges in the Nervous System

As with clinical treatments, the primary focus of biomimetics in the nervous system has been to enhance regeneration or to restore function following injury. In the PNS, despite the ability to regenerate, clinical functional recovery rates typically approach only 80% for gaps requiring autologous nerve graft repair (15). In addition, slow regeneration rates require a long rehabilitation and recovery period. Biomimetic devices designed for the peripheral system have targeted improvements in recovery rates.

The CNS has provided a greater challenge for biomimetic development. First, unassisted functional regeneration does not occur; therefore, biomimetic devices are designed to promote recovery. Regeneration with the aid of external intervention, in the form of a peripheral nerve graft, was first reported by Ramón y Cajal in 1928 (16). This strategy was not investigated, however, until Aguayo et al. (17) repeated the experiment in 1980 (18). Since that time, the number of researchers examining CNS regeneration has greatly increased, but results have been mixed (19,20). Second, it has been shown that regenerating fibers in the CNS will neither grow into nor make contacts with PNS tissue without additional support, such as cellular additives (21). Several independent researchers have attempted transplantation with fetal tissue and cells (22–24). Despite the fact that fetal tissue has been shown to generate new nervous system tracts, these tracts do not integrate with the host synaptic pathways (25). As evidenced from this work, the greatest challenges in CNS regeneration are creating permissive environments and interfacing between the CNS and PNS. Biomimetics for the CNS must engender regeneration while supporting the PNS–CNS interface.

III. BIOMIMETIC APPROACHES TO ENHANCE NERVE REGENERATION

The challenges presented by nerve injury provide fertile ground for the development of devices that enhance the natural regeneration environment. Currently, researchers are focusing efforts on devices that mimic native nerve and the ECM as closely as possible. Such devices take advantage of mechanical, chemical, and electrical effects that occur in the body to produce enhanced regeneration. Already mechanical and electrical cues have been incorporated into regeneration assist devices, such as nerve guidance channels, patterned substrates, and artificial ECMs. In addition, chemical cues, such as neurotrophins, cells, anti-inhibitory molecules, and proteins, have been added to these devices, enhancing homology to the native nerve and its environment. For the future, combined approaches lead the way to improved nerve regeneration.

A. Haptotactic Cues in Biomimetics

Some of the earliest attempts to enhance regeneration provided a physical structure for the regenerating nerve. Physical structure was identified as a necessary component for regeneration based on the ground-breaking work of Harrison in 1914 (27). Harrison reported that neurites do not extend when cells float freely in media. This led to the development of the "contact action" theory described by Weiss (28) in 1941. Weiss elaborates that growing neurons mechanically interact with their environment through surface tensions and that tension is needed for the extension of neurites. The incorporation of physical, or haptotactic, cues spurred the development of the most important biomimetic device used in nerve regeneration: the nerve guidance channel.

1. Nerve Conduit Properties

The nerve guidance channel, or conduit, is designed to span the gap created by nerve injury. The ideal guidance channel should display several properties. The material should be flexible but should not kink. Rigid channels have been shown to irritate the nerve, inducing pain in the patient (1). In addition, the conduit must be manufactured into a cylindrical form. Next, the ideal guidance channel should be biodegradable. Permanent materials may invoke a chronic immune response or irritate the nerve. Furthermore, the ideal conduit must be sterilizable (1). Finally, stimulatory cues that actively promote regeneration can also be incorporated into the guidance channel as a means to better mimic the native nerve graft (Fig. 3). These advanced modifications are described in more detail below.

2. Modified Nerve Conduits

Early modern work has focused on silicone guidance channels (e.g., 29) or other readily available synthetic polymers (30). [For a review of materials used in nerve guidance channels see Schmidt et al. (30).] Initial results of these studies demonstrated some success in enhancing peripheral nerve

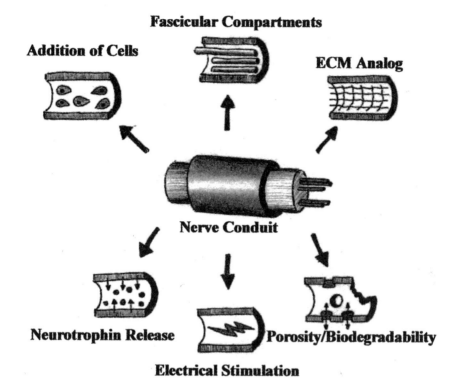

Figure 3 Nerve guidance channels and modifications to enhance nerve regeneration. Nerve guidance channels provide mechanical guidance for the regenerating axon. They may be functionalized with cells, fascicular compartments, ECM components, or neurotrophins. They may also be altered to enhance electrical conductivity or biodegradability and porosity. (Adapted from TW Hudson, et al. Clin Plast Surg 26:626, 1999. Drawn by Timothy Liu, University of Texas, Austin, TX.)

regeneration (30), but limited or no effect in the CNS. Recently, efforts have focused on creating conduits that are more representative of the actual nerve environment. Researchers have attempted to duplicate the fascicular nature of a nerve by creating longitudinal compartments within the guidance channel (31). Individual compartments encourage the formation of separate axon bundles within a single nerve, similar to natural nerve which contains multiple fascicles in each nerve cable. Also, compartments dramatically increase the surface area of the conduit, augmenting the area available for soluble factors or cell adherence.

Other groups have altered the conduit in other ways. Researchers have tried to duplicate the fibrin bridge, formed in the earliest stages of nerve regeneration, using conduits filled with fibers (32,33). Polyamide fibers placed inside a silicone conduit have been used to create a "bioartificial nerve graft." The graft demonstrated regeneration across gaps as long as 15 mm in rats (32). However, the regenerating axons did not interface with the fibers, indicating that the fibers did not provide the mechanical guidance that had been anticipated. Also, the graft was more successful than an empty tube only in gaps greater than 10 cm (33). Yet another approach includes the development of a spongy poly(lactic-glycolic) acid (PLGA) scaffold seeded with neural stem cells (34). The sponge allows axons and support cells to migrate through the pores while providing mechanical support (Fig. 4). Neural stem cells enhance the chemical environment, providing growth factors and other support molecules.

To enhance neuron–substrate interaction, others have focused on natural substrates, particularly collagen. Grafts with magnetically aligned longitudinal collagen have demonstrated increased nerve regeneration both in vitro and in vivo as compared with an unaligned collagen graft (35,36). This increase most likely results from the ability of collagen to serve as a scaffold for nerve regeneration. Other groups have combined collagen-filled conduits with laminin- and fibronectin-coated collagen fibers (37). Increased regeneration was demonstrated over a 1-cm defect in a rat. Yet another approach enhances collagen's mechanical structure by adding polyglycolic acid (PGA) mesh to the conduit (38). Collagen gel was deposited around the mesh and polymerized in situ. In preliminary results, the conduits bridged gaps of up to 8 cm in dogs. Based on the current understanding of conduit research, future biomimetic development will continue to focus on enhancing conduit–nerve homology through the incorporation of physical components and through the use of natural materials.

3. Patterned Biomimetic Systems

Mechanical cues have also been employed in other types of biomimetic systems; most notably to explore the effects of cell migration in vitro. Several researchers have used the technique pioneered by Hammarback et al. in 1985 (39) to pattern substrates with specific regions of biological activity. Briefly, a nonadherent substrate, such as silicon, is coated with the biological material of interest. Then a photolithographic mask is applied. Etching through the mask exposes the nonadherent substrate in selected locations. The mask is then removed revealing patterned regions (Fig. 5).

Microlithography and photomasking have been used to examine collagen (40), laminin (41,42), ECM peptides (43), and amine complexes (44)

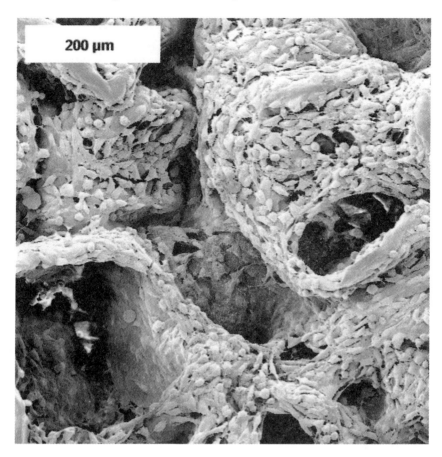

200 µm

Figure 4 Neural stem cells seeded on poly(lactic-glycolic) acid (PLGA) sponge. A SEM image shows a PLGA sponge that has been seeded with the murine NSC clone, C17.2, courtesy of Evan Snyder. The average pore size of the sponge is 250–500 µm. (Photo courtesy of Erin Lavik and Robert Langer, Massachusetts Institute of Technology, Boston, MA.)

as substrates. Studies have shown that collagen (40) and laminin (41) increase neurite outgrowth and that performance can be dependent on stripe spacing (42). Isolated 2-µm stripes of biomolecules successfully promoted neurite extension along the patterned area. On the other hand, groups of 2-µm stripes with 2-µm spacings did not encourage extension along stripes. This suggests that the regular parallel alignment of endoneurial collagen

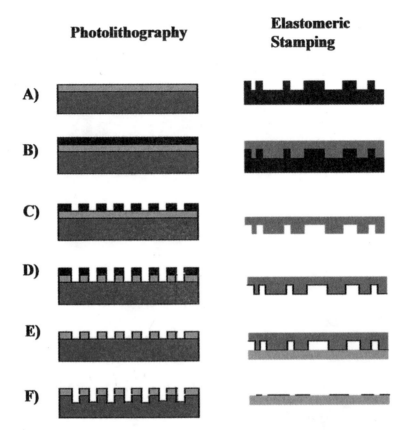

Figure 5 Photolithography v. elastomeric stamping. Photolithography: (a) A substrate is coated with the biomolecule of interest. (b) Photoresist is applied above the biomolecule. (c) A mask is applied (typically using deep UV) to the resist leaving a pattern behind. (d) The pattern is etched into the biomolecule of interest. (e) The photoresist is removed. (f) Further etching can be applied to create pillars or wells, if desired. Elastomeric stamping: (a) A substrate pattern is developed using lithographic techniques. (b) An elastomeric polymer is placed over the substrate and polymerized. (c) The polymer is removed from the substrate. (d) Biomolecule "ink" is applied to the stamp. (e) The stamp is applied to the cell growth substrate. (f) The stamp is removed leaving the patterned biomolecules behind. (Drawn by Timothy Liu, University of Texas, Austin, TX.)

may repel extending neurites (42). Patterned synthetic ECM, developed using peptides, may help elucidate this mechanism further (43).

In addition to microlithography, several other patterning techniques have been explored, including laser ablation (45) and laser printing (46).

More recent developments in printing include elastomeric stamping and elastomeric stenciling. Elastomeric stamping, a technique based in microlithography, uses a polydimethylsiloxane (PMDS) stamp, molded in photoresist, to print molecules onto a surface (47). Once on the surface, the molecules form a self-assembled monolayer (SAM) (Fig. 5). Alternatively, a stencil may be fabricated instead of a stamp. The stencil is pressed onto the surface. Cells are placed in the stencil during seeding, and the stencil is removed after attachment (48). [For a review of SAM techniques and elastomeric stamping, see Whitesides et al. (49).] The technique is advantageous over traditional photolithography-based methods because it allows for multiple proteins to be patterned on the same surface. Further, elastomeric stamping has been shown to be as effective as photolithographic techniques in promoting adhesion while reducing the exposure of delicate proteins to harsh chemicals required for photolithography (50). Some of the first applications of microcontact printing were demonstrated in 1993 by Whitesides et al. (51), who used the method to pattern gold surfaces with alkanethiolates for cell adhesion. Later work used microcontact printing and SAMs to pattern aminosilanes for nerve extension studies (52).

Although much work has focused on adhesion to biomolecule-coated surfaces, patterned surfaces (Fig. 6) have also been used to investigate the effect of substrate physical structure on cell adhesion and proliferation. In experiments using lithographically grooved quartz, hippocampal neurons in serum-free media interacted strongly with grooved areas (53). Axons grew perpendicular to the grooves, which were substantially narrower than the

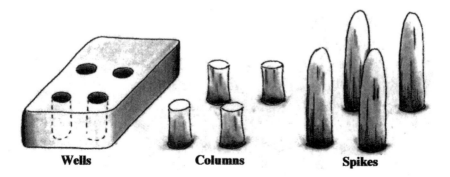

Wells   **Columns**   **Spikes**

Figure 6 Wells, columns, and spikes. Scale drawing of surface modifications shows relative dimensions of each feature. Wells and columns are approximately 1 µm in depth/height. Spikes are approximately 2.7 µm in height. All features are 0.5–2.0 µm in width and spaced by 0.5–5.0 µm. (Drawn by Timothy Liu, University of Texas, Austin, TX.)

axon width. Dendrite extensions were aligned parallel to the grooves. It is clear that mechanical cues alone can guide developing axons, and these results have sparked interest in the patterning of pillars and wells for migration studies. Using microlithographic techniques, barriers were shown to affect the attachment and migration of astrocytes and hippocampal cells. Glial cells have been shown to preferentially attach to pillars over wells (54). Another study, investigating the effect of silicon columns and spikes of various sizes, showed that glial cells and hippocampal neurons preferred columnar and spiked regions to smooth regions (Fig. 7) (55). The exact mechanism for this preferential growth is unclear but supports the premise that haptotactic cues can be used to guide cell migration.

B. Chemotactic Cues in Biomimetics

Although mechanical cues have been used to promote nerve regeneration in biomimetic devices, many other types of cues have been studied. The most active area of research has centered on chemical and biochemical cues, with recent work in factors such as neurotrophins, cells, and anti-inhibitory molecules. Factors may be used alone, but are more commonly incorporated into an existing device, such as a conduit. This is especially true in the PNS, where the use of channels is well established. The addition of factors is believed to enhance the benefit provided by mechanical guidance alone.

1. Neurotrophins

Some of the first additives studied were the neurotrophins, or proteins that promote nerve regeneration. The existence of neurotrophins was debated until experiments performed in the 1940s by Weiss and Taylor "seemingly" disproved the neurotrophic effect. Using aortic y chambers, they showed that nerves exhibit no preference for regenerating toward the distal stump versus another site (56). As a result, the study of neurotrophins was abandoned for more than 40 years. However, more recent work, using silicone y chambers, has conclusively shown that neurotrophic factors do play a role in guiding and enhancing nerve regeneration (57,58). It is believed that the misleading results of Weiss and Taylor were a result of neurotrophic factors present in the aortic y chambers themselves, which encouraged regeneration regardless of the distal target (57,58). Since this time, a number of neurotrophic factors have been identified, enhancing nerve growth in both the PNS and CNS. [These are reviewed by Terenghi (59), Bixby and Harris (60), Aguayo et al. (61), and Müller et al. (62).] One of the earliest neurotrophic factors identified was nerve growth factor (NGF), and experiments incorporating this factor in silicone conduits have

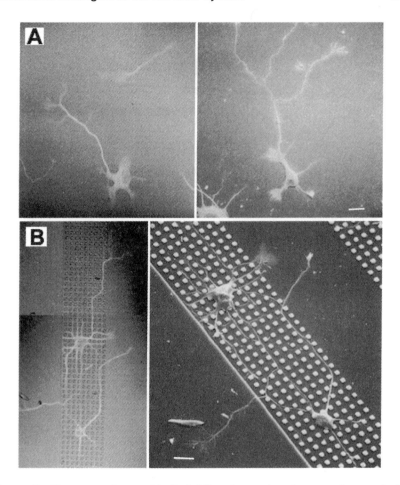

Figure 7   Fluorescent images [A, B (left)] and scanning electron micrographs [B (right)] show rat hippocampal neurons (E18) growing on silicon surfaces after 1 day in vitro. Neurons are shown on smooth and unmodified (A) and topographically modified (B) silicon substrates. The surface in (B) has been modified to have smooth regions and regions of 2-μm-wide pillars, 1 μm high separated by a distance of 3.5 μm. Polylysine has been applied uniformly to all surfaces. Axons, the long thin processes, grow on the unmodified smooth surfaces in (A) with a characteristic large growth cone at the distal end. The topographically modified surface guides axonal outgrowth and the axons grow faster, as much as two times faster, with a much smaller growth cone when the distal end is in the pillared region. Bars equal 5 μm. (These images are part of research performed in the NSF-supported Nanobiotechnology Center. Photo courtesy of Natalie Dowell, James Turner, and William Shain, Wadsworth Center, Albany, NY and Andrea Perez-Turner, and Harold Craighead, Cornell University, Ithaca, NY.)

demonstrated increased peripheral nerve regeneration over a conduit alone (63).

A great challenge in the use of neurotrophic factors is the method of delivery. The body metabolizes trophic factors in days. Since nerve regeneration can take up to weeks or months, consistent delivery is crucial. Several approaches have been developed to address this problem. Researchers have incorporated neurotrophic factors into Gelfoam, a commercially available matrix (64), as well as fibronectin (65) and collagen (66), naturally occurring ECM components. Factors have also been delivered by constant injection, using an internal minipump (67).

2. Cellular Additives

The difficulty in delivery of neurotrophic factors has led some researchers to develop a different approach altogether. Using genetic engineering, researchers have modified cells to deliver factors directly (68,69). [For a review of genetic engineering techniques for drug delivery, see Tresco et al. (70).] Also, some cells naturally produce neurotrophic factors, and direct cell seeding has been attempted in these cases. Typically, cells are isolated from tissue, cultured, and suspended in a gel or other material that fills the conduit. Schwann cells, olfactory ensheathing cells, and macrophages have all been investigated. Initially, conduits incorporated Schwann cells, which were selected for their ability to myelinate axons and for their role in guiding regeneration (71). As in native nerve repair, the transplanted Schwann cells formed bands of Bünger, which guided the axons to distal targets. [For review of Schwann cells in PNS repair, see Kemp et al. (72).] The success of Aguayo et al. in 1980 using peripheral nerve grafts in the CNS (17) made Schwann cells an attractive candidate for CNS repair as well. Schwann cells have been added to peripheral nerve grafts (73) and synthetic polymer conduits (74) for implantation into the CNS. Such grafts have been successful and have prompted the development of Schwann cell implantation techniques that do not require conduits. Schwann cell fibers (75) and solid grafts (76) have been developed for CNS implantation. Fibers were created by dragging a micropipette across the wound area while releasing Schwann cells. Solid grafts were prepared by placing cells in a conduit and applying suction to compact the cells. The conduit was then removed, leaving behind a solid Schwann cell graft. Schwann cell implantation has resulted in regeneration in the implant in all cases. However, regeneration in the transition zone, between the implant and the distal end of the host spinal cord, is limited (76).

The success of Schwann cell grafts has encouraged interest in other types of glial cells. In the olfactory system of the CNS, axons continue to grow throughout adulthood, unlike other CNS tissues. One noted difference in the olfactory system is the presence of olfactory ensheathing cells as the primary glial cell. Olfactory ensheathing cells, which span both the CNS and PNS of the olfactory system, display behaviors similar to those of glial cells from the CNS and PNS (77). The results of olfactory ensheathing cell transplantations surpass those of Schwann cell transplantations. Histological (78–82), electrophysiological (79), and some functional recovery (78,80–82) has been demonstrated. Most notably, olfactory ensheathing cell transplants have been shown to promote growth of axons across the CNS–PNS interface (80,81), thus addressing one of the major concerns in CNS research. This technique has also been applied to peripheral nerves (83) and has demonstrated success in this environment as well.

While Schwann cells and olfactory ensheathing cells are attractive components of biomimetic devices due to their roles in myelination and axon guidance, macrophages and other phagocytotic cells perform the critical function of debris clearance. The presence of myelin debris is inhibitory to regeneration (8), and early removal is essential for regeneration to proceed. Therefore, the addition of peripheral macrophages to the CNS, where macrophage infiltration is typically delayed (11), has been investigated as a method of enhancing regeneration. PNS tissue receives ample infiltration by phagocytotic cells due to the lack of a blood–spine barrier. Therefore, this type of graft is rarely used in PNS tissue.

Macrophages were first injected directly into severed optic nerve (84) and later studied in severed spinal cord (85). Intriguingly, phagocytotic activity in the CNS was enhanced by incubation of peripheral macrophages with a peripheral nerve segment prior to transplantation. This indicates that CNS injury alone may not sufficiently alter macrophage protein expression (84). Another study examined native CNS phagocytotic cells (microglia) and demonstrated that addition of these cells also increases nerve regeneration (86). Ironically, these results are in contrast with other studies demonstrating that depletion of macrophages benefits nerve function (87). Depletion of macrophages reduces swelling, and may reduce secondary injury, thereby increasing patient function. These contradictory results require further investigation. It is possible that the benefit of macrophages is time dependent, with an initial harmful phase that results in increased swelling, followed by a beneficial phase that gives rise to debris elimination. Future development is needed to take advantage of the positive effects of macrophage debris clearance, while minimizing the risk of secondary injury.

3. Anti-Inhibitory Molecules

One of the main benefits of macrophage addition to nerve grafts is enhanced clearance of inhibitory debris, but other methods for countering these effects have also been investigated. Certain ECM proteins, such as tenascin (88), proteoglycans such as chondroitin sulfate (88,89), myelin (8), and the myelin-derived proteins NI-250 and myelin-associated glycoprotein (MAG) (89) have all demonstrated inhibitory tendencies in the CNS. However, the effect is not clearly understood; in some forms these molecules can encourage axon growth, especially in development. More research is needed to elucidate the role of inhibitory compounds in the CNS. [For an excellent review of the current understanding of these molecules, see Fawcett et al. (89).]

Nonetheless, some exciting research has been conducted using antibodies to inhibit these molecules. Schwab et al. have developed an antibody (IN-1) to the myelin associated inhibitory protein NI-250. Treatment of transected spinal cord with this antibody increases sprouting from the injury site (90). Expanding on this approach, vaccines have been developed that stimulate the patient's immune systems to produce antibodies to myelin. This method resulted in "extensive regeneration of large numbers of axons" in mice (91).

4. Natural Biomaterials and ECM Analogs

While chemical additives have shown promise for enhancing nerve regeneration, combined approaches, adding both mechanical and chemical cues, are expected to surpass these in efficacy. In particular, many attempts have been made to form biomimetics that directly duplicate the material surrounding an axon, the ECM. The ECM in this location consists of basal lamina components, such as laminin, fibronectin, and collagen. All three of these molecules have been shown to enhance regeneration in vitro (92,93) and are prime conduit additive candidates. [For a review of ECM components and their regeneration-promoting behavior, see Bixby and Harris (60).] However, ECM components are primarily contained in hydrated tissue composed of glycosaminoglycan (GAG) polymer chains. Biomimetic development has focused on providing ECM components in a more representative mechanical environment.

Natural materials have been examined for this purpose, including tendon (94) and collagen coated with laminin and fibronectin (37,38), but the primary focus of study has been highly cross-linked hydrated polymers, known as hydrogels. Natural hydrogels have been developed from collagen-GAG (i.e., chondroitin sulfate) copolymers (95,96) and hyaluronic acid (HA) (97,98). Both HA and chondroitin sulfate are major components of the ECM and appear to play roles in wound healing. Also, both materials enhance nerve regeneration when implanted in gel form.

Synthetic hydrogels, on the other hand, allow for a greater selection of mechanical and physical properties than are available with natural materials. Gel porosity is a critical factor to nerve extension (99). Low-porosity gels can provide considerable resistance to regenerating neurons, whereas highly porous gels may not have the physical structure necessary for axon guidance. A careful balance, such as that evidenced in Fig. 8, is required for optimum neurite extension.

Agarose and acrylamide synthetic gels are commonly studied (100), as they are readily available, but they are not as effective as gels that include ECM proteins (101). Therefore, gels have been functionalized with laminin (102,103), collagen (103), fibronectin (104), growth factors (105,106), and laminin-derived peptides (107–109), all of which have been shown to

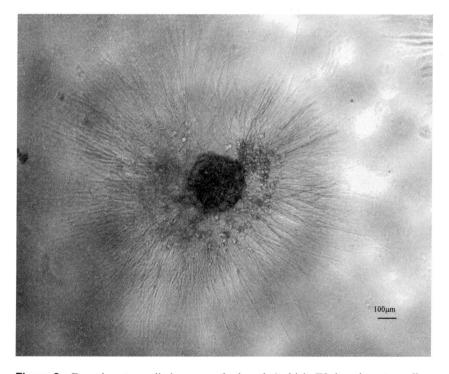

100μm

Figure 8 Dorsal root ganglia in agarose hydrogel. A chick, E9 dorsal root ganglion was cultured in 1% agarose gels for 3 days. Neurites extend radially from the ganglion cell. (Photo courtesy of Ryan Gilbert, Xiaojun Yu and Ravi Bellamkonda, Case Western Reserve University, Cleveland, OH.)

enhance nerve regeneration. Several commercial gels are available, of which Matrigel is the most popular. Matrigel is composed of laminin, collagen, elastin, and heparan sulfate proteoglycan. Comparative tests have found that Matrigel outperforms any of these components alone in promoting nerve regeneration (110).

In another method, used to mimic ECM in peripheral nerve, nerve tissue is treated in such a way as to render it "decellularized." This is accomplished by various techniques, but the most prominent are to repeatedly freeze and thaw tissue (111,112), to irradiate tissue (113), or to expose tissue to specific chemicals (112). The process is termed *decellularization* because all cells the nerve tissue are destroyed. The guiding principle behind this approach is that the major antigenic components are found on the cells; therefore, by removing the cells, foreign nerve tissue can be utilized as graft material without the danger of immunological rejection. In addition, the ECM and basal laminae tubes are preserved to a great extent (112), providing the preferred physical structure for regenerating neurons. Also, the proteins composing the basal lamina (e.g., collagen and laminin) form substrates on which axons naturally adhere and propagate. Thus, a decellularized graft of peripheral nerve tissue can provide the same physical structure and protein surface as an allograft with a minimized or negligible immune response.

C. Electrical Cues in Biomimetics

In addition to chemical and mechanical signals, nerves respond to electrical cues (114). In 1979, Jaffe and Poo showed that nerves exposed to electrical fields of $70-140 \, mV/mm$ extend neurites preferentially toward the cathode. Although the mechanism for this movement is unclear, one possible theory links the growth to migration of receptors for neurotrophic factors (114). Additional theories result from experimental evidence showing that inhibition of electrically induced growth occurs with the application of several substances known to affect Ca^{2+} concentrations and cytoskeleton organization (115). One possible explanation is that electric fields increase the hydrolysis of phosphatidylinositol biphosphate (PIP_2), a membrane protein and signaling molecule. The dissociation of this complex results in the release of profilactin and profilin. Profilactin increases levels of actin, a cytoskeleton component. Then, profilin encourages actin assembly and, therefore, axon migration. Another proposed theory suggests that Ca^{2+} levels are increased by the activation of voltage-sensitive Ca^{2+} channels. Then, Ca^{2+} up-regulates gelsolin, a cytoskeletal protein that encourages actin reorganization and growth cone migration (115).

Several biomimetic devices have capitalized on this approach, providing electric fields to regenerating nerves. Polyvinylidene fluoride (PVDF) piezoelectric conduits were used to study peripheral nerve regeneration in vitro (116) and in rats (117). Piezoelectric conduits are attractive for electrical delivery because charge is created by mechanical deformation of the device and does not require a power source. However, one drawback is that charge delivery is sporadic and not controllable or tunable. A separate study examined the effects of constant surface charge delivery using polytetrafluoroethylene (PTFE) electrets (118). In this case, regeneration was most enhanced by positive charge, with negative tubes showing intermediate values between those of the positive tubes and controls.

Electrically conducting polymers, such as polypyrrole, have also been developed as nerve guidance channels (119). These electrically active biomimetics have been further enhanced with chemical factors to take advantage of multiple techniques. Hyaluronic acid (HA), an ECM component, has been shown to promote nerve regeneration, wound healing, and angiogenesis (120). HA has been added to polypyrrole conduits to create a composite, electrically conductive biomaterial promoting both nerve extension and angiogenesis (120).

Alternatively, charged hydrogels have been created to duplicate the ECM, providing electrical stimulation and providing a charged substrate (121). Charged polysaccharides, such as chitosan (+) and alginate (−), were covalently coupled to agarose to produce cationic and anionic hydrogels. Nerves regenerated preferentially in cationic hydrogels.

D. The Future of Biomimetics for Nerve Regeneration

Devices designed to enhance regeneration in the nervous system are subject to many challenges. There are several techniques that show enhancement in regeneration rates, but no single technique has emerged from the field. Consequently, biomimetic development is moving toward combined approaches. We have already seen some evidence of these approaches, including surfaces patterned with biological molecules, cellular delivery of neurotrophins, artificial ECM development, and combined electrical and chemical cues. It is not surprising that multiple approaches are required in biological mimicry, as the body responds to a variety of signal types. We are only beginning to understand the complexity underlying wound healing in the body, but combined approaches provide a first approximation of natural regeneration processes.

IV. BIOMIMETIC APPROACHES TO REPLACE NERVE FUNCTION

The second major class of neurobiomimetics under development is aimed at replacing neural function rather than enhancing nerve repair. Devices currently being researched attempt to replace spinal cord or brain tissue function, while successful neural prosthetic devices already exist for retinal and auditory deficits. Biomimetics for spinal function began with the development of the microelectrode array, a collection of micrometer-sized electrodes patterned on a substrate. Recently, prosthetic development has expanded to field effect transistors (FETs), devices that carry charge in the presence of a voltage potential. Design improvements include the use of perforated devices to directly interface with regenerating nerve fibers. One of the major hurdles for biomimetic devices aimed at functional replacement is the ability of a biomimetic electronic circuit to approximate biological and ionic nerve response. Much recent work has focused on this area. Building on the successful design of the retinal and cochlear implants, biomimetics for replacement of CNS function are a distinct possibility for the future.

A. Microarray Biomimetics

There is an indisputable need for prosthetics to replace nerve function, but execution has progressed slowly. In 1979, one of the first attempts at prosthetic technology used fixed gold conductors mounted on a glass surface to interface with neurons in culture (122). This was the first successful application of photolithography in the development of a neuroprosthetic device. Microelectrode array technology, as it came to be called, has continued to advance. These initial arrays were constructed on a substrate, usually glass, using photolithography to pattern squares of conducting material, typically gold. The squares were connected to patterned wires, which were covered with a dielectric material. Electrical signals could be read from the array by connecting a probe to each patterned wire. Early arrays interacted with cells in culture, not real tissue, and the interaction was only one way: the array read from the cell only. Later arrays created interfaces with tissue sections, such as hippocampal slices, and stimulated neurons directly (123). In addition, the number of electrodes has increased and biocompatibility has been demonstrated (124).

Microarrays have shown significant promise but also have limitations, such as the inability to precisely position on the array and to control cell migration. Cells must be carefully positioned on array electrodes in order to make contact with the array. If cells migrate away from the contacts, the recording or stimulating interface is lost. One method to alleviate this difficulty is the incorporation of biorecognition molecules onto the array surface through hydrostatic bonding (125). When peptides, such as the laminin peptide YIGSR, were added, cell adhesion was greatly enhanced, although the improvement in signal quality was unclear. In addition, YIGSR molecules have been added to neural probes, i.e., electrodes that are inserted directly into the cortex (Fig. 9) (126). The incorporation of peptides increased attachment of neuroblastoma cells in vitro, suggesting an increased interaction between the device and neural tissue. Also, neural probes have been modified with conducting polymers, such as polypyrrole, to enhance the electrical interface between the probe and neural tissue (126).

Recent work in our laboratory has also used peptides and antibodies to situate quantum dots, nanometer-sized semiconductors, on nerve cell receptors (126a). Using multiple small semiconductor particles to interact directly with a nerve cell allows for the development of a multielectrode array that interacts with a single cell. In addition, microarray technologies have spawned a commercial device, the Neurochip (127), designed to interface with hippocampal neurons and promote neural networks. Nonetheless, microarray technology is still a long way from providing a prosthetic device to compensate for lost neural function.

B. Regeneration Microelectrode Arrays

The regeneration array is an adaptation of the microelectrode array that uses perforated chips to interact with regenerating nerve fibers. Regeneration is primarily a PNS phenomenon; but this device also has potential applications in treating spinal cord-injured patients. Fibers regenerate through the device, and individual axons make contact with electrodes in the array. Then, the array "reads" changes in membrane potential of the axons. The regeneration array can then transmit signals to a robotic controller allowing amputees control of their limbs. The device was first executed before the advent of photolithography, using teased nerve fibers regenerating through tubes containing electrodes (128). The advent of microarray technology greatly enhanced the efficacy of these devices (129). Arrays manufactured using silicon-based technologies have recorded signals up to 13 months after implantation; however, signal collection requires surgery to expose the wound site or leads that trail outside the body (130).

A major issue in the development of regeneration arrays has been optimal pore size. The pores must be large enough to allow unimpeded passage of regenerating axons but should be intimate to maximize electrical contact. Techniques have been developed to manufacture devices with varying geometries (131), and experiments have determined that devices must have holes greater than $50\,\mu m$ to allow regeneration (132).

(a)

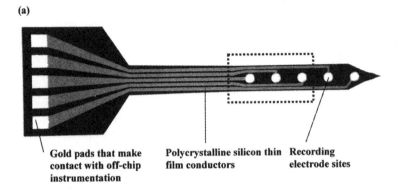

Gold pads that make   Polycrystalline silicon thin   Recording
contact with off-chip   film conductors   electrode sites
instrumentation

(b)

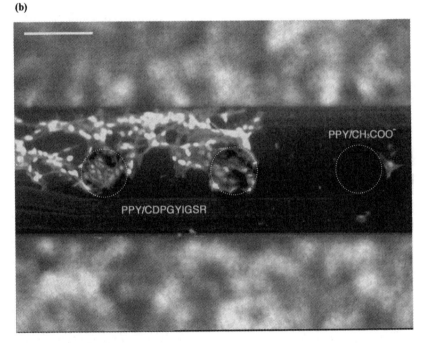

Figure 9 Neural probe coated with CDPGYIGSR peptide. (a) Neural probe construction. The neural probe consists of recording sites, coated with polypyrrole (PPY) and CDPGYIGSR peptide or polypyrrole and CH_3COO^- chemical. Thin film conductors transmit the signal to gold pads, which make contact with external instrumentation. (b) Close-up of recording region of neural probe. Probe contacts were coated with both PPY/CPDGYIGSR and PPY/CH_3COO^-. Increased neuroblastoma cell attachment occurred in the CPDGYIGSR-coated region. PPY, an electrically conducting polymer, was added for conductivity enhancement. (Photo courtesy of Xinyan Cui, David Martin, University of Michigan, Ann Arbor, MI.)

Furthermore, the incorporation of proteins, such as the laminin-like pronectin L, can be used to increase the number of axons regenerating through the array (133). The clinical potential of regeneration arrays has also been investigated, using externally generated signals sent through the spinal cord, and then interpreted with the array. A stimulation source was attached directly to the spinal cord to induce controlled signals. The signals then propagated down the cord, through the peripheral nerve, to the regeneration array. This method allowed researchers to visualize action potentials created from the spinal cord; however, intrinsic signals have yet to be evaluated (134).

C. FET Biomimetics

Another biomimetic prosthetic device developed recently uses field effect transistors (FETs) instead of microelectrodes to interact with the nerve cell. Field effect transistors are micrometer-sized transistors that consist of a source, a drain, an insulating oxide layer, and a gate. The source and drain are composed of either positively (p) or negatively (n) doped silicon, depending on the desired direction of current flow. A gate separates the source and drain and is usually doped with material of the opposite charge as the source and drain. An insulating layer, usually of silicon oxide, covers the FET surface. When a voltage is applied to the gate, opposite charges are attracted to the surface of the gate region. This allows current to flow. Fromherz and colleagues pioneered the technique in which a Retzius leech nerve cell is placed on the gate region of a p-channel FET (135). When the cell fires an action potential, the charge density of the gate region changes, inducing a current. Classical nerve behavior, as described by Hodgkin and Huxley (136), was measured and confirmed using this technique (137). The nerve demonstrated an inward cellular Na^+ current, followed by an outward cellular K^+ current.

FETs can also be used to excite the cell (138). As a voltage is passed through the FET, the membrane responds with a corresponding change in voltage. If the voltage is strong enough, the cell produces an action potential. Coupling between the transistor and the nerve cell is largely capacitive, as the gate oxide and cell membrane are highly insulating. The primary advantage of the FET technique over standard microarray technology is improved interfacing between the cell and device. FET devices separate the cell and gate region with a dielectric, usually silicon oxide, whereas standard arrays require cell–metal contact. It is believed that oxide is a more natural substrate for the cell. This technique has also been extended to mammalian cells and has been used in array form to interact with multiple neurons simultaneously (139). However, mammalian cells present several difficulties. For extended studies, cells must have low division and migration rates. Also, many mammalian cells require glial support cells, but glial cells insulate neurons from the device. Glial cells can be excluded by the use of serum-free media and the addition of a laminin-like synthetic peptide to promote cell adhesion (139).

D. Electronic Circuits

One of the greatest difficulties associated with biomimetic neural prostheses is the integration and interpretation of neural signals. Despite progress in emulating the behavior of a single neuron, researchers are still searching for circuitry to describe the behavior of multiple neurons working in conjunction (140). Initially, circuits focused on modeling biological response through traditional digital computing, instead of analogue computing, which is more representative of actual nerve signals. The difference between digital models and faithful neural replicates is vast. Digital computing stores data using 1's and 0's. The decision of a nerve to fire a potential is not based on a combination of 1's and 0's but comes directly from the circuit itself, through the integration of multiple signal inputs that are either inhibitory or excitatory (141). In digital computing, noise is eliminated at each calculation step by conversion of data into a 1 or a 0 to pass to the next stage. Neurons do not convert data between stages. Instead, multiple inputs are processed to a single "average" output. Fidelity of signal is ensured by a high number of inputs that should outnumber the sources of noise (140). In addition, calculations in digital computing occur in serial, one before the other, whereas nerves process signals in parallel, multiple calculations occurring simultaneously (141). Duplicating neural signaling requires more than a change in circuitry; it requires a paradigm shift in signal processing. Nonetheless, recent successes in analogue computing, at a minimum of cost and power usage (142), have encouraged researchers to develop faithful neural equivalents (143,144).

E. Successful Prosthetics

Several successful neural prosthetics have already been developed. The cochlear implant, designed to promote auditory function, and the retinal implant, improving visual acuity, serve as examples for future biomimetics. These devices are largely based on array technology, using electrodes to directly stimulate underlying neurons. Both devices restore function by interacting with the native environment at the earliest possible level. Using the success of these devices, researchers look to the future for improved biomimetics.

1. Prosthetics for Auditory Function

Among successful neuroprosthetic devices, the cochlear implant has been used for more than 20 years (145). The cochlear implant restores sound perception to profoundly deaf patients, using existing architecture. In the undamaged ear, sounds are converted from pressure waves to mechanical waves by the eardrum, and finally to electrical waves by auditory hair cells and auditory neurons in the cochlea. Many cases of deafness result from deficiencies of pressure-mechanical conversion, leaving the auditory neurons intact. Cochlear implants take advantage of remaining neurons to transmit sounds, as electrical signals, to the brain (146). A cochlear implant uses a microphone to pick up sounds and a signal processor to interpret them. An electrode array passes an electrical signal from the signal processor to the auditory neurons. The signal processor and microphone are usually contained in a small exterior device, which uses radio signals to send the desired output to a transmitter (Fig. 10). The transmitter may be located just outside the ear or may be implanted. The transmitter then sends signals to the electrode array, which stimulates the nerve cells (145).

Only some patients may successfully integrate cochlear implants. First, candidates must have sufficient surviving neurons to allow for electrode interfacing. Fortunately, many causes of deafness leave neurons intact (145). Second, cochlear implants are much more successful when implanted in patients who became deaf following the onset of language skills. Learning to interpret and create speech signals is an important part of development, which requires sound feedback. If the device is to be implanted in individuals with prelingual onset deafness, younger patients (about 2 years through adolescence) tend to perform better (145). At best, the device is expected to "provide at least 90% speech discrimination to at least 45% of profoundly deaf individuals" (147); however, actual success rates are lower.

Nonetheless, for the profoundly deaf, the future is constantly improving. Research has extended beyond the cochlear implant to a possible auditory brain stem implant. This implant is targeted at another class of deaf patients, those with few surviving neurons in the cochlea. Using the same concepts as the cochlear implant, the device bypasses auditory neurons altogether to make direct connections with neurons in the brain stem (148). The device has been successful. Following correct positioning during surgery, patients have been able to discern sounds with the aid of lip reading (148).

2. Prosthetics for Visual Function

Although still in early development, retinal implants offer a promising prosthetic solution for individuals with retinal diseases, such as retinal

Microphone · Receiver · Cochlea

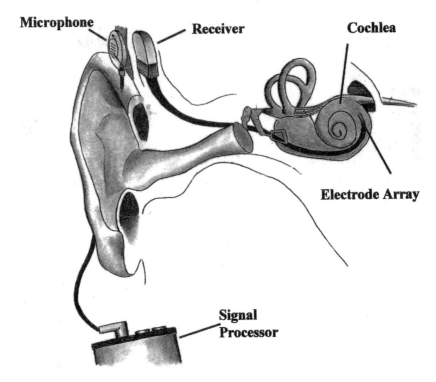

Electrode Array

Signal Processor

Figure 10 Cochlear implant. An external device contains the microphone and signal processor. The signal is then transmitted to the receiver, which relays it to an electrode array. The array stimulates auditory hair cells in the cochlea, and the signal is transmitted to the brain. (Adapted from Dallas Otarlaryngology Cochlear Implant Team. http://dallascochelar.com/clarion.htm, May 2001. Drawn by Stephen Liu, University of Texas, Austin, TX.)

pigmentosa and macular degeneration. The concept of the retinal implant began with research showing that visual responses could be elicited downstream of the retina. Responses were formed by stimulating the visual cortex (149) or from stimulating the retina itself (150). Implants to stimulate the visual cortex have several surgical drawbacks, including the need for brain surgery. On the other hand, retinal implants are easily implanted using existing surgical procedures. Retinal implants provide the most direct form of stimulation, interacting with the underlying ganglia cells and bypassing the photoreceptors. The development of specific prosthetic devices has resulted in two forms of retinal implants (Fig. 11). The epiretinal prosthetic is situated above the retina and elicits responses from retinal ganglia cells

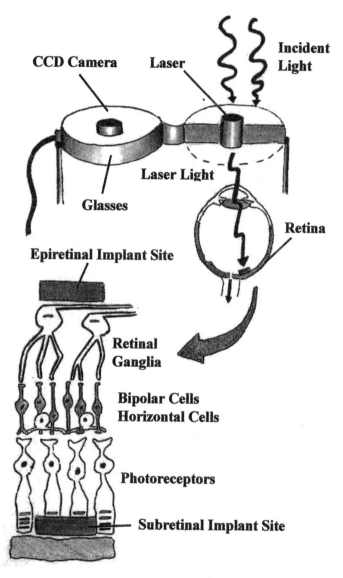

Figure 11 Retinal implant. Incident light enters a CCD camera located on a pair of eyeglasses. A laser mounted in the eyeglasses reproduces the incident light pattern with increased intensity. The laser light is collected by the implant, which may be located near the retinal ganglia (epiretinal) or near the photoreceptors (subretinal). (Adapted from J Wyatt et al. IEEE Spect May:50, 1996 and P Heiduschka, et al. Prog Neurobiol 55:450, 1998. Drawn by Timothy Liu, University of Texas, Austin, TX.)

and their axons. The implant consists of a photodiode array that interacts with a stimulation source, exciting individual neurons (151). Arrays may be designed to mimic the actual visual field, with several overlapping inputs for the same area (152). The subretinal implant places electrodes below the retina, in the location usually occupied by photoreceptors. The subretinal implant replaces functions at the earliest possible level, a significant advantage for signal processing (153,154). [For a short review of retinal implants, see Nadig (155).]

However, retinal implants have several drawbacks. The photodiodes currently used are too weak to respond with sunlight alone. Alternative designs circumvent this problem using laser beams, mounted in eyeglasses worn by the user, to increase the signal (151). The laser is modulated by a CCD camera that interprets optical data (151). However, this design can only be used with epiretinal implants due to the possibility of retinal damage associated with laser light (151). In addition, epiretinal input signals occur significantly downstream from that of normal vision, as much as two neuron levels away (151). One possible method of duplicating neuronal integration and response includes the use of neuromorphic analogue circuits, such as those developed by Mead et al. (156). Subretinal implants may have negative interactions with the layer of epithelial cells that underlie the retina. Also, electrochemical interactions (e.g., oxidation) could occur at the electrode sites, interfering with stimulation (151).

F. Future Biomimetics as Neural Prostheses

Following the success of retinal and cochlear implants, devices to provide movement to spinal cord–injured victims are not far behind. Some initially promising results have been demonstrated using stimulation at the root ganglia to provide movement (157). Spinal cord stimulation will continue to be an area of vigorous research over subsequent years. As silicon technologies become more advanced, prosthetics directly interfacing with nerve cells will become more prevalent in the field.

The success of these biomimetics depends on a few critical factors. First, any prosthetic implanted in the body must remain biocompatible over the life of the device. The environment in the body is an aqueous, electrolytic solution (151), i.e., not the optimal environment for silicon devices. Second, prosthetic devices should replace function at the earliest possible neurological level. Neural processing in the brain is not well understood at this time; therefore, the device should interact with the earliest level of remaining neural circuitry (151). Finally, biomimetic devices must try to imitate the nerve as closely as possible. There are vast differences between traditional digital computing and the analogue processes in the brain (141). Neural prostheses have already provided treatment for blind and deaf patients; certainly, the future will include mobility-impaired individuals as well.

V. THE FUTURE OF BIOMIMETICS IN THE NERVOUS SYSTEM

The nervous system presents several challenges to the development of biomimetics. The PNS displays the ability to regenerate on its own, but slowly. The CNS does not regenerate successfully on its own. Devices applicable to the PNS may not apply to the CNS. Despite many similarities, both systems display different native cell types and different responses to injury. Furthermore, the functional nervous system is not replicated using traditional digital computing; instead, neural circuitry is analogue.

Successful devices must navigate the obstacles presented by the nervous system. Nonetheless, tissue mimetics and neural prosthetics have already been developed to enhance nerve regeneration and to replace lost neural function. Regeneration devices have incorporated mechanical cues, neurotrophins, cells, anti-inhibitory molecules, ECM elements, and electrical cues to enhance homology to native nerve. While each of these individual factors promotes some regeneration, there is no single component that permits complete success. Thus, future devices must strive to further imitate nerve by combining various approaches. Neural prostheses have utilized advancements in silicon technology to create electrical devices that can interface with nerve directly. Although these devices have had success, future approaches should promote long-term biocompatibility and more directly duplicate neural architecture.

REFERENCES

1. EJ Furnish, CE Schmidt. Tissue engineering of the peripheral nervous system. In: CW Patrick, AG Mikos, LV McIntire, eds. Frontiers in Tissue Engineering. New York: Elsevier Science, 1998, pp 514–535.
2. JW McDonald. Repairing the damaged spinal cord. Sci Am Sep 1999: 64–73.
3. W DeMyer. Neuroanatomy. Philadelphia: Harwal Publishing, 1988, pp 59–62.
4. AV Waller. A new method for the study of the nervous system. London J Med 43:609–625, 1852.
5. V Chaudhry, JD Glass, JW Griffin. Wallerian degeneration in peripheral nerve disease. Neurol Clin 10(3):613–627, 1992.
6. FP Girardi, SN Kahn, FP Cammisa Jr, TJJ Blanck. Advances and strategies for spinal cord regeneration. Orthop Clin N Am 31(3):465–471, 2000.

7. G Stoll, JW Griffin, CY Li, D Trapp. Wallerian degeneration in the peripheral nervous system: participation of both Schwann cells and macrophages in myelin degradation. J of Neurocyt 18(5):671–683, 1989.

8. P Caroni, T Savio, ME Schwab. Central nervous system regeneration: oligodendrocytes and myelin as non-permissive substrates for neurite outgrowth. In: DM Gash, JR Sladek Jr, eds. Progress in Brain Research. New York: Elsevier Science, 1988, pp 363–370.

9. JM Schröder, R May, J Weis. Perineurial cells are the first to traverse gaps of peripheral nerves in silicone tubes. Clin Neurol Neurosurg 95(Suppl):S78–S83, 1993.

10. S Jacobsen, L Guth. An electrophysiological study of the early stages of peripheral nerve regeneration. Exp Neurol 11:48–60, 1965.

11. AM Avellino, D Hart, AT Dailey, M MacKinnon, D Ellegala, M Kliot. Differential macrophage response in the peripheral and central nervous system during Wallerian degeneration of axons. Exp Neurol 136:183–198, 1995.

12. A Castaño, MD Bell, VH Perry. Unusual aspects of inflammation in the nervous system. Neurol Aging 17(5):745–751, 1996.

13. VW Wu, JP Schwartz. Cell culture models for reactive gliosis: new perspectives. J Neurol Res 51:675–681, 1998.

14. JW Streilein. Unraveling immune privilege. Science 270:1158–1159, 1995.

15. DT Chiu. The development of autogenous venous nerve conduit as a clinical entity. In: P and S Medical Review, Vol 3, Issue 1. Columbia-Presbyterian Medical Center, Dec. 1995.

16. S Ramón y Cajal. Degeneration and Regeneration of the Nervous System. New York: Hafner, 1928, pp 738–744.

17. PM Richardson, UM McGuinness, AJ Aguayo. Axons from CNS neurons regenerate into PNS grafts. Nature 284:264–265, 1980.

18. PJ Horner, FH Gage. Regenerating the damaged central nervous system. Nature 407:963–970, 2000.

19. SJA Davies, MT Fitch, SP Memberg, AK Hall, G Raismann, J Silver. Regeneration of adult axons in white matter tracts of the central nervous system. Nature 390:680–683, 1997.

20. H Cheng, Y Cao, L Olsen. Spinal cord repair in adult paraplegic rats: partial restoration of hind limb function. Science 273:510–513, 1996.

21. T Carlstedt. Nerve fiber regeneration across the peripheral-central transition zone. J Anat 190(Pt 1):51–61, 1997.

22. A Espinosa de los Monteros, MS Zhang, M Gordon, M Aymie, J de Vellis. Transplantation of cultured premyelinating oligodendrocytes into normal and myelin-deficient rat brain. Dev Neurol 14(2):98–104, 1992.

23. SM Onifer, SR Whittemore, VR Holets. Variable morphological differentiation of a Raphé-derived neuronal cell line following transplantation into the adult rat CNS. Exp Neurol 122:130–142, 1993.

24. EA Zompa, DP Pizzo, CE Hulsebosch. Migration and differentiation of PC12 cells transplanted in the rat spinal cord. Int J Dev Neurol 11:535–544, 1993.

25. JJ Bernstein, WJ Goldberg. Experimental spinal cord transplantation as a mechanism of spinal cord regeneration. Paraplegia 33:250–253, 1995.
26. H Millesi, G Meissl, A Berger. The interfascicular nerve-grafting of the median and ulnar nerves. J Bone Joint Surg 54A:727, 1972.
27. RG Harrison. The reaction of embryonic cells to solid structures. J Exp Zool 17(4):521–545, 1914.
28. P Weiss. Nerve patterns: the mechanics of nerve growth. Third Growth Symposium 5:163–203, 1941.
29. G Lundborg, LB Dahlin, N Danielsen, RH Gelberman, FM Longo, HC Powell, S Varon. Nerve regeneration in silicone chambers: influence of gap length and of distal stump components. Exp Neurol 76:361–375, 1982.
30. TW Hudson, GRD Evans, CE Schmidt. Engineering strategies for peripheral nerve repair. Orthop Clin N Am 31(3):485–497, 2000.
31. T Hadlock, J Elisseeff, R Langer, J Vacanti, M Cheney. A tissue-engineered conduit for peripheral nerve repair. Arch Otol Head Neck Surg 124:1081–1086, 1998.
32. G Lundborg, L Dahlin, D Dohi, M Kanje, N Terada. A new type of "bioartificial" nerve graft for bridging extended defects in nerves. J Hand Surg (Br) 22B(3):299–303, 1997.
33. G Lundborg, M Kanje. Bioartificial nerve grafts. Scand J Plast Reconstr Hand Surg 30:105–110, 1996.
34. E Lavik, YD Teng, D Zurakowski, X Qu, E Snyder, R Langer. Functional recovery following spinal cord hemisection mediated by a unique polymer scaffold seeded with neural stem cells. Materials Research Society Symposium Proceedings, Boston, Fall 2000.
35. D Ceballos, X Navarro, N Dubey, G Wendelschafer-Crabb, WR Kennedy, RT Tranquillo. Magnetically aligned collagen gel filling a collagen nerve guide improves peripheral nerve regeneration. Exp Neurol 158:290–300, 1999.
36. N Dubey, PC Letourneau, RT Tranquillo. Guided neurite elongation and Schwann cell invasion into magnetically aligned collagen in simulated peripheral nerve regeneration. Exp Neurol 158:338–350, 1999.
37. X Tong, K Hirai, H Shimada, Y Mizutani, T Izumi, N Toda, P Yu. Sciatic nerve regeneration navigated by laminin-fibronectin double coated biodegradable collagen grafts in rats. Brain Res 663:155–162, 1994.
38. K Matsumoto, K Ohnishi, T Kiyotani, T Sekine, H Ueda, T Nakamura, K Endo, Y Shimizu. Peripheral nerve regeneration across an 80-mm gap bridged by a polyglycolic acid (PGA) collagen tube filled with laminin-coated collagen fibers: a histological and electrophysiological evaluation of regenerated nerves. Brain Res 868:315–328, 2000.
39. JA Hammarback, SL Palm, LT Furcht, PC Letourneau. Guidance of neurite outgrowth by pathways of substratum-adsorbed laminin. J Neurosci Res 13:213–220, 1985.
40. T Matsuda, T Sugawara, K Inoue. Two-dimensional cell manipulation technology: an artificial neural circuit based on surface microphotoprocessing. ASAIO J Forum 8:M243–M247, 1992.

41. M Matsuzawa, P Liesi, W Knoll. Chemically modifying glass surfaces to study substratum-guided neurite outgrowth in culture. J Neurosci Res 69:189–196, 1996.
42. P Clark, S Britland, P Connolly. Growth cone guidance and neuron morphology on micropatterned laminin surfaces. J Cell Sci 105:203–212, 1993.
43. S Saneinejad, MS Shoichet. Patterned glass surfaces direct cell adhesion and process outgrowth of primary neurons of the central nervous system. J Biomed Mater Res 42:13–19, 1998.
44. D Kleinfeld, KH Kahler, PE Hockberger. Controlled outgrowth of dissociated neurons on patterned substrates. J Neurosci 8(11):4098–4120, 1988.
45. JM Corey, BC Wheeler, GJ Brewer. Micrometer resolution silane-based patterning of hippocampal neurons: critical variables in photoresist and laser ablation processes for substrate fabrication. IEEE Tran Biomed Eng 43(9):944–955, 1996.
46. RJ Klebe. Cytoscribing: a method for micropositioning cells and the construction of two- and three-dimensional synthetic tissues. Exp Cell Res 179:362–373, 1988.
47. BC Wheeler, JM Corey, GJ Brewer, DW Branch. Microcontact printing for precise control of nerve cell growth in culture. J Biomech Eng 121:73–78, 1999.
48. A Folch, BH Jo, O Hurtado, DJ Beebe, M Toner. Microfabricated elastomeric stencils for micropatterning cell cultures. J Biomed Mater Res 52:346–353, 2000.
49. C Chen, E Ostuni, GM Whitesides, DE Ingber. Using self-assembled monolayers to pattern ECM proteins and cells on substrates. In: C Streuli, M Grant, eds. Methods in Molecular Biology, Vol 139. Totowa, NJ: Humana Press, 2000, pp 209–219.
50. DW Branch, JM Corey, JA Weyenmeyer, GJ Brewer, BC Wheeler. Microstamp patterns of biomolecules for high-resolution neural networks. Med Bio Eng Comp 36:135–141, 1998.
51. GP López, MW Albers, SL Schreiber, R Carroll, E Peralta, GM Whitesides. Convenient methods for patterning the adhesion of mammalian cells to surfaces using self-assembled monolayers of alkanethiolates on gold. J Am Chem Soc 115:5877–5878, 1993.
52. DA Stenger, JJ Hickman, KE Bateman, MS Ravenscroft, W Ma, JJ Pancrazio, K Shaffer, AE Schaffner, DH Cribbs, CW Cotman. Microlithographic determination of axonal/dendritic polarity in cultured hippocampal neurons. J Neurosci Meth 82:167–173, 1998.
53. AM Rajnicek, S Britland, CD McCaig. Contact guidance of CNS neurites on grooved quartz: influence of grooved dimensions, neuronal age, and cell type. J Cell Sci 110:2905–2913, 1997.
54. AMP Turner, N Dowell, SWP Turner, L Kam, M Isaacson, JN Turner, HG Craighead, W Shain. Attachment of astroglial cells to microfabricated pillar arrays of different geometries. J Biomed Mater Res 51:430–441, 2000.

55. HG Craighead, SW Turner, RC Davis, C James, AM Perez, PM St John, MS Isaacson, L Kam, W Shain, JN Turner, G Banker. Chemical and topographical surface modification for control of central nervous system cell adhesion. Biomed Microdev 1(1):49–64, 1998.
56. P Weiss, AC Taylor. Further experimental evidence against 'neurotropism' in nerve regeneration. J Exp Zool 95:233–257, 1944.
57. G Lundborg, LB Dahlin, N Danielsen, AK Nachemson. Tissue specificity in nerve regeneration. Scand J Plast Reconstr Surg 20:279–283, 1986.
58. M Ochi, T Matsuda, Y Ikuta, S Yonehara. Further experimental evidence of selective nerve regeneration in aortic y-chambers. Scand J Plast Reconstr Surg 28:137–141, 1994.
59. G Terenghi. Peripheral nerve regeneration and neurotropic factors. J Anat 194:1–14, 1999.
60. JL Bixby, WA Harris. Molecular mechanisms of axon growth and guidance. Annu Rev Cell Biol 7:117–159, 1991.
61. TN Jelsma, AJ Aguayo. Trophic factors. Curr Opin Neurobiol 4(5):717–725, 1994.
62. CC Stichel, HW Müller. Experimental strategies to promote axonal regeneration after traumatic central nervous system injury. Prog Neurobiol 56:119–148, 1998.
63. KM Rich, TD Alexander, JC Pryor, JP Hollowell. Nerve growth factor enhances regeneration through silicone chambers. Exp Neurol 105:162–170, 1989.
64. J Ye, JD Houle. Treatment of chronically injured spinal cord with neurotrophic factors can promote axonal regeneration from supraspinal neurons. Exp Neurol 143:70–81, 1997.
65. IH Whitworth, RA Brown, CJ Doré, P Anand, CJ Green, G Terenghi. Nerve growth factor enhances nerve regeneration through fibronectin grafts. J Hand Surg 21B(4):514–522, 1996.
66. DA Houweling, AJ Lankhorst, WH Gispen, PR Bar, EAJ Joosten. Collagen containing neurotropin-3 (NT-3) attracts regrowing injured corticospinal axons in the adult rat spinal cord and promotes partial functional recovery. Exp Neurol 153:49–59, 1998.
67. XM Xu, V Guénard, N Kleitman, P Aebischer, MB Bunge. A combination of BDNF and NT-3 promotes supraspinal axonal regeneration into Schwann cell grafts in adult rat thoracic spinal cord. Exp Neurol 134:261–272, 1995.
68. R Grill, K Murai, A Blesch, FH Gage, MH Tuszynski. Cellular delivery of neurotropin-3 promotes corticospinal axonal growth and partial functional recovery after spinal cord injury. J Neurosci 17(14):5560–5572, 1997.
69. Y Liu, D Kim, BT Himes, SY Chow, T Schallert, M Murray, A Tessler, I Fischer. Transplants of fibroblasts genetically modified to express BDNF promote regeneration of adult rat rubrospinal axons and recovery of forelimb function. J Neurosci 19(11):4370–4387, 1999.
70. PA Tresco, R Biran, MD Noble. Cellular transplants as sources for therapeutic agents. Adv Drug Del Rev 42:3–27, 2000.

71. V Guénard, N Kleitman, TK Morrissey, RP Bunge. Syngeneic Schwann cells derived from adult nerves seeded in semipermeable guidance channels enhanced peripheral nerve regeneration. J Neurosci 12(9):3310–3320, 1992.

72. SP Frostick, Q Yin, GJ Kemp. Schwann cells, neurotropic factors, and peripheral nerve regeneration. Microsurgery 18(7):397–405, 1998.

73. CE Dumont, LM Bolin, VR Hentz. A composite nerve graft system: extracted rat peripheral nerve injected with cultured Schwann cells. Muscle Nerve 19:97–99, 1996.

74. XM Xu, V Guénard, N Kleitman, MB Bunge. Axonal regeneration into Schwann cell-seeded guidance channels grafted into transected adult rat spinal cord. J Comp Neurol 351:145–160, 1995.

75. G Raisman. Use of Schwann cells to induce repair of adult CNS tracts. Revue Neurol 153(8–9):521–525, 1997.

76. JD Guest, A Rao, L Olsen, MB Bunge, RP Bunge. The ability of human Schwann cell grafts to promote regeneration in the transected nude rat spinal cord. Exp Neurol 148:502–522, 1997.

77. A Ramón-Cueto, J Avila. Olfactory ensheathing glia: properties and functions. Brain Res Bull 46(3):175–187, 1998.

78. Y Li, PM Field, G Raisman. Repair of adult rat corticospinal tract by transplants of olfactory ensheathing cells. Science 277:2000–2002, 1997.

79. T Imaizumi, KL Lankford, JD Kocsis. Transplantation of olfactory ensheathing cells or Schwann cells restores rapid and secure conduction across the transected spinal cord. Brain Res 854:70–78, 2000.

80. A Ramón-Cuerto, GW Plant, J Avila, MB Bunge. Long-distance axonal regeneration in the transected adult rat spinal cord is promoted by olfactory ensheathing glia transplants. J Neurosci 18(10):3803–3815, 1998.

81. Y Li, PM Field, G Raisman. Regeneration of adult rat corticospinal axons induced by olfactory ensheathing cells. J Neurosci 18(24):10514–10524, 1998.

82. A Ramón-Cuerto, MI Cordero, FF Santos-Benito, J Avila. Functional recovery of paraplegic rats and motor axon regeneration in their spinal cords by olfactory ensheathing glia. Neuron 25:425–435, 2000.

83. E Verdú, X Navarro, G Gudiño-Cabrera, FJ Rodríguez, D Ceballos, A Valero, M Nieto-Sampedro. Olfactory bulb ensheathing cells enhance peripheral nerve regeneration. Neuroreport 10(5):1097–1101, 1999.

84. O Lazarov-Spiegler, AS Solomon, AB Zeev-Brann, DL Hirschberg, V Lavie, M Schwartz. Transplantation of activated macrophages overcomes central nervous system regrowth failure. FASEB J 10:1296–1302, 1996.

85. R Franzen, J Schoenen, P Leprince, E Joosten, G Moonen, D Martin. Effects of macrophage transplantation in the injured rat spinal cord: a combined immunocytochemical and biochemical study. J Neurosci Res 51:316–327, 1998.

86. AG Rabchevsky, WJ Streit. Grafting of cultured microglial cells into lesioned spinal cord of adult rats enhances neurite outgrowth. J Neurosci Res 47:34–48, 1997.

87. D Guilian, C Robertson. Inhibition of mononuclear phagocytes reduces ischemic injury in the spinal cord. Ann Neurol 27(1):33–42, 1990.
88. MT Fitch, J Silver. Glial cell extracellular matrix: boundaries for axon growth in development and regeneration. Cell Tiss Res 290:379–384, 1997.
89. JW Fawcett, RA Asher. The glial scar and central nervous system repair. Brain Res Bull 49(6):377–391, 1999.
90. M Thallmair, GAS Metz, WJ Z'Graggen, O Raineteau, GL Kartje, ME Schwab. Neurite growth inhibitors restrict plasticity and functional recovery following corticospinal tract lesions. Nat Neurol 1(2):124–131, 1998.
91. DW Huang, L McKerracher, PE Braun, S David. A therapeutic vaccine approach to stimulate axon regeneration in the adult mammalian spinal cord. Neuron 24:639–647, 1999.
92. R Martini. Expression and functional roles of neural cell surface molecules and extracellular matrix components during development and regeneration of peripheral nerves. J Neurocytol 23:1–28, 1994.
93. KA Venstrom, LF Reichardt. Extracellular matrix 2: Role of the extracellular matrix molecules and their receptors in the nervous system. FASEB J 7:996–1003, 1993.
94. J Brandt, LB Dahlin, G Lundborg. Autologous tendons used as grafts for bridging peripheral nerve defects. J Hand Surg (Br) 24(3):284–290, 1999.
95. LJ Chamberlain, IV Yannas, H-P Hsu, GR Strichartz, M Spector. Near-terminus axonal structure and function following rat sciatic nerve regeneration through a collagen-GAG matrix in a ten-millimeter gap. J Neurosci Res 60:666–677, 2000.
96. DL Ellis, IV Yannas. Recent advances in tissue synthesis in vivo by the use of collagen-glycosaminoglycan copolymers. Biomaterials 17:291–299, 1996.
97. KK Wang, IR Nemeth, BR Seckel, DP Chakalis-Haley, DA Swann, JW Kuo, DJ Bryan, CL Cetrulo, Jr. Hyaluronic acid enhances peripheral nerve regeneration in vivo. Microsurgery 18(4):270–275, 1998.
98. BR Seckel, D Jones, KJ Hekimian, KK Wang, DP Chakalis, PD Costas. Hyaluronic acid through a new injectable nerve guide delivery system enhances peripheral nerve regeneration in the rat. J Neurosci Res 40:318–324, 1995.
99. R Bellamkonda, JP Ranieri, N Bouche, P Aebischer. Hydrogel-based three-dimensional matrix for neural cells. J Biomed Mater Res 29:663–671, 1995.
100. S Woerly, P Petrov, E Syková, T Roitbak, Z Simonová, AR Harvey. Neural tissue formation within porous hydrogels implanted in brain and spinal cord lesions: ultrastructural, immunohistochemical, and diffusion studies. Tiss Eng 5(5):467–488, 1999.
101. ST Carbonetto, MM Gruver. Nerve fiber growth on defined hydrogel substrates. Science 216:897–899, 1982.
102. RD Madison, C Da Silva, P Dikkes, RL Sidman, T Chiu. Peripheral nerve regeneration with entubulation repair: comparison of biodegradable nerve guides versus polyethylene tubes and the effects of a laminin-containing gel. Exp Neurol 95:378–390, 1987.

103. RD Madison, CF DaSilva, P Dikkes. Entubulation repair with protein additives increases the maximum nerve gap distance successfully bridged with tubular prostheses. Brain Res 447:325–334, 1988.

104. SP Baldwin, CE Krewson, WM Saltzman. PC12 cell aggregation and neurite growth in gels of collagen, laminin, and fibronectin. Int J Dev Neurosci 14(3):351–364, 1996.

105. MR Wells, K Kraus, DK Batter, DG Blunt, J Weremowitz, SE Lynch, HN Antonaides, HA Hansson. Gel matrix vehicles for growth factor application in nerve gap injuries repaired with tubes: a comparison of biomatrix, collagen, and methylcellulose. Exp Neurol 146:395–402, 1997.

106. X Yu, GP Dillon, RV Bellamkonda. A laminin and nerve growth factor-laden three-dimensional scaffold for enhanced neurite extension. Tiss Eng 5(4):291–304, 1999.

107. JC Schense, J Bloch, P Aebischer, JA Hubbell. Enzymatic incorporation of bioactive peptides into fibrin matrices enhances neurite extension. Nat Biotechnol 18:415–419, 2000.

108. JP Ranieri, R Bellamkonda, EJ Bekos, TG Vargo, JA Gardella Jr, P Aebischer. Neuronal cell attachment to fluorinated ethylene propylene films with covalently immobilized laminin oligopeptides YIGSR and IKVAV II. J Biomed Mater Res 29:779–785, 1995.

109. M Borkenhagen, JF Clémence, H Sigrist, P Aebischer. Three-dimensional extracellular matrix engineering in the nervous system. J Biomed Mater Res 40:392–400, 1998.

110. DA Tonge, JP Golding, M Edbladh, M Kroon, PER Edström, A Edström. Effects of extracellular matrix components on axonal outgrowth from peripheral nerves of adult animals in vitro. Exp Neurol 146:81–90, 1997.

111. P Weiss, AC Taylor. Repair of peripheral nerves by grafts of. frozen-dried nerve. Proc Soc Exp Biol Med 52:326–328, 1943.

112. SM Hall. Regeneration in cellular and acellular autografts in the peripheral nerve. Neuropathol Appl Neurobiol 12:27–46, 1986.

113. JB Campbell, CAL Bassett, J Böhler. Frozen-irradiated homografts shielded with microfilter sheaths in peripheral nerve surgery. 22nd Annual Session of the American Association for the Surgery of Trauma, Homestead, Hot Springs, VA, Oct. 29–31, 1962.

114. LF Jaffe, MM Poo. Neurites grow faster towards the cathode than the anode in a steady field. J Exp Zool 209:115–128, 1979.

115. CD McCaig, AM Rajnicek. Electrical fields, nerve growth, and nerve regeneration. Exp Phys 76:473–494, 1991.

116. RF Valentini, TG Vargo, JA Gardella Jr, P Aebischer. Electrically charged polymeric substrates enhance nerve fibre outgrowth in vitro. Biomaterials 13(3):183–190, 1992.

117. P Aebischer, RF Valentini, P Dario, C Domenici, PM Galletti. Piezoelectric guidance channels enhance regeneration in the mouse sciatic nerve after axotomy. Brain Res 436:165–168, 1987.

118. RF Valentini, AM Sabatini, P Dario, P Aebischer. Polymer electret guidance channels enhance peripheral nerve regeneration in mice. Brain Res 480:300–304, 1989.

119. CE Schmidt, VR Shastri, JP Vacanti, R Langer. Stimulation of neurite outgrowth using an electrically conducting polymer. Proc Natl Acad Sci USA 94:8948–8953, 1997.

120. JH Collier, JP Camp, TW Hudson, CE Schmidt. Synthesis and characterization of polypyrrole-hyaluronic acid composite biomaterial for tissue engineering applications. J Biomed Mater Res 50:574–584, 2000.

121. GP Dillon, X Yu, A Sridharan, JP Ranieri, RV Bellamkonda. The influence of physical structure and charge on neurite extension in a 3D hydrogel scaffold. J Biomat Sci Polym Ed 9(10):1049–1069, 1998.

122. G Gross. Simultaneous single unit recording in vitro with a photoetched laser deinsulated gold multimicroelectrode surface. IEEE Trans Biomed Eng 26(5):276–279, 1979.

123. JL Novak, BC Wheeler. Multisite hippocampal slice recording and stimulation using a 32 element microelectrode array. J Neurosci Meth 23:149–159, 1988.

124. P Connolly, P Clark, ASG Curtis, JAT Dow, CDW Wilkinson. An extracellular microelectrode array for monitoring electrogenic cells in culture. Biosens Bioelec 5:223–234, 1990.

125. SA Makohliso, P Aebischer, L Giovangrandi, HJ Bühlmann, M Dutoit. A biomimetic materials approach towards the development of a neural cell-based biosensor. Proceedings of the 18th Annual International Conference of the IEEE Engineering in Medicine and Biology Society, Amsterdam, pp 81–82.

126. X Cui, VA Lee, Y Raphael, JA Wiler, JF Hetke, DJ Anderson and DC. Martin. Surface modification of neural recording electrodes with conducting polymer biomolecule blends. J Biomed Mater Res 56(2):261–272, 2001.

126a. JO Winter, TY Liu, BA Korgel, CE Schmidt. Biomolecule-directed interfacing between semiconductor quantum dots and nerve cells. Advanced Materials 13:1673–1677, 2001.

127. MP Maher, J Pine, J Wright, YC Tai. The neurochip: a new microelectrode device for stimulating and recording from cultured neurons. J Neurosci Meth 87:45–56, 1999.

128. A Mannard, RB Stein, D Charles. Regeneration electrode units: implants for recording from single peripheral nerve fibers in freely moving animals. Science 183:547–549, 1974.

129. DJ Edell. A peripheral nerve information transducer for amputees: long-term multichannel recordings from rabbit peripheral nerves. IEEE Trans Biomed Eng 33:203–214, 1986.

130. GTA Kovacs, CW Storment, JM Rosen. Regeneration microelectrode array for peripheral nerve recording and stimulation. IEEE Trans Biomed Eng 39:893–902, 1992.

131. GTA Kovacs, CW Storment, M Halks-Miller, CR Belczynski Jr, CCDella Santina, ER Lewis, NI Maluf. Silicon-substrate microelectrode arrays for parallel recording of neural activity in peripheral and cranial nerves. IEEE Trans Biomed Eng 41:567–576, 1994.

132. Q Zhao, J Drott, T Laurell, L Wallman, K Lindström, LM Bjursten, G Lundborg, L Montelius, N Danielsen. Rat sciatic nerve regeneration through a micromachined silicon chip. Biomaterials 18:75–80, 1997.

133. AF Mensinger, DJ Anderson, CJ Buchko, MA Johnson, DC Martin, PA Tresco, RB Silver, SM Highstein. Chronic recording of regenerating VIII nerve axons with a sieve electrode. J Neurophys 83:611–615, 2000.

134. L Wallman, A Levinsson, J Schouenborg, H Holmberg, L Montelius, N Danielsen, T Laurell. Perforated silicon nerve chips with doped registration electrodes: in vitro performance and in vivo operation. IEEE Trans Biomed Eng 46:1065–1073, 1999.

135. P Fromherz, A Offenhäusser, T Vetter, J Weis. A neuron-silicon junction: a Retzius cell of the leech on an insulated-gate field-effect transistor. Science 252:1290–1293, 1991.

136. AL Hodgkin, AF Huxley. A quantitative description of membrane current and its application to conduction and excitation in nerve. J Physiol 117:500–544, 1952.

137. R Schätzhauer, P Fromherz. Neuron–silicon junction with voltage-gated ionic currents. Eur J Neurosci 10:1956–1962, 1998.

138. P Fromherz, A Stett. Silicon–neuron junction: capacitive stimulation of an individual neuron on a silicon chip. Phys Rev Lett 75(8):1670–1673, 1995.

139. A Offenhäusser, C Sprössler, M Matsuzawa, W Knoll. Field-effect transistor array for monitoring electrical activity from mammalian neurons in culture. Biosens Bioelec 12(8):819–826, 1997.

140. R Douglas, M Mahowald, C Mead. Neuromorphic analogue VLSI. Annu Rev Neurosci 18:255–281, 1995.

141. A Watson. Why can't a computer be more like a brain? Science 277:1934–1936, 1997.

142. M Mahowald, R Douglas. A silicon neuron. Nature 354:515–518, 1991.

143. C Rasche, RJ Douglas. Silicon synaptic conductances. J Comput Neurosci 7:33–39, 1999.

144. C Breslin, LS Smith. Silicon cellular morphology. Int J Neur Syst 9(5):491–495, 1999.

145. P Heiduschka, S Thanos. Implantable bioelectronic interfaces for lost nerve functions. Prog Neurobiol 55:433–461, 1998.

146. PC Loizou. Introduction to cochlear implants. IEEE Eng Med Biol 18(1):32–42, 1999.

147. JT Rubinstein, CA Miller. How do cochlear prostheses work? Curr Opin Neurobiol 9:399–404, 1999.

148. DE Brackmann, WE Hitselberger, RA Nelson, J Moore, MD Waring, F Portillo, RV Shannon, FF Telischi. Auditory brainstem implant: I Issues in surgical implantation. Otol Head Neck Surg 108(6):624–633, 1993.

149. EM Schmidt, MJ Bak, FT Hambrecht, CV Kufta, DK O'Rourke, P Vallabhanath. Feasibility of a visual prosthesis for the blind based on intracortical microstimulation of the visual cortex. Brain 119:507–522, 1996.

150. MS Humayun, E de Juan Jr, G Dagnelie, RJ Greenberg, RH Propst, DH Phillips. Visual perception elicited by electrical stimulation of retina in blind humans. Arch Ophthalmal 114:40–46, 1996.

151. J Wyatt, J Rizzo. Ocular implants for the blind. IEEE Spectrum May 1996, 47–53.

152. R Eckmiller. Learning retina implants with epiretinal contacts. Ophthalmal Res 29:281–289, 1997.

153. AY Chow, VY Chow. Subretinal electrical stimulation of the rabbit retina. Neurosci Lett 225:13–16, 1997.

154. E Zrenner, A Stett, S Weiss, RB Aramant, E Guenther, K Kohler, K-D Miliczek, MJ Seiler, H Haemmerle. Can subretinal microphotodiodes successfully replace degenerated photoreceptors? Vis Res 39:2555–2567, 1999.

155. MN Nadig. Development of a silicon retinal implant: cortical evoked potentials following focal stimulation of the rabbit retina with light and electricity. Clin Neurophys 110:1545–1553, 1999.

156. MA Mahowald, C Mead. The silicon retina. Sci Am May 1991, 76–82.

157. DN Rushton, N de N Donaldson, FMD Barr, VJ Harper, TA Perkins, PN Taylor, AM Tromans. Lumbar root stimulation for restoring leg function: results in paraplegia. Artif Organs 21(3):180–182, 1997.

13

Tissue Engineering Strategies for Axonal Regeneration Following Spinal Cord Injury

Xudong Cao
Harvard University, Boston, Massachusetts

Molly S. Shoichet
University of Toronto, Toronto, Ontario, Canada

I. INTRODUCTION

This chapter focuses on tissue engineering strategies for axonal regeneration, and in particular spinal cord injury (SCI) repair strategies. Since the peripheral nerve has been shown to provide a permissive environment for axonal regeneration in the central nervous system (CNS), a short description of regenerative strategies in the peripheral nervous system (PNS) is provided as a prelude to those in the CNS. As will become clearer, the complexity of the CNS requires that a multifaceted approach be integrated into the design of a biomimetic nerve guide. This chapter starts with a discussion on the differences between the CNS and PNS after injury, followed by a brief summary of the current strategies to overcome spinal cord injury, and ends with our proposal for a biomimetic device. The chapter emphasizes regenerative strategies that use chemical cues, such as haptotactic and chemotactic signals. Other strategies, such as electrical stimulation for regeneration, are described in the review paper by Winters and Schmidt. This chapter discusses neither neuroprotection of secondary injury and neural protective agents nor animal models of SCI.

I. THE NERVOUS SYSTEM AND NERVOUS SYSTEM INJURIES

A. The Nervous System

The human nervous system is separated anatomically into two regions: the CNS and the PNS. The distinct separation between the two systems has functional and physiological ramifications.

1. The Central Nervous System

The CNS consists of the brain and the spinal cord. The brain mainly operates in an integrative manner and is divided into several regions: medulla oblongata, pons, cerebellum, midbrain, diencephalon, and cerebrum. The brain is the most complex and unknown organ in the body, controlling sensory and motor functions, storing memory, and generating emotions, among others. The spinal cord is the most caudal part of the CNS (1). It functions not only as a channel for many nervous pathways to and from the brain, but also as a mediator to coordinate many subconscious activities (2). The spinal cord serves as the communication pathway between the periphery and the brain. The spinal cord is composed of gray matter in the core and white matter in the periphery that surrounds the gray matter. The gray matter is where the neuronal cell bodies are located. Peripheral spinal nerves connect to the spinal cord through the dorsal and ventral roots.

The CNS is an immunoprivileged site, where a barrier of three cellular membranes separate brain tissue and cerebrospinal fluid from direct contact with blood. This blood–brain barrier (BBB) is formed mainly from endothelial cells of brain capillaries in conjunction with astrocytic projections. This barrier protects the brain and spinal cord from fluctuations in the periphery, such as fluctuations in extracellular ion concentration or the influx of growth-promoting or inhibiting factors, which may cause CNS neurons to malfunction or die. The BBB also prevents passive diffusion across it, including that of ions, non-lipid-soluble molecules, and immune system cells.

2. The Peripheral Nervous System

The PNS consists of nerve fibers that receive information from the external environment and carry signals to and from the brain and spinal cord. It has two divisions: (a) the somatic division, which includes sensory neurons from the body to the dorsal root of the spinal cord and motor neurons from the ventral root of the spinal cord projecting to skeletal muscles; and (b) the autonomic division, which comprises the motor neurons for the smooth muscles and exocrine glands (2).

B. Nervous System Injuries

Physical injury to the nervous system, such as crush or transection, represents one of the major causes of nervous system injury. As mature neurons are nonproliferative, injury to the cell bodies leads to neuron death and consequently to loss of function. Similarly, injury to axons results in a disconnect in the communication pathway between cell bodies of the brain and periphery as well as in loss of function below the injury site.

1. Peripheral Nerve Injury

Severing the major nerve trunks in the PNS normally causes a total loss of function in the muscles and sensory organs innervated by these nerves. However, often damage to peripheral nerves is at least partially reversible. The severed processes spontaneously regenerate by extending axons through nerve bundles from proximal to distal ends.

Wallerian degeneration, which takes place during the first several days after injury (3), in conjunction with macrophage invasion, stimulates Schwann cells in the distal stump to proliferate within their lamina tubes (4,5), forming bands of Büngner (6). This proliferation lasts about 2 weeks during which the Schwann cells form aligned conduits that guide regenerating axons to their targets (7,8). Thus, permissive haptotactic cues for PNS nerve regeneration are provided by the extracellular matrix (ECM) and cell adhesion molecules (CAM) overexpression (cf. Section II.A) and aligned, conduit-forming Schwann cells (9). There are other factors present in the PNS that promote regeneration, as will be elaborated upon in II.A.

2. Spinal Cord Injury

Injury to the mature CNS is characterized by the inability of the axons to repair or regenerate by themselves. Functional recovery from such injuries is limited or nonexistent, as is true for patients with SCI. Although palliative measures are currently available to improve the quality of a patient's daily life, there is no accepted treatment to restore impaired sensory or motor function, leaving patients permanently paralyzed below the site of injury. Causes of SCI include motor vehicle accidents, violence, accidental falls, and sports injuries (10). It has been estimated that there are between 250,000 to 400,000 people who live with SCI in North America and that the cost of care of these patients exceeds $10 billion annually (11).

Trauma in the CNS extends beyond the primary injury site, as secondary processes often cause greater damage to the adjacent tissues of the brain and spinal cord. Local ischemia and edema lead to necrosis and inflammation, releasing membrane breakdown products (i.e., leukotrienes, thromboxane), cations, excitatory amino acids, monoamines, and neuropeptides (12). This secondary cascade leads to scar formation and further neuronal death, and, perhaps most importantly, prevents axonal regeneration.

II. NERVE REGENERATION STRATEGIES

As will become clearer, the biologies of the PNS and CNS differ, and thus the approaches required to achieve regeneration of the PNS and CNS are different. In the following text, we will emphasize the differences between the PNS and CNS in terms of their glial environments where regenerative attempts take place after injury. This will set the stage for the discussion of nerve regeneration strategies, emphasizing new biomimetic device designs to promote nerve regeneration after traumatic injury to the CNS and specifically after SCI.

A. PNS Regeneration Strategies

In the PNS, the severed processes spontaneously regenerate by extending axons through nerve bundles from proximal to distal ends, which can result in successful regeneration and functional recovery. However, a major problem in PNS regeneration is that the efficacy of healing is limited to very short gaps (13). For repair of large gaps (i.e., longer than 5 mm), nerve autografts are currently accepted as the standard of care (14). However, donor site morbidity and insufficient donor tissue availability complicate the autograft approach (15). Moreover, recovery following nerve graft repair is limited by incomplete and nonspecific regeneration (16). To overcome the limitations associated with the autograft approach, we (17) and others (18–20) have engineered biomimetic artificial grafts to augment peripheral nerve regeneration, especially over long gaps. Most of the strategies have focused on using a conduit that is filled with either a matrix, such as dilute collagen or Matrigel, or neurotrophic factors to promote regeneration. Despite much research, the autograft remains the gold standard for repair. For a more detailed description of PNS regeneration strategies, we suggest that interested readers consult two recent excellent reviews (21,22) and/or Chapter 12 of this volume. We will focus on CNS nerve regeneration strategies.

B. CNS Regeneration Strategies

Although it was once believed that mature CNS neurons intrinsically lack the ability to regenerate, this view was disproved by Aguayo and colleagues (23), who elegantly demonstrated that mature retinal ganglion cells (RGCs), a type of CNS neuron, could regenerate their axons through fragments of peripheral nerve grafts. This was perhaps the first experiment that clearly demonstrated that mature CNS axons had the intrinsic ability to regenerate. Furthermore, it provided the promise that SCI could be overcome by manipulating the local CNS environment for regeneration. A significant number of approaches have been taken toward this goal and they will be reviewed later in the text.

1. CNS vs. PNS: The Glial Reaction to Injury

Perhaps the most important question to be answered for SCI regeneration is why the nerve regeneration in the adult mammalian CNS is so elusive whereas that in the adult PNS and that in the developing mammalian CNS are spontaneous and relatively robust. Answers to this question may be the key to better understanding CNS regeneration and designing strategies to overcome the currently irreversible and often devastating effects of SCI. Recent research in this area has revealed that the disparity between the CNS and PNS regenerative abilities can be explained, at least partially, by glial differences in CNS and PNS. CNS glia (i.e., astrocytes, oligodendrocytes, and microglia) and PNS glia (i.e., Schwann cells) respond differently to injury (14), and this difference ultimately gives rise to multiple elements that in turn differentiate the regenerative ability of the CNS and PNS. For example, whereas PNS Schwann cells help to promote neuronal survival after injury, it is uncertain whether CNS glia help to rescue CNS neurons (25). PNS glia strongly enhance growth of regenerating axons by up-regulating the syntheses of neurotrophic factors (e.g., nerve growth factor), permissive extracellular matrices (e.g., laminin and collagen), and cell adhesive molecules and receptors, including L1, γ1 integrins, and the neural cell adhesion molecule (N-CAM) (25). Conversely, CNS glia appear to actively inhibit axonal regeneration by forming a "reactive glial scar," which presents both physical and chemical barriers to regeneration (26). These two hypotheses for limited regeneration—i.e., the physical and chemical barriers presented by the glial scar—are expanded upon below.

a. Physical Barrier to Regeneration in the CNS
The cellular and molecular events following CNS injury are dramatically different from those in the PNS. Within hours of injury, macrophages (which enter from the bloodstream when the BBB is compromised by injury)

and resident microglia arrive at the site of injury, followed by a large number of oligodendrocyte precursors from the surrounding tissue. The final structure of the evolving scar tissue around the injury is predominantly composed of reactive astrocytes, the processes of which are closely apposed to one another, thus forming tight junctions. This limited extracellular space is believed to present a physical barrier for nerve fiber growth and therefore impedes regeneration through it (9).

b. *Chemical Barrier to Regeneration in the CNS*
When Aguayo disproved the dogma that CNS axons could not regenerate by demonstrating that adult CNS axons regrew in the permissive environment of a peripheral nerve graft, he found that the CNS axons would not leave the permissive PNS environment for the apparently nonpermissive environment of the CNS (23,27). Interestingly, PNS neurons were also shown to abort neurite outgrowth in CNS tissues (28,29). Taken together, these results led researchers to question what about the CNS environment was different from that of the PNS and, in particular, what was inhibitory about the CNS milieu. It is now widely accepted that nonpermissive molecules in CNS white matter myelin significantly prevent axonal outgrowth in injured CNS tissue (30–33).

Several inhibitory molecules present in the CNS white matter and reactive glial scar have been identified, such as NI-35/250 (30), myelin-associated glycoprotein (MAG), primarily expressed by oligodentrocytes (34,35), and chondroitin sulfate proteoglycans (CSPGs), mainly produced by subpopulations of activated astrocytes (9). Orginally isolated from CNS myelin and differentiated oligodendrocytes of rats, NI-35/250 [NI-250 is also known as Nogo-A (36)] is perhaps the most studied inhibitory factor. It has been shown to inhibit neurite outgrowth both in vivo and in vitro (30). Since NI-35/250-related activities were also found in the spinal cords of other higher vertebrates, such as bovine (37) and human (38), but not in myelinated fish axons (39), it is speculated that the rigorously regenerative capacity seen in some fish species could be explained in part by the lack of the NI-35/250-related inhibitory effects. Thus, the inhibitory glial environment in the injured CNS likely presents a hostile environment and a significant chemical barrier to regenerating axons.

2. Overcoming the Glial Scar

The inhibitory environment of the injured CNS (including both physical and chemical barriers) must be overcome in order to allow repair of spinal cord injury. To this end, a number of ideas have been explored. Given the physically limited extracellular space that the reactive astrocytes form in the glial scar tissue, bridging grafts, such as tubular structures (40) and peripheral nerve tissue (41), are being investigated to provide a permissive pathway across the site of injury. To reduce the chemically inhibitory CNS glial environment, several strategies are being investigated: (a) the glial cells that produce the inhibitory molecules are removed from the site of injury using high-energy irradiation (32); (b) the inhibitory molecules are blocked by delivering neutralizing antibodies (42,43); (c) inhibitory molecules syntheses are reduced or their degradation accelerated (44,45). Although these attempts to reduce the inhibitory environment (both physical and chemical) in the CNS have improved nerve sprouting and regeneration after injury to the CNS, the extent of the regeneration is greatly limited and impaired. For example, delivery of IN-1, the monoclonal antibody against the most potent inhibitory molecule NI-250, allowed less than 10% of axons to regrow after injury in mice (42,46). The limited regeneration observed may reflect an inadequate delivery strategy: IN-1 was delivered from IN-1-secreting hybridoma cells that were injected into the site of injury. This underlines the importance of engineering design to regenerative strategies; the full potential of IN-1 therapy may not have been realized due to its complex and ill-defined delivery modality. Despite the encouraging results with IN-1, there is likely no "magic bullet" in CNS repair, and a multifaceted approach is required for greater success.

3. Current CNS Regeneration Strategies

Nerve regeneration in the mature CNS is a net result of a dynamic equilibrium between the limited intrinsic ability to regenerate and the inhibitory glial environment where regeneration must occur (47,48). Usually the inhibitory glial environment overwhelms the regenerative power of adult mammalian CNS neurons, resulting in abortive regeneration attempts observed in the mature CNS. To shift the regeneration–degeneration equilibrium in favor of regeneration in the CNS, two general approaches are being pursued: (a) providing the regenerating neurons with a growth-permissive local environment to promote axonal regeneration; and (b) eliminating the inhibitory environment in the CNS to encourage regeneration. These were elaborated upon in Section II.B, and interested readers are encouraged to read the references cited therein as well as recent reviews by Schwab (36), Steeves (45), and Filbin (49).

One strategy involves stem cell transplantation to replace injured neurons and glial cells with new healthy cell populations, and to activate endogenous cells to provide "self-repair" (50). Being multipotent, stem cells have the ability to propagate in vitro and to differentiate into different neural and glial subspopulations once transplanted into the CNS, in response to the local environment (51,52). Although recently some advances have been made to address CNS regeneration after traumatic injury (53,54), clear and indisputable evidence for adult functional regeneration remains to be seen.

In another strategy, peripheral nerve grafts or Schwann cell-populated three-dimensional hydrogels (55,56) have been implanted into the adult CNS in an attempt to mimic the permissive regenerative environment of the PNS and thereby promote axonal regeneration in the CNS. Similarly, olfactory ensheathing glia (OEG), unique CNS glial cells that exhibit axonal growth-promoting properties (57), have been transplanted into the transected adult rat spinal cord to circumvent the hostile CNS milieu so as to allow regeneration (57,58). In addition, neurotrophic factors, such as nerve growth factor (NGF) (59), neurotrophic-3 (NT-3) (60–62), brain-derived neurotrophic factor (BDNF) (63,64), and the combination of NT-3 and BDNF (65), have been administered using a minipump into the CNS to promote nerve fiber regeneration after injury. While effective in delivering factors to the spinal cord, minipump delivery is not site specific and likely not the optimal method to promote regeneration. Furthermore, it is unlikely that axons will regenerate significantly in response to one stimulus. Building on this notion, Olson reported that the combined approach of nerve bridges with growth factor delivery was most beneficial for regeneration. Specifically, completely transected spinal cord gaps were bridged with multiple intercostal nerve grafts that were aligned to direct axons from white matter to the noninhibitory gray matter of the spinal cord. The peripheral nerve grafts were immobilized with fibrin glue from which acidic fibroblast growth factor (a-FGF) was released at the site of injury. This multifaceted approach resulted in progressive functional recovery in adult paraplegic rats after 6 months (41). These results, while very exciting, have been difficult to reproduce (66). Furthermore, the clinical implications of this strategy are unrealistic: multiple intercostal or other nerves would have to be harvested from the patient, creating additional nerve injury and possibly painful neuromas. Thus, the method of harvesting peripheral nerve grafts to repair spinal cord injury is inherently flawed.

Promising as they may appear, the current CNS regeneration strategies have been insufficient for functional recovery, as reentry of regenerating axons into the distal CNS environment has been largely abortive. As shown in Fig. 1, Schwann cell transplants have been used to induce axon regrowth across a complete transection and beyond (67). Three weeks after transplantation into completely transected adult rat thoracic spinal cords, prominent inhibitory chondroitin sulfate proteoglycans immunoreactivity was observed, especially at the caudal end of the graft–cord interface. This localized inhibitory molecular barrier could explain, at least in part, the failure of descending axons to reenter the caudal host cord,

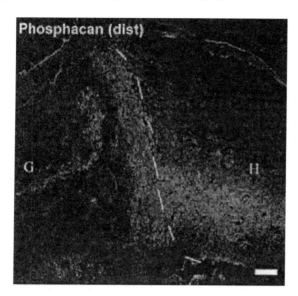

Figure 1 Distribution of phosphacan, a specific antibody to condroitin sulfate proteoglycan (CSPG) in the host–distal spinal cord–Schwann cell/Matrigel graft. It is evident that the distal cord–graft interface shows a dramatic increase in immunoreactivity of CSPG, which has been identified as one of the inhibitory molecules produced by reactive astrocytes after traumatic injury to the CNS. The intense immunostaining between the distal host spinal cord and the graft clearly demonstrates the substantially inhibitory chemical barrier at this interface. This may explain, at least in part, why regenerating nerve fibers are unable to enter the distal cord, as observed in almost all SCI regeneration therapies. H, host; G, Schwann cell/ Matrigel graft. The dashed line indicates the graft–host interface (bar = 100 μm). (From Ref. 67 with permission from Academic Press.)

an abortive regeneration attempt observed with most of the current CNS regeneration strategies. This observation may warrant delivery of neutralizing molecules specifically to the graft–host interface to encourage regrowth of the nerve fibers across and beyond the injury site.

Alternative strategies using synthetic conduits that present a regenerative environment offer great promise (40) but have yet to be proven efficacious. Such biomimetic grafts consist of polymeric materials imbibed with growth factors and/or cell adhesion molecules and/or populated with growth-promoting/supporting cells. The central premise is that these grafts can be designed to present the most desirable conditions for regeneration in the nonpermissive and hostile environment of the CNS. The remainder of this chapter will focus on the design of biomimetic devices for enhanced CNS axonal regeneration.

C. Biomimetic Grafts for CNS Regeneration

Combining principles of tissue engineering, drug delivery, and biomaterial science, biomimetic grafts promise a new horizon for CNS axonal regeneration strategies. By providing the appropriate pathway for regeneration, a synthetic nerve guide obviates the need for a nerve autograft, thereby overcoming the limited tissue availability and the incomplete regeneration associated with autograft strategies. To achieve regeneration beyond that achieved with the peripheral nerve graft, the biomimetic graft must enhance regeneration both within the graft and into the CNS tissue. Designing such a graft provides hope for SCI repair.

1. General Considerations

We have hypothesized that a synthetic biomimetic graft that incorporates chemotactic and heptotactic cues distributed along a cell-invasive scaffold will stimulate regeneration of spinal cord axons. Furthermore, we have hypothesized that incorporating a gradient of neurotrophic factors within the graft will promote nerve fiber extension over greater lengths and possibly stimulate axonal growth and entry into the CNS tissue, as we have demonstrated in vitro (69). Ultimately, a biomimetic graft will incorporate molecules that either neutralize the inhibitory molecules in the CNS or accelerate degradation of the reactive glial scar (or both). This will allow axons to penetrate into and beyond the site of injury and into the CNS, thereby reestablishing nerve connection. The delivery of molecules to the CNS to counteract the inhibitory environment may warrant the use of a drug delivery system to specifically deliver the neutralizing molecules (e.g., IN-1) in a controlled and desired manner. We propose a graft design that consists of a polymeric hollow-fiber membrane (or porous tube) that is filled with haptotactic and chemotactic cues for axonal regeneration plus molecules to promote regeneration into CNS tissue, beyond the site of injury. This design is illustrated in Fig. 2.

2. Design of a Polymeric Hollow-Fiber Membrane Guidance Channel

Non-nerve biological tissue and biodegradable materials have served as bridges for neural repair for over a century in the PNS (70). Multiple biological and synthetic conduits have been attempted, including the use of arteries and veins (71,72), muscle (73–75), collagen (76,77), polyglycolic acid

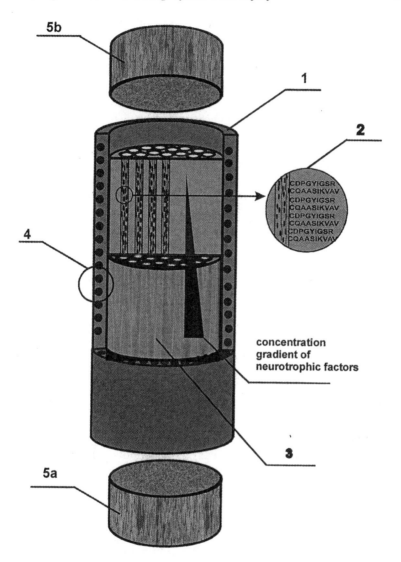

Figure 2 Design of a biomimetic device that may enhance nerve regeneration after SCI. The design can be divided into four main components: (1) The hollow-fiber membrane guidance channel; (2) the haptotatic cues to regeneration incorporated within (3) a cell-invasive scaffold that also comprises chemotactic cues, such as concentration gradients of neurotrophic factors; and (4) the walls of the HFM, which can be used as a drug delivery system to deliver neutralizing molecules or neurotrophic factors. The severed ends of the nerve cable (5a and 5b) are inserted into either end of guidance channel (1).

(PGA) (78,79), and silicon (80,81). While some of these strategies have been moderately successful in the PNS, none has shown viable utility in the CNS. Nevertheless, these previous attempts have accumulated a wealth of data that can be utilized to design and prepare a new generation of polymeric guidance channels for axonal regeneration in the CNS.

The guidance channel itself is critical to the success of the biomimetic graft. The physical properties of the channel, such as modulus and diffusion properties, have been shown to dramatically affect the extent and quality of regeneration inside the channel (22). Yet only limited attention has been given to designing a guidance channel with the physical properties that match those of the tissue. For example, the spinal cord generally has a much lower modulus than peripheral nerve tissue, yet the same poly(acrylonitrile-co-vinyl chloride) [P(AN/VC)] tubes have often been implanted in both sites (55,82). Conversely, we have implanted hydrogel tubes of poly(2-hydroxyethyl methacrylate-co-methyl methacrylate) [P(HEMA/MMA)] in both the PNS and CNS; however, the Young's modulus of those implanted in the PNS ($\sim 1000\,\mathrm{kPa}$) was significantly greater than those implanted in the CNS ($\sim 200\,\mathrm{kPa}$), thereby matching the modulus of the nerve tissues in which they were implanted (i.e., PNS and CNS), respectively (83,84).

The design and fabrication of the channel itself can be accomplished by a number of techniques: phase inversion of an extruded polymer through a spinneret, casting the polymer in a mold, coating a mandrel through sequential immersion in a polymer solution followed by a polymer nonsolvent or a newly invented technique termed *centrifugal spinning*. Phase inversion of a polymer solution via a spinneret is a well-established technique and has been used to create the P(AN/VC) hollow-fiber membranes (HFMs) used in PNS and SCI repair strategies. Tubes created by casting have relatively thick walls, which limits oxygen and nutrient diffusion to regenerating cells and tissue within the tube (85). Biodegradable poly(lactic-co-glycolic acid) (PLGA) tubes have been created by sequentially dipping a mandrel in a polymer solution and then a nonsolvent (86). Although simple, controls over the permeability and the mechanical properties of these tubes are elusive.

We recently invented the centrifugal spinning technique, which relies on phase separation during centrifugation to create tubular structures (87). Synthesis of HFMs using centrifugal forces is a highly dynamic process; by controlling phase separation kinetics, membrane properties such as elastic modulus (87) and permeability (88) can be finely tuned to a specific application or implantation site. This versatile technique is applicable to a spectrum of polymeric materials, such as cross-linked polymers, and may not require the use of organic solvents, thereby allowing incorporation into the wall structure of bioactive molecules, such as growth factors or neutralizing antibodies, and their delivery to CNS tissue. The HFM provides the physical pathway for regeneration yet is insufficient for functional recovery alone. To serve as an effective guidance channel, the HFM must promote regeneration, which may be achieved by incorporating haptotactic and chemotactic signals.

3. Haptotatic Cues

Haptotactic cues are modulated by the substrate via cell–surface or cell–cell receptors. The haptotactic cues in healthy neuronal tissue consist of ECM molecules, such as laminin, collagen, and fibronectin. To create a permissive environment within the tubes, many researchers have focused on creating a cell-adhesive environment using proteins or peptides. The rationale for this approach is derived from in vivo recovery paradigms in the PNS and the apparent lack of permissive terrain for axonal outgrowth (89,90).

Schwann cells have been exploited to promote regeneration in vitro and in vivo in model systems for SCI repair. While Schwann cells are not present in normal CNS tissue, they are integral to the healing process in the PNS where they form the aligned bands of Büngner and up-regulate the expression of ECM, cell adhesion molecules, and neurotrophic factors. In vivo strategies using Schwann cell–populated HFMs have promoted axonal outgrowth within the guidance channel but not beyond the channel into the tissue, presumably due to the inhibitory environment in the CNS (67). Schwann cells have also been shown to align along magnetically oriented collagen fibers in vitro, forming structures reminiscent of bands of Büngner, which may extend nerve fibers over greater distances (91). While the inclusion of cells within nerve guidance channels has provided exciting results, the design is inherently complex and its efficacy has yet to be proven.

a. Topographical and Chemical Cues for Guided Regeneration
Axonal growth and orientation have been modulated by either well-controlled topographical cues, such as patterned grooves, or chemical cues, such as ECM molecules or cell adhesion moieties thereof (92). A number of microfabrication and patterning techniques have been developed to facilitate the creation of topographical cues, such as photolithography (93), microcontact printing (94), and microfluidic technology (95). For example, 20-μm laminin stripes were created on a glass coverslip by photolithography and shown to guide dorsal root ganglion (DRG) neurite outgrowth (96). Recently, oriented Schwann cell growth was successfully demonstrated on a micropatterned biodegradable poly(D,L-lactic acid) substrate, using both grooves for topographical signals and patterned laminin as chemical signals (97). Fig. 3 shows the groove structures, the

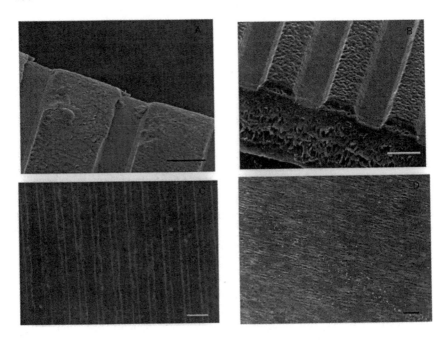

Figure 3 Scanning electron microscope micrographs of (A) image of solvent-cast PDLA film with patterns of dimensions (groove/spacing/depth) of 10:20:3.3 in μm (bar = 10 μm) before degradation; (B) solvent-cast PDLA films with initial dimensions of 10:10:3.3 μm after 2 weeks in culture (bar = 10 μm); (C) Fluorescent image of the adsorbed laminin coated on to the patterned film with initial dimensions 10:20:3.3 μm (bar = 30 μm); and (D) Schwann cells align along the microgrooves (10:20:1.5 μm) after 2 days in culture (bar = 50 μm). (From Ref. 97 with permission from Elsevier Science.)

pattern of the adsorbed laminin in the grooves, and the alignment of Schwann cells along the microgrooves.

We also demonstrated that alternating regions of cell-adhesive CGYIGSR or CSIKVAV and cell-nonadhesive polyethylene glycol (PEG) guided hippocampal neuron cell adhesion and neurite outgrowth. Interestingly, the nonadhesive region was critical for neurites to be confined to the cell-permissive regions, thereby mimicking the in vivo guidance cues, which include both attractive and repulsive cues to guide axonal outgrowth (98). These two-dimensional in vitro model systems provide insights for three-dimensional devices for implantation.

To combine both topographical and chemical guidance cues, we have modified expanded poly(tetrafluoroethylene) (ePTFE) fibers with CDPGYIGSR and CQAASIKVAV peptides (99). The curvature of the synthetic fibers provides physical guidance by constraining the cellular cytoskeleton, while the peptides provide the chemical cues for adhesion and growth. Preliminary results indicate that DRG processes align with the fiber, depending on the fiber diameter, and that cell adhesion and neurite outgrowth is greatest on fibers modified with both peptide sequences, as we previously demonstrated (100). Peptide-modified fibers aligned within the lumen of the biomemitic graft (*cf.* Fig. 2) will provide both more surface area and better directional guidance for regenerating nerve fibers, possibly mimicking the bands of Büngner formed by Schwann cells. While these and other strategies for guided regeneration along a physical scaffold in the lumen are promising, transferring in vitro results to an implantable device for in vivo evaluation is nontrivial. For example, aligning the fibers within the device can be difficult and if not properly done may impede axonal outgrowth by presenting a physical barrier (17).

b. Scaffolds Within the Tube for Regeneration
It has been hypothesized that the CNS conduit gap may be partially overcome by including within the lumen of the HFM matrix or scaffold that is both conducive to and inducive for axonal regeneration, such as an inner gel matrix (101). If properly designed, this inner matrix would confer structural stability to the tube, provide a growth supportive environment that favors cellular invasion, and act as a medium in which to suspend materials that augment surface area, thereby promoting axonal regeneration.

The gel matrix that has been studied in greatest depth is collagen. Due to its low immunogenicity, collagen has been the material of choice in biomedical applications, such as skin grafts, wound dressings, three-dimensional cell culture constructs, drug delivery devices, and nerve guidance tubes (77,81). Recently, a self-assembling peptide (sapeptide) hydrogel was reported as one of the potential gel matrices that could be used (102). The polypeptide consists of alternating repeat units of positively charged lysine or arginine and negatively charged aspartate or glutamate. The sapeptide spontaneously self-assembles in the presence of millimolar concentrations of monovalent salts (i.e., NaCl and KCl), at levels that are found in physiological solution and thereby forms a weak scaffold in situ. Carbohydrate hydrogels, particularly agarose, have also been studied as the inner matrix that fills the lumen. While agarose itself is nonadhesive to cells and neurites, it can be modified with cell-adhesive ligands via the primary hydroxyl groups in its molecular backbone. Laminin-modified agarose promotes neurite outgrowth from PC12 cells and DRGs in a three-dimensional cell culture construct and may ultimately be useful as a biosynthetic three-dimensional bridge to promote regeneration across severed nerve gaps (101).

Synthetic biocompatible hydrogels, such as poly[N-(2-hydroxypropyl)methacrylamide] (PHPMA) modified with the cell-adhesive peptide, Arg-Gly-Asp (RGD), were synthesized to promote axonal outgrowth in the injured adult and developing rat spinal cord in vivo (103). Axons grew within the PHPMA-RGD constructs, and supraspinal axons migrated into the reconstructed cord segment. We too are developing a cell-invasive scaffold. By synthesizing poly(2-hydroxyethyl methacrylate-*co*-methyl methacrylate) (PHEMA-MMA) under centrifugal force, cell-invasive PHEMA-MMA was created with an oriented, bicontinuous, interconnected, open porous structure. This oriented scaffold, once modified with cell-adhesive ligands, may provide the inner matrix to both support and guide axonal regeneration by topographical and chemical cues (104).

4. Chemotactic Cues

It has been recognized since Cajal's pioneering work that axons from a severed nerve exhibit tropism, i.e., the tendency to extend across a gap toward and into the denervated distal stump. Only recently has it been verified and widely accepted that developing and regenerating axons are guided to their targets by a combination of contact-mediated and diffusible cues that are either attractive or repulsive (105). The view now is supported by a wealth of observations both in vivo and in vitro. For example, in the developing vertebrate nervous system, netrin-1 acts as a chemoattractant for commissural axons both in vivo and in vitro (106,107). Furthermore, experiments show that during PNS regeneration, the regenerating axons respond to tropic cues (108) and grow back preferentially toward the target organ that they originally innervated (8). Recently, Kuffler confirmed this finding using a frog sciatic nerve injury model where he demonstrated unequivocally that denervated distal stump tissues release both trophic and tropic factors that guide nerve reinnervation (109). At the nerve fiber terminus, the growth cone is believed to guide the axon by sampling the environment for either positive or negative signals using filopodial and lamellar protrusions (110–112). This sampling, comparing, and decision-making procedure is believed to be a concentration gradient–dependent action (113), which evokes a set of intracellular events involving cytoplasmatic second messenger (114). A gradient of the cytoplasmatic second messenger may signal the preferential incorporation of new plasma membrane material and asymmetrical cytoskeleton reorganization at the growth cone that is required for the appropriate orientation of neurites (115). Recently, we used a well-defined diffusion chamber to study the effect of a NGF concentration gradient on the guidance of PC12 cell neurites. We determined that there was a minimum NGF concentration gradient required to guide PC12 cell neurites. We determined that there was a minimum NGF concentration gradient required to guide PC12 cell neurite outgrowth over a maximum effective distance (69), as shown in Fig. 4. Furthermore, when concentration gradients of NGF and NT-3 were used together, a synergistic guidance effect was observed to guide axons of chick dorsal root ganglion cells (DRGs) (116).

Axons of developing neurons depend on both contact-mediated and diffusible cues to navigate to their targets (111). Contact-mediated cues are provided by ECM molecules expressed by other cells (or neurons), while diffusible cues are provided by target tissues (111). These cues act synergistically to precisely navigate growth cones over long distances (112). Recently, Bahr et al. (117) showed that regenerating axons regain some of their developing stage characteristics and may also rely on both cues to reinnervate their targets. This view is shared by Woolford (118),

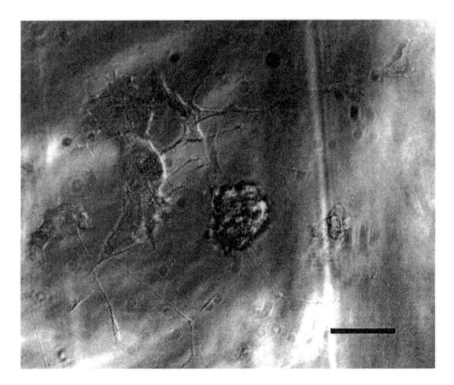

Figure 4   Neurite outgrowth of PC12 cells by a NGF concentration gradient was evident. Note the preferential directional growth towards the right hand side of the micrograph (bar = 100 μm).

Houwelling (60), and Bregman (105) who demonstrated that neurotrophic factors exerted a neurotropic influence on injured, mature CNS axons. Chemotactic cues are likely important to CNS regeneration strategies, and an inner matrix loaded with such cues may provide a vital addition to current device designs that are intended to augment CNS axonal regeneration. However, simply incorporating growth factors into a device is likely insufficient for guidance. A neurotrophic factor gradient is required for guidance. Furthermore, when growth factors are simply incorporated in a matrix, bioavailability is unknown; the growth factor may diffuse out of the device, be taken up by other cells, or simply degrade before impacting regeneration. Thus, there are significant challenges to overcome prior to useful clinical application of growth factors. For example, the diffusible concentration gradient that we created in our model diffusion chamber is not stable and will become a homogeneous concentration of growth factor over an extended period of time. To overcome this problem, we are currently investigating ways to create a concentration gradient of chemotactic cues within our biomimetic graft design.

III. CONCLUSIONS

Injury to the CNS leads to a cascade of reactions that results in axonal death and retraction. Since the view that mature CNS neurons instrinsically lack the ability to regenerate was disproved two decades ago (23), our understanding of the CNS has provided us with insight into strategies to reverse devastating and traumatic injury. To overcome SCI, the delicate balance between the strong inhibitory glial environment and the limited regenerative capacity of the mature CNS neurons has to be reversed with judicious intervention, such as with the biomimetic regeneration device. Currently a variety of regenerative strategies are being actively pursued: (a) neurotrophic factors are being delivered alone or within a nerve guidance channel; (b) neutralizing molecules are being delivered by minipump; and (c) guidance channels filled with one or a combination of matrix, cells (i.e., Schwann and olfactory ensheathing glia), haptotactic (i.e., cell-adhesive ligands) or chemotactic (i.e., neurotrophic factors) cues. The complexity of the CNS requires that multiple strategies be pursued in unison. While peripheral nerve grafts offer promise for SCI repair, they alone are insufficient for functional recovery. A multifaceted approach is required, and the key "ingredients" are still to be defined. However, a strategy that provides a pathway with chemotactic and haptotactic cues plus a way to overcome the glial scar is promising. Furthermore, the possibility of incorporating stem cell (51–53) and gene therapies (119) into the device design may provide even greater hope for successful regeneration.

ACKNOWLEDGMENTS

We thank Dr. Rajiv Midha (Sunnybrook and Women's College Health Science Center and University of Toronto) and Dr. Charles Tator (University Health Network and University of Toronto) for reviewing this manuscript. We are grateful to the Ontario Neurotrauma Foundation and the Whitaker Foundation for financial support.

REFERENCES

1. ER Kandel, JH Schwartz, TM Jessell. Principles of Neural Science, 3rd ed. Norwalk, CT: Appleton & Lange, 1991, pp. 5–32.
2. AC Guyton. Basic Neuroscience: Anatomy and Physiology. Philadelphia: W.B. Saunders, 1987, pp. 8–54.
3. JL Salzer, RP Bunge. Studies of Schwann cell proliferation I: an analysis in tissue culture of proliferation during development, Wallerian degradation and direct injury. J Cell Biol 84:739–752, 1980.
4. JL Salzer, AK Williams, L Glaser, RP Bunge. Studies of Schwann cell proliferation II: characterization of the stimulation and specificity of the response to a neurite membrane fraction. J Cell Biol 84:753–766, 1980.
5. RP Bunge. Some observations on the role of the Schwann cells in the peripheral nerve regeneration. In: DL Jewet, ed. Nerve Repair and Regeneration: Its Clinical and Experimental Basis. St. Louis: C V Mosby Co, 1980, pp. 58–64.
6. YJ Son, WJ Thompson. Schwann cell processes guide regeneration of peripheral axons. Neuron 14:125–132, 1995.
7. G Terenghi. Peripheral nerve regeneration and neurotrophic factors. J Anat 194:1–14, 1999.
8. JL Bixby, J Lilien, LF Reichardt. Indentification of the major proteins that promote neuronal process outgrowth on Schwann cells in vitro. J Cell Biol 107:353–361, 1988.
9. JW Fawcett, R Asher. The glial scar and the central nervous system repair. Brain Res Bull 49:377–391, 1999.
10. RA Philipp, BA Green. Spinal cord injury: epidemiological studies, diagnosis, and classification. In: PL Petersen, JW Phillis, eds. Novel Therapies for CNS Injuries: Rationales and Results. Boca Raton: CRC Press, 1995, pp. 13–27.
11. M Berkowitz, PK O'Leary, DL Kruse, C Harvey. Spinal Cord Injury: An Analysis of Medical and Social Costs. New York: Demos Medical, 1998, pp. 1–7.

12. ME Schwab, D. Bartholdi, Degeneration and regeneration of axons in the lesioned spinal cord. Physiol Rev 76:319–370, 1996.

13. RDG Evans. Challenges to nerve regeneration. Seminars Surg Oncol 19:312–318, 2000.

14. G Lundborg. Nerve Injury and Repair. New York: Churchill Livingstone, 1988, pp. 196–216.

15. ME Ortiguela, MB Wood, DR Cahill. Anatomy of the sural nerve complex. J Hand Surg Am 12:1119–1123, 1987.

16. L de Medinaceli, RR Rawlings. Is it possible to predict the outcome of peripheral nerve injuries? A probability model based on prospects for regenerating neurites. Biosys 20:243–258, 1987.

17. R Midha, SM Shoichet, PD Dalton, X Cao, CA Munro, J Nobel, MKK Wong. Tissue engineered alternatives to nerve transplantation for repair of peripheral nervous system injuries. Transplant Proc 33:613–615, 2001.

18. LJ Chamberlian, IV Yannas, A Arrizabalaga, H-P Hsu, TV Norregarrd, M Spector. Early peripheral nerve healing in collagen and silicone tube implants: myofibroblasts and the cellular response. Biomaterials 19:1393–1403, 1998.

19. N Danielsen, LR Williams, LB Dahlin, S Varon, G Lundborg. Peripheral nerve regeneration in Gore-rex chambers. Scand J Plast Reconstr Surg Hand Surg 22:207–210, 1988.

20. G Lundborg, LB Dahlin, N Danielsen, HA Hansson, A Johanneseson, FM Longo, S Varon. Nerve regeneration across an extended gap: a neurobiological view of nerve repair and the possible involvement of neurotrophic factors. J Hand Surg Am 7:580–587, 1982.

21. CA Health, GE Rutkowski. The development of bioartificial nerve grafts for peripheral-nerve regeneration. Trends Biotech 16:163–168, 1998.

22. TW Hudson, RDG Evans, CE Schmidt. Engineering strategies for peripheral nerve repair. Clin Plast Surg 26:617–628, 1999.

23. S David, AJ Aguayo. Axonal elongation into peripheral nervous system "bridges" after central nervous system injury in adult rats. Science 214:931–933, 1981.

24. BA Barres. Neuron-glial interactions. In: WM Cowan, TM Jessell, SL Zipursky, ed. Molecular and Cellular Approaches to Neural Development. New York: Oxford University Press, 1997, pp. 64–107.

25. JL Goldberg, BA Barres. The relationship between neuronal survival and regeneration. Annu Rev Neurosci 23:579–612, 2000.

26. JL Goldberg, BA Barres. Nogo in nerve regeneration. Nature 403:369–370, 2000.

27. AJ Aguayo, GM Bray, M Rasminsky, T Zwimpfer, D Carter, M Vidal-Sanz. Synaptic connections made by axons regeneration in the central nervous system of adult mammals. J Exp Biol 153:199–224, 1990.

28. N Giftochristos, S David. Immature optic nerve glia of rat do not promote axonal regeneration when transplanted into peripheral nerve. Brain Res 467:149–153, 1988.

29. SM Hall, AP Kent. The response of regenerating peripheral neurites to grafted optic nerve. J Neurocytol 16:317–331, 1987.
30. P Caroni, ME Schwab. Two membrane protein fractions from rat central myelin with inhibitory properties for neurite growth and fibroblast spreading. J Cell Biol 106:1281–1288, 1988.
31. BP Niederost, DR Zimmermann, ME Schwab, CE Bandtlow. Bovine CNS myelin contains neurite growth-inhibitory activity associated with chondroitin sulfate proteoglycans. J Neurosci 19:8979–8989, 1999.
32. T Savio, ME Schwab. Lesioned corticospinal tract axons regenerate in myelin-free rat spinal cord. Proc Natl Acad Sci USA 87:4130–4133, 1990.
33. T Savio, ME Schwab. Rat CNS white matter, but not gray matter, is nonpermissive for neuronal cell adhesion and fiber outgrowth. J Neurosci 4:1126–1133, 1989.
34. L McKerracher, S David, DL Jackson, V Kottis, RJ Dunn, PE Braun. Identification of myelin-associated glycoprotein as a major myelin-derived inhibitor of neurite growth. Neuron 13:805–811, 1994.
35. G Mukhopadhyay, P Doherty, FS Walsh, PR Crocker, MT Filbin. A novel role for myelin-associated glycoprotein as an inhibitor of axonal regeneration. Neuron 13:757–767, 1994.
36. CE Bandtlow, ME Schwab. NI-35/250/Nogo-A: a neurite growth inhibitor restricting structural plasticity and regeneration of nerve fibers in the adult vertebrate CNS. Glia 29:175–181, 2000.
37. AA Spillmann, CE Bandtlow, F Lottspeich, F Keller, ME Schwab Identification and characterization of a bovine neurite outgrowth inhibitor (bNI-220). J Bio Chem 273:19283–19293, 1998.
38. AA Spillmann, VR Amberger, ME Schwab. High molecular weight protein of human central nervous system myelin inhibits neurite outgrowth: an effect which can be neutralized by the monoclonal antibody IN-1. Eur J Neurosci 9:549–555, 1997.
39. M Wanner, DM Lang, CE Brandlow, ME Schwab, M Bsatmeyer, CA Stuermer. Reevaluation of the growth-permissive substrate properties of goldfish optic nerve myelin and myelin proteins. J Neurosci 15:7500–7508, 1995.
40. G Lundborg, J Drott, L Wallman, M Reimer, M Kanje. Regeneration of axons from central neurons into microchips at the level of the spinal cord. Neuroreport 9:861–864, 1998.
41. H Cheng, Y Cao, L Olson. Spinal cord repair in adult paraplegic rats: partial restoration of hind limb function. Science 273:510–513 1996.
42. BS Bregman, E Kunkel-Bagden, L Schell, HN Dai, D Gao, ME Schwab. Recovery from spinal cord injury mediated by antibodies to neurite growth inhibitors. Nature 378:498–501, 1995.
43. DW Hunag, L Mckerracher, PE Braun, S David. A therapeutic vaccine approach to stimulate axon regeneration in the adult mammalian spinal cord. Neuron 24:639–647, 1999.

44. J Zuo, D Neubauer, K Dyess, TA Ferguson, D Muir. Degradation of chondroitin sulfate proteoglycan enhances the neurite promoting potential of spinal cord tissue. Exp Neurol 154:654–662, 1998.

45. J McGraw, GW Hiebert, JD Steeves. Modulating astrogliosis after neurotrauma. J Neurosci Res 63:109–115, 2001.

46. L Schnell, ME Schwab. Axonal regeneration in the rat spinal cord produced by an antibody against myelin-associated neurite growth inhibitors. Nature 343:269–272, 1990.

47. H Bomze, KR Bulsara, BJ Iskandar, P Caroni, JH Skene. Spinal axon regeneration evoked by replacing two growth cone proteins in adult neurons. Nat Neurosci 4:38–43, 2001.

48. C Woolf. Turbocharging neurons for growth: accelerating regeneration in the adult CNS. Nat Neurosci 4:7–9, 2001.

49. J Qiu, D Cai, MT Filbin. Glial inhibition of nerve regeneration in the mature mammalian CNS. Glia 29:166–174, 2000.

50. FH Gage. Mammalian neural stem cells. Science 287:1433–1438, 2000.

51. S Weiss, BA Reynolds, AL Vescovi, C Morshead, CG Graig, D van der Kooy. Is there a neural stem cell in the mammalian forebrain? Trends Neurosci 19:387–393, 1996.

52. A Villa, EY Snyder, A Vescovi, A Martinez-Serrano. Establishment and properties of a growth factor-dependent, perpetual neural stem cell line from the human CNS. Exp Neurol 161:67–84, 2000.

53. S Liu, Y Qu, TJ Stewart, MJ Howard, S Chakrabortty, TF Holekamp, JW McDonald. Embryonic stem cells differentiate into oligodendrocytes and myelinate in culture and after spinal cord transplantation. PNAS 97:6126–6131, 2000.

54. PJ Horner, FH Gage. Regenerating the damaged central nervous system. Nature 407:963–970, 2000.

55. JD Guest, A Rao, L Olson, MB Bunge, RP Bunge. The ability of human Schwann cell grafts to promote regeneration in the transected nude rat spinal cord. Exp Neurol 148:502–522, 1997.

56. GW Plant, TV Chirila, AR Harvey. Implantation of collagen IV/poly(2-hydroxyethyl methacrylate) hydrogels containing Schwann cell into the lesioned rat optic tract. Cell Transplant 7:381–391, 1998.

57. A Ramon-Cueto, MI Cordero, F Santos-Benito, J Avila. Functional recovery of paraplegic rats and motor axon regeneration in their spinal cords by olfactory enshealthing glia. Neuron 25:425–435, 2000.

58. G Raisman. Olfactory ensheathing cells—another miracle cure for spinal cord injury? Nat Rev Neurosci 2:369–374, 2001.

59. M Oudega, T Hagg. Nerve growth factor promotes regeneration of sensory axons in adult rat spinal cord. Exp Neurol 140:218–229, 1996.

60. DA Houwelling, AJ Lankhorst, WH Gispen, PR Bar, EA Joosten. Collagen containing neurotrophin-3 attracts regrowing injured corticospinal axons in the adult rat spinal cord and promotes partial functional recovery. Exp Neurol 153:49–59, 1998.

61.   L Schnell, R Schneider, R Kolbeck, YA Barde, ME Schwab. Neurotrophin-3 enhances sprouting of corticospinal tract during development and after spinal cord lesion. Nature 367:170–173, 1994.

62.   R Grill, K Murai, A Blesch, FH Gage, MH Tuszynski. Cellular delivery of neurotrophin-3 promotes corticospinal axonal growth and partial functional recovery after spinal cord injury. J Neurosci 17:5560–5572, 1997.

63.   P Menei, C Montero-Menei, SR Whittemore, RP Bunge, MB Bunge. Schawnn cells genertically modified to secrete human BDNF promote enhanced axonal regrowth across transected adult rat spinal cord. Eur J Neurosci 10:607–621, 1998.

64.   J Namiki, A Kojima, CH Tator. Effect of brain-derived neurotrophic factor, nerve growth factor, and neurotrophin-3 on functional recovery and regeneration after spinal cord injury in adult rats. J Neurotrauma 17:1219–1231, 2000.

65.   XM Xu, V Guenard, N Kleitman, P Aebischer, MA Bunge. Combination of BDNF and NT-3 promotes supraspinal axonal regeneration into Schwann cell grafts in adult rat thoracic spinal cord. Exp Neurol 134:261–271, 1995.

66.   JW Fawcett, HM Geller. Regeneration in the CNS: optimism mounts. Trends Neurosci 21:179–180, 1998.

67.   GW Plant, ML Bates, MB Bunge. Inhibitory proteoglycan immunoreactivity is higher at the caudal than the rostral Schwann cell graft-transected spinal cord interface. Mol Cell Neurosci 17:471–487, 2001.

68.   SJA Davies, MT Fitch, SP Memberg, AK Hall, G Raisman, J Silver. Regeneration of adult axons in white matter tracts of the central nervous system. Nature 390:680–683, 1997.

69.   X Cao, MS Shoichet. Defining the concentration gradient of nerve growth factor for guided neurite outgrowth. Neurosci 103:831–840, 2001.

70.   VB Doolabh, MC Hertl, SE Mackinnon. The role of conduits in nerve repair: a review. Rev Neurosci 7:47–84, 1996.

71.   RL Walton, RE Brown, WE Matory, GL Borah, JL Dolph. Autogenous vein graft repair of digital nerve defects in the finger: a retrospective clinical study. Plast Reconstr Surg 84:944–952, 1989.

72.   JB Tang. Vein conduits with interposition of nerve tissue for peripheral nerve defects. J Reconstr Microsurg 11:21–26, 1995.

73.   RW Norris, MA Glasby, JM Gattuso, RE Bowden. Peripheral nerve repair in humans using muscle autografts: a new technique. J Bone Joint Surg Br 70:530–533, 1988.

74.   MA Glasby, SE Gschmeissner, CL Huang, BA de Souza. Degenerated muscle grafts used for peripheral nerve repair in primates. J Hand Surg Br 11:347–351, 1986.

75.   S Hall. Axonal regeneration through acellular muscle grafts. J Anat 190:57–71, 1997.

76.   SJ Archibald, C Krarup, J Shefner, ST Li, RD Madison. A collagen-based nerve guide conduit for peripheral nerve repair: an electrophysiological study

of nerve regeneration in rodents and nonhuman primates. J Comp Neurol 306:685–696, 1991.

77. EAJ Joosten, PR Bar, WH Gispen. Directional regrowth of lesioned corticospinal tract axons in adult rat spinal cord. Neuroscience 69:619–626, 1995.

78. SE Mackinnon, AL Dellon. Clinical nerve reconstruction with a bioabsorbable polyglycolic acid tube. Plast Reconstr Surg 85:419–424, 1990.

79. AL Dellon, SE Mackinnon. An alternative to the classical nerve graft for the management of the short nerve gap. Plast Reconstr Surg 82:849–856, 1988.

80. LR Williams, NA Azzam, AA Zalewski, RN Azzam. Regenerating axons are not required to induce the formation of a Schwann cell cable in a silicone chamber. Exp Neurol 120:49–59, 1993.

81. DA Abernethy, A Rud, PK Thomas. Neurotrophic influence of the distal stump of transected peripheral nerve on axonal regeneration: absence of topographic specificity in adult nerve. J Anat 180:395–400, 1992.

82. P Aebischer, V Guenard, RF Valentini. The morphology of regenerating peripheral nerves is modulated by the surface microgeometry of polymeric guidance channels. Brain Res 531:211–218, 1990.

83. H Millesi, G Zoch, R Reihsner. Mechanical properties of peripheral nerves. Clinical Orthopaedics and Related Research 314:76–83, 1995.

84. TK Hung, GL Chang, HS Lin, FR Walter, L Bunegin. Stress–strain relationship of the spinal cord of anesthetized cats. J Biomechanics 14:269–276, 1981.

85. FT Gentile, EJ Doherty, DH Rein, MS Shoichet, SR Winn. Polymer science for macroencapsulation of cells for central nervous system transplantation. React Polym 25:207–227, 1995.

86. MF Meek, WF Den Dunnen, JM Schakenraad, PH Robinson. Long-term evaluation of functional nerve recovery after reconstruction with a thin-walled biodegradable poly (DL-lactide-epsilon-caprolactone) nerve guide, using walking track analysis and electrostimulation tests. Microsurgery 19:247–253, 1999.

87. PD Dalton, MS Shoichet. Creating porous tubes by centrifugal forces for soft tissue application. Biomaterials 22:2661–2669, 2001.

88. Y Luo, PD Dalton, MS Shoichet. Investigating the properties of novel poly(2-hydroxethyl methacrylate-co-methyl methacrylate) hydrogel hollow fiber membranes. Chem Mater 13:4087–4093, 2001.

89. SA Lipton. Growth factors for neuronal survival and process regeneration. Implications in the mammalian central nervous system. Arch Neurol 46:1241–1248, 1989.

90. L Olson. Regeneration in the adult central nervous system: experimental repair strategies. Nat Med 3:1329–1335, 1997.

91. N Dubey, PC Letourneau, RT Tranquillo. Guided neurite elongation and Schwann cell invasion into magnetically aligned collagen in simulated peripheral nerve regeneration. Exp Neurol 158:338–350, 1999.

92. A Curtis, C Wilkinson. Topographical control of cells. Biomaterials 18:1573–1583, 1997.
93. RS Kane, S Takayama, E Ostuni, DE Inger, GW Whitesides. Patterning proteins and cells suing soft lithography. Biomaterials 20:2363–2376, 1999.
94. N Patel, R Padera, GHW Sanders, SM Cannizzaro, MC Davies, R Langer, CJ Roberts, SJB Tendler, PM Williams, KM Shakesheff. Spatially controlled cell engineering on biodegradable polymer surfaces. FASEB J 12:1447–1454, 1998.
95. HG Craighead, SW Turner, RC Davis, C James, AM Perez, PM St. John, MS Isaacson, L Kam, W Shain, JN Turner, G Banker. Chemical and topographical surface modification for control of central nervous system cell adhesion. Biomed Microdev 1:49–64, 1998.
96. HC Tai, HM Buettner. Neurite outgrowth and growth cone morphology on micropatterned surfaces. Biotechnol Prog 14:364–370, 1998.
97. C Miller, H Shanks, A Witt, G Rutkowski, S Mallapragada. Orientated Schwann cell growth on micropatterned biodegradable polymer substrates. Biomaterials 22:1263–1269, 2001.
98. S Saneinejad, MS Shoichet. Patterned poly(chlorotrifluoroethylene) guides primary nerve cell adhesion and neurite outgrowth. J Biomed Mater Res 50:464–474, 2000.
99. D Shaw, MS Shoichet. Peptide surface modification of poly(tetrafluorethylene) fibers for guided neurite outgrowth. Trans 27th Annual Meeting of Society for Biomaterials, St Paul, 2001, p 276.
100. YW Tong, MS Shoichet. Enhancing the neuronal interaction on fluoropolymer surfaces with mixed peptides or spacer group linker. Biomaterials 22:1029–1034, 2001.
101. X Yu, GP Dillon, RV Bellamkonda. A laminin and nerve growth factor-laden three imensional scaffold for enhanced neurite extension. Tissue Eng 5:219–304, 1999.
102. TC Holmes, S Lacalle, X Su, G Liu, A Rich, S Zhang. Extensive neurite outgrowth and active synapses formation on self-assembling peptide scaffolds. PNAS 97:6728–6733, 2000.
103. S Woerly, E Pinet, L de Robertis, VD Diep, M Bousmina. Spinal cord repair with PHPMA hydrogel containing RGD peptides (NeuroGel™). Biomaterials 22:1095–1111, 2001.
104. PD Dalton, EC Tsai, S Sanghavi, C Tator, MS Shoichet. Oriented hydrogel scaffold for neuronal tissue engineering. Trans 27th Annual Meeting of Society for Biomaterials, St Paul, 2001, p 240.
105. BS Bregman, M McAfee, HN Dai, PL Kuhn. Neurotrophic factors increase axoanl growth after spinal cord injury and transplantation in the adult rat. Exp Neurol 148:475–494, 1997.
106. TE Kennedy, T Serafini, JR Torre, M Tessier-Lavigne. Netrins are diffusible chemotropic factors for commissural axons in the embryonic spinal cord. Cell 78:425–436, 1994.

107. T Sarafini, SA Colamarino, ED Leonardo, H Wang, R Beddington, WC Skarnes, M Tessier-Lavigne. Netrin-1 is required for commissural axon guidance in the developing vetebrate nervous system. Cell 87:1001–1014, 1996.

108. X Gu, PK Thomas, RHM King. Chemotropism in nerve regeneration studied in tissue culture. J Anat 186:153–163, 1995.

109. M Zhang, D Kuffler. Guidance of regenerating motor axons in vivo by gradients of diffusible peripheral nerve-derived factors. J Neurobiol 42:212–219, 2000.

110. JQ Zheng, JJ Wan, MM Poo. Essential role of filopodia in chemotropic turning of nerve growth cone induced by a glutamate gradient. J Neurosci 16:1140–1149, 1996.

111. CS Goodman. Mechanisms and molecules that control growth cone guidance. Annu Rev Neurosci 19:341–377, 1996.

112. BK Mueller. Growth cone guidance: first steps towards a deeper under-standing. Annu Rev Neurosci 22:351–388, 1999.

113. CA Parent, PN Devreotes. A cell's sense of direction. Science 284:765–770, 1999.

114. HJ Song, MM Poo. Signal transduction underlying growth cone guidance by diffusible factors. Curr Opin Neurobiol 9:355–363, 1999.

115. R Keynes, GM Cook. Axon guidance molecules. Cell 83:161–169, 1995.

116. X Cao, MS Shoichet. Guiding neurite outgrowth by neurotrophic factor concentration gradients. Trans 27th Annual Meeting of Society for Biomaterials, St Paul, 2001, p 550.

117. M Bahr, ME Schwab. Antibody that neutralizes myelin-associated inhibitors of axon growth does not interfere with recognition of target specific guidance information by rat retinal axons. J Neurobiol 30:281–291, 1996.

118. TJ Woolford. The enhancement of nerve regeneration using growth factors. J Long Term Effects Med Implants 5:19–26, 1995.

119. LL Jones, M Oudega, MB Bunge. Neurotrophic factors, cellular bridges and gene therapy for spinal cord injury. J Physiol 533:83–89, 2001.

14
Micropatterning Biomimetic Materials for Bioadhesion and Drug Delivery

Mark E. Byrne, David B. Henthorn, Yanbin Huang, and Nicholas A. Peppas
Purdue University, West Lafayette, Indiana

I. INTRODUCTION: SURFACE MODIFICATION OF POLYMERIC MATERIALS

Polymer surfaces in contact with biological fluids, cells, or cellular components are normally tailored to provide specific recognition properties or to resist binding depending on the intended application and environment. The specific surface chemistry and topography directly influence a favorable recognition event (1). Engineering the molecular design of biomaterials by controlling recognition and specificity is the first step in coordinating and duplicating complex biological and physiological processes (2,3).

Modification of polymer surfaces by chemical reaction, grafting, and so forth can create a desirable surface for an intended application. The design of surfaces for cellular recognition and adhesion, analyte recognition, and surface passivity encompass a number of techniques, such as surface grafting (ultraviolet radiation, ionizing radiation, electron beam irradiation) (4), photoinitiated grafting (visible or ultraviolet light) (5), and plasma polymerization (6–8). These techniques, while not exhaustive, can change the chemical nature of surfaces and produce areas of differing chemistry, such as micropatterning. They can also produce surfaces and polymer matrices with binding regimes for a given analyte, termed molecular imprinting or microimprinting. Surface grafting, micropatterning, and microimprinting are presented and discussed in this work.

II. SURFACE-GRAFTED POLYMERS FOR BIOADHESION

The surface interaction between biomaterials and various types of tissues, cells, and biomacromolecules is essential for their performance. Therefore, the surface modification of biomaterials has been under intensive investigation since the beginning of biomaterials science. However, until recently most of the studies focused on the design of nonthrombogenic or nonfouling surfaces, i.e., anti-adhesive surfaces (9,10). As typical examples, synthetic polymers such as poly(ethylene glycol) (PEG) and biopolymers such as heparin and dextran were grafted on various surfaces to prevent protein adsorption (11,12). In particular for the PEG-tethered surface, numerous studies have made progress on the design of tethered layers (13,14) and the molecular reason why PEG but not other hydrophilic polymers is effective for adsorption prevention (10).

On the other hand, the application of tethered polymers to produce an adhesive biomaterial surface has attracted increased interest. The incorporation of bioactive groups on the surface through flexible polymer chains has been used to achieve the recognition of special proteins or regulate cell surface behavior (15–18). Among these studies, the most widely used ideas are the inclusion of antibodies to achieve targeting ability (15) and the incorporation of cell adhesion peptides [such as RGD oligopeptide (arginine, glycine, aspartic acid sequence)] to achieve regulated cell adhesion (17,19). These bioactive groups on the surface are specifically recognized by the protein or cellular receptors.

Thus, the design of biorecognitive surfaces has two major areas of interest: (a) a desire to increase specific interactions between the active groups compared to other environment components; and (b) a reduction of nonspecific adhesion to a minimum at the material surface. Therefore, optimal performance can be achieved by a designed surface-tethered structure consisting of chains with both bioactive groups and the polymers previously used in the nonfouling surfaces (Fig. 1). The intensive study of surface-tethered polymers in polymer science (20,21) enables us to predict the effect of various system parameters on the tethered layer structure. By changing the relative length and surface coverage of the two polymers, the nonspecific adhesion can be minimized without affecting the accessibility of the bioactive groups (15,22). The use of designed surfaces, such as self-assembled monolayers as model surfaces, to find optimal surface structures also is becoming increasingly important in designing novel structures and elucidating molecular mechanisms (23,24).

This tethered structure adhesion is regarded as a biomimetic approach. Most biological adhesions, such as those between cells and substrates or bacteria and tissues, are based on interactions among surface-tethered

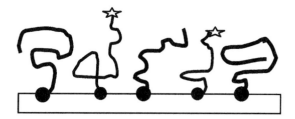

Figure 1 A mixed layer of tethered polymers on the biomaterial surface. The star symbols represent the bioactive groups attached to the end of some polymers on the surface. The function of these modified polymers is to enable biorecognition and enhance bioadhesion, whereas the other polymers are used to decrease nonspecific adhesion.

adhesion receptors (25). These tethered biopolymers are attached to the membranes and play important roles in cell–cell recognition and adhesion (25–27). The use of tethered receptors instead of short-ranged surface forces provides versatility of surface structures and more control ability.

Recently, studies of synthetic heteropolymers as artificial receptors have attracted increased attention (18,28,29). From a polymer science point of view, proteins with biorecognition ability are nothing more than heteropolymers, which are made of multitype chemical groups with different hydrophobic, hydrogen binding, and electrostatic properties. The special topology of these chemical groups along the chain gives them specific three-dimensional structures (30) and interaction with other molecules or surfaces (31). Recent progress of heteropolymer theories (32,33) calls for additional experimental studies on designed heteropolymers as artificial proteins. After the successful synthesis of these polymers with recognition ability, a biorecognitive surface can be constructed by grafting them onto the surface.

Recently, our group studied the application of tethered polymers as adhesion promoters in mucoadhesive drug delivery systems (34,35). Mucus is the viscous layer that covers and protects epithelial cells in the gastrointestinal tract and is the primary tissue surface with which the orally delivered drug carriers interact. Mucous layers can be modeled as a highly expanded hydrogel formed by the self-association of mucins. By introducing strong adhesion between the drug-carrying synthetic hydrogel and the mucous gel, drug carriers will have a longer residence time in the gastrointestinal tract, and hence a better drug adsorption profile can be obtained (36). The idea of using tethered polymers to enhance mucoadhesion is based on the assumption that these tethered polymers will penetrate into the mucous layer, form more adhesive interactions, and resist

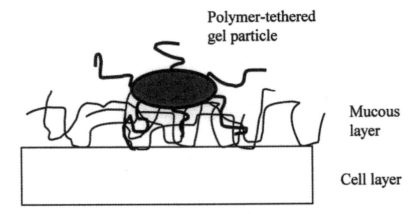

Figure 2 Schematic representation of the surface-grafted polymer chains penetrating into the mucous layer.

separation (Fig. 2). The surface tethered layer extends the planar surface adhesion into a three-dimensional interfacial interaction. More importantly, and similar to biological surfaces, the tethered polymers provide more control of the surface properties and allow the bulk structure to be optimized separately.

The choice of tethered polymer chemical structures is essential for chain penetration. We have developed a molecular thermodynamic method to model the interaction between the tethered polymer layer and the mucous layer. Fig. 3 shows that the system free energy changes with distance from the interface between the substrate gel and the mucous gel for four different tethered polymers (35). We discovered that if no attraction between tethered polymers and mucins exists, the tethered polymer layer makes a repulsive barrier for the gel/mucus adhesion, which reminds us of the tethered polymer in the nonfouling surface structure. However, by using other polymers that possess attraction with mucins, the gel/mucus adhesion becomes a favorable process and the tethered polymers spontaneously penetrate into the mucous layer as desired. Recently, the surface force apparatus has been used to test the interaction between tethered PEG chains and adsorbed mucin layers (37) as the first experimental attempt to test the approach.

In summary, it has been shown that a surface structure with desirable properties can be designed by starting with tethered polymer layers. The success of such surface structures will depend on progress in the following areas: (a) the theoretical prediction of the effects of design variables on the

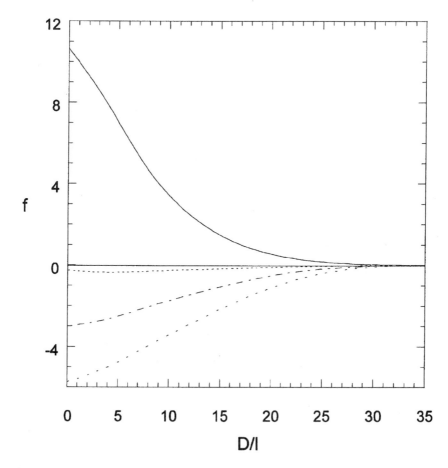

Figure 3 The system free energy per tethered polymer as a function of the gel–mucus distance D for four tethered polymers with different polymer–mucin attraction $\chi = 0.0$ (solid line), -0.2 (dotted line), -0.25 (dotted-dashed line), and -0.3 (dashed line). Parameter l is the segment length of the tethered polymer. In all cases, tethered polymers have 100 segments and the volume fraction of the gel is 0.3. (From ref. 35.)

structure at the molecular level; (b) the synthesis method to prepare the polymers and the construction of the tethered structure; (c) the understanding of the interaction between tethered polymers and the proteins or cells at the molecular level; and (d) the application of new characterization methods such as atomic force microscopy (38) and the surface force apparatus (39).

III. MICROPATTERNING

Spatial control of the grafting procedure permits development of a new class of devices. By micropatterning a surface, it is possible to create domains on the size of a few micrometers, each able to maintain different interactions with the environment (Fig. 4). The substrate material is modified, thereby allowing a layer of molecules to be covalently bound or adsorbed on the surface. Controlling where the binding reaction occurs creates a patterned surface. For example, a biosensor may be constructed with microdomains that selectively bind analyte molecules. Because of the small size, it is possible to make an array of these domains on a single chip. Another possible application of micropatterning is in the directed proliferation of cells. Surfaces may be modified with cell adhesion promoters, such as RGD oligopeptide, in order to promote cell growth in a specific direction or pattern. In the future, micropatterning for cell or protein recognition will allow for the creation of rapid screening and diagnostic devices.

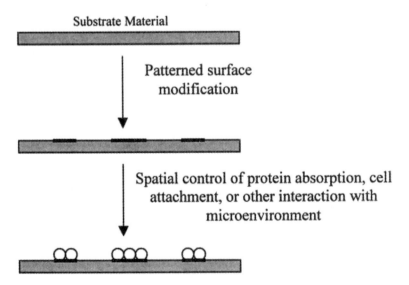

Figure 4 Description of micropatterned device structure. The surface of a material is modified in a precise pattern to promote interaction between the material and surrounding medium.

A. Micropatterning Techniques

In order for a surface to be micropatterned, there must be a means to spatially control the chemical reaction used to modify the surface. The reaction must be adequately controlled at the resolution necessary to fit the design of the device (e.g., micropatterning a device for cell adhesion may require resolution on the order of a few micrometers, the diameter of a cell). Various techniques have been developed to achieve this fine level of control.

1. Photolithographic Techniques

Photolithographic techniques, first developed for the production of integrated circuits (40), have formed the most basic step in micropatterning. First, a photomask is created by depositing an opaque material, such as chromium, on the surface of a flat, transparent quartz plate. Once the mask is made, it may be used for repeated exposures. The photomask is placed on the surface and exposed to UV light. Transparent areas of the mask allow light to reach the surface, where a chemical reaction triggered by irradiation can then occur (Fig. 5). In this manner, the rest of the surface is protected from reaction. Careful control of this technique may lead to resolution of 1 μm or less. In the production of silicon wafers, a photoresist, which is a

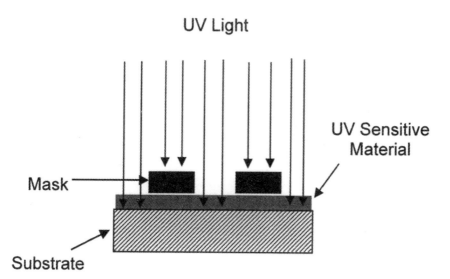

Figure 5 Production of a patterned surface using photolithographic techniques.

polymeric material that undergoes cleavage when exposed to UV light, is spread on the surface of the silicon substrate. Subsequent irradiation through the mask leaves regions of degraded polymer, which is then removed with an appropriate solvent leaving an unprotected surface. Modification of the exposed surface may be done in one of several ways; a metal may be deposited, molecules may be covalently bound, or the surface may be etched. Following modification, a strong solvent is used to remove the remaining intact photoresist. This process is repeated a number of times until all desired features are created.

Photolithography has been used in a number of distinctly different ways to create micropatterned surfaces. The first, and most direct, is photoablation. First, the surface of the substrate is laminated with a protective sheet. Irradiation through a photomask ablates the protective laminate in selected areas only, leaving behind exposed substrate. Molecules may then be adsorbed onto the laminate–substrate surface. Following adsorption, the laminate is removed. Schwarz et al. (41) used this technique to pattern the surface of polymer substrates with avidin. Other research by Girault (42,43) has focused on the ablation of polymeric materials for the production of microsensors.

Recently, several groups created patterned polymeric surfaces using a class of initiators known as iniferters (44). The iniferter technique allows a classical free-radical polymerization to serve as a living polymerization because of a reversible termination reaction. Iniferter molecules are first covalently attached to the substrate surface. The procedure used by de Boer et al. (45) involved modifying iniferter molecules such that an organosilane group could be used to covalently couple the molecule to a glass or silicon surface. In contrast, Ward et al. (46) used iniferter molecules to polymerize a substrate material from its monomers, thus directly incorporating the iniferter molecules. A substrate material could then be chosen to fit the needs of the application. In this study, hydrophobic substrate materials, such as poly(methyl methacrylate) and poly(styrene), as well as hydrophilic cross-linked PEG substrates [formed by reacting poly(ethylene glycol) dimethacrylate (PEGDMA) and poly(ethylene monomethacrylate) (PEGMA) together] were investigated.

After an iniferter molecule was bound to the substrate, a thin film of monomer was placed on the surface and subsequently irradiated with UV light through a photomask. Surface-bound iniferter molecules initiated the reaction, allowing for a covalent bond to be formed between the surface and raised polymer domain. Unreacted monomer was then washed away, leaving polymer covalently bound to the substrate surface. Well-defined regions, with resolution of less than $5\,\mu m$ and high aspect ratios, were produced (Fig. 6).

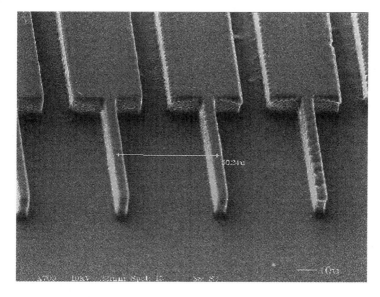

Figure 6 SEM micrograph of polymeric patterned surface. Substrate layer produced by reacting PEGDMA (average MW of PEG chain 200 g/mol) to form a cross-linked PEG-rich network. Micropatterned layer consists of 50% PEG200DMA and 50% PEG200MA. Height of patterned layer is approximately 40 μm, as determined with profilometry. Scale bar is 10 μm.

2. Soft Lithography

A different approach involves the use of soft lithography (47). First, a stamp is created (Fig. 7) using an elastomer, usually poly(dimethylsiloxane) (PDMS). A PDMS solution is cast on a silicon wafer patterned by conventional photolithographic techniques. The stamp may then be used in one of several techniques to produce a micropatterned surface. In the case of microcontact printing, the stamp is "inked" (Fig. 8), usually by contacting with a self-assembled monolayer (48). The inked stamp is then brought into contact with a surface and molecules are transferred from stamp to surface in the desired pattern. Besides microcontact printing, microfluidics (49) may be used to pattern a surface. Solution is flowed through channels formed when stamp and substrate are brought into contact. Molecules from the solution may absorb on the surface, but only in the channel regions. Aside from the creation of the silicon wafer used to produce the stamps, soft lithography avoids costly and difficult photolithographic procedures. Reviews of these soft lithographic techniques discussing patterned surface

Cast PDMS

PDMS Stamp

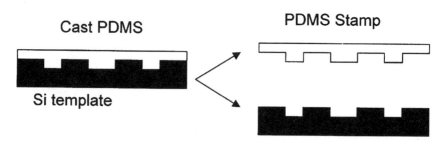

Si template

Figure 7 Creation of a PDMS stamp used in soft lithography. PDMS is first cast on a patterned silicon wafer. After separation, the template may be reused.

PDMS Stamp

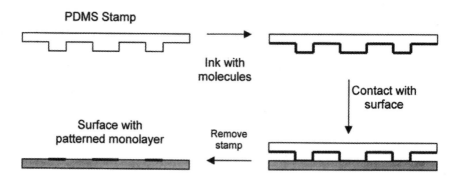

Ink with
molecules

Contact with
surface

Surface with
patterned monolayer

Remove
stamp

Figure 8 Method of creating a patterned monolayer by microcontact printing. Stamp is first inked with the desired molecule. The inked stamp is then brought into contact with the surface, transferring molecules only in the desired pattern.

creation (48,50) as well as their application for microfluidics devices (51) were recently published.

IV. MICROIMPRINTING: MOLECULAR IMPRINTING

Design and synthesis of artificial molecular structures capable of specific molecular recognition of biological molecules is inherently classified and fundamentally defined by the term *biomimetic materials*. These macromolecular networks with precise chemical architecture often possess enhanced mechanical, thermal, and recognition properties in comparison with their biological counterparts (52). However, it is difficult to rival nature's biological recognition, and few systems demonstrate better affinity and specificity (53,54). Numerous reviews describe the evolving field of designed molecular recognition and molecular imprinting (52,55–60). Molecular imprinting creates stereospecific three-dimensional binding cavities based on the biological compound of interest. However, efforts for the imprinting of larger molecules and proteins have focused on two-dimensional surface imprinting (61,62), a method of recognition at a surface rather than within a bulk polymer matrix. More recently, by using an epitope approach and imprinting a short peptide chain representing an exposed fragment of the total protein, three-dimensional imprinting of proteins within a bulk matrix has demonstrated moderate success (63). Molecular imprinting involves forming a prepolymerization complex between the molecule of interest, named the *template* or *imprint*, and functional monomers or functional oligomers (or polymers) (64) with specific chemical structures designed to interact with the template. This interaction can involve covalent (56) or non-covalent chemistry (self-assembly) (57,58), or both (65,66). Once the prepolymerization complex is formed, the polymerization reaction occurs in the presence of a cross-linking monomer and an appropriate solvent. Once the original imprint is removed, the result is a polymer matrix with specific recognition elements for the imprint molecule.

With non-covalent techniques, the solvent choice is a determining factor in effective imprint success, and it is the preferred synthesis scheme with biological applications since an easy binding/nonbinding template switching method is needed (i.e., no harsh conditions to remove template). Imprinting success, correlating to high binding affinity and specificity, depends on the relative amount of cross-interaction between the solvent and the intended non-covalent interactions (hydrogen bonding, hydrophobic interactions, $\pi - \pi$ orbital interactions, ionic interactions, and van der Waals forces) employed during complex formation. If the solvent interferes or competes with any of these interactions, a less effective recognition polymer will be formed. Naturally, these constraints have led to less polar organic synthesis routes for non-covalent aqueous recognition systems, which demonstrate orders of magnitude weaker binding affinity and decreased selectivity in polar, aqueous solvents (60,67). However, proper tuning of non-covalent interactions, such as increasing macromolecular chain hydrophobicity (68), or including stronger hydrogen bond donors and acceptors (69), or including strong ionic directed recognition sites with hydrophobic domains (70), has been shown to enhance binding in aqueous media and achieve selective recognition in aqueous solutions. Analysis of the free-energy contributions of ligand–receptor binding outlines the thermodynamic importance of directed tuning of these parameters in non-covalent recognition (71,72).

Fundamentally, mutual solubility regimes must exist between all monomers, templates, and polymerization initiators as solvent-resolved interaction strengths limit template choice. From a polymer science perspective, solvent must be present in the synthesis scheme because the composition and relative amount of solvent controls the overall polymer morphology and macroporous structure. Cross-linking in dilute polymer solutions minimizes physical entanglements and heterogeneity within the polymer network (73).

A. Imprinted Macromolecular Network

The nature of the imprinted polymer network is of considerable interest and has not yet been fully explored. The heteropolymer network structure depends on the type of monomer chemistry (anionic, cationic, neutral, amphiphilic), the association interactions between monomers, and the relative amounts of monomer species in the structure. Most molecular imprinting techniques suggest a significant amount of cross-linking monomer to produce three-dimensional receptor sites of adequate specificity. The rationale behind high cross-linking ratios is to produce a very stiff polymer network and thereby limit the movement of the molecular memory site via macromolecular chain relaxation, swelling phenomena, etc. As an increase in cross-linking monomer content leads to a decrease of the average molecular weight between cross-links (M_c), the macromolecular chains become more rigid. In less cross-linked systems, movement of the macromolecular chains or, more specifically, of the spacing of functional groups will inherently change as the network expands or contracts depending on the chosen rebinding solvent (thermodynamic interaction parameters characterizing the segment–solvent interaction) or application solution environment (Fig. 9). This fully reversible process will transiently affect the binding behavior and lead to sites with varying affinity and decreased selectivity (74–76). Variations on the adsorption process can also involve template–template intermolecular interactions and possible template aggregation, which can also create areas of differing affinity (77). By the same argument, but in regard to monomer type and composition, as the cross-linking monomer is increased in molecular weight, the length of the functional monomer or monomers should increase accordingly to avoid similar behavior (i.e., loss of possible binding regimes) irrespective of swelling or shrinking phenomena (Fig. 10). Therefore, there is an optimum cross-linking to functional monomer molecular weight ratio, which directly depends on the size of the template. Considerations of template structure and molecular rigidity (i.e., must possess sufficient functionality and must be

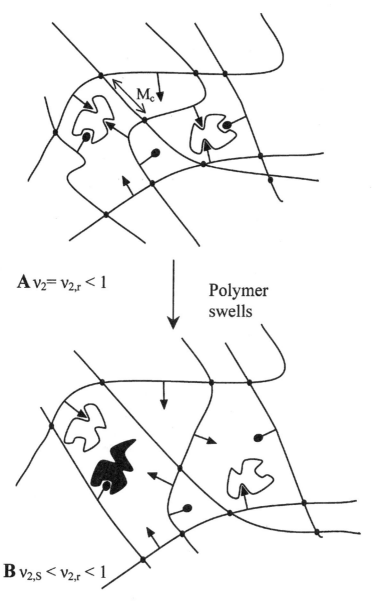

Figure 9 Ideal imprinted macromolecular network. (A) Ideal network after imprinting in original solvent. (B) Swelling behavior of macromolecular network demonstrating reduced affinity (different binding behavior of varying affinity) and selectivity. (Dark molecules are different molecules other than imprint and circles and triangles represent different functional monomers.)

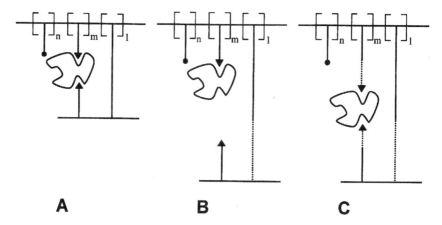

Figure 10   Ideal imprinted macromolecular network highlighting functional and cross-linking monomer molecular weight ratio. (A) Appropriately sized cross-linking monomer and functional monomers. (B) An increase in cross-linker molecular weight corresponding to an increased length without an equivalent change in functional monomer size. (C) An increase in length of both cross-linking and functional monomers produces a binding regime for the analyte.

appropriately rigid) are also important considerations in the overall design to mimic biological binding behavior (71,72).

It is also important to examine the nature of the network morphology on a molecular level. Compositional effects, such as an increase in the cross-linking monomer relative to other monomers, will greatly influence polymerization kinetics, the types of macromolecular chains formed, and the overall network properties. Types of chains formed with high cross-linking monomer ratios consist of primary copolymer chains of cross-linker and functional monomer and other secondary chains of cross-linking monomer that connect each macromer unit (73). It is widely accepted that selective molecularly imprinted polymers must be sufficiently cross-linked (54,56,57). However, lower cross-linked (19–22%) molecularly imprinted polymers are effective and adequate specificity can occur, albeit at a lower level compared to higher cross-linked systems (78,79). Recently, new directions and formulations involving imprinted functional polymers have produced selective imprinted recognition and lowered the cross-linking percentage further (64).

Therefore, in conclusion, an optimal system would consist of (a) functionalized sites with correct spatial geometry, (b) strong non-covalent forces with more than two points of binding (54,56), (c) dynamic recognition capability (i.e., rigid enough to provide stability and decreased binding of similar analytes, but equally able to reconform slightly to bind the intended molecule), and (d) bonding moieties without interfering sites of questionable and reduced selectivity.

B. Biological Recognition: Peptides as Functional Monomers

With proteins, and more specifically enzymes, function and activity arise from conformation, which is the three-dimensional arrangement of atoms in the structure. Since proteins are composed of a linear sequence of amino acids, it is this sequence that will dictate the conformation of the final protein. There are 20 possible amino acids that can be incorporated into the sequence with each amino acid having a unique residue (side chain) group. These residues can be hydrophilic or hydrophobic, have positive charge, have negative charge, can be hydrogen bond donors and acceptors, can be bulky or small groups, etc. It is the interaction of these groups with the solvent, each other, and other molecules (e.g., cofactors, etc.) that influence the folding of a protein into a three-dimensional arrangement. For example, in an aqueous environment, a polypeptide chain will fold spontaneously to bury hydrophobic groups (they are thermodynamically more stable here) and place polar, charged groups on the surface. However, some proteins need a hydrophobic exterior and are designed differently from aqueous proteins [integral membrane proteins need a hydrophobic outer layer to easily penetrate and traverse biological membranes (80)]. Nature can choose among the different amino acids to neatly fill the interior of a protein and maximize stabilizing interactions. Therefore, thermodynamics dictate the constraints placed on a protein or enzyme to have a precise three-dimensional shape. Influencing the conformational shape by solvent-induced conformational changes and subsequently exposing the protein to a template and then cross-linking (or freeze drying), proteins can be manipulated to form new memory for ligands (81,82). In effect, processes of this type, termed *bioimprinting*, have been shown to work in anhydrous organic solvents but completely lose selectivity in aqueous environments (81). It is expected that advances in the fields of protein folding and protein–enzyme ligand recognition will stimulate developments in molecular imprinting.

C. Applications of Molecularly Imprinted Polymers

Creating artificial receptor molecules with specific recognition has application in separation processes (chromatography, capillary electrophoresis, solid phase extraction, membrane separations), catalysis and artificial enzymes, immunoassays and antibody mimics, and biosensor recognition elements (55). However, it also has direct application as recognition elements in intelligent drug delivery devices, in targeted drug delivery applications, and in controlled tissue engineering applications as well as micropumps and microactuators in microfluidics devices.

D. Molecularly Imprinting D-Glucose

Our work in this area is developing on two fronts: (a) gaining a fundamental understanding of the imprinting polymerization process by characterizing imprinted gel structures and (b) creating biomimetic molecularly imprinted polymer gels for various biologically active molecules and incorporating them as recognition elements in novel controlled drug delivery, targeted drug delivery, and tissue engineering. One template, D-glucose, will be highlighted and briefly discussed below.

Producing tailor-made particles with recognition sites for glucose is the first step in the development of a novel intelligent polymer device for the modulated release of insulin or specific diabetes drugs. As expected, it also has application outside the realm of drug delivery to a number of problems requiring the separation or sensing of glucose in aqueous systems.

Current glucose-sensitive intelligent polymeric devices that incorporate glucose-specific proteins or glucose-binding moieties either are not glucose-specific (83–85), are limited by inherent immunogenicity (86–93), or operate far from physiological conditions (94,95). Development of a modulated insulin delivery device based on triggering of the delivery mechanism by the concentration of glucose in the blood or subcutaneous tissue has become a significant research interest. Development of a truly modulated insulin delivery device is still years away mainly because of the lack of biocompatible glucose-sensing molecules. Thus, more specific and biocompatible glucose-binding molecules are needed in the development of glucose biosensors and intelligent implantable polymeric devices for the modulated (i.e., autoregulated) release of insulin.

A literature review analyzing glucose binding methods has rather few alternatives for the molecular recognition of glucose. These include molecular imprinting methods (non-covalent and covalent) (64,94–99); protein recognition methods [glucose-binding proteins: concanavalin A, lectins, genetically engineered proteins (86,87,92,93,100)]; active enzyme recognition [glucose oxidase (88–91)]; and inactive enzyme recognition [apoglucose oxidase by removal of FAD cofactor (101)]. Molecular imprinting methods either are not suited for biological saccharide recognition (covalent approaches) or do not work well in aqueous environments or under the conditions of biological recognition in vivo (non-covalent approaches). However, analyzing and properly mimicking glucose protein binding sites might provide insight into appropriate non-covalent interactions.

Study of various polysaccharide-binding proteins reveals planar polar side chains (carboxylic acids and amines) that are hydrogen bond donors and acceptors (102,103). Analyzing these sites has provided invaluable insight into the development of appropriate polymerization moieties for successful imprinting of glucose. It has been suggested that the main interaction providing glucose specificity in an aqueous environment is hydrogen bonding (glucose-binding protein provides 13 hydrogen bonds) as well as hydrophobic interactions (glucose pyranose ring is hydrophobic on both faces) (102). The amino acids involved in multiple hydrogen bonding are aspartate (Asp), glutamate (Glu), and asparagine (Asn), which provide hydrogen bond donors and acceptors (carboxylic acid–Asp, Glu; and amine group–Asn). The amino acids phenylalanine (Phe) and tryptophan (Trp) each have aromatic rings that enhance binding by providing hydrophobic interactions with both sides of the glucose pyranose ring.

Our group has synthesized novel glucose-binding molecules based on non-covalent interactions formed via molecular imprinting techniques within an aqueous environment (polar, protic solvent). The benefit of these molecules compared to current intelligent polymer devices and polymer-binding systems is their affinity and selectivity in an aqueous environment, robust nature, and nonantigenic properties.

Polymer films were prepared by UV free-radical polymerization in an appropriate solvent with mutual solubility of monomers and imprint. Polymers differing in imprint, cross-linker (% mol/mol monomers), and functional monomer ratios were synthesized.

Polymers were allowed to dry at ambient conditions and then were crushed and sieved. The resulting particle sizes ranged from 300 to less than 150 μm. Particles were vortexed and resuspended within a wash solvent multiple times to remove template and unreacted monomer. Testing of these materials via kinetic, equilibrium, and competitive binding assays involves conventional analytical methods of analyte detection, such as high-performance liquid chromatography (HPLC), enzymatic assays, and colorimetric methods.

Equilibrium binding studies were conducted using cell culture plates and a titer plate shaker to provide continuous mixing. A known glucose solution was added to a known amount of polymer particles and equilibrium binding results were quantitatively calculated by HPLC measurements of the resulting supernatant (HPX-87H column, 0.005 M H_2SO_4 mobile phase, 0.8 mL/min flow rate, temperature 65°C, L-3350

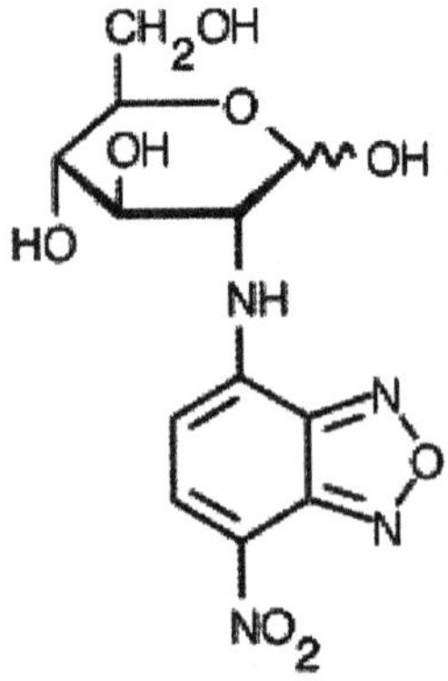

Figure 11   Fluorescent D-glucose analogue: 2-NBDG (Molecular Probes, Inc.).

refractive index detector). Qualitative equilibrium binding results were obtained using the fluorescent glucose analogue 2-(N-(7-nitrobenz-2-oxa-1,3-diazol-4-yl)amino)-2-deoxyglucose (2-NBDG, Molecular Probes). 2-NBDG (Fig. 11) was added to vials containing a known amount of polymer (maximum absorption 466 nm; maximum emission 542 nm). A Nikon Labophot fluorescent microscope with a FITC filter set was used to visualize binding of the glucose analogue. Images were acquired with an Optronics 470T CCD camera and captured using MetaMorph software from Universal Imaging.

Our results qualitatively and quantitatively demonstrate effective glucose-binding polymers. Competitive binding studies between glucose and 2-NBDG yielded conclusive results that glucose is bound to our polymers and not the additional fluorescent group in 2-NBDG. Fig. 12 shows equilibrium binding of fluorescent glucose analogue to a D-glucose molecularly imprinted polymer with a 48% cross-linking ratio (% mol/mol monomers). Increased fluorescence of the imprinted polymer demonstrates increased recognition and binding in comparison with that of control polymers. Fig. 13, which shows the same monomer types but differing compositions, demonstrates different binding behavior when cross-linking monomer percentage is lowered to 11%. These polymers swelled significantly in aqueous solution and have lost effective recognition in certain areas of the gel. However, a few regions demonstrate effective recognition possibly introduced by inhomogeneities in the matrix. The specificity and control of these systems are the subject of further study in our laboratory.

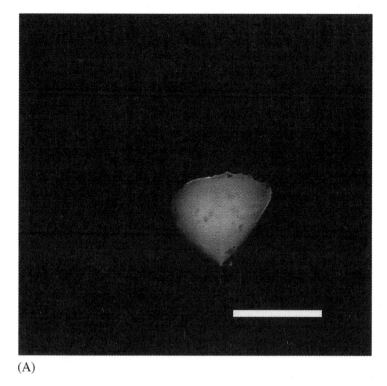

(A)

Figure 12 Fluorescent glucose analogue equilibrium binding to D-glucose molecularly imprinted polymer with 48% cross-linking ratio (% mol/mol monomers). (A) Imprinted polymer, (B) nonimprinted polymer. Increased fluorescence demonstrates increased recognition and affinity compared to control polymers. Scale bar is 100 μm.

V. CONCLUSIONS

Developments in the field of biomimetic micropatterned and microimprinted structures are still in their infancy. Up to now work has concentrated mostly on modification of polymer surfaces to attach desirable tethers or grafted chains with specific characteristics. Over the past 10 years, such synthetic techniques have led to a wide range of new polymer systems, but without much focus on the associated molecular recognition. In fact, only recently have such efforts been made in the micropatterning field.

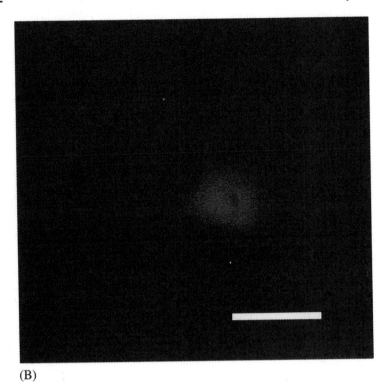

(B)

Figure 12 Continued.

Although microimprinting has been a field of research for more than 20 years, there has been little effort to use it in biomimetic systems. Thus, in the next 10 years we expect that the field is going to grow and to focus on ingenious solution of actual biomimetic problems. Developments of particular interest to the field are expected to be wide and far reaching, such as recognition of undesirable biologicals, nanoscale patterning and recognition of proteins, site-specific interaction with tissues, etc.

Yet for best achievement of these goals, our molecular methods of patterning or imprinting have to become more specific to the environment. Also, development of self-assembled polymer structures with specific characteristics for recognition of biological compounds might be needed. Clearly, in this regard, the field is in its infancy.

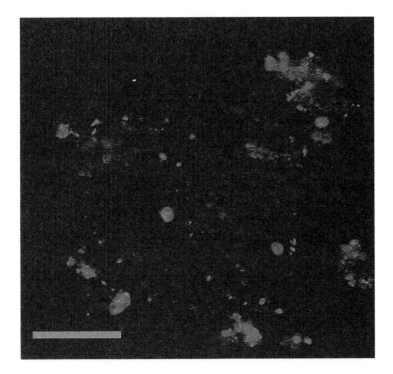

Figure 13 Fluorescent glucose analogue equilibrium binding to D-glucose molecularly imprinted polymer with 11% cross-linking ratio (% mol/mol monomers). Note the monomers are the same as in Figure 12. The imprinted polymer demonstrates drastically different binding behavior in comparison with higher crosslinking ratios. Scale bar is 100 μm.

ACKNOWLEDGMENTS

The work presented here was supported by grants from the National Science Foundation (DGE-99-72770, BES-9706538) and the National Institutes of Health (GM56231, GM43337). M. E. Byrne and D. B. Henthorn are NSF IGERT Fellows.

REFERENCES

1. JM Schakenraad. Cells: their surfaces and interactions with materials. In: BD Ratner, AS Hoffman, FJ Schoen, JE Lemons, eds. Biomaterials Science: An

Introduction to Materials in Medicine. San Diego: Academic Press, 1996, pp 141–147.

2. NA Peppas, R Langer. New challenges in biomaterials. Science 263:1715–1720, 1994.

3. BD Ratner. The engineering of biomaterials exhibiting recognition and specificity. J Mol Recognit 9:617–625, 1996.

4. BD Ratner, AS Hoffman. Thin films, grafts, and coatings. In: BD Ratner, AS Hoffman, FJ Schoen, JE Lemons, eds. Biomaterials Science: An Introduction to Materials in Medicine. San Diego: Academic Press, 1996, pp 105–118.

5. VH Thom, G Altankov, T Groth, K Jankova, G Jonsson, M Ulbricht. Optimizing cell-surface interactions by photografting of poly(ethylene glycol). Langmuir 16:2756–2765, 2000.

6. BD Ratner, A Chilkoti, GP Lopez. Plasma deposition and treatment for biomedical applications. In: R D'Agostino, ed. Plasma Deposition, Treatment and Etching of Polymers. San Diego: Academic Press, 1990, pp 463–516.

7. A Ohl, K Schroder. Plasma-induced chemical micropatterning for cell culturing applications: a brief review. Surf Coat Tech 116–119:820–830, 1999.

8. CM Chan, TM Ko, H Hiraoka. Polymer surface modification by plasmas and photons. Surf Sci Rep 24:1–54, 1996.

9. SW Kim. Nonthrombogenic treatments and strategies. In: BD Ratner, AS Hoffman, FJ Schoen, JE Lemons, eds. Biomaterials Science: An Introduction to Materials in Medicine. San Diego: Academic Press, 1996, pp 297–307.

10. AS Hoffman. Non-fouling surface technologies. J Biomater Sci Polym Ed 10:1011–1014, 1999.

11. M Morra, E Occhiello, F Garbassi. Surface modification of blood contacting polymers by poly(ethyleneoxide). Clin Mater 14:255–265, 1993.

12. JH Lee, HB Lee, JD Andrade. Blood compatibility of polyethylene oxide surfaces. Prog Polym Sci 20:1043–1079, 1995.

13. I Szleifer, MA Carignano. Tethered polymer layers: phase transitions and reduction of protein adsorption. Macromol Rapid Commun 21:423–448, 2000.

14. A Halperin, DE Leckband. From ship hulls to contact lenses: repression of protein adsorption and the puzzle of PEO. C R Acad Sci Paris IV 1:1171–1178, 2000.

15. VP Torchilin. Affinity liposomes in vivo: factors influencing target accumulation. J Mol Recogn 9:335–346, 1996.

16. AK Dillow, M Tirrell. Targeted cellular adhesion at biomaterial interfaces. Curr Opin Solid State Mater Sci 3:252–259, 1998.

17. JA Hubbell. Bioactive biomaterials. Curr Opin Biotech 10:123–129, 1999.

18. KE Healy. Molecular engineering of materials for bioactivity. Curr Opin Solid State Mater Sci 4:381–387, 1999.

19. RG Lebaron, KA Athanasiou. Extracellular matrix cell adhesion peptides: functional applications in the orthopedic materials. Tissue Eng 6:85–103, 2000.

20. A Halperin, M Tirrell, TP Lodge. Tethered chains in polymer microstructures. Adv Polym Sci 100:31–71, 1992.
21. I Szleifer, MA Carignano. Tethered polymer layers. Adv Chem Phys 94:165–260, 1996.
22. Y Dori, H Bianco-Peled, SK Satija, GB Fields, JB McCarthy, M Tirrell. Ligand accessibility as means to control cell response to bioactive bilayer membrane. J Biomed Mater Res 50:75–81, 2000.
23. M Mrksich, GM Whitesides. Using self-assembled monolayers to understand the interactions of man-made surfaces with proteins and cells. Annu Rev Biophys Biomole Struct 25:55–78, 1996.
24. W Knoll, M Matsuzawa, A Offenhausser, J Ruhe. Tailoring of surfaces with ultrathin layers for controlled binding of biopolymers and adhesion and guidance of cells. Israel J Chem 36:357–369, 1996.
25. DA Hammer, M Tirrell. Biological adhesion at interfaces. Annu Rev Mater Sci 26:651–691, 1996.
26. N Sharon. Bacterial lectins, cell-cell recognition and infection disease. FEBS Lett 217:145–157, 1987.
27. TR Neu, KC Marshall. Bacterial polymers: physiochemical aspects of their interactions at interfaces. J Biomater Appl 5:107–133, 1990.
28. M Jozefowicz, J Jozefonvicz. Randomness and biospecificity: random copolymers are capable of biospecific molecular recognition in living systems. Biomaterials 18:1633–1644, 1997.
29. M Mammen, S Choi, GM Whitesides. Polyvalent interactions in biological systems: implications for design and use of multivalent ligands and inhibitors. Angew Chem Int Ed 37:2754–2794, 1998.
30. D Baker. A surprising simplicity to protein folding. Nature 405:39–42, 2000.
31. AJ Golumbfskie, VS Pande, AK Chakraborty. Simulation of biomimetic recognition between polymers and surfaces. Proc Natl Acad Sci USA 96:11707–11712, 1999.
32. VS Pande, AY Grosberg, T Tanaka. Heteropolymer freezing and design: towards physical models of protein folding. Rev Mod Phys 72:259–314, 2000.
33. AK Chakraborty. Disordered heteropolymers: models for biomimetic polymers and polymers with frustrating quenched disorder. Phys Rep 342:1–61, 2001.
34. Y Huang, W Leobandung, A Foss, NA Peppas. Molecular aspects of muco- and bioadhesion: tethered structures and site-specific surfaces. J Controlled Release 65:63–71, 2000.
35. Y Huang, I Szleifer, NA Peppas. Gel-gel adhesion by tethered polymers. J Chem Phys 114:3809–3818, 2001.
36. NA Peppas, PA Buri. Surface, interfacial and molecular aspects of polymer bioadhesion on soft tissues. J Controlled Release 2:257–275, 1985.
37. NV Efremova, Y Huang, NA Peppas, DE Leckband. Direct measurement of interactions between tethered PEG chains and adsorbed mucin layers. Langmuir 18(3): 836–845, 2002.

38. VJ Morris, AR Kirby, AP Gunning. Atomic Force Microscopy for Biologists. London: Imperial College Press, 1999.

39. DE Leckband. The surface force apparatus—a tool for probing molecular protein interactions. Nature 376:617–618, 1995.

40. M Madou. Fundamentals of Microfabrication. Boca Raton: CRC Press, 1997.

41. A Schwarz, JS Rossier, E Roulet, N Mermod, MA Roberts, HH Girault. Micropatterning of biomolecules on polymer substrates. Langmuir 14:5526–5531, 1998.

42. BJ Seddon, Y Shao, HH Girault. Printed microelectrode array and amperometric sensor for environmental monitoring. Electochim Acta 39:2377–2386, 1994.

43. JS Rossier, P Bercier, A Schwarz, S Loridant, HH Girault. Topography, crystallinity and wettability of photoablated PET surfaces. Langmuir 15:5173–5178, 1999.

44. T Otsu, M Yoshida. Role of initiator-transfer agent-terminator (iniferter) in radical polymerizations: polymer design by organic disulfides and iniferters. Makromol Chem Rapid Commun 3:133–140, 1982.

45. B de Boer, HK Simon, MPL Werts, EW van der Wegte, G Hadziioannou. Living free radical photopolymerizations initiated from surface-grafted iniferter monolayers. Macromolecules 33:349–356, 2000.

46. JH Ward, R Gomez, R Bashir, NA Peppas. UV free-radical polymerization for micropatterning poly(ethylene glycol)–containing films. Proceedings of SPIE—The International Society for Optical Engineering, Vol 4097, Bellingham, WA, 2000, pp 221–228.

47. A Kumar, GM Whitesides. Features of gold having micrometer to centimeter dimensions can be formed through a combination of stamping with an elastomeric stamp and an alkanethiol ink followed by chemical etching. Appl Phys Lett 63:2002–2004, 1993.

48. R Jackman, J Wilbur, GM Whitesides. Fabrication of submicron features on curved substrates by microcontact printing. Science 269:664–666, 1995.

49. E Kim, Y Xia, GM Whitesides. Polymer microstructures formed by molding in capillaries. Nature 376:581–584, 1995.

50. R Kane, S Takayama, E Ostuni, DE Ingber, GM Whitesides. Patterning protein and cells using soft lithography. Biomaterials 20:2363–2376, 1999.

51. JC McDonald, DC Duffy, JR Anderson, DT Chiu, H Wu, OJ Schueller, GM Whitesides. Fabrication of microfluidics systems in poly(dimethylsiloxane). Electrophoresis 21:27–40, 2000.

52. RJ Ansell, K Mosbach. Molecularly imprinted polymers: New tools for biomedical science. Pharmaceut News 3(2):16–20, 1996.

53. G Vlatakis, LI Andersson, R Muller, K Mosbach. Drug assay using antibody mimics made by molecular imprinting. Nature 361:645–647, 1993.

54. F Flam. Molecular Imprints make a mark. Science 263:1221–1222, 1994.

55. T Takeuchi, J Haginaka. Separation and sensing based on molecular recognition using molecularly imprinted polymers. J Chromatogr B 728:1–20, 1999.

56. G Wulff. Molecular imprinting in cross-linked materials with the aid of molecular templates—a way towards artificial antibodies. Angew Chem Int Ed Engl 34:1812–1832, 1995.

57. K Mosbach, O Ramstrom. The emerging technique of molecular imprinting and its future impact on biotechnology. Biotechnol 14:163–170, 1996.

58. B Sellergren. Noncovalent molecular imprinting: antibody-like molecular recognition in polymeric network materials. Trends Anal Chem 16(6):310–320, 1997.

59. T Takeuchi, J Matsui. Molecular imprinting: an approach to "tailor made" synthetic polymers with biomimetic functions. Acta Polym 47:471–480, 1996.

60. K Mosbach, K Haupt. Some new developments and challenges in noncovalent molecular imprinting technology. J Mol Recogn 11:62–68, 1998.

61. H Shi, W Tsai, MD Garrison, S Ferrari, BD Ratner. Template-imprinted nanostructured surfaces for protein recognition. Nature 398:593–597, 1999.

62. H Shi, BD Ratner. Template recognition of protein-imprinted polymer surfaces. J Biomed Mater Res 49:1–11, 2000.

63. A Rachkov, N Minoura. Towards molecularly imprinted polymers selective to peptides and proteins. The epitope approach. Biochim Biophys Acta 1544:255–266, 2001.

64. W Wizeman, P Kofinas. Glucose specific polymeric molecular imprints. Polym Preprints 41(2):1632, 2000.

65. MJ Whitcombe, ME Rodriguez, P Villar, EN Vulfson. A new method for the introduction of recognition site functionality into polymers prepared by molecular imprinting: synthesis and characterization of polymeric receptors for cholesterol. J Am Chem Soc 117:7105–7111, 1995.

66. N Kirsch, C Alexander, M Lubke, MJ Whitcombe, EN Vulfson. Enhancement of selectivity of imprinted polymers via post-imprinting modification of recognition sites. Polymer 41:5583–5590, 2000.

67. LI Andersson, R Muller, G Vlatakis, K Mosbach. Mimics of the binding sites of opiod receptors obtained by molecular imprinting of enkephalin and morphine. Proc Natl Acad Sci USA 92:4788–4792, 1995.

68. C Yu, O Ramstrom, K Mosbach. Enantiomeric recognition by molecularly imprinted polymers using hydrophobic interactions. Anal Lett 30(12):2123–2140, 1997.

69. C Yu, K Mosbach. Molecular imprinting utilizing an amide functional group for hydrogen bonding leading to highly efficient polymers. J Org Chem 62:4057–4064, 1997.

70. K Haupt. Noncovalent molecular imprinting of a synthetic polymer with the herbicide 2, 4-dichlorophenoxyacetic acid in the presence of polar protic solvents. In: RA Bartsch, M Maeda, eds. Molecular and Ionic Recognition with Imprinted Polymers. ACS Symposium Series 703. Washington, DC: American Chemical Society, 1998, pp 135–142.

71. IA Nicholls. Towards the rational design of molecularly imprinted polymers. J Mol Recog 11:79–82, 1998.

72. IA Nicholls. An approach toward the semiquantitation of molecular recognition phenomena in noncovalent molecularly imprinted polymer systems: consequences for molecularly imprinted polymer design. Adv Mol Cell Bio 15B:671–679, 1996.

73. RA Scott, NA Peppas. Compositional effects on network structure of highly cross-linked copolymers of PEG-containing multiacrylates with acrylic acid. Macromolecules 32:6139–6148, 1999.

74. C Alvarez-Lorenzo, O Guney, T Oya, Y Sakai, M Kobayashi, T Enoki, Y Takeoka, T Ishibashi, K Kuroda, K Tanaka, G Wang, AY Grosberg. Reversible adsorption of calcium ions by imprinted temperature sensitive gels. J Chem Phys 114(6):2812–2816, 2001.

75. C Alvarez-Lorenzo, O Guney, T Oya, Y Sakai, M Kobayashi, T Enoki, Y Takeoka, T Ishibashi, K Kuroda, K Tanaka, G Wang, AY Grosberg, S Masamune, T Tanaka. Polymer gels that memorize elements of molecular conformation. Macromolecules 33:8693–8697, 2000.

76. T Enoki, K Tanaka, T Watanabe, T Oya, T Sakiyama, Y Takeoka, K Ito, G Wang, M Annaka, K Hara, R Du, J Chuang, K Wasserman, AY Grosberg, S Masamune, T Tanaka. Frustrations in polymer conformation in gels and their minimization through molecular imprinting. Phys Rev Lett 85(23):5000–5003, 2000.

77. A Katz, ME Davis. Investigations into the mechanisms of molecular recognition with imprinted polymers. Macromolecules 32:4113–4121, 1999.

78. Y Cong, K Mosbach. Influence of mobile phase composition and cross-linking density on the enantiomeric recognition properties of molecularly imprinted polymers. J Chromatogr A 888:63–72, 2000.

79. E Yilmaz, K Mosbach, K Haupt. Influence of functional and cross-linking monomers and the amount of template on the performance of molecularly imprinted polymers in binding assays. Anal Commun 36:167–170, 1999.

80. L Stryer. Biochemistry, 3rd ed. New York: WH Freeman, 1988, pp 29–30.

81. K Dabulis, AM Klibanov. Molecular imprinting of proteins and other macromolecules resulting in new adsorbents. Biotechnol Bioeng 39:176–185, 1992.

82. M Stahl, U Jeppsson-Wistrand, MO Mansson, K Mosbach. Induced stereoselectivity and substrate selectivity of bio-imprinted alpha-chymotrypsin in anhydrous organic media. J Am Chem Soc 113:9366–9368, 1991.

83. D Shiino, K Kataoka, Y Koyama, M Yokoyama, T Okano, Y Sakurai. A self-regulated insulin delivery system using boronic acid gel. J Intel Mater Syst Struct 5(3):311–314, 1994.

84. K Kataoka, H Miyazaki, M Bunya, T Okano, Y. Sakurai. Totally synthetic polymer gels responding to external glucose concentration: their preparation and application to on-off regulation of insulin release. J Am Chem Soc 120:12694–12695, 1998.

85. H Miyazaki, G Sasagawa, T Okano, Y Sakurai, K Kataoka. Novel glucose sensitive phase transition gel of N-isopropylacrylamide with 3-acrylamido-

phenylboronic acid group as command moiety. Fifth World Biomaterials Congress, Toronto, Canada, May 29–June 2, 1996, p 875.

86. S Lee, K Park. Synthesis and characterization of sol-gel phase-reversible hydrogels sensitive to glucose. J Mol Recogn 9:549–557, 1996.

87. A Obaidat, K Park. Characterization of protein release through glucose-sensitive hydrogel membranes. Biomaterials 18:801–806, 1997.

88. K Podual, FJ Doyle, NA Peppas. Glucose-sensitivity of glucose oxidase-containing cationic copolymer hydrogels having poly(ethylene glycol) grafts. J Controlled Release 67:9–17, 2000.

89. K Podual, FJ Doyle, NA Peppas. Preparation and dynamic response of cationic copolymer hydrogels containing glucose oxidase. Polymer 41:3975–3983, 2000.

90. K Podual, FJ Doyle, NA Peppas. Dynamic behavior of glucose oxidase-containing microparticles of poly(ethylene glycol)-grafted cationic hydrogels in an environment of changing pH. Biomaterials 21:1439–1450, 2000.

91. F Ghodsian, JM Newton. Simulation and optimisation of a self-regulating insulin delivery system. J Drug Target 1:67–80, 1993.

92. E Kokufata, Y Zhang, T Tanaka. Saccharide-sensitive phase transition of a lectin-loaded gel. Nature 351:302–304, 1991.

93. K Nakamae, T Miyata, A Jikihara, AS Hoffman. Formation of poly (glucosyloxyethyl methacrylate)-concanavalin A complex and its glucose sensitivity. J Biomater Sci Polym Ed 6(1):79–90, 1994.

94. C Chen, G Chen, Z Guan, D Lee, FH Arnold. Polymeric sensor materials for glucose. Polym Preprints 37(2):216–217, 1996.

95. S Streigler. Molecularly imprinted polymers using metal coordination for selective binding interactions in water. 1st International Workshop on Molecular Imprinting, Cardiff, UK, July 3–5, 2000, p 49.

96. AG Mayes, LI Andersson, K Mosbach. Sugar binding polymers showing high anomeric and epimeric discrimination by non-covalent molecular imprinting. Anal Biochem 222:483–488, 1994.

97. G Wulff, J Haarer. Enzyme-analogue built polymers. The preparation of defined chiral cavities for the racemic resolution of free sugars. Makromol Chem 192:1329–1338, 1991.

98. G Wulff, D Oberkobusch, M Minarik. Enzyme-analogue built polymers. Chiral cavities in polymer layers coated on wide-pore silica. React Polym 3:261–275, 1985.

99. C Malitesta, I Losito, PG Zambonin. Molecularly imprinted electrosynthesized polymers: new materials for biomimetic sensors. Anal Chem 71(7):1366–1370, 1999.

100. L Tolosa, I Gryczynski, LR Eichhorn, JD Dattelbaum, FN Castellano, G Rao, JR Lakowicz. Glucose sensor for low-cost lifetime-based sensing using a genetically engineered protein. Anal Biochem 267:114–120, 1999.

101. S D'Auria, P Herman, M Rossi, JR Lakowicz. The fluorescence emission of the apo-glucose oxidase from Aspergillus niger as probe to estimate glucose concentrations. Biochem Biophys Res Commun 263:550–553, 1999.

102. T Li, H Lee, K Park. Comparative stereochemical analysis of glucose-binding proteins for rational design of glucose specific agents. J Biomater Sci Polym Ed 9(4):327–344, 1998.
103. FA Quiocho. Protein carbohydrate interactions: basic molecular features. Pure Appl Chem 61:1293–1306, 1989.

15
Bioinspired Engineering of Intelligent Drug Delivery Systems and Protein–Polymer Conjugates

Patrick S. Stayton, Allan S. Hoffman, Niren Murthy, Chantal Lackey, Charles Cheung, Tsuyoshi Shimoboji, Zhongli Ding, Jean S. Campbell, Nelson Fausto, Themis R. Kyriakides, and Paul Bornstein
University of Washington, Seattle, Washington

Oliver W. Press
Fred Hutchinson Cancer Research Center, Seattle, Washington

Fiona Black
Illumina, Inc., San Diego, California

I. INTRODUCTION

One of the hallmarks of biological systems is their ability to change important properties in response to environmental cues. The molecular mechanisms that biological molecules utilize to sense and respond provide interesting paradigms for the development of biomaterials that display "smart" properties. There are numerous technologies in which responsive material properties have proven useful or have important potential, including controlled release/drug delivery, tissue engineering, biomedical materials, diagnostics, affinity separations, microfluidic devices, and chip/array devices. In addition, responsive biomolecular components that reversibly exist in two distinct physical states might represent potential device elements for information storage and read/write technologies. In this chapter, we review our work on hybrid polymer–biomolecule systems that are designed to have environmentally responsive properties and function. These systems merge the impressive recognition and biofunctional properties of biomolecules, with the impressive responsiveness and chemical versatility of functional polymers.

II. BIOMIMETIC DELIVERY OF BIOMOLECULAR THERAPEUTICS

A. Delivery Challenge and General Design of Carriers

The biotechnology and pharmaceutical industries have developed a wide variety of potential therapeutics based on the molecules of biology: DNA, RNA, and proteins. While these therapeutics have tremendous potential, effectively formulating and delivering them has also been a widely recognized challenge. There are a variety of difficult barriers, including drug stability, tissue penetration, and transport. While a number of creative delivery systems show significant potential for overcoming these problems with biomolecules that act at the extracellular membrane, a widespread barrier for those that function intracellularly is cytoplasmic entry (1,2). Passive or receptor-mediated endocytosis results in localization of biomolecules to the endosomal compartment, where the predominant trafficking fate is fusion with lysosomes and subsequent degradation (3).

One of the most significant barriers for the delivery of biomolecular therapeutics that function inside the cell is thus the endosomal barrier (Fig. 1). For therapeutics such as plasmid DNA, antisense oligonucleotides, ribozymes, and immunotoxins, their ability to reach their target is

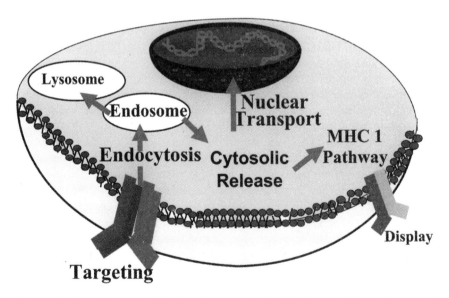

Figure 1 Schematic model of pathways involved in intracellular delivery of biomolecular therapeutics and vaccines, including key barriers.

dependent on their initial ability to reach the cytoplasm from the endosomal compartment. Similarly, the delivery of plasmid-based or protein/peptide-based molecular vaccines is also dependent on getting the plasmid to the nucleus, or the peptides or proteins into the cytoplasm, for entry into the protein processing and display pathways. The magnitude of this challenge for the delivery field can easily be seen in a comparison of viral versus nonviral gene delivery, where the relative efficiencies can be conservatively compared as 4–6 orders of magnitude.

How did viruses and pathogenic organisms get so good at intracellular delivery of DNA or proteins? They have evolved wonderfully sophisticated proteins that enhance transport of DNA or proteins from the endosome. Their most important property ties together the sensing of pH changes to membrane destabilizing activity. The endosome develops one of the few large chemical gradients found in biology through the proton pumping activity of membrane-bound ATP-dependent proton pumps. As a result, the pH of these compartments drops during endosomal development to values of 5.5 or lower. This pH drop serves as a trigger for a conformational change and exposure of a membrane-active domain in viral proteins such as hemagglutinin (4).

These membrane-active domains control membrane fusion and transport, and their activity is "smart" because the biopolymers sense the low-pH environment of the endosome and reversibly change their properties in response to this external cue. Several types of pathogenic organisms, including *corynebacterium diphtheriae* (5), have also evolved protein domains that sense the lower pH environment of the endosome and aid transport across the endosomal barrier. Hemagglutinin and toxin share a common pH-sensing strategy, where the protonation equilibria of carboxylate-containing side chains are tied to the pH-dependent conformational change that results in membrane destabilizing activity (6). When the pH has dropped sufficiently to protonate key carboxylate residues, the conformational equilibria are shifted toward the membrane-active state by the loss of these electrostatic charges.

The use of these proteins, and peptides displaying similar activities, as endosomal releasing agents in gene and protein delivery systems has been investigated (7–9). The GALA peptide family from Szoka and coworkers (10,11) was designed as a consensus sequence to display the key properties of naturally occurring endosomal releasing peptides (EDPs). The GALA repeating sequence contains the glutamic acid carboxylate as a pH sensor, whose average pK_a is set by the local environment of alkyl side chains. GALA peptides of the appropriate length show excellent activity as EDPs, with the desirable pH-dependent properties. While these peptides demonstrate that endosomal disrupting components can significantly increase the efficacy of some carrier systems, they potentially suffer from problems of stability, immunogenicity, and low activity.

Inspired by the principle behind these biological strategies, we have been designing and investigating synthetic polymers that contain similar constituent pH-sensing chemical functionalities as new endosomal releasing components to enhance the intracellular delivery of biomolecules. We have constructed new pH-responsive polymeric carrier systems that incorporate biomolecular drugs and also enhance their delivery to the cytoplasm from the endosomes. These polymeric carrier systems are designed like viruses and pathogenic proteins to have modular components with different functional properties. Ringsdorf first noted the potential of grafted polymers to serve as multifunctional delivery vehicles (12).

The carriers have a targeting element that directs uptake into specific cells, a versatile conjugation or complexation element that allows biomolecules to be incorporated, a pH-responsive component that enhances membrane transport selectively in the low-pH environment of the endosome, and a masking component as necessary to evade uptake by the reticuloendothelial system and optimize circulation stability. An important design element is that the carrier can be built to break down into these individual components in the low-pH environment of the endosome, leaving the membrane-disruptive element to enhance the delivery of the free functional biomolecule into the cytoplasm. In an important sense, then, we are attempting to synthesize modular polymeric carriers that mimic the important elements of viruses and pathogenic organisms.

B. Membrane-Disruptive Properties of pH-Responsive Polymers

It is the pH-responsive polymeric element that represents the most important new component to these carrier systems. Initial work was also inspired by the pioneering work of Tirrell and coworkers, who first described the pH-dependent disruptive properties of poly(ethylacrylic acid) (PEAA) with lipid vesicles (13,14). PEAA destabilizes model lipid bilayers at pHs within the range of endosomal acidification (pH 5.5–6.5). These properties suggested that related polymers could serve as endosomal releasing agents with biological membranes. We thus investigated a larger chemistry space, where the carboxylate group was surrounded by a variety of alkyl groups (Fig. 2). In addition, we also designed copolymers that combined acrylic acid with monomers that contained different alkyl substituents.

The polymers and copolymers were initially screened in a red blood cell hemolysis assay to determine the concentration dependence and pH

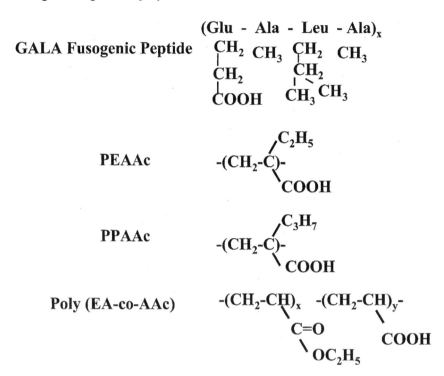

Figure 2 Chemical compositions of pH-responsive biopolymers.

profiles for membrane disruption (Fig. 3) (15). PEAA is inactive at physiological pH and becomes strongly hemolytic with a sharp transition around pH 6.3. PEAA is approximately as active as the membrane-disruptive peptide mellitin in this hemolysis assay. We next looked at poly(propylacrylic acid) (PPAA), which differs from PEAA by the addition of a single methylene unit. PPAA exhibited a surprising increase over PEAA in hemolytic efficiency at low pH, as well as a shift to the membrane-active state at higher pH (Fig. 3). PPAA was more efficient at hemolysis by approximately an order of magnitude in comparison with PEAA (15).

The addition of another methylene unit with poly(butylacrylic acid) shifted the pH profile for membrane disruption even further toward physiological pH. We envision some potential delivery uses for this polymer because it is membrane active at physiological pH, and it can also be activated by ultrasound at concentrations below where it is hemolytic (16). The general shift in the pH profiles is consistent with the trend expected for making the alkyl group longer and more hydrophobic. The concentration

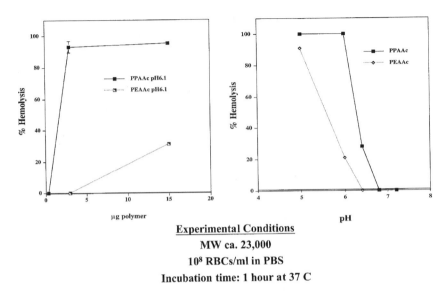

Experimental Conditions
MW ca. 23,000
10^8 RBCs/ml in PBS
Incubation time: 1 hour at 37 C

Figure 3 Model red blood cell disrupting properties of PPAA and PEAA to compare concentration dependencies (left) and pH profiles (right).

dependencies and pH profiles are also dependent on the polymer molecular weight, and it must be noted that these comparisons are for similar molecular weights. In general, the profiles are shifted to higher pH transitions as molecular weight increases, and higher polymer concentrations are required to achieve the same degree of hemolysis as molecular weight decreases.

These results suggested that random 1:1 copolymers of acrylic acid and alkylacrylates, which contain the same carboxylate and related ethyl pendent groups in a different steric and spatial orientations, could also serve as pH-responsive membrane-disrupting agents. Random copolymers of acrylic acid with either ethylacrylate or butylacrylate were synthesized and their membrane disruptive properties assessed in the hemolysis assays. The activities (concentration dependence) of the copolymers were dependent on both the nature of the alkylacrylate monomer and on the relative proportion of the alkylacrylate monomer relative to the acrylic acid monomer. The best of the ethyacrylate and acrylic acid copolymers were nearly as effective at membrane disruption as PEAA, and the copolymer of butylacrylate and acrylic acid at approximately a 50:50 ratio was more effective.

C. Enhancement of Gene Transfection with PPAA

The initial red blood cell membrane disruption studies suggested that PPAA was particularly active and might serve as an endosomal releasing agent. We thus first tested whether PPAAc could enhance gene transfection in a model lipoplex delivery system (Fig. 4). Ternary particles of the cationic lipid DOTAP, the pCMV β-galactosidase reporter plasmid, and PPAA were formulated at a variety of solution charge ratios. In these lipoplexes, the PPAA was designed to serve in analogous fashion to the fusogenic peptides that have previously been incorporated into gene delivery systems. The quantities of β-galactosidase activity were subsequently measured after transfection of NIH 3T3 fibroblast cells, with the ternary lipoplex transfection levels compared to a control of DOTAP/DNA (Fig. 5). The PPAA-containing lipoplexes displayed a significant increase in transfection efficiencies. Transfections with PMAA or PEAA of molecular weights comparable to that of PPAA showed only minimal increase in gene expression compared with PPAA, implying that the added hydrophobicity of PPAA is essential for transfection enhancement.

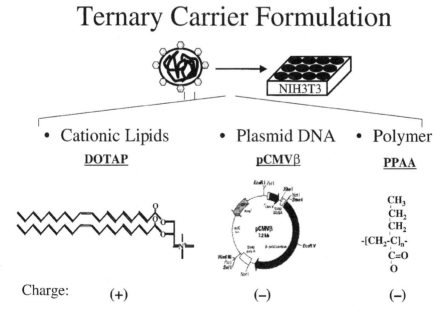

Figure 4 Schematic of experimental gene delivery system for assessing activity of PPAA in NIH 3T3 fibroblast cell culture.

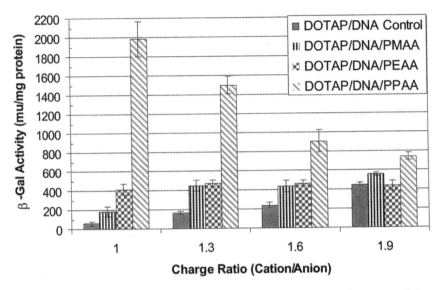

Figure 5 β-Galactosidase transfection levels for ternary complexes containing PMAA, PEAA, and PPAA versus the control binary DOTAP/plasmid alone.

Cationic lipoplexes are often inactivated by interactions with serum proteins (17), and so the ability of PPAA to increase the serum stability of DOTAP/DNA lipoplexes was investigated. The DOTAP/DNA lipoplex was inactivated in media containing as little as 10% fetal bovine serum (FBS), while the DOTAP/DNA/PPAA particles exhibited high levels of transfection throughout the entire range of serum levels tested (Fig. 6). Nearly 70% of the transfection levels were preserved with DOTAP/DNA/PPAA particles at 50% FBS. Histological staining of the fibroblast cells for β-galactosidase activity confirmed the absence of transfection with DOTAP/DNA alone, whereas a significant number of stained cells were evident after transfection with DOTAP/DNA/PPAA (Fig. 6).

These results in cell culture suggested that the PPAA could provide significant transfection enhancements and serum stability for in vivo applications. We have thus carried out initial animal studies using a local delivery scheme in a mouse model of wound healing (Fig. 7). This model is based on previous studies that demonstrated that excisional wound healing is accelerated in thrombospondin-2 (TSP2)–null knockout animals (18). Without TSP2, the excisional wounds exhibit an irregular deposition of extracellular matrix and enhanced vascularization that is associated with significantly accelerated wound healing. These results with the knockout

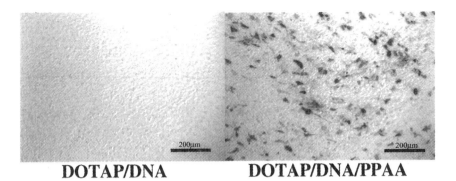

DOTAP/DNA   DOTAP/DNA/PPAA

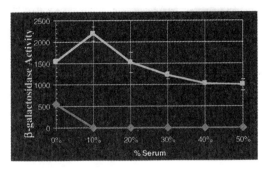

Figure 6 Enhancement of gene transfection by PPAA in the presence of serum. The upper panels represent the staining of adherent NIH 3T3 fibroblast cells for β-galactoside activity in 10% serum using the same ternary complexes of Figure 5. The bottom panel compares the transfection efficiencies of the ternary PPAA complex to the control DOTAP/plasmid in the presence of increasing serum levels.

mouse model suggested that delivery of a plasmid encoding an antisense oligonucleotide to inhibit TSP2 expression could enhance healing in the wild-type mouse (T. R. Kyriakides et al., submitted for publication). In addition, delivery of a plasmid encoding for TSP2 should reverse the TSP2-null phenotype as a built-in control of the delivery and of the mechanism.

The deposition of TSP2 in wild-type mouse wounds was found to be absent during the early inflammatory phase and peaking on day 10, coinciding with the period of maximal vascular regression (19). The DOTAP-DNA-PPAA formulations were thus tested in a protocol where wounds were injected on days 4, 8, and 12, with evaluation of the wounds at day 14. In the TSP2-null mice, the DOTAP-DNA-PPAA formulations resulted in significantly higher TSP2 expression in comparison with DOTAP-DNA controls (Fig. 8).

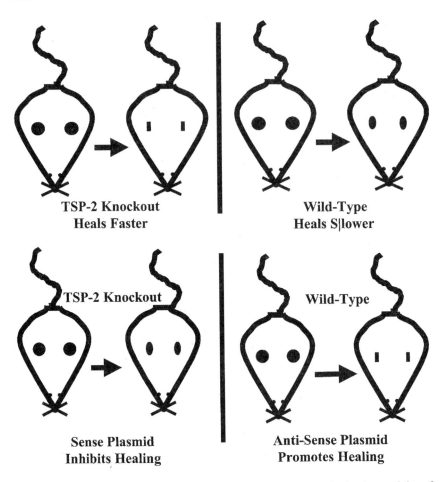

Figure 7 Schematic of the mouse wound model used to test the in vivo activity of PPAA.

In the wild-type mice, the PPAA-containing lipoplexes with the antisense-encoding plasmid resulted in significantly enhanced disorganization of the wound extracellular matrix, resembling that seen with the TSP2-null wound healing process. Immunohistochemical analysis of wound sections for the endothelial cell marker PECAM1 demonstrated that PPAA addition to the lipoplexes also resulted in significantly greater vascularization, again similar to that seen in the TSP2-null wounds. Taken together, the experiments with the knockout and wild-type mice demonstrate that inclusion of PPAA in the lipoplex plasmid formulations greatly enhanced

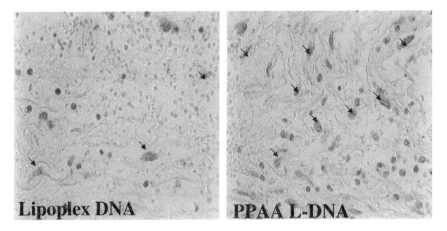

Lipoplex DNA   PPAA L-DNA

Figure 8 Histological analysis of the expression of transfected TSP-2 in the TSP-2 knockout mouse model. Significant increases in the level of TSP-2 were observed in wounds treated with the PPAA-containing lipoplexes.

transfection and resulted in the localized modulation of the wound healing response.

D. Intracellular Delivery of Proteins with pH-Responsive Polymers

There are many other biomolecular therapeutics in development that require intracellular delivery. In particular, the delivery of proteins to the cytoplasmic compartment represents a significant barrier for the development of many protein therapeutics and vaccines. Thus, we have investigated whether PPAA could also enhance the delivery of proteins to the cytoplasm (C. Lackey et al., manuscript submitted). The immunotoxins represent a good model therapeutic system where drug action requires translocation from vesicular compartments to the cytoplasm. In initial studies, we have asked the question whether PPAA can enhance the cytoplasmic delivery of an immunoconjugate that utilizes a targeting antibody previously used in immunotoxin studies. The monoclonal antibody (MoAb) 64.1 is an anti-CD3 antibody that has been extensively characterized as a T-cell lymphoma targeting agent (20). MoAb 64.1 is rapidly localized to the lysosome after receptor-mediated endocytosis (21) and thus serves as an excellent model for endosomal release (Fig. 9).

Moab 64.1 was biotinylated and complexed with streptavidin, along with a biotinylated PPAA oligomer (Fig. 10). The PPAA did not alter the

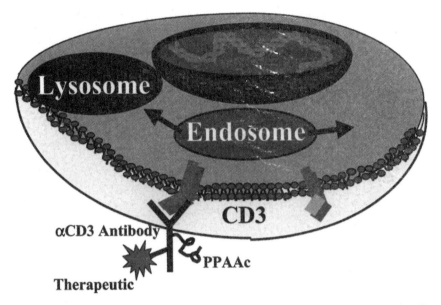

Figure 9 Schematic illustration of the anti-CD3 delivery system for the Jurkat T-cell lymphoma model that tests the ability of PPAA to enhance the cytoplasmic delivery of the antibody-targeted immunoconjugate.

uptake of the MoAb 64.1–streptavidin complex into the Jurkat T-cell lymphoma cell line, as demonstrated by fluorescence-activated cell sorting (FACS) analysis. The trafficking fates of the antibody–streptavidin

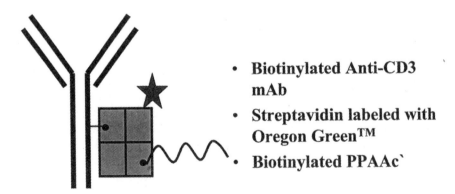

- **Biotinylated Anti-CD3 mAb**
- **Streptavidin labeled with Oregon Green™**
- **Biotinylated PPAAc**

Figure 10 Schematic model of the antibody-streptavidin-PPAA bioconjugate that was used to test the activity of PPAA in enhancing the endosomal release of therapeutic antibodies.

complexes were initially characterized by laser scanning confocal micro-scopy using fluorescein-labeled streptavidin. Without the PPAA, the antibody–streptavidin complex was localized in vesicular compartments (e.g., endosome/lysosome) as shown by the punctate fluorescence emission patterns (Fig. 11). In contrast, a broadly diffuse fluorescence emission was observed after 4-h incubation of the Jurkat cells with the PPAA-containing complexes. This diffuse fluorescence indicates that the polymer is aiding escape of the streptavidin to the cytoplasm. Because the nucleus becomes visible as a darkened region after the appearance of the diffuse cytoplasmic fluorescence, it is likely the fluorophore is still attached to streptavidin (which does not diffuse to the nucleus).

More direct confirmation of the endosomal releasing activity of PPAA was obtained by Western blotting analysis after Jurkat cell fractionation. An anti-MoAb 64.1 was used to assay for the presence of the intact MoAb 64.1 in total-cell homogenates as opposed to isolated cytoplasmic fractions (Fig. 12). Without PPAA, there was no detectable amount of the antibody released into the cytoplasm in the absence of the polymer, but it was clearly taken up into the cells as evidenced by the intact antibody band in the total cell homogenate. However, when PPAA was added to the MoAb 64.1–

with PPAAc-biotin   without PPAAc

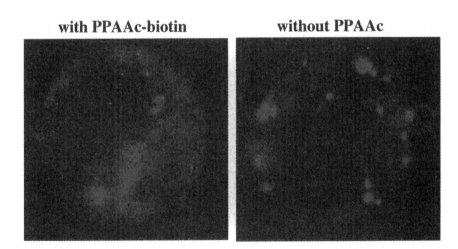

Figure 11 Confocal microscopy analysis of intracellular localization of the antibody–streptavidin bioconjugates. The panel on the left shows the diffuse, cytoplasmic staining of the fluorescently labeled streptavidin when PPAA is complexed (note the dark appearance of the cell nucleus that becomes visible as the cytoplasm is illuminated). The panel on the right shows the punctate distribution typical of endosomal/lysosomal localization when PPAA is absent.

Whole Cell Cytosol Whole Cell Cytosol Whole Cell Cytosol

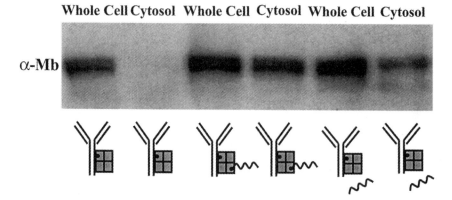

α-Mb

Figure 12 Western blot analysis of the cytoplasmic subcellular fractions using anti-antibody detection of the targeting monoclonal antibody (4-h timepoint). The first two panels show that the antibody is not released to the cytoplasm in significant levels without PPAA, but is released when PPAA is complexed (middle two panels) and to a lesser extent when PPAA is added in trans (right two panels).

streptavidin complex, the cytoplasmic band displayed 73% of the staining intensity of the crude homogenate band. The free PPAA (nonbiotinylated) also displayed significant activity when physically mixed with the MoAb 64.1–streptavidin complex, with 29% of the total intracellular staining intensity observed in the cytoplasmic fraction. The Western blotting analysis also verifies that the protein detected in the cytoplasm has not been degraded, as the molecular weight of the cytoplasmic band is identical to that detected in the crude homogenate. These results suggest that EDPs could be applicable to a wide range of protein/peptide intracellular delivery needs, including both direct therapeutics and vaccine development.

E.   Encrypted pH-Responsive Polymeric Carriers for Bimolecular Therapeutics

The interesting properties of the polymers described above suggested that other designs could also incorporate pH-responsive elements that provide membrane-disruptive capabilities in the endosome. We have thus developed a new class of polymers that incorporate a membrane disruptive backbone that is masked by grafted hydrophilic oligomers, such as polyethylene glycol (PEG) (Fig. 13). These hydrophilic oligomers are grafted through a pH-degradable linkage that can degrade in the low-pH environment of the endosome to release the active backbone. In addition, there are several

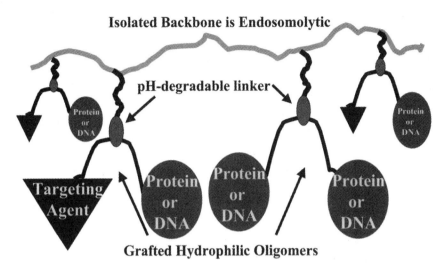

Figure 13 Schematic illustration of the "encrypted" polymers that carry biomolecular therapeutics and cell targeting molecules via pH-degradable bonds. The backbone is membrane disruptive when unmasked by the hydrolysis of PEGylated grafts, which releases the therapeutics to the cytosol.

linkage routes to incorporating targeting agents and biomolecular drugs such as oligonucleotides and proteins/peptides that are also released as free therapeutics (or PEGylated therapeutics).

These polymers are thus designed as self-contained carriers that incorporate the primary functionalities of viruses and toxins: targeting agents that direct receptor-mediated endocytosis, a pH-responsive element that selectively disrupts the endosomal membrane, and the biomolecular component which is delivered as a free and active agent into the cytoplasm. We have termed these polymers "encrypted" by analogy to encrypted domains in biological proteins. Active domains of several extracellular and matricellular proteins are initially masked but become exposed and activated by proteolytic processing at controlled timepoints (22). Similarly, the encrypted polymers contain a masked membrane-disruptive element that is activated in the low-pH environment of the endosome.

The first example of an encrypted polymer is the terpolymer of dimethylaminoethyl methacrylate (DMAEMA), butyl methacrylate (BMA), and styrene benzaldehyde (Fig. 14). This backbone was chosen as a membrane-disruptive element on the basis of our previous work with copolymers discussed in the prior sections. The PEG grafts were attached to this backbone through acid-degradable acetal linkers. The acetal linkages

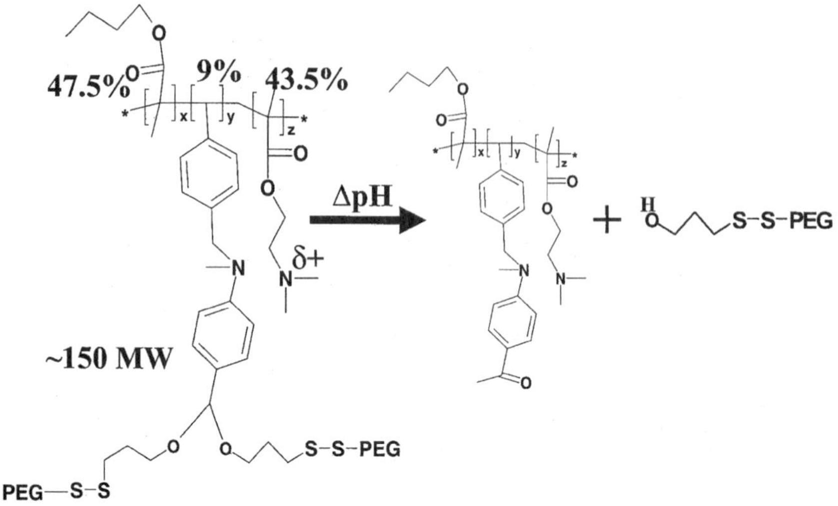

Figure 14 Chemical composition of the encrypted polymer.

degrade at rates that are proportional to the hydronium ion concentration and therefore will hydrolyze 250 times faster at pH 5.0 than at pH 7.4. The rate constants can also be controlled over a wide range of time scales to optimize the degradation properties for specific delivery requirements (23). The PEG grafts were chosen on the basis of their well-characterized biocompatibility as well as their ability to improve stability and biodistribution properties by minimizing clearance.

The hydrolysis of PEG grafts from the terpolymer shown in Fig. 15 exhibited a half-life of 15 min at pH 5.4, with only 38% of the PEG grafts hydrolyzed after 12 h at pH 7.4 (Fig. 15). These kinetics match the general time frame for trafficking of internalized biomolecules to the lysosome. The hydrolysis properties matched the hemolysis properties, with about 1 μg/mL of this polymer achieving 100% hemolysis of 10^8 red blood cells after a 20-min. incubation at pH 5.0 (Fig. 16). No hemolysis was observed after incubation at pH 7.4. As a first cultured cell system for testing the general carrier capabilities, we investigated whether the encrypted polymer could enhance the cytoplasmic delivery of oligonucleotides to hepatocytes (Fig. 17). The polymer incorporated lactose for targeting of the asialoglycoprotein receptor, which is known to rapidly direct lysosomal localization, and thus represents a tough model system to ask whether our polymer can escape this trafficking fate.

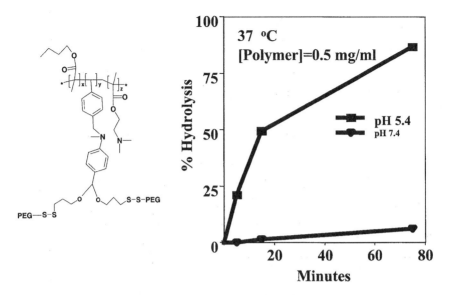

Figure 15 Hydrolysis of the PEG grafts from the encrypted polymer as a function of pH.

Hexalysine was linked to approximately 20% of the PEG grafts, which then was used to physically complex the rhodamine-labeled oligonucleotides. After a 3-h incubation of this carrier with hepatocytes, a striking localization of the rhodamine fluorescence was observed in the cell nuclei (Fig. 18). In contrast, hepatocytes incubated with the oligonucleotides alone exhibited a punctate vesicular localization. These results demonstrate that the encrypted polymer enhances escape of lysosomal trafficking, resulting in cytoplasmic delivery of the oligonucleotides (where they can subsequently diffuse rapidly to the nucleus). These results suggest that they could provide a direct route to enhancing antisense ODN therapeutic delivery. They are also well suited to carry peptides and proteins for vaccine delivery, through the versatile linkage chemistries available with this platform design.

III. SMART POLYMER–PROTEIN CONJUGATES

A hallmark of biological regulation is the allosteric modulation of protein activity. The binding or catalytic activities of many proteins can be modulated by the binding of regulatory molecules that are cooperatively

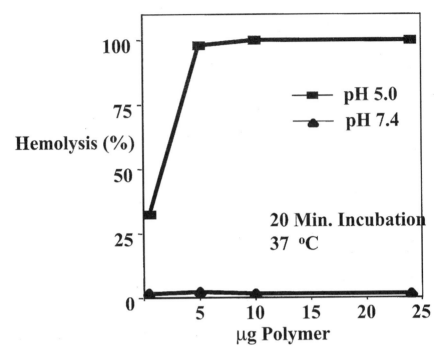

Figure 16 Hemolytic activities of the encrypted polymers before and after hydrolysis of the PEG grafts.

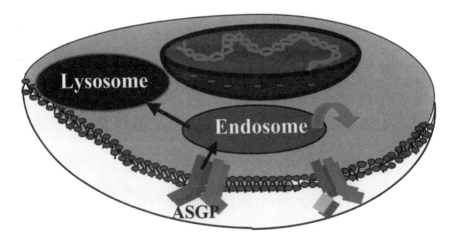

Figure 17 Schematic of the hepatocyte delivery model system with targeting of the asialoglycoprotein (ASGP) receptor using conjugated galactose.

ODN ionically-complexed
with encrypted polymer

Control:
ODN only

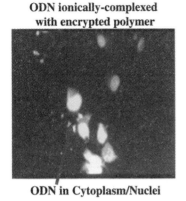

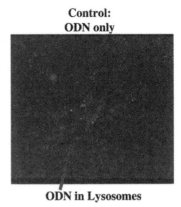

ODN in Cytoplasm/Nuclei

ODN in Lysosomes

Figure 18 Fluorescence microscopy analysis of the intracellular localization of rhodamine-labeled oligonucleotides that were electrostatically complexed with the encrypted polymers and targeted with galactose. The panel on the right shows that the encrypted polymers enhanced the cytoplasmic delivery of the oligonucleotides as they have diffused into the nucleus, while the control oligonucleotides are taken up into punctate endosomes/lysosomes.

coupled to the active site of primary function. While these energetic couplings provide a mechanistic paradigm for regulating protein activities in the device environment, they do not usually provide a direct route to controlling activity. More standard routes involve altering protein molecular recognition properties through changes in environmental conditions, such as pH, ionic strength, or temperature. For example, in affinity separations, low pH is often used to release target antigens from immobilized antibodies. These environmental changes may affect protein structure, alter the magnitude of electrostatic interaction energies, lower the activation barrier to dissociation of capture protein and target, and/or alter the catalytic barriers to control enzyme kinetics.

For many affinity separation, diagnostic, biosensor, biochip, and bioprocessing technologies that utilize biomolecular recognition properties, there is a continuing need for better control routes. Many of the current environmental methods are relatively harsh and can lead to damage of biomolecules and cells. In addition, the environmental signals are typically large, general solution changes and thus not targeted to selective recognition components. We have thus been investigating a new approach to reversibly controlling protein recognition properties that is more selective, like allosteric regulation, and relies on small changes in environmental conditions or signals. This approach utilizes "smart" polymers that

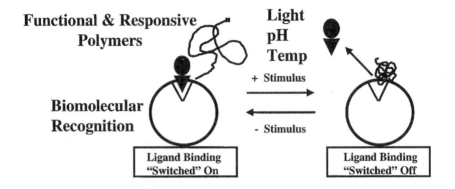

Functional & Responsive Polymers

Light
pH
Temp
+ Stimulus

Biomolecular Recognition

- Stimulus

| Ligand Binding "Switched" On | | Ligand Binding "Switched" Off |

Smart Switches Could Control:
Target Capture and Release
Enzyme Activity/Substrate Selectivity
Nanopatterning in Array Technologies
Controlled Release of Therapeutics

Figure 19 Schematic illustration of the smart polymer–protein conjugate concept that utilizes the environmentally responsive properties of the polymer as a switch to regulate protein activity.

reversibly change their physical properties in response to small and controllable changes in pH, temperature, and light (Fig. 19).

These smart polymers reversibly cycle between an extended and hydrophilic random coil, and a collapsed, hydrophobic state that is reduced in average volume by about threefold (24). We attach the smart polymers at defined protein side chains, typically by genetically engineering cysteine or lysine residues, at a controlled distance from the protein active site (Fig. 20). The polymers serve as environmental sensors and differentially control access of ligands or substrates to binding or catalytic sites as a function of their expanded or collapsed states. The collapse of the smart polymers can also result in allosteric regulation of ligand affinity. This general approach targets mild environmental signals to specific polymer–protein conjugates, thus, for example, allowing differential control of different antibodies in a device by using conjugated polymers that are sensitive to different signals (e.g., antibody 1 with pH, antibody 2 with temperature, antibody 3 with light).

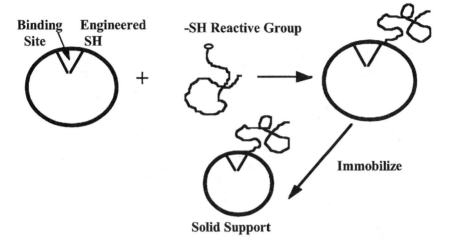

Figure 20 Schematic of the conjugation strategy to attach the stimuli-responsive polymer to a specific site on the target recognition protein.

A. "Smart" Temperature-Responsive Polymer–Protein Affinity Switches

We have utilized streptavidin as our primary model system for developing environmentally responsive polymer–protein conjugates. In addition to its broad technological relevance, the high-resolution structural database for streptavidin has facilitated the design of conjugates and the interpretation of their activities. One of the most striking structural elements connected to biotin binding is the flexible binding loop (Fig. 21). This loop is open and in a disordered conformation in the absence of biotin, but it closes and a hinge side chain forms a hydrogen bond to biotin in the biotin-bound state (25,26). This loop can be viewed as a swinging door that is open in the ligand-free state to allow biotin association and closes upon ligand binding. We thus chose to first conjugate the temperature-responsive poly(N-isopropylacrylamide) (pNIPAAm) onto this loop, with the goal of controlling the opening and closing of the door differentially with the extended versus collapsed states of the polymer (27).

The pNIPAAm was first synthesized to have a single thiol-reactive endgroup, in conjunction with the genetic engineering of streptavidin to substitute a cysteine side at amino acid position for asparagine (N49C) on the binding loop. Streptavidin is a tetramer of four identical subunits, each contributing one biotin-binding pocket. The stoichiometry of the conjuga-

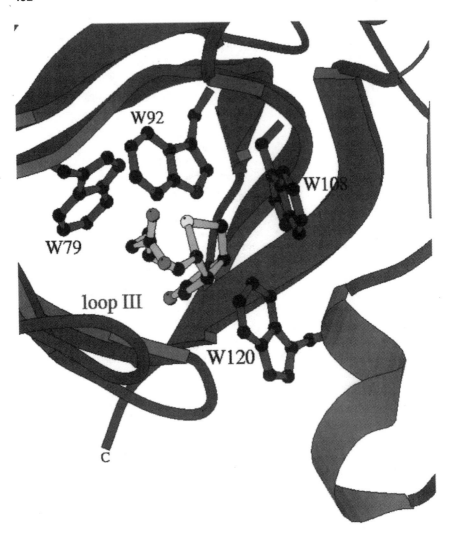

Figure 21 Molecular model of the streptavidin binding site that shows the spatial relationships of the important tryptophan contacts to biotin.

tion was thus controlled to a maximum of one polymer chain per subunit at the prescribed cysteine position on the binding loop (streptavidin does not contain cysteine in the native sequence). The pNIPAAm–streptavidin conjugate was immobilized and a radiolabeled-biotin used to characterize the binding activity as a function of temperature. The binding activity of the conjugate was identical to wild-type and N49C streptavidin controls when the pNIPAAm was in its extended state at 4°C. When the temperature was raised above the lower critical solution temperature (LCST) of the free pNIPAAm at 37°C, the conjugate displayed an 84% blocking of biotin association. The temperature dependence of biotin gating follows the behavior of that polymer, with a similar midpoint. This correlation demonstrates that it is indeed the physical state of the polymer that leads to molecular switching.

The pNIPAAm conjugation at position 49 served as an efficient gate of biotin association, but if biotin was prebound, the polymer collapse did not lead to ligand dissociation. The molecular switching capabilities will depend on parameters such as the polymer's composition and attachment site, the magnitude of the conformational and physical change, and the size of the ligands or substrates. We therefore designed a second conjugation at a solvent-accessible site near an important biotin binding contact residue at position 120 (Fig. 21). Site-directed mutagenesis studies had demonstrated that Trp120 plays a particularly important energetic role in biotin affinity (28). We thus chose position Glu116 to introduce a new cysteine (E116C) that lies at the nearest solvent-accessible position relative to Trp120. In addition, to increase the steric alterations induced by the polymer, a pNIPAAm derivative that had pendant reactive groups at positions along the backbone was designed to increase the number of subunits which were conjugated to single oligomers (29).

This conjugate displays reversible binding and release of biotin when the temperature is cycled below and above the LCST. The conjugate binds biotin at 4°C where the polymer is hydrated and releases a significant fraction of bound biotin at 37°C where the polymer is collapsed (Fig. 22). With combined temperature cycling and washing at 37°C, all of the bound biotin can be released. The precise mechanism by which the polymer phase change leads to a change in biotin affinity and dissociation rate is very difficult to determine experimentally. The most likely mechanism involves a coupling between the steric conformation of the Trp120 loop and the physical change of the polymer. It is known from mutagenesis studies that relatively small changes in the Trp120 side chain can result in large changes in the biotin off-rate, so that it is reasonable that the changes induced by the collapse of the hydrophobic pNIPAAm could result in an unfavorable steric alteration at Trp120. The pendant polymer may also attach at more than one position, which likely plays an important role in transmitting steric alterations to the protein. Other recent experiments with a different thermally responsive polymer have demonstrated that conjugation away from the binding pocket does not lead to switching activity (30). These composite results have demonstrated that both the choice of conjugation

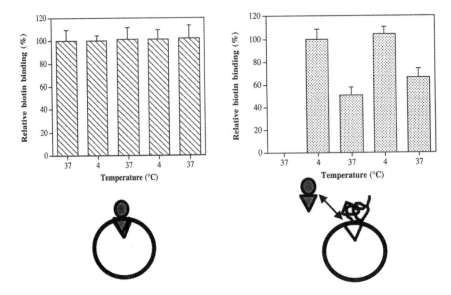

Figure 22   The biotin-releasing activity of the E116C streptavidin–pNIPAAm conjugate. The temperature-independent binding of biotin to the control E116C streptavidin is shown on the left panel, with the temperature-dependent switching activity of the polymer–protein conjugate on the right panel.

site and the type of polymer are very important in determining the molecular switching properties.

B.   "Smart" pH-Responsive Polymer-Protein Affinity Switches

A second important environmental signal in current technologies that rely on modulation of protein recognition is pH. Changes in pH can alter molecular electrostatic and hydrogen bonding interaction energies, but the disruption of biomolecular complexes often requires extreme changes in pH that can lead to an unwanted protein denaturation. We were thus interested in developing pH-responsive polymer–protein conjugates that again utilize the polymer to sense a mild change in pH and respond by modulating protein activity.

Smart polymers have been developed that display pH sensitivity over relatively narrow ranges around physiological pH that would not lead to protein destabilization. A series of NIPAAm and acrylic acid (AAc) copolymers were synthesized and characterized with regard to their joint temperature and pH responsiveness (31). At the isothermal temperature of 37°C, a copolymer with 5.5 mol % AAc content reversibly cycled between a water soluble state at pH 7.4 and an insoluble state at pH 4.0. This polymer had appropriate properties for serving as a pH-responsive switch at 37°C, and a vinyl sulfone endgroup was linked to one end to provide a thiol-reactive derivative. A different type of pH-responsive switch that relies on chemical modification of a binding site side chain has also been developed by Wilchek and coworkers (32).

This polymer was conjugated to the E116C streptavidin mutant, and the biotin blocking and release properties of the conjugate were characterized. The conjugate exhibited a strong dependence of biotin blocking and release on pH at 37°C, whereas neither wild-type streptavidin or the unconjugated E116C mutant controls exhibited any change in bound biotin when the pH is cycled between pH 4.0 and 7.4 at 37°C (Fig. 23). The pH profile for blocking of biotin association was distinct from the pH profile for biotin release, indicating that there are interesting mechanistic differences between the blocking effect and the release effect. The blocking efficiency increased between pH 6 and pH 4, whereas the release effect was

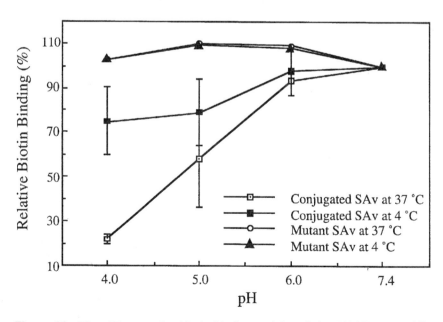

Figure 23 The pH-responsive biotin binding activity of the E116C streptavidin bioconjugate.

largely maximized by pH 6, and did not increase substantially between pH 6 and pH 4.

There was also a lesser but real pH-dependent switching activity at 4°C, indicating that at these lower temperatures the copolymer exhibits a smaller pH-dependent change in physical state. The copolymer will be most collapsed at the lowest pH (4.0) and highest temperature (37°C), and most expanded and hydrated at the highest pH (7.4) and lowest temperature (4°C). Repulsion of the ionized carboxyl groups at pH 7.4 promotes the expansion of the polymer beyond a random coil. Because NIPAAm is the major component of the copolymer, the conformation is likely more sensitive to temperature than to pH, leading to more condensed conformations at any particular pH and 37°C compared with the same pH and 4°C.

There are several reasons for combining both pH and temperature sensitivity in the copolymer characterized here. First, the phase transition behavior of these copolymers can be controlled by more than one environmental variable, thus increasing the opportunities for designing polymer compositions with temperature, pH, and ionic strength responses that meet the requirements for a particular application. Second, there is a potential cooperative effect of (lowered) pH and (raised) temperature on the phase transition of these copolymers due to H bonding between the AAc and NIPAAm components. This mutual influence can be used to design polymer systems with pH-controlled temperature sensitivity and/or with temperature-controlled pH sensitivity.

C. "Smart" Light-Responsive Polymer–Protein Affinity Switches

For device development, the use of light to control biomolecular recognition processes could offer significant new advantages. We have thus also designed photoresponsive polymer–protein conjugates to provide a general approach to the development of photo-switchable proteins, whose functions are reversibly controlled by external light signals. We have recently described two types of stimuli-responsive polymers that display joint temperature and photoresponsiveness (Shimoboji et al., manuscript submitted). These polymers are N,N-dimethylacrylamide (DMA)-co-4-phenylazophenylacrylate ("AZAA") copolymer (DMAA) (MW. 18 kDa; AZAA; 5.9 mol %) and DMA-co-N-4-phenylazophenylacrylamide (AZAAm) copolymer (DMAAm) (MW. 10 kDa; AZAAm; 9.6 mol %) (Fig. 24). The photoresponsiveness of both polymers depends on temperature, and similarly the temperature-responsive properties depend on whether the diazo chromophore is in the cis or trans state. The maximal difference in the degree of precipitation for each polymer under UV versus

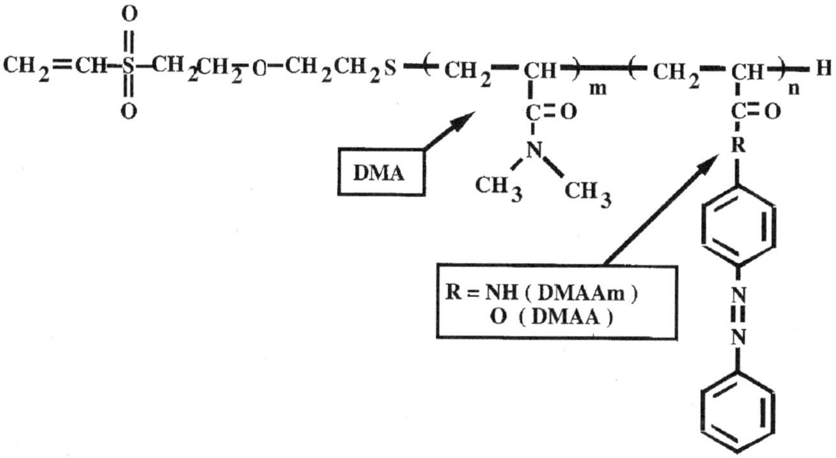

$$CH_2=CH-\overset{\overset{\displaystyle O}{\|}}{\underset{\underset{\displaystyle O}{\|}}{S}}-CH_2CH_2-O-CH_2CH_2S-\left(CH_2-CH\right)_m\left(CH_2-CH\right)_n H$$

DMA

$$\underset{CH_3}{\overset{C=O}{\underset{\diagdown}{\overset{|}{N}}}}\underset{CH_3}{\diagup}$$

$$\overset{C=O}{\underset{R}{|}}$$

R = NH (Dmaam)
O (DMAA)

Figure 24 The chemical structure of the photoresponsive copolymer of DMA and the diazobenzene-containing monomers.

visible illumination occurs at slightly greater than 40°C, and the two polymers displayed opposite photoresponses to UV and visible irradiation (Fig. 25).

The polymers were each synthesized with a vinylsulfone terminus for site-specific end-conjugation to the E116C SA. The biotin binding properties of the E116C conjugates were determined under UV versus visible illumination at 40°C where the difference in physical polymer states was approximately maximal (Fig. 26). The SA-DMAA conjugate exhibited a 47% greater blocking and releasing activity under visible irradiation, while the SA-DMAAm conjugate showed a 38% greater effect effect on blocking and release under UV irradiation. The photo-switching of biotin recognition thus follows the different photoresponsiveness of the polymers, which collapse and expand differentially under UV/visible photocycling. Neither SA alone, physical mixtures of SA and the polymers, or a conjugate of the azobenzene monomer with SA displayed any blocking or releasing photoresponsiveness.

These results demonstrate that photoresponsive polymers can regulate the association of biotin as a function of their physical state. The DMAA and DMAAm polymers display opposite collapse and expansion properties in response to UV versus visible irradiation, and these polymer properties are mirrored in the switching activities of the streptavidin conjugates. The release of bound biotin proceeds at a similar off-rate as free streptavidin at

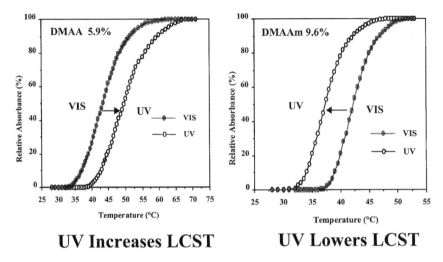

UV Increases LCST   UV Lowers LCST

Figure 25 The relationship between temperature and the photoresponse of the DMAA and DMAAM polymers, showing the opposite directions of the LCST shift under UV illumination.

this temperature, and thus the dissociation must be tied to the inability of released biotin to rebind with the polymer in the collapsed state. The diazo monomers are not capable of modulating the access of biotin to the pocket

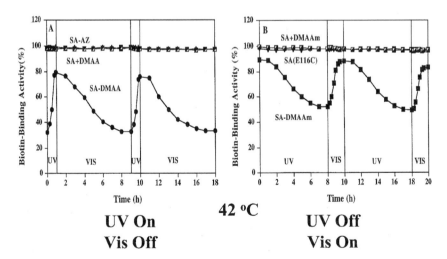

                                        42 °C
UV On   UV Off
Vis Off   Vis On

Figure 26 The opposite photoresponsive properties of the DMAA– and DMAAM–streptavidin bioconjugates.

when conjugated to E116C SA, consistent with the need for the larger polymer to achieve this steric blocking mechanism.

D. "Smart" Molecular Shields for Size-Selective Control of Ligand Binding

In the previous examples, the stimuli-responsive polymers controlled the binding of biotin at the same streptavidin subunit and binding pocket where it was conjugated. The polymer switches allowed the binding of the small ligand biotin in the expanded state but blocked and/or released biotin when in the collapsed state. We recently discovered that the stimuli-responsive polymers block the access of larger biotinylated proteins in either the expanded or collapsed state at the binding pocket where they are conjugated (33). This discovery opened the interesting opportunity to develop the concept of smart "molecular shields," where the polymer is conjugated at a greater (but still defined) distance from a protein recognition pocket. In the expanded state, the hydrated polymer occupies sufficient volume to block the recognition site, but when it is collapsed back to the more distant site of conjugation, the recognition pocket is unmasked and opened to binding of the target macromolecule.

The streptavidin tetramer displays approximate C_{222} symmetry that gives rise to two distinct biotin binding faces, with each binding face presenting two biotin-binding pockets that are separated by approximately $20\,\text{Å}$. One binding face exposes two binding pockets when streptavidin is immobilized, and we have found that only one stimuli-responsive polymer can be conjugated per binding face due to steric constraints (although the conjugation of an additional very small molecular weight oligomer to the second binding pocket cannot be ruled out). Because the polymer blocks the binding of biotinylated proteins in either the collapsed or expanded states at the pocket where it is conjugated, each binding face has a maximal potential to bind one biotinylated protein at the unconjugated pocket that is about $20\,\text{Å}$ distant. However, if the conjugated polymer has sufficient volume to sterically block this nearby pocket, then the biotinylated protein will be unable to associate with streptavidin. Depending on the size of the polymer and the target biotinylated protein, both the expanded and collapsed states could block association, or the expanded state could block while the collapsed state unblocked, or both the expanded and collapsed states could be too small to block the access of smaller biotinylated proteins.

The potential for developing these molecular shields was first discovered by characterizing the binding of biotinylated bovine serum albumin (BSA) to a smart polymer–streptavidin conjugate. The polymer designed for this purpose was PDEAAm, which displays nearly identical

LCST behavior to the previously described PNIPAAm but which can be synthesized with significantly more narrow polydispersity by group transfer polymerization. A new streptavidin mutant was also constructed, with two very solvent-accessible positions at amino acid Glu51 and Asn118 chosen to introduce lysine residues. This E51K/N118K streptavidin mutant was designed to enhance conjugation efficiency by placing reactive primary amine groups on the exposed binding face of streptavidin. Radiolabeled biotin binding experiments demonstrated that only polymer could be conjugated per streptavidin binding face (i.e., per two subunits/binding pockets).

The PDEAAm-streptavidin conjugate (average PDEAAm M of 12.8 kDa) displayed low levels of biotinylated BSA binding below the LCST of PDEAAm, but as the temperature was increased through the phase transition temperature of the polymer, the conjugate was unmasked and biotinylated BSA could bind. The correlation between the unmasking of the approximately 20 Å distant binding pocket and the phase transition of the PDEAAm is shown in Fig. 27. This result suggested that the expanded

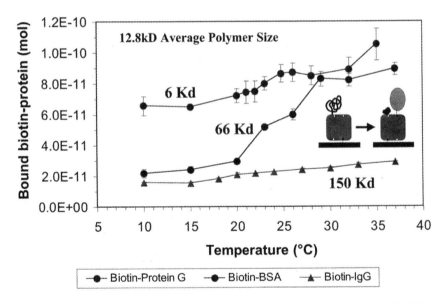

Figure 27 Dependence of the molecular shield activity on target protein size. The smaller protein G binds relatively well at all temperatures, the larger IgG antibody is largely blocked at all temperatures, and the mid-sized BSA shows a strong temperature dependence that correlates with the LCST transition of the PDEAAm.

polymer was of sufficient size to block BSA association, but that the collapsed polymer was small and distant enough to unmask the binding site for BSA association.

To test the dependence of this shielding activity on target size, the smaller biotinylated protein G (MW 6.2 kDa) and larger biotinylated IgG antibody (MW 150 kDa) were characterized. The ability of the 12.8-kDa PDEAAm polymer to shield the 20-Å distant pocket was found to be strongly dependent on the size of the biotinylated protein target. Protein G binds efficiently both above and below the LCST of PDEAAm, and thus is small enough to access the nearby binding pocket when PDEAAm is in either the expanded or collapsed state (Fig. 27). Conversely, the biotinylated IgG was large enough to be blocked from accessing the binding pocket when the PDEAAm was in either the expanded or collapsed state, so that IgG binding was low over the entire temperature range. These results are summarized in Fig. 28.

To further confirm this steric shielding mechanism, we synthesized PDEAAm oligomers that were biotinylated at one end. The biotinylated PDEAAm (average MW 12.8 kDa) was then complexed directly at one biotin-binding pocket, and steric constraints limited the stoichiometry to

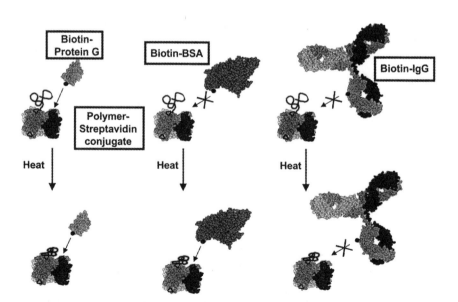

Figure 28 Molecular models illustrating the proposed mechanism of the molecular shielding activity.

one polymer per immobilized streptavidin tetramer. The temperature-dependent binding of BSA, protein G, and IgG to this PDEAAm–streptavidin complex (polymer again at about 20 Å from the nearby unoccupied binding site) was very similar to the covalent PDEAAm–streptavidin conjugates. The BSA showed a temperature dependence that closely followed the phase transition behavior of PDEAAm, whereas the protein G bound well and the IgG poorly at all temperatures.

The dependence of the shielding activity on the size of the biotinylated target proteins suggested that different polymer sizes could also be used to control the size selectivity of the shields. PDEAAm oligomers were thus synthesized with smaller average molecular weights and covalently coupled to streptavidin. At 10°C below the LCST of the PDEAAm, the quantity of bound biotinylated BSA increases as the PDEAAm MW decreases (Fig. 29). This finding supports the steric hindrance mechanism for shielding because smaller polymer chains allow greater access of the target biotinylated proteins. It also suggests that the polymer size could be selected to allow the binding of a certain size range of target proteins while blocking larger target proteins above the size cutoff. Proof of this concept was achieved by measuring the ability of the 12.8-kDa PDEAAm–streptavidin conjugates to

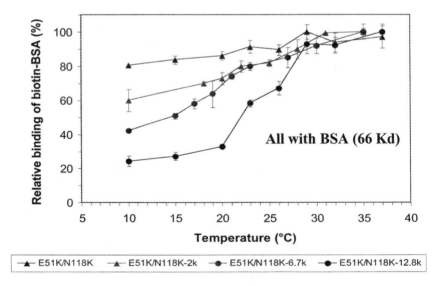

Figure 29   The dependence of molecular shielding of BSA as a function of polymer molecular weight. As the polymer molecular weight is decreased, the binding of BSA becomes higher, supporting a steric blocking mechanism.

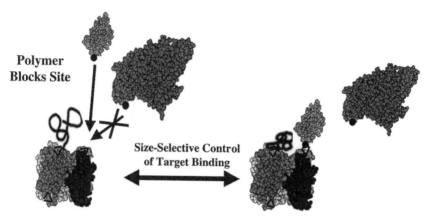

Figure 30 Schematic molecular model showing that the polymer molecular weight can be chosen to control protein access in a mixture on the basis of size.

discriminate between biotinylated protein G and biotinylated BSA together in solution (Fig. 30). Protein G was found to associate at the same quantity measured when it was the only protein in solution, whereas the association of biotinylated BSA was blocked. The PDEAAm shields can thus be used to discriminate access to protein-binding pockets on the basis of size.

The concept of the smart molecular shield should in principle be applicable to any protein active site and is complementary to the smart switches that control binding directly at the active site (Fig. 31). The responsive polymer must be conjugated at an appropriate distance from the ligand binding site so that its collapse unmasks the site to target ligands of a defined size range. The specificity and selectivity of these molecular shields should be controllable by matching the sizes of the polymer to those of the targets, and the polymers can be designed to be pH or light responsive in addition to temperature (as shown above). We envision applications in affinity separations and diagnostics through control of capture and release steps. The shields should also be applicable to enzyme bioprocesses, where the control of polymer coil size near the active site in response to temperature, pH, or light signals could favor the enzymatic transformation of smaller substrates, due to "gating" (shielding) of large substrates. Finally, the shielding and unshielding of recognition sites on surfaces with the responsive polymers through spatially defined light signals could provide new "read/write" avenues for biomolecular array technologies.

Smart Molecular Switches   Smart Molecular Shields

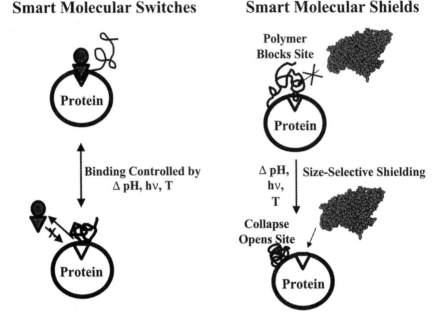

Figure 31 Schematic illustrating the use of stimuli-responsive polymers as molecular switches and shields.

ACKNOWLEDGMENTS

This work was supported by research grants from the NIH (NIGMS Grant No. R01-GM53771 to ASH and PSS, R01-CA55596 to OP), NSF (EEC-9529161), the NSF IGERT program DGE-9987620 (Graduate Fellowship to CL and NM), the Office of Technology Transfer at University of Washington, the Washington Technology Center, and the Washington Research Foundation.

REFERENCES

1. J Zabner, AJ Fasbender, T Moninger, KA Poellinger, MJ Welsh. Cellular and molecular barriers to gene transfer by a cationic lipid. J Biol Chem 270:18997–19007, 1991.
2. OW Press, PJ Martin, PE Thorpe, ES Vitetta. Ricin A-chain containing immunotoxins directed against different epitopes on the CD2 molecule differ in their ability to kill normal and malignant T cells. J Immunol 141:4410–4417, 1988.

3. S Mukherjee, RN Ghosh, FR Maxfield. Endocytosis. Physiol Rev 77:759–803, 1997.

4. DC Wiley, JJ Skehel. The structure and function of the hemagglutinin membrane glycoprotein of influenza virus. Annu Rev Biochem 56:365–394, 1983.

5. FM Hughson. Structural characterization of viral fusion proteins. Curr Biol 5:265–274, 1995.

6. J Ren, JC Sharpe, RJ Collier, F London. Membrane translocation of Charged Residues at the Tips of Hydrophobic Helices in the T Domain of Diphtheria Toxin. Biochem. 38:976–984.

7. E Wagner, C Plank, K Zatloukal, M Cotten, ML Birnstiel. Influenza virus hemagglutinin HA-2 N-terminal fusogenic peptides augment gene transfer by transferrin-polylysine-DNA complexes: toward a synthetic virus-like gene-transfer vehicle. Proc Natl Acad Sci USA 89:7934–7938, 1992.

8. C Plank, B Oberhauser, K Mechtler, C Koch, E Wagner. The influence of endosome-disruptive peptides on gene transfer using synthetic virus-like gene transfer systems. J Biol Chem 269:12918–12924, 1994.

9. VV Tolstikov, R Cole, H Fang, SH Pincus. Influence of endosome-destabilizing peptides on efficacy of anti-HIV immunotoxins. Bioconj Chem 8:38–43, 1997.

10. NK Subbarao, RA Parente, FCJ Szoka, L Nadasdi, K Pongracz. pH-Dependent bilayer destabilization by an amphipathic peptide. Biochemistry 26:2964–2972, 1987.

11. RA Parente, S Nir, FCJ Szoka. pH-dependent fusion of phosphatidylcholine small vesicles. J Biol Chem 263:4724–4730, 1988.

12. H Ringsdorf. J Polym Sci Symp 51:135, 1985.

13. JL Thomas, DA Tirrell. Polyelectrolyte-sensitized phospholipid vesicles. Acc Chem Res 25:336–342, 1992.

14. JL Thomas, SW Barton, DA Tirrell. Membrane solubilization by a hydrophobic polyelectrolyte: surface activity and membrane binding. Biophys J 67:1101–1106, 1994.

15. N Murthy, JR Robichaud, DA Tirrell, PS Stayton, AS Hoffman. The design and synthesis of polymers for eukaryotic membrane disruption. J Controlled Release 61:137–143, 1999.

16. PD Mourad, N Murthy, TYM Porter, SL Poliachik, LA Crum, AS Hoffman, PS Stayton. Focused ultrasound and poly(2-ethylacrylic acid) act synergistically to disrupt lipid bilayers in vitro. Macromolecules 34:2400–2401, 2001.

17. H Du, P Chandaroy, SW Hui. Grafted poly-(ethylene glycol) on lipid surfaces inhibits protein adsorption and cell adhesion. Biochim Biophys Acta 1326:236–248, 1993.

18. TR Kyriakides, YN Zhu, LT Smith, SD Bain, Z Yang, MT Lin, KG Danielson, RV Iozzo, M LaMarca, CE McKinney, EI Ginns, P Bornstein. Mice that lack thrombospondin 2 display connective tissue abnormalities that are associated with disordered collagen fibrillogenesis, an increased vascular density, and a bleeding diathesis. J Cell Biol 140:419–430, 1998.

19. TR Kyriakides, JW Tam, P Bornstein. (1999) Accelerated wound healing in mice with a disruption of the thrombospondin 2 gene. J Invest Dermatol 113:782–787, 1999.

20. OW Press, JA Hansen, A Farr, PJ Martin. Endocytosis and degradation of murine anti-human CD3 monoclonal antibodies by normal and malignant T-lymphocytes. Cancer Res 48:2249–2257, 1988.

21. F Geissler, SK Anderson, O Press. Intracellular catabolism of radiolabeled anti-CD3 antibodies by leukemic T cells. Cell Immunol 137:96–110, 1991.

22. D Pei, SJ Weiss. Furin-dependent intracellular activation of the human stromelysin-3 zymogen. Nature 375:244–247, 1995.

23. RW Taft, MM Kreevoy. The evaluation of inductive and resonance effects on reactivity. I hydrolysis rates of acetals and non-conjugated aldehydes and ketones. J Am Chem Soc 77:5590, 1955.

24. C Wu, XH Wang. Globule-to-coil transition of a single homopolymer chain in solution. Phys Rev Lett 80:4092–4094, 1998.

25. PC Weber, DH Ohlendorf, JJ Wendoloski, FR Salemme. Structural origins of high-affinity biotin binding to streptavidin. Science 243:85–88, 1989.

26. S Freitag, I Le Trong, LA Klumb, PS Stayton, R Stenkamp. Structural studies of the streptavidin binding loop. Protein Sci 6:1157–1166, 1997.

27. PS Stayton, T Shimoboji, C Long, A Chilkoti, G Chen, JM Harris, AS Hoffman. Control of protein-ligand recognition using a stimuli-responsive polymer. Nature 378:472–474, 1995.

28. A Chilkoti, PS Stayton. Molecular origins of the slow streptavidin–biotin dissociation kinetics. J Am Chem Soc 117:10622–10628.

29. Z Ding, LJ Long, Y Hayashi, EV Bulmus, AS Hoffman, PS Stayton. Temperature control of biotin binding and release with a streptavidin-poly(N-isopropylacrylamide) site-specific conjugate. Bioconj Chem 10:395–400, 1999.

30. T Shimoboji, Z Ding, S Stayton, AS Hoffman. Mechanistic investigation of smart polymer–protein conjugates. Bioconj Chem 12:314–319, 2001.

31. V Bulmus, Z Ding, CJ Long, PS Stayton, AS Hoffman. Conjugation of a pH- and temperature-sensitive polymer to a specific site on streptavidin for pH-controlled binding and triggered release of biotin. Bioconj Chem 11:78–83, 1999.

32. E Morag, EA Bayer, M Wilchek. Immobilized nitro-avidin and nitro-streptavidin as reusable affinity matrices for application in avidin-biotin technology. Anal Biochem 243:257–263, 1996.

33. Z Ding, RB Fong, CJ Long, PS Stayton, AS Hoffman. Nature (in press).

16

Implantable Drug Delivery Devices
Design of a Biomimetic Interfacial Drug Delivery System

Thomas D. Dziubla and Anthony M. Lowman
Drexel University, Philadelphia, Pennsylvania

Marc C. Torjman and Jeffrey I. Joseph
Jefferson Medical College, Thomas Jefferson University, Philadelphia, Pennsylvania

I. INTRODUCTION

Over the last decade, research on implantable interfacial drug delivery devices coupled with significant advances in micro- and nanoscale technology have brought new ideas to the fields of pharmacology and controlled release. Perhaps these devices' greatest potential in clinical medicine lies in their ability to provide superior drug delivery kinetics for the treatment of certain chronic diseases. A dosing regimen offering the necessary precision for the delivery of drugs in a continuous or pulsatile fashion with rapid uptake, coupled with improved patient compliance as well as convenience, has brought important potential advantages to implantable drug delivery. Ongoing research focused on the development of closed-loop delivery systems, particularly that of an artificial pancreas for use in insulin-dependent diabetes, has demonstrated some of the complexities related to long-term functionality of the implants and the difficulties in maintaining healthy surrounding tissue (1–4). Therefore, the immense potential behind implantable drug delivery is still overshadowed by our lack of understanding of the numerous factors relating to implantation biology, specifically the biomaterial–tissue interaction. It is important for the success of an implantable drug delivery device that this interaction be carefully evaluated so that the long-term function of future devices will not be limited but rather be enhanced by the tissue reaction. Focusing our efforts on techniques (and technologies) adopted from biomimetics could lead to a harmonious incorporation of the implant into the host environment, and should therefore be a primary consideration in the design of these new implantable drug delivery systems.

In this chapter we will discuss some of the key concepts in the field of implantable drug delivery from controlled delivery to the foreign body response, some of the designs currently being developed, and the work we have done in developing an interface for an implantable drug delivery system.

II. CONTROLLED DRUG RELEASE

The difficulty with routine injections and/or oral administrations is that the resulting peaks and exponential decays in drug concentrations may cause undesirable physiological responses (Fig. 1) (5–7). This presents several problems. First, there is a "window" of effectiveness that must be obtained in order for the drug to be pharmacologically active without becoming toxic. The peak concentration typically associated with injections and oral administrations could easily overshoot this window and result in acute

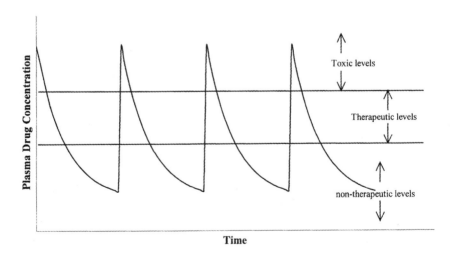

Figure 1 Plasma drug concentrations resulting from multiple injections and/or oral administrations.

toxic levels. During the decay phase, the active concentration could easily drop below the window and no longer be therapeutically effective. For example, drugs such as colchicine, which is used for the treatment of severe gout, require tight monitoring due to a narrow therapeutic window (8). The purpose of controlled drug delivery is to sustain a specific drug concentration within the body for an extended period of time (9–11). A device that provides a sustained release of drug can maintain desired drug concentrations while minimizing concern about toxic or ineffective doses. Moreover, controlled release is a more cost-effective way of delivering expensive medications. Since the amount of drug delivered is equal to the area under the concentration versus time curve, it is apparent that the amount of drug delivered is not being optimally utilized. By delivering just the amount of drug needed, patient care is improved in a cost-effective manner.

The idea of continuous release describes a steady-state system with a time-independent delivery scheme, also known as zero-order kinetics. However, this is just a subset of the actual goal. The primary aim of controlled drug delivery is complete optimization, i.e., the ability to deliver to the desired location a precise therapeutic dose for a finite period of time (5–7). With such a system, one could achieve high bioavailability with minimal side effects and drug exposure. This definition calls not only for responsive systems, but also systems that can deliver drug locally with rapid uptake. The advantage to implantable drug delivery devices is that they can be designed to meet any and all of these aims in controlled drug delivery. But without considering the potential effects of the tissue response to the implant, the clinical results can vary from reduced delivery rates to impaired uptake to complete device failure.

III. FOREIGN BODY RESPONSE

Implants, including implantable drug delivery devices, are foreign bodies that will invoke the natural defense mechanism against such intrusions, i.e., the inflammatory response. Typically this response is split into two categories: acute and chronic (12,13). During the acute phase of inflammations an influx of fluid, plasma proteins, and neutrophils enters the wound/implantation site (14). These neutrophils accumulate at the site of implantation and start to phagocytize any small debris or bacteria that is present. Phagocytosis can be activated when the neutrophil comes into contact with activating factors called opsonins (12). If an implant surface absorbs opsonins, as in IgG, the neutrophil will try to engulf the implant, but the neutrophil to implant size disparity prevents this process from occurring. This leads to an event known as "frustrated phagocytosis," whereby the neutrophils dump the contents of lysosomes into the extracellular matrix (ECM) (15). This presents a problem if the drug being delivered is destroyed by the lysozymes. After the neutrophils have entered the area and cleared away any debris, granulation tissue begins to form, and the natural wound healing response continues. At this point, the response can split into either a chronic inflammatory response or a foreign body reaction of the acute type (13). If there is a consistent chemical or physical irritation (as in free movement of implant), the chronic inflammatory response occurs (16). If there are no negative chemical or physical signals, a normal foreign body response occurs. Typically, this response results in three characteristic layers (13). A primary layer of macrophages and/or foreign body giant cell formations surrounds the implant. These cells secrete the second layer composed of dense fibrous tissue 30–100 μm in thickness. A third layer of highly vascularized tissue—granulation tissue—surrounds this fibrous wall. This response is indefinitely stable except for a decrease in cellularity of the primary layer. The dense nature of the fibrous layer greatly impedes the diffusion of most chemical species, hence the lag time to rendering any implanted drug delivery device inoperable (17). Even biodegradable polymers are susceptible to fibrous tissue encapsulation (18).

One technique that has been used to prevent this fibrous capsule formation is the addition of a tissue implant intermediary (19,20). In 1989, Lipsky and Lamberton developed a polyurethane sponge for neovascularization (21). They noted that this vascular tissue interface would be an effective way to deliver drugs systemically (22). If a material possesses a continuous porous structure 8–10 μm or greater, macrophages are capable of invading the device (23,24). Under these conditions, vascularized tissue may grow into the implant, preventing the occurrence of the foreign body response. With such a porous structure, the implant material is able to mimic the ECM. The ECM provides structure to tissue and provides signals to the cells, which helps dictate growth and maintenance (25,26). It is important that the implant material be nonimmunogenic, nonteratogenic, and nontoxic in order for this vascularized tissue to remain healthy in the long term (27).

IV. TYPES OF IMPLANTABLE DELIVERY DEVICES

A. Passive Depot Delivery Systems

The original concept for an implantable drug delivery device is a depot of drug that is released slowly over a given length of time (11). All of the passive depot systems rely on diffusion of drug through an implant material that is nondegradable to control the rate of drug release. Silicone, poly(ethylene-*co*-vinyl acetate), polyacrylates, and ceramics are used as the nondegradable implant material (9,28,29). These depot systems can be categorized into two main types: encapsulated reservoir systems and matrix-loaded systems.

In the encapsulated reservoir system, a polymer membrane surrounds a core of drug. The diffusion of drug through this membrane becomes the rate-limiting step to drug release. By tailoring the thickness of the membrane and the diffusion coefficients, the rate at which drug is delivered can be controlled. During the time when the drug concentration inside and outside the polymer membrane is in equilibrium, drug release will be zero order. Currently, Norplant, an implantable 5-year contraceptive, is based on the passive depot delivery method. It consists of a flexible implant with six capsules containing levonorgesterol (LNG) (30,31). The main drawback to this method is that if the membrane is ruptured, there will be a sudden dumping of drug into the body (Fig. 2). Moreover, the diffusion of larger bioactive substances is typically extremely slow in polymeric membranes (32).

In matrix systems, instead of a concentrated core of drug, the drug is evenly dispersed throughout the entire polymer. As in the reservoir system, release from the matrix system is diffusion controlled. However, the release profiles for these systems are drastically different. Two of the advantages of this type are that they are easier to manufacture and are not susceptible to the rupturing that can occur with reservoir systems. Moreover, release of proteins becomes more feasible because factors that affect the microstructure, such as the loading concentration, can greatly increase the diffusion coefficients (33). The main drawback to matrix loading is their more complex release mechanism. It is difficult to create systems that possess zero-order drug release (10). Some of the matrix systems being developed and used are polymethyl methacylate (PMMA) containing varying types of drugs for the treatment of osteomyelitis (34,35).

B. Biodegradable/Bioerodable Systems

The primary disadvantage to the passive depot delivery system is after all drug is delivered, a second surgical procedure is required to remove the spent polymer. A more novel approach is the use of biodegradable/bioerodable polymers. In these systems, the polymer contains bonds that are susceptible to hydrolysis or some enzymatic cleavage. There are several advantages to and concerns about this type of implantable drug delivery device. We no longer need to use diffusion as the controlling mechanism of delivery. It may be possible to better obtain the desired release rates by

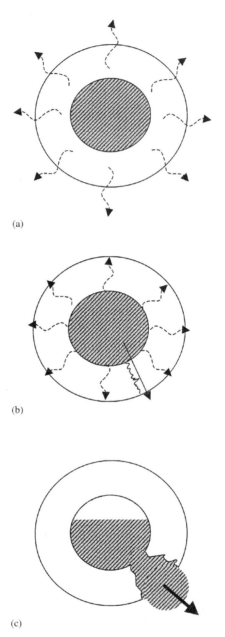

(a)

(b)

(c)

Figure 2 (a) Drug delivery from functioning reservoir system. Cracks in shell (b) can cause incorrect delivery rates, while tears (c) can cause dumping of entire contents.

controlling the degradation kinetics along with diffusional release (10). Unlike passive depots where a shrinking concentration gradient prevents total release, degradable networks are not subject to a decreasing release rate and can deliver 100% of the loaded drug. Also, it is possible to deliver high molecular weight drugs, such as proteins, when diffusion of these molecules would be too slow. Because the system degrades with time there will be no residual material to be removed; however, the biocompatibility and toxicity of the degradation products also become an important consideration.

One group of biodegradable polymers are polyesters. Some of the more popular polyesters being evaluated as a biomaterial are poly(lactic acid-*co*-glycolic acid) (PLGA). The most recent of such work has been the development of injectable systems that allow for the long-term delivery of proteins while being minimally invasive. Some research in this area include PLGA-based microspheres for the delivery of biologically active compounds such as insulin, vascular endothelial growth factor, insulin-like growth factor, and recombinant human growth factor (36–45). Moreover, there have been developments of PLGA-containing networks that are thermo-gelling (46,47). This system consists of a injectable liquid that gels under physiological conditions. This gel then slowly degrades over time, delivering the drug at a controlled rate. The degradation products of this polymer are lactic acid and glycolic acid, which are natural cellular metabolites and are eliminated through natural means. The hydrolysis of the lactic acid repeating unit occurs much faster than that of the glycolic acid repeating unit, which are both acid-catalyzed reactions. Therefore, the rate of degradation can be controlled by changing the copolymer ratio or by adding acidic groups to the polymer networks. This polymer undergoes bulk decomposition, which is when the degradation occurs uniformly throughout the entire sample (48). Hence, over time the structural integrity of the network decreases, and the result could be the production of tiny irregularly shaped particles.

Polyanhydrides are another type of biodegradable polymer. One advantage of this polymer class is that their degradation is typically dominated by surface erosion (49,50). This is advantageous because the design of proper kinetics becomes much easier, and the structural integrity of the delivery network is maintained for the lifetime of the device (51). Currently, poly[bis(*p*-carboxyphenoxy)propane-co-sebacic acid] is being used as an implantable carrier for taxol for local delivery after an excised brain tumor (52,53). Some of the more exciting polyanhydrides include salicylic acid (aspirin)–derived polymers (54). Upon degradation, these networks release aspirin as one of the degradation products. This polyaspirin type of polymer is part of a class of drug delivery devices called prodrugs (55). Hence, the drug being delivered does not need to be just matrix loaded but part of the polymer network. In this form there would be no release of drug by diffusion easing the design of delivery. Also, bioactive agents attached covalently to polymers have been shown to increase the half-life of the activity of these drugs.

Surface-eroding polymers tend to degrade much more rapidly than that of bulk-degrading polymers. Hence, the duration of drug release can be a limiting factor when using surface-eroding polymers. By creating a composite release system of polyanhydride coated in a polylactic acid shell, Goepferich showed that it is possible to obtain drug release duration three times longer than that of a typical surface erosion scheme with drug release still remaining diffusion controlled (51,56).

C. Active Delivery Systems

Mazer shown that for a somatostatin derivative, a zero-order release is the best pharmacokenetic pathway for the suppression of growth hormone secretion (57,58). The previously mentioned types of implantable drug delivery devices are ideal for such a system. However, for a gonadotropin-releasing hormone, a pulsatile delivery is most effective at stimulating the pituitary (58,59). For such a demand, a passive implantable drug delivery device might not be the best alternative. There needs to be some delivery mechanism that can give varying amounts of drug based on demand. For this reason, there has been growing research on active delivery systems. Fig. 3 depicts the idealization of an active delivery system. As shown, drug is only delivered at times of need and is turned off instantly when the demand has been met. One type of active system that is currently being developed is the drug array implant. This device is a silicon chip with many tiny reservoirs filled with drug or a microporous membrane in which the drug is held (60). In one system, the reservoirs are coated in a thin nonporous metal layer. If a voltage is sent across the metal layer, it ruptures open thus delivering the drug (61,62). This design holds great promise, as it is capable of rapid on/off delivery. Also, the reservoirs can be filled with many different types of drugs, allowing for complex drug delivery schemes to be achieved. Another type of active delivery device is the drug delivery micropump. Currently, some diabetes patients use an external pump connected to a subcutaneous catheter (63,64). The pump is set to deliver basal levels of insulin and can give bolus injections to meet demands during meal times. However, due to miniaturization of the systems, there is a push to make these pumps fully implantable. All of these devices can be connected to a sensing mechanism and microcontroller, thus creating an implantable closed-loop drug delivery device, one of the ultimate goals of

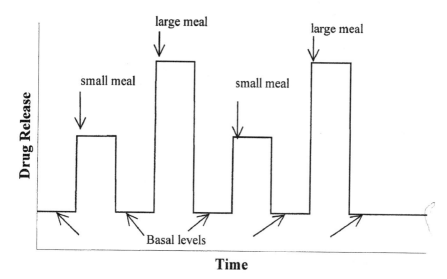

Figure 3 An active delivery system would be able to dynamically control the amount of insulin needed based on demand.

controlled drug delivery. Such a system would be capable of demand-based instant on/off delivery. However, this instant on/off control is only possible if rapid, systemic insulin uptake can occur. This might be achieved in the presence of a high density of blood vessels near the delivery port of the catheter tip.

One device in development that falls into this category is the artificial pancreas. This device can be broken down into three components: the glucose sensor that monitors blood glucose levels, the control mechanism that determines rates of delivery based on the physiological data obtained from the control mechanism, and the delivery pump and catheter that is the active system delivering insulin to the body. Determined through several clinical trials, the most common cause of device failure was due to tissue inclusion at the catheter port of delivery caused by the foreign body response (3,4,63–67). Hence, a biomimetic layer that would allow vascular tissue ingrowth rather than fibrotic tissue inclusion could be a potential solution to this problem.

V. DEVELOPMENT OF TISSUE–IMPLANT INTERFACE

Previous studies have reported on the use of porous hydroxyapatite ceramics as drug delivery devices because they allow the ingrowth of tissue.

These ceramics are easily manufactured and have shown to be both biocompatible and osteoconductive (68,69). For this reason, efforts have been made to use them as carriers for vaccines, antibiotics, hormones, and anticancer drugs (28,70–72). The first work done with a tissue interface for catheter delivery was with a silicone rubber tissue cage (73). In this setup a cage was implanted and given eight weeks for the tissue regeneration to occur. After that time, drug was infused through the lumen of the tissue cage, and systemic drug levels were monitored. They found that it was possible to maintain continual drug levels through the device; however, there was a 40-min lag time. This was attributed to the actual size of the lumen, which acted as a diffusional barrier between the catheter port and the vascular tissue. A tissue intermediary for an implantable catheter drug delivery system must possess an interconnected pore structure of 8–10 μm or larger in order for vascularized tissue to penetrate the material (Fig. 4) (19,23,27). For this work a hydrogel-based tissue intermediary is proposed. Hydrogels are three-dimensional hydrophilic structures that are capable of absorbing a large amount of water (74,75). These swollen networks have been of considerable interest in biomaterials as well as drug delivery

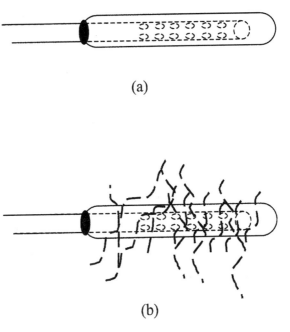

(a)

(b)

Figure 4   (a) Interconnected macropores coating the tip of the implanted catheter allow for (b) the ingrowth of vascularized tissue.

applications due to their higher water content and softness. In the hydrated state, these polymers mimic soft tissue in that they have a similar mechanical behavior and water content.

Poly(2-hydroxyethyl methacrylate) (PHEMA) is a hydrogel that can be easily synthesized into a macroporous, spongy material. Unlike traditional hydrogels, which are transparent homogeneous networks with a porous structure measured in nanometers, these spongy hydrogels are actually a two-phase opaque system with a micrometer-sized macroporous structure. The first uses were pursued in the late 1960s for breast augmentation and nasal cartilage replacement (76–78). In the 1980s, some work was done with pancreatic islet sequestering using PHEMA sponges (79,80). While the hydrogels sponge performed well as an immunoisolation device, long-term viability of the islets was not achieved.

The synthesis of these hydrogel sponges has been well documented (77,81–83). Sponge formation is dependent on the interaction between two phases: the polymer phase and the aqueous phase (83). Since these phases are not the same density, longer reaction times would allow for settling of the two phases. This would result in a porous network that could have an inhomogeneous porous structure. Prior investigations demonstrated that a water layer periodically formed on top of the hydrogel, indicative of this settling polymer phase (81,82). For this reason, reactions were performed at higher temperatures than previous work and also involved the use of sonication to act as a mixing aide during the reaction (84). Sonication adds agitation to the system by means of cavitation. It has been used in microsphere and microemulsion preparations to aid in the homogeneity and the uniformity of microsphere size distribution (85,86). To avoid the potential problem of focusing the wave propagation, a low-frequency bath sonicator was used (44–48 kHz).

To characterize the synthesized scaffolds, mercury porosimetry and SEM analysis were performed. In order for these techniques to be employed, samples were freeze-dried. Although samples were handled carefully to prevent gross alterations of porous structure, this process could further reduce pore sizes compared to the hydrated state. One concern with using mercury porosimetry was the alteration of intrusion data from compressibility of the sponge. If a sample compresses during the study, then the volume of mercury entering the sample would no longer be equal to the volume of the pores, resulting in inaccurate readings for the pore size distribution and porosity. Samples were tested for compressibility by running compression-corrected blank using a nonporous dried PHEMA hydrogel. As the compression corrected data varied by 1.2% or less for all materials, it was concluded that compressibility had a negligible effect on the porosity analyses (84).

A. Surface Pore Structure (Shell Effect)

It was found that sonication had no strong effect on the pore size distribution but did reduce the occurrence of the "shell" that can form at the mold–polymer interface (Fig. 5) (83). The smaller pore size of the shell would hinder the ability of tissue to penetrate the internal porous structure. Since tissue/vascular penetration is dependent on the presence of the interconnected pore structure, these shelled samples are not of any significant use. Moreover, the fact that the presence of the shell greatly influences the information obtained from mercury porosimetry must be considered when interpreting the data. The dense shell formation contains sparsely located pores that allow access to the internal porous structure. When the porosimeter reaches a pressure that would allow for the intrusion of mercury, the mercury starts to flow into the inner structure of the sponge, resulting in porosimetry data that may be different from what is actually present.

B. Internal Pore Structure

Porosity is the ratio of pore volume to total volume. This is useful for us to consider because the greater the porosity the greater the likelihood that there exists an interconnected pore structure. From Fig. 6 it is clear that as we increased the amount of water, the porosity increased. The reason for this is that a portion of the water acted to swell the polymer phase, and the remaining water served as the pore-forming agent. Since the water was present in such excess, we expected the majority of the water to behave as the pore-forming agent. As a result, a nearly 1:1 ratio of the initial water volume content and the porosity in the final sponge was observed. Moreover, SEM micrographs shown in Fig. 7 exhibited a good indication that there is a uniform, interconnected porous structure for sponges with 80% water content.

Fig. 8 shows the results of pore size and pore distribution. Volume average pore sizes varied from 6 to 15 µm as the reacting solution water content increased from 60% to 90%. The important point to note is that these data show a slight discrepancy in terms of previously published literature. This is assumed to be a result of the elevated reaction temperature used. The phase separation of PHEMA and water is based on PHEMA's negative temperature dependence, and at higher temperatures it is less soluble.

Using mercury porosimetry, both volume average and area average pore sizes were calculated. Volume average pore size weighted the averaging based on the volume of mercury penetrated, thus favoring larger pores. The

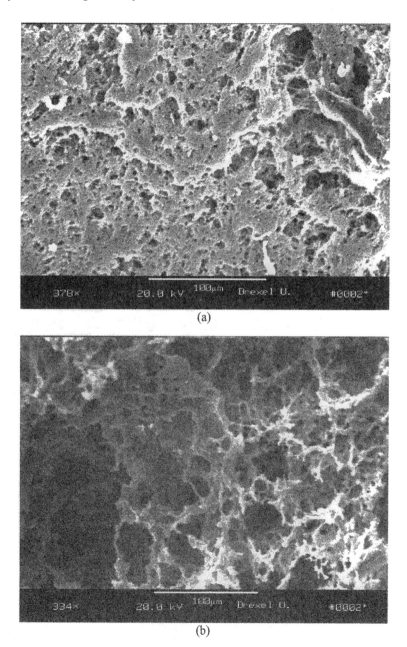

Figure 5 Surface of (a) unsonicated and (b) sonicated sponges prepared from reaction mixture containing 90% water. (From Ref. 84.)

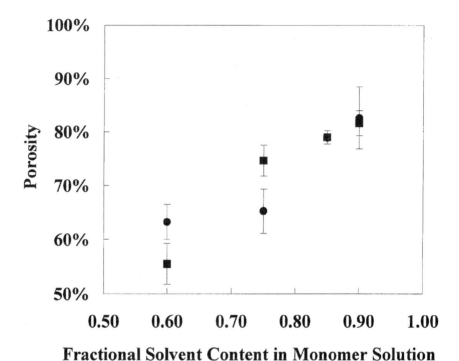

Fractional Solvent Content in Monomer Solution

Figure 6   Porosity of the (■) sonicated and (•) unsonicated sponge networks as a function of solvent content in the reaction mixture ($n = 4 \pm$ SE). (From Ref. 84.)

area average pore size was based on pore surface area. As the smaller pores have a greater surface area per weight of polymer, this averaging favored the smaller pores. To account for the dispersity of the pore sizes, a pore size distribution index was defined as the ratio of the volume average pore size over the area average pore size. In Fig. 9, the pore size distribution index is shown as a function of solvent content in the reaction mixture for both the sonicated and unsonicated samples. Although it appears that the sonicated samples had a greater dispersity than the unsonicated, we must consider that the unsonicated samples possessed a shell with periodic intermittent large pores; unsonicated samples also possessed a dense shell around the internal structure. In mercury porosimetry, the pressure is incrementally increased over a range of pressures. For each pressure increment, the volume of mercury that penetrates the sample is measured. It is theorized that every pressure increment relates to a specific pore size. Shelled sponges possess fewer smaller pores externally than is present internally. When the

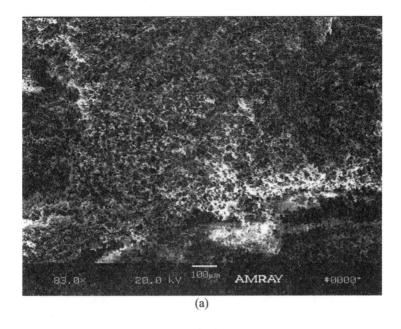

(a)

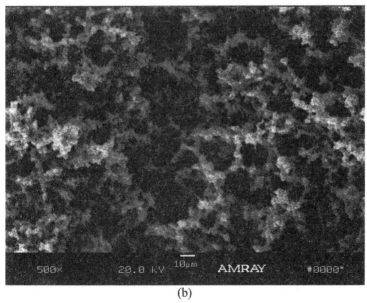

(b)

Figure 7 Eighty vol % water PHEMA networks exhibited a regular porous interconnected structure. (a) 83 ×, (b) 500 ×. (From Ref. 84.)

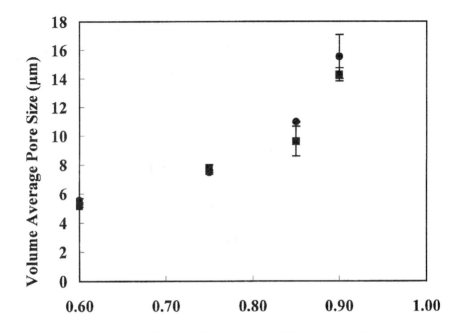

Fractional Solvent Content in Monomer Solution

Figure 8 Volume average pore size of the (■) sonicated and (•) unsonicated sponge networks as a function of solvent content in the reaction mixture ($n = 4 \pm$ SE). (From Ref. 84.)

porosimeter reached a pressure that would allow for the intrusion of mercury through these exterior smaller pores, the mercury would start to flow into the inner structure of the sponge, resulting in porosimetry data that may be artificially more monodisperse.

C. In Vivo Insulin Infusion Kinetics

In order to determine the efficacy of PHEMA sponges as a tissue intermediary, preliminary in vivo studies were performed on Sprague-Dawley rats. Briefly, catheter tubes coated in the sonicated 75 vol % water PHEMA sponge were implanted into the rats. Five months postimplantation, the catheter's proximal end was exteriorized and connected to a microinfusion pump. Blood insulin levels increased rapidly with 5 minutes postinfusion and remained elevated for 30 min for both mesenteric and subcutaneous infusions (Fig. 10a). The mean plasma insulin concentrations

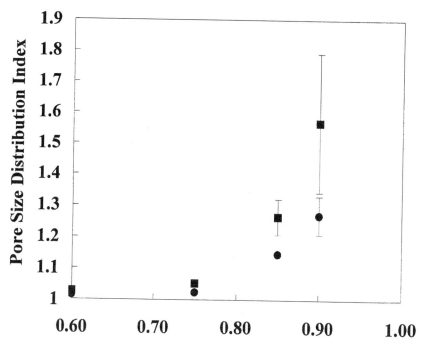

Figure 9 Pore size distribution of the (■) sonicated and (•) unsonicated sponge networks as a function of solvent content in the reaction mixture ($n = 4 \pm SE$). (From Ref. 84.)

rose to near 300 μIU/mL, which was beyond the standard range (3–200 μIU/mL) of the assay. Blood glucose concentrations decreased in proportion to increasing insulin concentrations (Fig. 10b). The high baseline glucose levels are attributable to a combination of the animals not having been fasted prior to the experiment and the effects of isoflurane anesthesia (suppression of insulin production).

D. Histological Evaluation of Catheter Sponge Explants

On explants of both subcutaneous and intraperitoneal catheters, gross examination of surrounding tissues appeared normal with no evidence of inflammation or encapsulation. Histological sections of implants and surrounding tissues (Fig. 11) supported these observations, revealing little to no lymphocyte infiltration peripheral to the hydrogel and only a thin

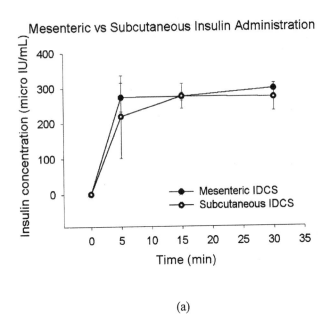

(a)

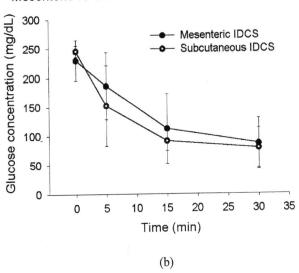

(b)

Figure 10 Systemic (a) human insulin concentration and (b) glucose response following infusion of human insulin from external pump, 5 months postimplantation. (From Ref. 84.)

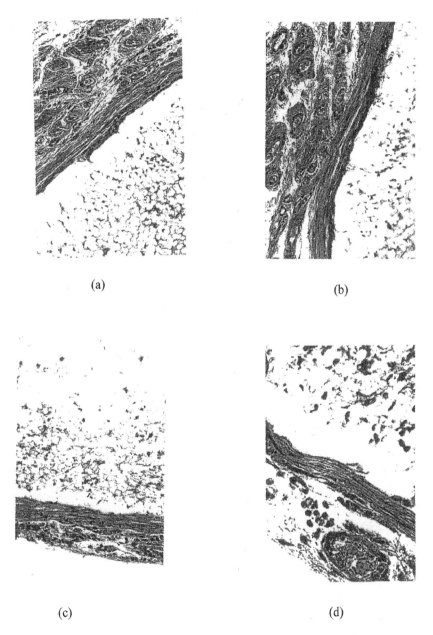

Figure 11 Histological slides of mesenteric implant: (a) 100 ×, (b) 200 ×; and subcutaneous implant: (c) 100 ×, (d) 200 ×. (From Ref. 84.)

(10–35 µm) connective tissue boundary (CTB) adjacent to the hydrogel. Although the CTB was richly vascularized, with the methods used it was not possible to ascertain the extent of vascularization into the gel scaffold. The tissue immediately adjacent to the CTB therefore provided a large surface area for insulin diffusion into the systemic (subcutaneous implant) or portal (mesenteric implant) circulation. Numerous capillaries of varying sizes can be seen as well as capillaries along the CTB.

VI. SUMMARY

The purpose of this work was to evaluate the efficacy of macroporous PHEMA sponges as interfacial drug delivery devices. Since it was possible to form networks with pore sizes greater than 8–10 µm, macroporous PHEMA sponges were determined to be excellent candidates for vascular tissue–implant intermediaries. Five months after implantation of sponge-coated catheters, insulin was infused into the devices from external pumps. Following administration, insulin absorption was observed in conjunction with dramatic lowering of blood glucose levels. From histological evaluation of explanted devices, highly vascularized tissue was observed surrounding the mesenteric implants. These results indicate that PHEMA sponges may be excellent candidates for tissue intermediation in long-term implantable drug delivery devices.

ACKNOWLEDGMENTS

Financial support for this work was provided by a grant from The Whitaker Foundation.

REFERENCES

1. CD Saudek, JL Selam, HA Pitt, K Waxman, RE Fischell, MA Carles. A preliminary insulin trial with the programmable implantable medication system for insulin delivery. N Engl J Med 320(9): 574–579, 1989.
2. E Renard, P Balder, MC Picot, D Jacques-Apostol, D Lauton, G Costalat, J Bringer, C Jaffiol. Catheter complications associated with implantable systems for peritoneal insulin delivery. Diabetes Care 18:300–306, 1995.
3. M Scavini, L Galli, S Reich, RP Eaton, MA Charles, FL Dunn. Catheter survival during long-term insulin therapy with an implanted programmable pump. Diabetes Care 20:610–613, 1997.

4. JL Selam, P Micossi, FL Dunn, DM Nathan. Clinical trial of programmable implantable insulin pump for type 1 diabetes. Diabetes Care 15:877–885, 1992.
5. BA Hertzog, C Thanos, M Sandor, V Raman, ER Edelman. Cardiovascular drug delivery systems. In: E Mathoiwitz, ed. Encyclopedia of Controlled Drug Delivery. New York: John Wiley and Sons, 1999.
6. K Leach. Cancer, drug delivery to treat—local and systemic. In: E Mathoiwitz, ed. Encyclopedia of Controlled Drug Delivery. New York: John Wiley and Sons, 1999.
7. MJ Groves. Parenternal drug delivery systems. In: E Mathoiwitz, ed. Encyclopedia of Controlled Drug Delivery. New York: John Wiley and Sons, 1999.
8. SB Kulkarni, M Singh, GV Betageri. Encapsulation, stability and in vitro release characteristics of liposomal formulations of colchicine. J Pharm Pharm 49:491–495, 1997.
9. LK Fung, WM Saltzman. Polymeric implants for cancer chemotherapy. Adv Drug Del Rev 26:209–230, 1997.
10. J Siepmann, A Goepferich. Mathematical modeling of bioerodible, polymeric drug delivery systems. Adv Drug Del Rev 48:229–247, 2001.
11. AK Dash, GC Cudworth II. Therapeutic applications of implantable drug delivery systems. J Pharmacal Toxical Meth 40:1–12, 1998.
12. JM Anderson. Mechanisms of inflammation and infection with implanted devices. Cardiovasc Pathol 2:33–41, 1993.
13. JM Anderson. Inflammatory response to implants. Trans Am Soc Artif Intern Organs 19:101–107, 1988.
14. H Malech, J Gallin. Current concepts: immunology. Neutrophiles in human diseases. N Engl J Med 317:687–694, 1987.
15. P Henson. Mechanisms of exocytosis in phagocytic inflammatory cells. Am J Pathol 101:494–511, 1980.
16. JI Galin, IM Golstein, R Snyderman. Inflammation: Basic Principles and Clinical Correlates. New York: Raven Press, 1988.
17. DW Scharp, NS Mason, RE Sparks. Islet immuno-isolation: the use of hybrid artificial organs to prevent islet tissue rejection. World J Surg. 8:221–229, 1984.
18. RE Marchant, A Hiltner, C Hamlin, A Rabinovitch, R Slobodkin, JM Anderson. In vivo biocompatibility studies. I. The cage implant system and a biodegradable hydrogel. J Biomed Mater Res 17:301–325, 1983.
19. JH Brauker, VE Carr-Brendel, LA Martinson, J Crudele, WD Johnston. Neovascularization of synthetic membranes directed by membrane micro-architecture. J Biomed Mater Res 29:1517–1524, 1995.
20. RL Walton, RE Brown. Tissue engineering of biomaterials for composite reconstruction: an experimental approach. Ann Plast Surg 30:105–110, 1993.
21. MH Lipsky, P Lamberton. Establishment of a neovascular bed in a collagen-impregnated polyurethane sponge. J Biomed Mater Res 23:1441–1452, 1989.
22. MH Lipsky, P Lamberton. Establishment of a neovascular bed in a collagen-impregnated polyurethane sponge. J Biomed Mater Res 23:1441–1452, 1989.

23. AG Mikos, G Sarakinos, MD Lyman, DE Ingber, JP Vacanti, R Langer. Prevascularization of porous biodegradable polymers. Biotech Bioeng 42:716, 1993.
24. SA Weslowski, CC Fries, KE Karlson, MD Bakey, PN Sawyer. Porosity: primary determinant of ultimate fate of synthetic vascular grafts. Surgery 50:91, 1961.
25. MW Long (ed). Tissue microenvironments. Tissue Engineering. Boca Raton: CRC Press, 1995.
26. GA Dunn (ed). Cell motility and tissue architecture. Tissue Engineering. Boca Raton: CRC Press, 1995.
27. DJ Mooney, RS Langer. Engineering biomaterials for tissue engineering: the 10–100 micron size scale. In: JD Bronzino, ed. The Biomedical Engineering Handbook. Boca Raton: CRC Press, 1995.
28. H Gautier, J Caillon, AM Le Ray, G Daculsi, C Merle. Influence of isotactic compression on the stability of vancomycin loaded with a calcium phosphate–implantable drug delivery device. J Biomed Mater Res 52:308–314, 2000.
29. P Kortesuo, M Ahola, S Karlsson, I Kangasnierni, A Yli-Urpo, J Kiesvaara. Silica xerogel as an implantable carrier for controlled drug delivery evaluation of drug distribution and tissue elects after implantation. Biomaterials 21:193–198, 2000.
30. CJ Munro, LS Laughlin, T VonSchalscha, DM Baldwin, BL Lasley. An enzyme immunoassay for serum and urinary levonorgestrel in human and nonhuman primates. Contraception 54:43–53, 1996.
31. I Chi. Intrauterine contraceptive device status report. Adv Drug Del Rev 17:165–178, 1995.
32. SP Baldwin, WM Saltzman. Materials for protein delivery in tissue engineering. Adv Drug Del Rev 33:71–86, 1998.
33. WM Saltzman, R Langer. Transport rates of proteins in porous polymers with known microgeometry. Biophys J 55:163–171, 1989.
34. DH Robinson, S Sampath. Release kinetics of tobramycin sulfate from polymethylmethacrylate implants. Drug Dev Ind Pharm 15:2339–2357, 1989.
35. F Greco, L Palma, N Specchia, S Jacobelli, C Gaggini. Poly methyl methacrylate-antiblastic drug compounds: an in vitro study assessing the cytotoxic effect in cancer cell lines—a new method for local chemotherapy of bone metastasis. Orthopedics 15:189–194, 1992.
36. YY Tang, TS Chung, NP Ng. Morphology, drug distribution, and in vitro release. Biomaterials 22:231–241, 2001.
37. TW King, CW Patrick, Jr. Development and in vitro characterization of vascular endothelial growth. J Biomed Mater Res 51:383–390, 2000.
38. M Dunne, OI Corrigan, Z Ramtoola. Influence of particle size and dissolution conditions on the degradation of polylactide-co-glycolide particles. Biomaterials 21:1659–1668, 2000.
39. JB Oldham, DB Porter, T-S Tan, H Brisby, BL Currier, AG Mikos, MJ Yaszemski. Influence of changes in experimental parameters on size of plga microspheres. J Biomech Eng 122:289–292, 2000.

40. ZR Shen, JH Zhu, Z Ma, F Wang, ZY Wang. Preparation of biodegradable microspheres of testosterone with poly(d,l-lactide-co-glycolide) and test of drug release in vitro. Artif Cells Blood Subs Immob Biotechnol 28:57–64, 2000.

41. X Cao, MS Shoichet. Delivering neuroactive molecules from biodegradable microspheres for application in central nervous system disorders. Biomaterials 20:329–339, 1999.

42. JL Cleland. Solvent evaporation processes for the production of controlled release biodegradable microsphere formulations for therapeutics and vaccines. Biotechnol Prog 14:102–107, 1998.

43. JL Cleland, OL Johnson, S Putney, AJS Jones. Recombinant human growth hormone poly(lactic-co-glycolic acid) microsphere formulation development. Adv Drug Del Rev 28:71–84, 1997.

44. JM Anderson, MS Shive. Biodegradation and biocompatibility of pla and plga microspheres. Adv Drug Del Rev 28:5–24, 1997.

45. S Cohen, L Chen, RN Apte. Controlled release of peptides and proteins from biodegradable polyester microspheres: an approach for treating infectious diseases and malignancies. React Polym 25:177–187, 1995.

46. B Jeong, MR Kibbey, JC Birnbaum, Y-Y Won, A Gutowska. Thermogelling biodegradable polymers with hydrophilic backbones. Macromolecules 33:8317–8322, 2000.

47. B Jeong, YH Bae, SW Kim. Thermoreversible gelation of PEG-PLGA-PEG triblock. Macromolecules 32:7064–7069, 1999.

48. R Langer, NA Peppas. Chemical and physical structure of polymers as carriers for controlled release of bioactive agents: a review. Rev Macromol Chem Phys C 23:61–126, 1983.

49. A Goepferich, R Langer. Modeling polymer erosion. Macromolecules 16:4105–4112, 1993.

50. J Tamada, R Langer. Erosion mechanism of hydrolytically degradable polymers. Proc Natl Acad Sci USA 90:552–556, 1993.

51. A Goepferich. Erosion of composite polymer matrices. Biomaterials 18:397–403, 1997.

52. WL Hunter, HM Burt, L Machan. Local delivery of chemotherapy: a supplement to existing cancer treatments a case for surgical pastes and coated stents. Adv Drug Del Rev 26:199–207, 1997.

53. KA Walter, MA Cahan, A Gr, B Tyler, J Hilton, OM Colvin, PC Burger, AJ Domb, H Brem. Interstitial taxol delivered from a biodegradable polymer implant against experimental malignant glioma. Cancer Res 54:2207–2212, 1994.

54. L Erdmann, KE Uhrich. Synthesis and degredation characteristics of salicylic acid–derived poly(anhydride esters). Biomaterials 21:1941–1946, 2000.

55. P Liso, M Rebuelta, J Roman, A Gallardo, A Villar. Polymeric drugs derived from ibuprofen with improved antiinflammatory profile. J Biomed Mater Res 32:553–560, 1996.

56. A Goepferich, R Langer. Modeling of polymer erosion in three dimensional rotationally symmetric devices. AICHE J 41:2292–2299, 1995.

57. NA Mazer. Pharmacokinetic and pharmacodynamic aspects of polypeptide delivery. J Controlled Release 11:343–356, 1990.

58. DD Breimer. Pharmacokinetic and pharmacodynamic basis for peptide drug delivery system design. J Controlled Release 21:5–10, 1992.

59. E Konobil. The neuroendocrine control of the menstrual cycle. Recent Prog Horm Res 36:53–88, 1980.

60. L Low, S Seetharaman, K He, MJ Madou. Microactuators toward microvalue for responsive controlled drug delivery. Sensors Actuators B 67:149–160, 2000.

61. MJ Tierney, CR Martin. New electrorelease systems based upon microporous membranes. J Electrochem Soc 137:3789–3793, 1990.

62. MJ Tierney, CR Martin. Electroreleasing composite membranes for delivery of insulin and other macromolecules. J Electrochem Soc 137:2005–2006, 1990.

63. CD Saudek. Future developments in insulin delivery systems. Diabetes Care 16:122–132, 1993.

64. KD Hepp. Implantable insulin pumps and metabolic control. Diabetologia 37:S108–S111, 1994.

65. CD Saudek. Novel forms of insulin delivery. J Clin Endocrinol Metab North Am 26:599–610, 1997.

66. JV Santiago, NH White, DA Skor. Mechanical devices for insulin delivery. In: M Nattrass, JV Santiago, eds. Recent Advances in Diabetes. Edinburgh: Churchill Livingstone, 1984.

67. G Knatterud, M Fisher. Report from the international study group on implantable insulin delivery devices. ASAIO Trans 34:148–149, 1988.

68. JE Lemons. Ceramics: past, present, and future. Bone 19:121s–128s, 1996.

69. Y Shinto, A Uchida, F Korkusuz, N Araki, K Ono. Calcium hydroxyapatite ceramic used as a drug system for antibiotics. J Bone Joint Surg 74B:600–604, 1992.

70. AK Walduck, JP Opdebeec, HE Benson, R Prankerd. Biodegradable implants for the delivery of veterinary vaccines: design, manufacture and antibody response in sheep. J Controlled Release 51:269–280, 1998.

71. DJA Netz, P Sepulveda, VC Pandolfelli, ACC Spadaro, JB Alencastre, MVLB Bentley, JM Marchetti. Potential use of gelcasting hydroxyapatite porous ceramic as an implantable drug delivery system. Int J Pharm 213:117–125, 2001.

72. JH Calhoun, JT Mader. Treatment of osteomyelitis with a biodegradable antibiotic implant. Clin Orthop Relat Res 341:206–214, 1997.

73. IP Thonus, AV De Lange-Macdaniel, CJ Otte, MF Michel. Tissue cage infusion: a technique for the achievement of prolonged steady state in experimental animals. J Pharm Meth 2:63–69, 1979.

74. N Peppas. Hydrogels in Medicine and Pharmacy, Vol. I, Fundamentals. Boca Raton: CRC Press, 1986.

75. AM Lowman, NA Peppas. Hydrogels. In: E Mathoiwitz, ed. Encyclopedia of Controlled Drug Delivery. New York: John Wiley and Sons, 1999.

76. Z Voldrich, Z Tomanek, J Vacik, J Kopecek. Long term experience with poly(glycol monomethacrylate) gel in plastic operations of the nose. J Biomed Mater Res 9:675–685, 1975.

77. BJ Simpson. Hydron: a hydrophilic polymer. Biomed Eng 4:65–68, 1969.
78. K Kliment, M Stol, K Fahoun, B Stockar. Use of spongy hydron in plastic surgery. J Biomed Mater Res 2:237–243, 1968.
79. GF Klomp, H Hashiguchi, PC Ursell, Y Takeda, T Taguchi, WH Dobelle. Macroporous hydrogel membranes for a hybrid artificial pancreas. II. Biocompatibility. J Biomed Mater Res 17:865–871, 1983.
80. SH Ronel, MJ D'Andrea, H Hashiguchi, GF Klomp, WH Dobelle. Macroporous hydrogel membranes for a hybrid artificial pancreas. I. Synthesis and chamber fabrication. J Biomed Mater Res 17:855–864, 1983.
81. AB Clayton, TV Chirila, X Lou. Hydrophilic sponges based on 2-hydroxyethyl methacrylate. V. Effect of crosslinking agent reactivity on mechanical properties. Polym Int 44:201–207, 1997.
82. AB Clayton, TV Chirila, PD Dalton. Hydrophilic sponges based on 2-hydroxyethyl methacrylate. III. Effect of incorporating a hydrophilic cross-linking agent on the equilibrium water content and pore structure. Polym Int 42:45–56, 1997.
83. TV Chirila, IJ Constable, GJ Crawford, S Vijayasekaran, DE Thompson, Y-C Chen, WA Fletcher, BJ Griffen. Poly(2-hydroxyethyl methacrylate) sponges as implant materials: in vivo and in vitro evaluation of cellular invasion. Biomaterials 14:26–38, 1993.
84. TD Dziubla, MC Torjman, JI Joseph, M Murphy-Tatum, AM Lowman. Evaluation of porous networks of poly(2-hydroxyethyl methacrylate) as interfacial drug delivery devices. Biomaterials 22:2893–2899, 2001.
85. PD Scholes, AGA Coombes, L Illum, SS Davis, M Vert, MC Davies. The preparation of sub-200nm poly(lactide-co-glycolide) microspheres for site specific drug delivery. J Controlled Release 25:145–153, 1993.
86. G Reich. Ultrasound-induced degradation of PLA and PLGA during microsphere processing: influence of formation variables. Eur J Pharm Biopharm 45:165–171, 1998.

17
Pharmacologically Active Biomaterials

Kristyn S. Masters and Jennifer L. West
Rice University, Houston, Texas

I. INTRODUCTION

Pharmacologically active materials offer the advantage of providing site-specific pharmacotherapy for prolonged periods of time. The use of biomaterials as drug delivery vehicles is a continuing area of research, due to the desire not only to provide localized drug therapy but to improve the body's acceptance of the implanted materials or initiate desired cell responses at the implantation site. However, it is also possible to covalently modify materials such that the "drug" remains attached to the biomaterial, providing a truly localized therapy, and is pharmacologically active for indefinite periods of time. In this manner, not only do the materials retain their biological activity, but the activity of the incorporated biological molecule or drug is often better preserved when bound to a substrate than when free in solution. Many pharmacological agents have extremely short half-lives in vivo. Attachment to materials often helps to stabilize the active substance while allowing it to interact with its environment and perform its intended functions. A wide range of biologically active molecules can be covalently attached to synthetic biomaterials in a manner such that the substance retains its bioactivity, and is sometimes more effective than its soluble counterpart.

Covalent modification of materials with pharmacologically active substances has been investigated for a number of applications. In many cases, the objective is simply to make a material more biocompatible; an example is the development of bioactive materials to improve hemocompatibility. Another aim in development of pharmacologically active materials can be the stimulation or inhibition of cellular events, such as proliferation or extracellular matrix production. In tissue engineering, combinations of biological signals can accelerate the adhesion, proliferation, or synthetic activity of cells; these can often be immobilized on synthetic polymers and retain their activity.

In this chapter, we have reviewed the synthesis and biological performance of several materials which have been modified to present various bioactive molecules. As already noted, the most common goal of these modifications has been to improve blood compatibility. The implantation of blood-contacting devices, ranging from vascular grafts to stents to artificial hearts, is constantly complicated by the thrombogenic nature of the materials used for these devices. Small-diameter vascular grafts inserted in low-flow blood vessels fail rapidly due to occlusion caused by thrombosis and fibrotic hyperplasia (1). Systemic anticoagulant therapy helps maintain the patency of larger diameter (>6 mm) vascular grafts but is ineffective for small diameter grafts (2). Prevention of vessel reocclusion, or restenosis, following balloon angioplasty is another active area in the development of antithrombotic materials (3,4). Stents constructed of metals such as stainless steel or titanium alloys have demonstrated a high rate of thrombosis (5). In all of these applications, platelets first adhere to an artificial surface or injured tissue via adsorbed proteins, then aggregate. Coagulation via the intrinsic and extrinsic pathways then produces a fibrin-rich thrombus (Fig. 1). In the intrinsic system, contact activation is followed

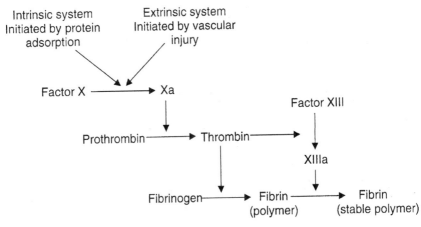

Figure 1 Coagulation can be initiated by either protein adsorption or tissue factor generation. Both situations lead to formation of a fibrin clot that can impair implant performance.

by activation of factor XII, which then initiates the activation cascade of several other clotting factors, ultimately leading to formation of factor Xa. The extrinsic system commences after the activation of factor VII by interaction with tissue factor, which becomes available following vascular damage. Factor VIIa, in turn, leads to formation of factor Xa from factor X, which is the starting point for the common coagulation pathway. Factor Xa joins with a cofactor, factor V, and, in the presence of calcium and platelet phospholipids, converts prothrombin to thrombin. Thrombin, in turn, cleaves both fibrinogen and factor XIII. The fibrin monomers assemble to form a gel, and factor XIIIa acts to create a tough, insoluble fibrin polymer (6). To improve hemocompatibility, biomaterials have been modified with pharmacological agents that prevent platelet adhesion and aggregation or inhibit the coagulation process.

II. POLYSACCHARIDES

A. Heparin

Heparin is commonly used as an anticoagulant and antiplatelet agent. Discovered in the 1960s to treat venous thromboembolism (7), it is composed of repeating units of heterogenously sulfated L-iduronic acid and D-glucosamine sugars, and ranges in molecular weight from 2 to 50 kDa, with an average molecular weight of 15 kDa and half-life of 0.6 h. The antithrombotic mechanism of heparin results from its binding and potent activation of antithrombin III. Antithrombin III (ATIII) is a natural inhibitor of coagulation; upon binding heparin, ATIII undergoes a conformational change that increases its binding affinity for thrombin and factor Xa. Thrombin, in turn, is neutralized by the interaction with ATIII, thereby preventing the catalysis and cleavage of fibrinogen to fibrin. Heparin is also capable of directly inhibiting clotting factors such as factor Xa. Heparin may also inhibit smooth muscle cell proliferation independently of its anticoagulant and antithrombotic properties (5). Although the antiproliferative mechanism is not completely understood, there is evidence that heparin prevents the cells from entering the S phase of mitosis and that this process is specific for smooth muscle cells.

   Site-specific delivery of heparin has been achieved through a variety of polymers, such as polyvinyl alcohol (PVA) (8), ethylenevinyl acetate (9), polyanhydrides (10), polyvinyl chloride (PVC) (11), polyurethane (PU) (12), polyhydroxyethyl methacrylate (13), and silicone (14). The uses of heparin-releasing materials have included periadventitially placed polymers, intraluminal coatings, and vascular grafts (5,15,16). However, a more prolonged treatment can be achieved through the immobilization of heparin onto blood-contacting materials. Covalently modified materials should exhibit thromboresistance for longer periods than systems incorporating dispersed or ionically bound heparin.

Synthesis of covalently heparinized materials often involves the use of a hydrophilic spacer molecule in order to increase the bioavailability of the bound heparin. Polyethylene oxide (PEO) is often used as a spacer, and is frequently coupled to a polymer surface and heparin through diisocyanate groups (Fig. 2). The use of PEO has several advantages for this application. In general, hydrophilic surfaces tend to be less thrombogenic. Thus, in addition to enabling heparin to retain its bioactivity, the PEO spacers themselves help to create a more hemocompatible material surface. Comparing the use of PEO with that of a more hydrophobic alkyl chain spacer molecule, heparin immobilized through PEO demonstrated increased bioactivity (17). The kinetics of thrombin and ATIII binding to immobilized heparin has been examined on styrene/p-amino styrene random copolymer surfaces (18,19). Tolylene diisocyanate–modified PEO was covalently coupled to the surface, followed by heparin immobilization. The free isocyanate on the PEO spacer was used to couple the heparin through a condensation reaction with heparin's pendant hydroxyl or amine groups. Heparin has also been immobilized on the styrene surfaces without a PEO spacer. It was found that heparin directly immobilized onto the surface bound only thrombin, whereas spacer-immobilized heparin retained the ability to bind both thrombin and ATIII, though to a somewhat lesser extent than soluble heparin. The molecular weight of the PEO spacer also affects heparin bioactivity, with increasing molecular weight leading to increased antithrombotic efficacy (19).

Heparin has also been immobilized to PU materials. PUs are used in a number of blood-contacting devices, such as catheters, heart assistance pumps, artificial hearts, and vascular grafts (20). PU surfaces have been treated with diisocyanate, then reacted with PEO or heparin (21). The addition of either PEO or heparin alone significantly increased the hydrophilicity of the material. Increasing the chain length of the PEO led to even greater increases in hydrophilicity and surface mobility. A corresponding trend was observed with the thrombogenicity, as modification with PEO or heparin alone led to decreased thrombogenicity (22), but their synergistic use resulted in the greatest enhancement of blood compatibility.

Although the blood compatibility of polyurethane has been improved by heparin immobilization, the surface densities attained have been quite low due to the restricted coupling sites. Various chemistries exist to accomplish the coupling of PEO-heparin to plasma-modified PU. Following plasma glow-discharge treatment, 1-acryloylbenzotriazole (AB) can be

a.)

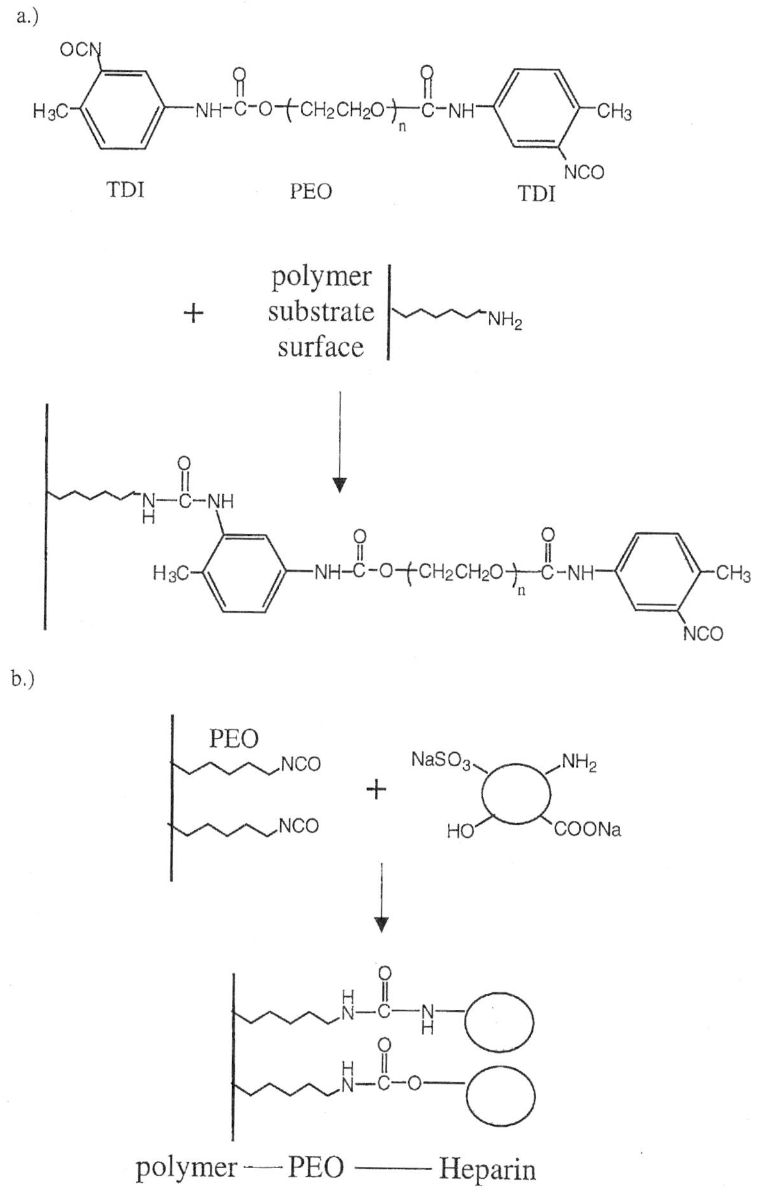

b.)

polymer —— PEO ——— Heparin

Figure 2 Immobilized heparin has been shown to be more effective when coupled via a PEO spacer. (a) Attachment of PEO functionalized with tolylene diisocyanate (TDI) to a polymer substrate to form a PEO spacer. (b) Coupling heparin to the PEO spacer.

grafted onto PU, and then further reacted with sodium hydroxide and ethylene diamine to form the carboxylic acid and primary amine groups needed for heparin immobilization (23,24). Thrombus formation was compared with glass control surfaces. On heparin-modified materials, thrombus formation was significantly suppressed (25% of that on glass controls), whereas the amount of thrombus on PU-AB materials (75% of that on glass controls) was much larger than that of even control PU (50%), indicating that AB grafted onto PU surfaces is not promising for the reduction of device thrombosis. The activated partial thromboplastin time (APTT) was prolonged by the immobilization of heparin (31 $\pm$ 1 s for PU, 38 $\pm$ 1 s for PU-heparin), suggesting the binding of ATIII to heparin, which led to suppressed thrombin activity. Platelet activation, as measured by serotonin release, was also significantly reduced on covalently heparinized surfaces.

Other approaches to dense heparinization of PU surfaces include surface grafting of several polyfunctional polymers (PFP), such as PVA, polyethyleneimine (PEI), and polyallylamine through diisocyanates to the surface of PU (25). The -OH and -NH$_2$ groups were then modified with diisocyanates and coupled to PEO (MW 4000). Heparin was then immobilized through free -NCO groups of the grafted polymers. The purpose of such a system is to amplify the number of potential heparin immobilization sites on the polymer. A twofold increase in immobilized heparin was achieved in comparison with heparin bound directly to the PU surface. In addition, increased bioactivity of heparin immobilized through PU-PFP-PEO was demonstrated through APTT and factor Xa activity assays when compared with heparin immobilized to PU-PFP or PU alone. The enhanced bioactivity of PU-PFP-PEO-heparin over PU-PFP-heparin materials is likely caused by the increased mobility and accessibility of heparin immobilized through hydrophilic and mobile PEO chains.

Several other classes of polymers have been used as substrates for heparin immobilization. Polyethylene terephthalate (PET; Dacron) is commonly used as a vascular graft material. This material has been treated with oxygen plasma glow discharge to form peroxides that catalyze the polymerization of acrylic acid on the surface; the resultant carboxylic acid groups can then be used to graft PEO spacers and heparin (26). Thrombus formation on the PET-PEO-heparin was approximately threefold less than on the PET control. The APTT was prolonged to 58 $\pm$ 1 s on PET-PEO-heparin versus 40 $\pm$ 1 s on PET alone, and the plasma recalcification time (PRT) was almost doubled on the heparinized surfaces. This decrease in thrombogenicity of the PET appears to be due to the action of the heparin, and not the PEO, as the PET-PEO modification did not cause a significant effect on platelet adhesion or activation.

Heparin has been immobilized on various other polymeric materials, such as PVA (27), polydimethylsiloxane (28), polypyrrole (29), and poly(D,L-lactide) (30) in order to create less thrombogenic surfaces. The need for a spacer molecule persists in all studies, as direct attachment of heparin does not always lead to a significant decrease in platelet adhesion over the polymer substrate alone (27,31).

In addition, heparin strongly interacts with basic fibroblast growth factor (bFGF), and modification of materials with heparin has been investigated to localize the growth factor. Photolithography has been used to achieve patterning of heparin on PET surfaces, as displayed in Fig. 3 (32). In this study, heparin was coupled with azidoaniline, cast as a film, and photoirradiated to graft it to the PET surface in the presence or absence of a photomask. Although the adherence of cells occurred independently of the pattern of heparin immobilization, the proliferation of fibroblasts was found to be enhanced only in the heparin-immobilized regions, indicating the localization of bFGF by heparin to induce cell growth. Similarly, albumin-heparin conjugates have been bound to CO_2 plasma–treated polystyrene to create a material that encourages the complexation with bFGF (33,34).

Heparin has also been covalently bound to cross-linked collagen to encourage endothelial cell growth through the binding of bFGF (35). The objective was to develop a vascular graft coating that would promote endothelialization. Cross-linking of collagen reduces the thrombogenicity of the material to a certain extent, although further modification is needed to prevent platelet adhesion and coagulation on the collagen coatings. Increasing amounts of heparin bound to the collagen led to binding of an increasing amount of bFGF, which, in turn, resulted in increased growth of endothelial cells on the collagen surface. However, another issue to be considered is that bFGF is a potent mitogen for smooth muscle cells and fibroblasts, and thus may have the potential to induce intimal hyperplasia.

Heparin has also been attached to fibrin matrices via covalently immobilized heparin-binding peptide sequences in order to provide controlled delivery of bFGF for the enhancement of nerve regeneration (36). In this study, a heparin-binding peptide (FAKLAARLYRKA) was covalently bound to fibrin matrices, and heparin was immobilized via electrostatic interactions with the peptide. The fibrin polymers were cross-linked using factor XIIIa, and peptides were synthesized to contain a factor XIIIa substrate site at the amino terminus, which allowed their attachment to the fibrin matrices, and a heparin-binding sequence derived from ATIII, which allowed for interactions with heparin. Heparin bound by the peptides then sequestered bFGF within the fibrin matrices, which was subsequently released by enzymatic or passive mechanisms. Neurite extension of dorsal root ganglia within bFGF-containing fibrin matrices was enhanced up to

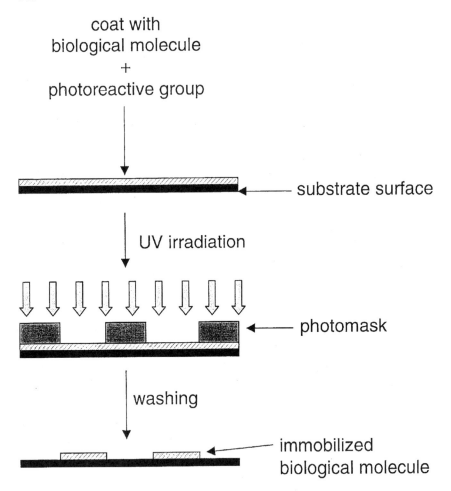

Figure 3 Procedure for photoimmobilization of biologically active molecules, such as heparin.

100% relative to unmodified fibrin. Incorporation of free bFGF into fibrin matrices that did not contain heparin resulted in no enhancement of neurite extension, indicating that sustained activity of bFGF bound to the material via heparin was necessary for increased neurite extension.

B. Hyaluronic Acid

Hyaluronic acid (HA) is an unbranched mucopolysaccharide composed of repeating disaccharide units of D-glucuronic acid and N-acetylglucosamine found in connective tissue. The most abundant natural occurrence of HA is in the cartilage and vitreous, where its primary functions include lubrication of body tissue and blockade of the spread of invading microorganisms. HA is used as a viscoelastic material in ophthalmologic surgery (37), and as an injectable solution for the treatment of joint disease in orthopedics (38). The remarkable viscoelastic properties of HA and its complete lack of immunogenicity have made it an attractive biomaterial. Its efficacy as a drug carrier matrix has been demonstrated through the vestibular delivery of gentamicin, ocular delivery of pilocarpine, intranasal insulin release, and vaginal delivery of calcitonin (39,40). In addition, HA possesses several pharmacological properties that make it attractive in vascular applications, as it inhibits platelet adhesion and aggregation, as well as stimulates angiogenesis (41).

Localized therapy using HA has been achieved via two mechanisms. First, materials can be functionalized with HA through surface modification. Modification schemes can be used that are similar to those described for heparinization. An alternative approach is to modify HA such that cross-linked hydrogels of HA can be formed. Cross-linking of HA has been performed using several different chemistries, such as cross-linking via divinylsulfone (42) or a glycidyl ether (43). Formation of HA hydrogels leads to materials with greater than 90% water content that rapidly biodegrade. More stable HA hydrogels may be synthesized using a water-soluble carbodiimide (WSC) that forms ester bonds between hydroxyl and carboxyl groups on HA (Fig. 4) (44). Amide bonds can also be introduced into the hydrogels by cross-linking in the presence of L-lysine methyl ester. This procedure was used to produce HA hydrogels with a lower water content that were more resistant to degradation (44).

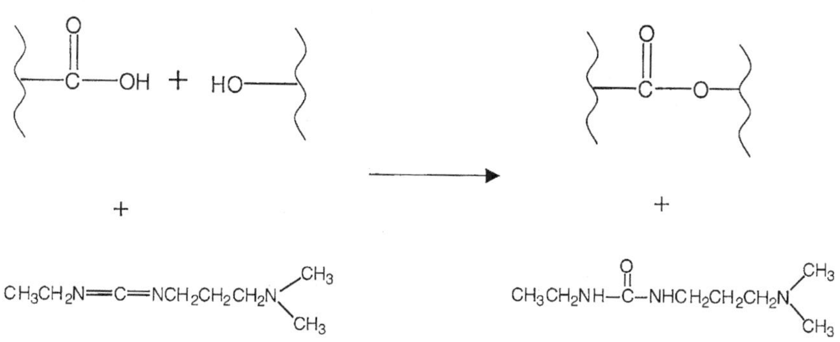

Figure 4 Mechanism of cross-linking hyaluronic acid via use of 1-ethyl-3-(3-dimethylaminopropyl)carbodiimide (EDAC), a commonly used water-soluble carbodiimide.

Binding sites for the covalent attachment of drugs to HA hydrogels can be created via a different HA cross-linking method (45). While drugs have previously been covalently attached to soluble HA, this is the first instance of covalent binding to cross-linked HA. To synthesize these materials, a WSC is used to couple adipic dihydrazide to the carboxylic acid functions of the glucuronic acid moieties on HA (45,46). Polyhydrazides were then used to cross-link the HA. The resulting hydrogels were stable over a range of pH values, as well as significantly less susceptible to degradation by hyaluronidase. Drug molecules may also be incorporated into the hydrogels through reaction with the polyhydrazide cross-linker chains. To illustrate this concept, hydrocortisone was immobilized to HA hydrogels via a polyhydrazide cross-linker (46). Hydrocortisone was released from the backbone of the HA hydrogels through cleavage by porcine liver esterase, whereas hyaluronidase did not affect the release of hydrocortisone.

HA has been shown to have antithrombotic activity, inhibiting platelet adhesion and aggregation. Stainless steel stents have been coated with HA in order to impart better blood compatibility to the metal surfaces (47). In arteriovenous shunts in baboons, coating of stents or stainless steel tubes with HA resulted in a significant reduction in platelet deposition on all coated surfaces. In the case of stents, $0.82 \pm 0.2 \times 10^9$ platelets adhered to coated stents, compared with $1.83 \pm 0.23 \times 10^9$ platelets on uncoated control surfaces. In addition, HA is inherently angiogenic and thus may encourage endothelialization of vascular implants (41).

PU vascular grafts have also been coated with a photopolymerizable form of HA (48). A photoreactive thyminated HA was prepared by the reaction of the tributylamine salt of HA with 1-(2-carboxyethyl)thymine. The photocurable HA was then cast on PU grafts and exposed to UV light. These grafts were implanted in the infrarenal abdominal aorta of dogs. However, the stability of the gel on the graft surface was not optimal, as thrombi formed in areas of the graft where the HA gel had either detached or not been evenly coated.

Sulfation of HA to form a compound referred to as HyalS has been performed to create antithrombogenic coatings upon vascular graft materials such as PET. The anticoagulant activity of HA is related to its degree of sulfation, where a high degree of sulfation leads to increasing anticoagulant performance (49). Similar to heparin, HyalS possesses the ability to inactivate thrombin and is repellent to platelets due to the high density of negative charges. HyalS has been immobilized on PET films in patterns by photolithography (32,49,50). To accomplish this, sulfated HA was coupled to azidoaniline using WSC, cast onto PET, and photoirradiated in the presence or absence of a photomask (Fig. 3). Following exposure to platelet-rich plasma, platelet adhesion occurred preferentially in areas without immobilized HyalS. In vitro thrombus formation on HyalS-modified PET was found to be significantly reduced (32,49). In addition, endothelial cells spread on these surfaces and tended to migrate to regions that contained immobilized HyalS (49). Due to the ability of the HyalS coating to impart hemocompatibility on the PET surface, as well as encourage endothelial cell attachment, its use as a vascular graft coating appears promising.

HA hydrogels also appear to stimulate angiogenesis. A hyaluronate-rich stroma often accompanies cell migration in developing or remodeling tissues (46). Vascular ingrowth in these tissues is associated with an increase in hyaluronidase and a decrease in hyaluronic acid concentration (46). Degradation fragments of hyaluronic acid ranging in length from 4 to 25 disaccharides have been shown to promote angiogenesis (41). Addition of HA oligosaccharides to a collagen gel stimulated the ingrowth of endothelial cells into the collagen and formation of capillary-like tubes in vitro (51). Stimulation of angiogenesis in vivo has been achieved with polypyrrole(PP)-hyaluronic acid composite materials (52). PP is an electrically conducting material that has been shown to support the growth of neural and endothelial cells in vitro (29,53). Electrical stimulation of neuron-like cells on a PP substratum resulted in a twofold enhancement of neurite outgrowth compared with unstimulated controls. The synthesis of PP requires the incorporation of a negatively charged dopant molecule, which facilitates the addition of the negatively charged HA to form PP-HA composites. Following in vivo subcutaneous implantation for 2 weeks, PP-HA films exhibited a twofold enhancement of vascularization in the vicinity of the implant compared with PP-poly(styrenesulfonate) (PP-PSS) controls. In addition, the blood vessels surrounding the PP-HA implants were significantly larger than those surrounding the control materials.

III. POLYPEPTIDES

A. Hirudin

Hirudin is a 65-amino-acid polypeptide originally derived from the salivary glands of the leech *Hirudo medicinalis* that acts as an anticoagulant through its ability to inhibit thrombin. Unlike heparin, hirudin is able to directly inhibit thrombin without interaction with ATIII. Thrombin that is already bound to clots or extracellular matrices can also be inactivated by hirudin, whereas heparin is ineffective in this situation (54). Hirudin, unlike heparin, is not inactivated by platelet factor 4, histidine-rich glycoprotein, or vitronectin. These advantages, coupled with the emergence of recombinant hirudin (rHir) and synthetic hirudin, have caused its gain in popularity as an anticoagulant.

Hirudin has been covalently attached to the surfaces of PET vascular grafts in order to improve their blood compatibility (55,56). To synthesize these materials, bovine serum albumin (BSA) was reacted with the heterobifunctional cross-linker sulfosuccinimidyl 4-(N-maleimidomethyl)cyclohexane-1-carboxylate (sulfo-SMCC). These BSA-SMCC complexes were then covalently bound to hydrolyzed PET via a water-soluble carbodiimide. rHir was modified to create sulfhydryl groups using Traut's reagent (2-iminothiolane hydrochloride) and then covalently linked to the PET-BSA-SMCC surfaces. Hirudin grafted to surfaces in this manner retained biological activity as determined by thrombin inhibition. Immobilization of hirudin to other vascular graft materials, such as PUs, has also been investigated (57–59). In these studies, hirudin was immobilized onto poly(carbonate urea)urethane grafts via the scheme described above for PET. The immobilized hirudin maintained its ability to bind and inhibit thrombin.

Covalent immobilization of rHir on poly(D,L-lactide-co-glycolide) (PLG) has also been achieved using glutaraldehyde as a coupling reagent (60). This system is unique in that PLG is a biodegradable polymer. This study aimed to create a blood-compatible, biodegradable material for use in applications where temporary reconstruction or stabilization of tissue or organs is needed, an example being vascular stents or stent coatings. Surface modification of PLG with rHir resulted in decreased platelet adhesion and activation, as well as slightly prolonged coagulation times (partial thromboplastin time) and a decreased clot formation rate of whole blood in contact with the modified polymer.

One concern that has arisen with the use of hirudin is the irreversible binding of hirudin to thrombin (60). This leads to loss of bioactivity of the immobilized peptide over time.

IV. ENZYMES

Although enzymes have many medical applications, their use is restricted by temperature sensitivity, pH limitations, and the possibility of inactivation by a variety of biological agents. The simple adsorption of enzymes to a material does not always alleviate these problems, as the adsorption is reversible, and the enzyme is often still susceptible to any deactivating influence, such as other enzymes or antibodies. Matrix entrapment of enzymes has also been explored, with the disadvantage that the catalytic activity appears to occur near the surface of the particles, indicating that most of the loaded enzyme is wasted (61). Enzyme immobilization offers many advantages over the use of free enzymes. Immobilization of enzymes results in enzyme stabilization and greater resistance to thermoinactivation and pH inactivation as well as decreased sensitivity to the action of endogenous inhibitors and proteases (62). In addition, immobilized enzymes often exhibit decreased toxicity and antigenicity.

A. Streptokinase

Streptokinase is a streptococcal protein that accelerates fibrinolysis and can thus be useful for thrombolytic therapy. Streptokinase catalyzes the conversion of inactive plasminogen to active plasmin (Fig. 5). Systemic use of free streptokinase as a fibrinolytic agent has been successful, although the foreign nature of the protein has elicited an adverse response (63).

Streptokinase has been immobilized to poly(methacrylic acid-*g*-ethylene oxide) [P(MAA-g-EO)] (64). Enzymes are typically more stable in a hydrophilic environment, making these polymers suitable for streptokinase immobilization. In addition, this material contains PEO, which has been shown to decrease the immunogenicity of enzymes, presumably by forming a hydrophilic steric barrier to shield the antigenic determinants of the enzyme (64). To immobilize streptokinase on P(MAA-g-EO), the carboxyl groups of MAA were activated using a WSC to form an *O*-acylisourea derivative that easily reacts with the terminal amine of the

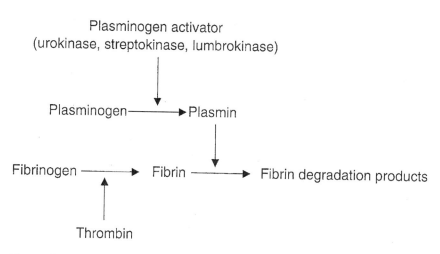

Figure 5   Urokinase, streptokinase, and lumbrokinase can initiate the fibrinolytic cascade.

enzyme to result in an amide bond linkage between the polymer and enzyme. The fibrinolytic activity of the materials was examined through a clot lysis assay, where increasing streptokinase content of the polymer led to a decrease in clot lysis time, indicating the maintenance of enzyme activity following immobilization.

B. Lumbrokinase

Lumbrokinase (LK) is another fibrinolytic enzyme. This enzyme is a plasminogen activator purified from the earthworm *Lumbricus rubellus* and can convert plasminogen to plasmin to cause fibrinolysis. Lumbrokinase is also capable of degrading fibrin directly in the absence of plasminogen.

Using polyallylamine as a photoreactive linker, lumbrokinase has been immobilized onto a PU total artificial heart valve (65). Polyallylamine was spray-coated onto PU valves and then exposed to UV light to induce the amine groups. A WSC was used to couple lumbrokinase to the aminated PU surface. Following implantation in lambs, treated valves exhibited fibrinolytic activity that was threefold that of unmodified PU. Overall, LK-treated valves led to decreased thrombus formation in vivo.

PU has also been modified with LK for the purpose of creating a more blood-compatible vascular graft surface (66–68). Methanol-extracted PU was coated with maleic anhydride methylvinyl ether copolymer (MAMEC) and incubated with a solution of LK. This reaction resulted in the stable immobilization of LK on the PU surface. Immobilized LK retained 34% of its activity, and was stable against thermal inactivation and degradation. Implantation of this LK-functionalized PU material in an ex vivo rabbit arterio-arterial shunt model demonstrated significantly prolonged occlusion time over control surfaces.

C. Urokinase

Urokinase is another enzyme that converts plasminogen to the active enzyme plasmin (Fig. 5). Urokinase may also inhibit platelet aggregation through mechanisms independent of the generation of plasmin (69). Urokinase has been investigated to increase the hemocompatibility of blood-contacting synthetic materials such as PU and expanded polytetra-fluoroethylene (ePTFE). Using MAMEC as a carrier, urokinase was immobilized on PU as described above for LK (70). In vitro analysis of these materials demonstrated no platelet adhesion to the modified surfaces and no significant adsorption of serum proteins, such as fibrinogen, fibronectin, and von Willebrand factor (vWF). The PU-urokinase surfaces catalyzed fibrinolysis as well as the digestion of clotting factors. Urokinase has been immobilized to ePTFE (71), PVC (72), poly(2-hydroxyethyl methacrylate) [p(HEMA)] (73), ethylene vinyl acetate (74), and collagen (75). Cross-linking urokinase to p(HEMA) via ^{60}Co irradiation resulted in greater pH and thermal stability of the enzyme, as well as more resistance to inactivation by plasma protease inhibitors (73). Furthermore, thrombus formation on these materials was greatly reduced. Urokinase-modified collagen was synthesized via activation of collagen carboxyl groups with acyl azide, and reaction with the amine groups of urokinase (75). This collagen solution can then be used as a coating on various materials, including polyethylene and polypropylene. Again, the immobilized urokinase was more stable than the free enzyme, and it retained its fibrinolytic properties.

D. Asparaginase

Asparaginase (ASNase) is an enzyme purified from *Escherichia coli* that has been found to be effective for the treatment of various leukemias. ASNase catalyzes the hydrolysis of L-asparagine into L-aspartic acid and ammonia. The cause of its antileukemic activity is the fact that L-asparagine is required for the proliferation of many types of leukemia cells, and ASNase depletes the blood of this essential amino acid. Normal cells are not as sensitive to this ASNase depletion, as they constitutively express asparagine synthetase, which catalyzes the synthesis of asparagine from aspartic acid. Due to its rapid blood clearance, frequent systemic injections of ASNase are required for effective therapy. In addition, the nature of its origin (from *E. coli*) often results in hypersensitivity reactions.

While ASNase has been coupled to many water-soluble polymers in order to prolong its half-life, ASNase can also be incorporated into an implantable hydrogel "bioreactor" (76,77). To synthesize these hydrogels, ASNase was combined with BSA and PEG-dinitrophenylcarbonate at a basic pH. After 50 days of incubation in vitro, the immobilized ASNase retained over 90% of its activity, compared with a half-life of 2 days for free ASNase. Peritoneal implantation of these hydrogels in rats decreased serum asparagine levels to an undetectable level for 6 days following implantation, at which time the hydrogels still retained 80% of their enzymatic activity (77).

V. GROWTH FACTORS

Polypeptide biological signals involved in the regulation of cell growth and differentiation, as well as in the control of specific metabolic processes, are known as growth factors. The term "growth factor" does not always accurately describe the function of these molecules, as they often do not promote growth. Instead, growth factors modulate cellular activities and often have varied effects in different cell types. They are capable of eliciting a wide variety of responses from an equally diverse array of tissues and cell types. Many different growth factors have been described in the literature (78), and they demonstrate potential for applications ranging from the acceleration of dermal wound healing to the induction of bone growth into implanted biomaterials (79). Modification of biomaterials with growth factors may target activity to the desired tissue and may maintain an effective dosage for a prolonged period of time.

A. Epidermal Growth Factor

Epidermal growth factor (EGF) is a 53-amino-acid, 6-kDa polypeptide that is mitogenic for many of the cell types involved in wound healing. It has been administered topically (79) and delivered from polymeric devices to achieve accelerated keratinocyte division and epidermal regeneration in vivo (80), in addition to increasing wound tear strength and collagen synthesis (81). The need for repeated applications of EGF limits its therapeutic use in wound healing, but its immobilization to biomaterials may provide a solution to this problem.

EGF has been covalently coupled to amine-modified glass via a star PEO spacer molecule (82). In this scheme, the EGF retained significant mobility and assumed its active conformation. The tethered EGF demonstrated bioactivity equivalent to soluble EGF, eliciting DNA synthesis and cell rounding responses in primary rat hepatocytes. In addition, the immobilized EGF was more effective than physically adsorbed EGF, which showed no activity.

EGF has also been immobilized to surface-hydrolyzed polymethyl methacrylate (PMMA) in order to examine its mitogenic activity while covalently bound to a solid substrate (83). Compared with unconjugated EGF and EGF bound to water-soluble polyacrylic acid, the immobilized EGF on PMMA exhibited maximal mitogenic effects.

EGF has also been immobilized on polystyrene surfaces in distinct patterns through a photoreaction (84). Photoreactive EGF was formed through reaction with polyallylamine coupled with N-[4-(azidobenzoyl)-oxy]succinimide. UV irradiation of the modified EGF on polystyrene resulted in the attachment of EGF to the polymer surface, and enhanced cell growth was observed on these materials.

B. Basic Fibroblast Growth Factor

Basic fibroblast growth factor (bFGF) is a potent mitogen for a variety of cell types and is involved in angiogenesis and wound healing. It is a single, 16-kDa, heparin-binding peptide that, along with its receptors, can be found in essentially all tissues in the body. Upon injection or ingestion into the body, bFGF is rapidly degraded. Diffusional delivery of bFGF from polymer matrices has resulted in a loss of 99% of its mitogenic activity (79). Because bFGF strongly binds heparin, covalently heparinized materials have been created to achieve complexation of bFGF to the material, thereby retaining the growth factor's activity and promoting the growth of endothelial cells (33,35,85,86). This approach has been specifically investigated for the endothelialization of vascular grafts. The extracellular matrix (ECM), particularly heparan sulfate proteoglycans, functions as a storage pool for bFGF, and tissue damage leads to the release of bFGF, inducing endothelial cell proliferation (87). Binding of bFGF to heparinized materials is thought to potentially mimic this mechanism for cell growth.

Heparin and bFGF have been coimmobilized on PU grafts either directly or through a cross-linked gelatin gel. Aortic implantation of the PU-gelatin-heparin-bFGF grafts resulted in significantly accelerated endothelial growth on the graft surface compared with PU-gelatin controls (85). The extent of endothelial cell coverage in heparin/bFGF grafts was $58.3 \pm 19.6\%$, compared with $29.4 \pm 9.8\%$ for controls. Perianastomotic migration of endothelial cells was significantly greater in heparin/bFGF grafts, as was the thickness of the neoarterial wall. This regeneration occurred via both perianastomotic and transmural tissue ingrowth.

C. Transforming Growth Factor β

The actions of transforming growth factor β (TGF-β) include the regulation of cellular proliferation, differentiation, and ECM metabolism. The active form of TGF-β is a homodimer of 12- to 15-kDa subunits linked by a disulfide bond. A conserved loci of seven cysteines within the sequence forms a rigid cysteine knot that provides stability for the protein structure (79).

One obstacle in the development of a tissue-engineered vascular graft is obtaining sufficient mechanical strength to prevent burst failure of the graft. The mechanical properties of vascular tissues are largely related to the amount and composition of ECM proteins in the tissue. TGF-β increases the ECM protein production of both smooth muscle cells and endothelial cells without affecting their proliferation (88). The proliferation of smooth muscle cells in this instance is not desirable, as it may lead to thickening of the graft wall. TGF-β has been covalently attached to PEG through reaction with acryloyl-PEG-N-hydroxysuccinimide with the amine terminus of TGF-β. This polymer was then blended with PEG-diacrylate derivatives and photopolymerized to form cross-linked hydrogels (89). Tethering this growth factor to photopolymerized PEG hydrogels actually increased the ability of TGF-β to stimulate ECM protein production by vascular smooth muscle cells relative to soluble TGF-β. This effect is believed to result from the ability of cells to interact with TGF-β via the appropriate receptors, while not being able to internalize it.

VI. HORMONES

A. Insulin

Insulin is a 51-amino-acid polypeptide composed of two chains linked by a disulfide bridge. It is synthesized and secreted exclusively by the β cells of the islets of Langerhans in the pancreas in response to elevated blood glucose levels. Initially, it is produced in the form of a large precursor called preproinsulin, then processed to the intermediate precursor, proinsulin, in order to finally obtain the mature form of insulin. Insulin decreases blood glucose by increasing the cellular uptake and utilization of glucose (78). Insulin also regulates the use and storage of molecules such as glucose, amino acids, fatty acids, and ketone bodies. An additional effect of insulin is its ability to stimulate cell proliferation by interaction with cell surface receptors. Immobilization of insulin onto biomaterials has been investigated as a means to increase cell growth.

The mitogenic effects of immobilized insulin on fibroblasts have been examined on surface-hydrolyzed PMMA films (90–95). Immobilized insulin exhibits 10- to 100-fold greater mitogenic activity than that observed for free insulin. In addition to the increase in efficacy, the duration of this effect is prolonged with the insulin-modified PMMA materials. Introduction of a α-ω-diaminopolyoxyethylene (POE) spacer molecule between the PMMA and insulin via reaction with a water-soluble carbodiimide resulted in further enhancement of cell growth (92). It is believed that the superior activity of immobilized insulin over free insulin is due to the prevention of internalization (93). Coimmobilization of insulin with fibronectin (92) or a cell-adhesive peptide sequence such as RGDS (91) has also resulted in enhanced mitogenic effects on fibroblasts. The synergistic effect of insulin and fibronectin together was evidenced by a threefold increase in growth rate over that of fibroblasts on unmodified materials, compared with only a 1.8-fold increase for immobilized insulin alone.

Insulin-immobilized PUs have been developed as another strategy to enhance vascular graft endothelialization. In one study, amine groups were introduced on the surface of PU via glow-discharge treatment in the presence of ammonia gas (96). These amine groups were then coupled to insulin using either dimethyl suberimidate (DMS) or WSC. DMS proved to be a better coupling agent choice, as insulin-modified PU produced by this method caused superior endothelial cell growth compared with materials prepared using the WSC. Cell growth was 1.4-fold higher on immobilized insulin materials than on materials with free insulin, and materials with immobilized insulin stimulated cell growth more so than materials to which insulin had been adsorbed. While the immobilization of collagen alone on these surfaces did not affect the endothelial cell growth, the coimmobilization of collagen with insulin may be necessary to maintain endothelial cells on the material surface for extended periods of time. The endothelial cells cultured on surfaces with both collagen and insulin exhibited a significant increase in prostacyclin production ($360 \pm 25 \, \text{pg}/10^5$ cells·days) versus insulin-immobilized ($336 \pm 25 \, \text{pg}/10^5$ cells·days) and control ($274 \pm 20 \, \text{pg}/10^5$ cells·days) materials.

It is also possible to attach insulin to PU via PEO spacer chains. Graft polymerization of acrylic acid on oxygen plasma glow-discharge–treated PU, and subsequent coupling with PEO and insulin results in an insulin-immobilized PU surface (26,97). These modifications not only increase the hydrophilicity of the material, thereby theoretically decreasing its thrombogenicity, but they also encourage fibroblast cell growth through the insulin immobilization. In the case of insulin, however, the length of the PEO spacer chain was not found to have an effect on cell proliferation.

PET has been covalently modified with insulin (98). The PET was partially hydrolyzed, and the insulin and adhesion factors were coimmobilized via reaction with a WSC. While fibroblast adhesion to the surfaces was enhanced by the adhesion factors alone, only the immobilization of insulin led to an acceleration of cell growth. Because fibronectin and polylysine were capable of promoting only cell adhesion, and insulin enhanced cell growth without affecting cell adhesion, it can be concluded that the mitogenic effect of immobilized insulin was due to the biospecific interaction of insulin with cell receptors.

B. Prostaglandins

Prostacyclin is a naturally occurring eicosanoid belonging to the prostaglandin family. Produced by endothelial cells, it acts as a vasodilator and reduces platelet aggregation. The anticoagulant action of prostaglandins is believed to stem from their ability to stimulate membrane-bound adenyl cyclase, thereby raising intracellular cAMP levels within platelets and inhibiting their adhesion and aggregation (99).

Due to the short half-life of soluble prostacyclin, immobilization is an attractive option for its use as an antithrombotic agent. Polyetherurethane urea (PEUU) has been coupled to a chemically stable prostacyclin analogue, 10,10 difluoro-13-dehydroprostacyclin (DF_2-PGI_2) (100). The PEUU was exposed to albumin, treated with plasma glow discharge, and then exposed to DF_2-PGI_2 in order to immobilize the prostacyclin. Negligible platelet adherence was observed on the surfaces, even in the presence of inducing agents such as fibrinogen, thrombin, and adenosine diphosphate.

The prostaglandin $PGF_{2\alpha}$ has been immobilized onto PVA hydrogels through the reaction of a $PGF_{2\alpha}$-polylysine adduct with gluteraldehyde (101), as well as to polystyrene (PS) using a diaminoalkane spacer molecule (102). However, as $PGF_{2\alpha}$ does not itself inhibit platelet adhesion and aggregation, it must be converted to the active yet hydrolytically unstable prostacyclin, PGI_2. Following this conversion, platelet adhesion to PS-PGI_2 was 6% of that on PS alone, and platelet aggregation on control PS surfaces was fourfold higher than on PS-PGI_2 (102). Another active form of prostacyclin, PGE_1, has been immobilized on polycarbonate (PC) surfaces (103). To bind PGE_1, albuminated PC was activated by the addition of glutaraldehyde and then reacted with PGE_1. These modifications reduced platelet adhesion on PC (1.4 ± 1 platelets/field of view for PC-PGE_1, compared with 7.0 ± 1.5 platelets/field of view for PC control), and also increased the PRT from 204 ± 5.5 s to 246.5 ± 6.5 s.

VII. NITRIC OXIDE DONORS

Constitutive nitric oxide synthase produced by endothelial cells (eNOS) converts L-arginine to L-citrulline and nitric oxide (NO) (104). NO acts as a vasodilator and also inhibits platelet activation, adhesion, and aggregation. NO activates soluble guanylate cyclase by binding to its heme moiety, thus leading to elevation of intracellular cyclic guanosine monophosphate (cGMP), which then activates a cGMP-dependent protein kinase (104). Activation of this second-messenger system prevents the platelets from becoming activated. Another result of NO synthesis is the impairment of intracellular calcium flux, which does not allow the conformational change of glycoprotein IIb/IIIa needed for fibrinogen binding and platelet aggregation (105). NO has also been shown to reversibly inhibit smooth muscle cell proliferation through a cGMP-dependent mechanism (106). The in vivo half-life of NO is approximately 0.1 s, and NO is capable of diffusing readily across biological membranes (107). Due to the multiple beneficial effects of NO, it is attractive for use as a therapeutic agent for the prevention of restenosis or for improvement of vascular graft or stent performance.

A number of compounds that spontaneously produce NO under physiologic conditions, called NO donors, have been identified and function to mimic the normal biological functions of endogenous NO. Several classes of NO donor molecules exist, including S-nitrosothiols and NO–nucleophile complexes (1-substituted diazen-1-ium-1,2-diolates, or NONOates) (108). Both diazeniumdiolate and S-nitrosothiol NO donors have demonstrated properties of increasing vasodilation (109), inhibiting platelet aggregation (110,111), and inhibiting smooth muscle cell migration (106). These donors have been administered systemically or locally via diffusional release from various polymers (112,113).

Diazeniumdiolates can be attached to pendant groups of a polymer or introduced into the polymer backbone itself to provide NO release for up to 5 weeks (114). Diazeniumdiolates attached to cross-linked PEI inhibited the in vitro proliferation of smooth muscle cells when added to cell culture media in powdered form. PTFE vascular grafts were also coated with the PEI-NO polymer and implanted in a baboon arteriovenous shunt model. Platelet adhesion to the NO-modified grafts was decreased almost fivefold compared with control materials. Cross-linked microspheres composed of NO-releasing PEI have also been formed and incorporated into PTFE vascular grafts (115). These microspheres remained entrapped within the graft, even following immersion and completion of NO release. Diazeniumdiolate NO donors have also been covalently bound to hydrophobic polymer films constructed from PU and PVC (116). NO release from these materials ranged from 10 to 72 h, and the NO-modified polymers successfully reduced platelet adhesion in vitro.

Hydrogels formed from copolymers of PEG with NO donors have also been synthesized to achieve NO delivery for periods of time ranging from hours to months (4). Poly(L-lysine) (DP = 5), diethylenetriamine (DETA), and cysteine (Cys) have been covalently attached to PEG through reaction with acryloyl-PEG-N-hydroxysuccinimide. The amine groups of Lys_5 and DETA react with NO gas to form diazeniumdiolates, and the thiol group on cysteine reacts with sodium nitrite at acidic pH to form S-nitrosocysteine. The polymers of PEG-Lys_5-NO, PEG-DETA-NO, or PEG-Cys-NO were then blended with PEG-diacrylate derivatives and photopolymerized under UV light to form cross-linked hydrogels. Exposure of blood to the NO-generating hydrogels resulted in decreased platelet adhesion to thrombogenic surfaces (Fig. 6), whereas smooth muscle cell growth was completely inhibited in the presence of the PEG-NO hydrogels. These types of materials can be formed as thin coatings on the luminal surface of arteries following

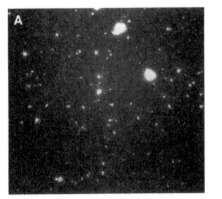
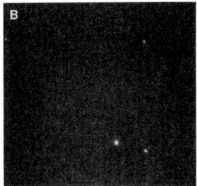

Figure 6   Fluorescence micrographs of platelets adherent to collagen I–coated glass after exposure to (A) PEG-diacrylate hydrogels or (B) PEG-Cys-NO hydrogels. (From Ref. 4.)

angioplasty or stent deployment to provide highly localized treatment for the prevention of thrombosis and restenosis (3).

VIII. DIPYRIDAMOLE

Dipyridamole is a potent, nontoxic inhibitor of platelet adhesion and aggregation, as well as an inhibitor of vascular smooth muscle cell proliferation. Vasodilation by dipyridamole occurs through several mechanisms, including direct stimulation of prostacyclin release from the vascular endothelium and potentiation of prostacyclin activity.

Dipyridamole (Persantin) has been immobilized onto PU materials for use as vascular grafts (117–120). It has been chemically derivatized with an arylazide photoreactive moiety, p-azidophenyl. Photoimmobilization of dipyridamole on PU then occurs upon exposure to UV light, where photochemical excitation of the p-azidophenyl group leads to formation of a cyclic heterocumulene structure that reacts with nucleophilic sites formed at the polymer surface, enabling covalent immobilization of the drug on the polymer. As in the case of heparin, use of a spacer molecule enhances the efficacy of dipyridamole. Modification of PU with dipyridamole has successfully decreased platelet adhesion and activation on these surfaces in vitro. The APTT times were significantly prolonged with modified materials (784–1279 s) compared with controls (569 s), and the thrombin concentration was reduced on dipyrimadole-modified surfaces (118). In addition, the coating appears to promote endothelialization of the graft surface (119). However, in vivo studies employing these materials were not as successful. Following implantation in goats for 10 weeks, dipyridamole-modified grafts did not exhibit an increase in graft patency over unmodified control surfaces.

IX. ANTINEOPLASTIC AGENTS

Daunomycin is an antineoplastic agent belonging to the anthracycline class of antibiotics isolated from cultures of *Streptomyces peucetius*. The use of daunomycin is limited by a chronic, cumulative, dose-related toxicity resulting in irreversible congestive heart failure (121). It is currently used as part of the treatment regimen for acute myeloid leukemia. Its antineoplastic action is due to its ability to intercalate into the stacked bases of DNA to inhibit cell replication.

Daunomycin can be incorporated into biodegradable polyaldehyde guluronate (PAG) hydrogels through a labile covalent bond (122). Adipic dihydrazide was used to graft the drug into the polymer backbone and then cross-link the polymer to form hydrogels. Hydrolysis of the covalent hydrazone linkage between drug and polymer results in sustained release of daunomycin, with maintenance of antitumor activity.

Adriamycin is also an antineoplastic antibiotic currently used in the chemotherapy treatment of several types of cancers, including breast cancer, ovarian cancer, thyroid cancer, and neuroblastoma (121). It has been shown that immobilization of adriamycin onto agarose through carbamate linkages for localized delivery results in a significant reduction in the toxic side effects of the drug, such as abdominal adhesions, inflammatory peritonitis, and cardiac toxicity (123). However, the immobilized drug remains active and can effectively kill rapidly dividing cells. The primary amine group on adriamycin also enables it to be coupled to other polymeric supports, such as PVA (124,125). Immobilization of adriamycin on PVA is more stable and leads to lower drug release rates than those found with agarose materials.

X. ANTI-INFLAMMATORY AGENTS

Salicylic acid, the active component of aspirin, is commonly used as an anti-inflammatory agent with a wide spectrum of medical applications. Polymers have been synthesized to incorporate salicylic acid into the polymer backbone (126–128). These polyanhydride esters are composed of alkyl chains linked by ester bonds to salicylic acid. Degradation occurs via cleavage of the ester bonds, thus yielding salicylic acid as a degradation product. This polymeric prodrug material has applications for use in Crohn's disease, a chronic inflammation of the intestine, or inflammatory bowel syndrome. In these conditions, release of salicylic acid from the polymer via degradation would be targeted to the lower intestine due to enhanced degradation in the basic pH environment. These polymers may also be used for wound closure or wound healing products, where they could not only release an anti-inflammatory agent, but also function as a biodegradable scaffold for cell adhesion and growth and tissue regeneration.

XI. CONCLUSIONS

The development of localized delivery systems of pharmacologically active substances is driven by many factors, including the desire to increase drug efficacy and decrease toxic systemic effects. As many substances are too toxic to administer systemically at therapeutic levels (i.e., antineoplastic agents), site-specific therapy provides a promising alternative. Local administration of antithrombotic agents, such as heparin and hirudin, may help avoid bleeding complications often seen when they are infused systemically. Schemes involving synthetic matrices that allow for diffusional release of biologically active molecules have been widely investigated, using endless combinations of polymers and active molecules. These drug delivery systems have often met with success in a variety of applications. However, the ability to immobilize the bioactive substance to a solid substrate frequently allows for increased drug stability, prolonged drug lifetime, and sometimes even increased drug activity. Materials covalently modified with pharmacologically active materials have displayed great potential for use in applications ranging from increasing hemocompatibility to the treatment of cancer and tissue engineering, and the development of additional material–drug combinations is an ongoing field of study.

REFERENCES

1. SK Williams. Endothelial cell transplantation. Cell Transplant 4:401–410, 1995.
2. GW Bos, AA Poot, T Beugeling, WG van Aken, J Feijen. Small-diameter vascular graft prostheses: current status. Arch Physiol Biochem 106:100–115, 1998.

3. JL Hill-West, SM Chowdhury, MJ Slepian, JA Hubbell. Inhibition of thrombosis and intimal thickening by in situ photopolymerization of thin hydrogel barriers. Proc Natl Acad Sci USA 91:5967–5971, 1994.

4. KS Bohl, JL West. Nitric oxide-generating polymers reduce platelet adhesion and smooth muscle cell proliferation. Biomaterials 21:2273–2278, 2000.

5. BR Landzberg, WH Frishman, K Lerrick. Pathophysiology and pharmacological approaches for prevention of coronary artery restenosis following coronary artery balloon angioplasty and related procedures. Prog Cardiovasc Dis 39:361–398, 1997.

6. SR Hanson, LA Harker. Blood coagulation and blood–materials interactions. In: BD Ratner, AS Hoffman, FJ Schoen, JE Lemons, eds. Biomaterials Science. San Diego: Academic Press, 1996, pp 193–199.

7. DW Barritt, SC Jordan. Anticoagulant drugs in the treatment of pulmonary embolism: a controlled trial. Lancet 1: 1309–1312, 1960.

8. T Okada, DM Bark, MR Mayberg. Localized release of perivascular heparin inhibits intimal proliferation after endothelial injury without systemic anticoagulation. Neurosurgery 25:892–898, 1989.

9. ER Edelman, DH Adams, MJ Karnovsky. Effect of controlled adventitial heparin delivery on smooth muscle cell proliferation following endothelial injury. Proc Natl Acad Sci USA 87:3773–3777, 1990.

10. D Teomim, I Fishbein, G Golomb, L Orloff, M Mayberg, AJ Domb. Perivascular delivery of heparin for the reduction of smooth muscle cell proliferation after endothelial injury. J Controlled Release 60:129–142, 1999.

11. CD Ebert, SW Kim. Heparin polymers for the prevention of surface thrombosis. Med Appl Controlled Release 2:77, 1984.

12. C Nojiri, KD Park, DW Grainger, HA Jacobs, T Okada, H Koyanagi, SW Kim. In vivo nonthrombogenicity of heparin immobilized polymer surfaces. ASAIO Trans 36:M168–M172, 1990.

13. C Ebert, J McRea, SW Kim. Controlled release of antithrombotic agents from polymer matrices. In: R Baker, ed. Controlled Release of Bioactive Materials. New York: Academic Press, 1980, pp 107–122.

14. CA Hufnagel, PW Conrad, JF Gillespie, R Pifarre, A Ilano, T Yokoyama. Characteristics of materials for intravascular application. Ann N Y Acad Sci 146:262–270, 1968.

15. M Chorny, I Fishbein, G Golomb. Drug delivery systems for the treatment of restenosis. Crit Rev Ther Drug Carr Sys 17:249–284, 2000.

16. G Golomb, M Mayberg, AJ Domb. Polymeric perivascular delivery systems. In: Domb AJ, ed. Polymeric Site-Specific Pharmacotherapy. New York: Wiley, 1994, p 205.

17. SW Kim. Nonthrombogenic treatments and strategies. In: BD Ratner, AS Hoffman, FJ Schoen, JE Lemons, eds. Biomaterials Science. San Diego: Academic Press, 1996, pp 297–307.

18. Y Byun, HA Jacobs, SW Kim. Heparin surface immobilization through hydrophilic spacers: thrombin and antithrombin III binding kinetics. J Biomater Sci Polym Ed 6:1–13, 1994.

19. Y Byun, HA Jacobs, SW Kim. Binding kinetics of thrombin and antithrombin III with immobilized heparin using a spacer. ASAIO J 38:M649–M653, 1992.

20. MD Lelah, SL Cooper. Polyurethane in Medicine. Boca Raton: CRC Press, 1986, pp 57–60.

21. DK Han, SY Jeong, YH Kim. Evaluation of blood compatibility of PEO grafted and heparin immobilized polyurethanes. J Biomed Mater Res 23:211–228, 1989.

22. DK Han, KD Park, KD Ahn, SY Jeong, YH Kim. Preparation and surface characterization of PEO-grafted and heparin immobilized polyurethanes. J Biomed Mater Res 23:87–104, 1989.

23. IK Kang, OH Kwon, YM Lee, YK Sung. Preparation and surface characterization of functional group-grafted and heparin-immobilized polyurethanes by plasma glow discharge. Biomaterials 17:841–847, 1996.

24. IK Kang, OH Kwon, MK Kim, YM Lee, YK Sung. In vitro blood compatibility of functional group-grafted and heparin-immobilized polyurethanes prepared by plasma glow discharge. Biomaterials 18:1099–1107, 1997.

25. AZ Piao, HA Jacobs, KD Park, SW Kim. Heparin immobilization by surface amplification. ASAIO J 38:M638–M643, 1992.

26. YJ Kim, IK Kang, MW Huh, SC Yoon. Surface characterization and in vitro blood compatibility of poly(ethylene terephthalate) immobilized with insulin and/or heparin using plasma glow discharge. Biomaterials 21:121–130, 2000.

27. CH Cholakis, MV Sefton. In vitro platelet interactions with a heparin-polyvinyl alcohol hydrogel. J Biomed Mater Res 23:399–415, 1989.

28. D Grainger, J Feijen, SW Kim. Poly(dimethylsiloxane)-poly(ethylene oxide)-heparin block copolymers, I: Synthesis and characterization. J Biomed Mater Res 22:231–242, 1988.

29. B Garner, B Georgevich, AJ Hodgson, L Liu, GG Wallace. Polypyrrole-heparin composites as stimulus-responsive substrates for endothelial cell growth. J Biomed Mater Res 44:121–129, 1999.

30. B Seifert, T Groth, K Herrmann, P Romaniuk. Immobilization of heparin on polylactide for application to degradable biomaterials in contact with blood. J Biomater Sci Polym Ed 7:277–287, 1995.

31. SW Tay, EW Merrill, EW Salzman, J Lindon. Activity toward thrombin–antithrombin of heparin immobilized on two hydrogels. Biomaterials 10:11–15, 1989.

32. Y Ito. Micropattern immobilization of polysaccharide. J Inorg Biochem 79:77–81, 2000.

33. GW Bos, NM Scharenborg, AA Poot, GHM Engbers, T Beugeling, WG van Aken, J Feijen. Proliferation of endothelial cells on surface-immobilized albumin-heparin conjugate loaded with basic fibroblast growth factor. J Biomed Mater Res 44:330–340, 1999.

34. GW Bos, NM Scharenborg, AA Poot, GHM Engbers, JG Terlingen, T Beugeling, WG van Aken, J Feijen. Adherence and proliferation of endothelial cells on surface-immobilized albumin-heparin conjugate. Tissue Eng 4:267–279, 1998.

35. MJB Wissink, R Beernink, AA Poot, GHM Engbers, T Beugeling, WG van Aken, J Feijen. Improved endothelialization of vascular grafts by local release of growth factor from heparinized collagen matrices. J Controlled Release 64:103–114, 2000.

36. SE Sakiyama-Elbert, JA Hubbell. Development of fibrin derivatives for controlled release of heparin-binding growth factors. J Controlled Release 65:389–402, 2000.

37. P Bulpitt, D Aeschlimann. New strategy for chemical modification of hyaluronic acid: preparation of functionalized derivatives and their use in the formation of novel biocompatible hydrogels. J Biomed Mater Res 47:152–169, 1999.

38. H Iwata. Pharmacologic and clinical aspects of intraarticular injection of hyaluronate. Clin Orthop 289:285–291, 1993.

39. NE Larsen, EA Balazs. Drug delivery systems using hyaluronan and its derivatives. Adv Drug Deliv Rev 7:279–293, 1991.

40. J Drobnik. Hyaluronan in drug delivery. Adv Drug Deliv Rev 7:295–308, 1991.

41. DC West, IN Hampson, F Arnold, S Kuman. Angiogenesis induced by degradation products of hyaluronic acid. Science 228:1324–1326, 1985.

42. EA Balazs, A Leshchiner. U.S. Patent 4,605,691, 1986.

43. T Malson, P Algvere, L Aivert, B Lindqvist, G Selen, S Stenkula. Cross-linked hyaluronate gels for use in vitreous surgery. In: A Pizzoferrato, PG Marchetti, A Ravaglioli, AJC Lee, eds. Biomaterials and Clinical Applications. Amsterdam: Elsevier, 1987, pp 345–348.

44. K Tomihata, Y Ikada. Crosslinking of hyaluronic acid with water-soluble carbodiimide. J Biomed Mater Res 37:243–251, 1997.

45. KP Vercruysse, DM Marecak, JF Marecek, GD Prestwich. Synthesis and in vitro degradation of new polyvalent hydrazide cross-linked hydrogels of hyaluronic acid. Bioconjug Chem 8:686–694, 1997.

46. GD Prestwich, DM Marecak, JF Marecek, KP Vercruysse, MR Ziebell. Controlled chemical modification of hyaluronic acid: synthesis, applications, and biodegradation of hydrazide derivatives. J Controlled Release 53:93–103, 1998.

47. S Verheye, CP Markou, MY Salame, B Wan, SB King, KA Robinson, NA Chronos, SR Hanson. Reduced thrombus formation by hyaluronic acid coating of endovascular devices. Arterioscler Thromb Vasc Biol 20:1168–1172, 2000.

48. H Kito, T Matsuda. Biocompatible coatings form luminal and outer surfaces of small-caliber artificial grafts. J Biomed Mater Res 30:321–330, 1996.

49. R Barbucci, A Magnani, R Rappuoli, S Lamponi, M Consumi. Immobilisation of sulphated hyaluronan for improved biocompatibility. J Inorg Biochem 79:119–125, 2000.

50. G Chen, Y Ito, Y Imanishi, A Magnani, S Lamponi, R Barbucci. Photoimmobilization of sulfated hyaluronic acid for antithrombogenicity. Bioconjug Chem 8:730–734, 1997.

51. R Montesano, S Kumar, L Orci, MS Pepper. Synergistic effect of hyaluronan oligosaccharides and vascular endothelial growth factor on angiogenesis in vitro. Lab Invest 75:249–262, 1996.

52. JH Collier, JP Camp, TW Hudson, CE Schmidt. Synthesis and characterization of polypyrrole-hyaluronic acid composite biomaterials for tissue engineering applications. J Biomed Mater Res 50:574–584, 2000.

53. CE Schmidt, VR Shastri, JP Vacanti, R Langer. Stimulation of neurite outgrowth using an electrically conducting polymer. Proc Natl Acad Sci USA 94:8948–8953, 1997.

54. SR Bailey. Local drug delivery: current applications. Prog Cardiovasc Dis 40:183–204, 1997.

55. RK Ito, MD Phaneuf, FW LoGerfo. Thrombin inhibition by covalently bound hirudin. Blood Coag Fibrinol 2:77–81, 1991.

56. MD Phaneuf, SA Berceli, MJ Bide, WC Quist, FW LoGerfo. Covalent linkage of recombinant hirudin to poly(ethylene terephthalate) (Dacron): creation of a novel antithrombin surface. Biomaterials 18:755–765, 1997.

57. MD Phaneuf, DJ Dempsey, MJ Bide, M Szycher, WC Quist, FW LoGerfo. Bioengineering of a novel small diameter polyurethane vascular graft with covalently bound recombinant hirudin. ASAIO J 44:M653–M658, 1998.

58. MD Phaneuf, M Szycher, SA Berceli, DJ Dempsey, WC Quist, FW LoGerfo. Covalent linkage of recombinant hirudin to a novel ionic poly(carbonate) urethane polymer with protein binding sites: determination of surface antithrombin activity. Artif Organs 22:657–665, 1998.

59. DJ Dempsey, MD Phaneuf, MJ Bide, M Szycher, WC Quist, FW LoGerfo. Synthesis of a novel small diameter polyurethane vascular graft with reactive binding sites. ASAIO J 44:M506–M510, 1998.

60. B Seifert, P Romaniuk, T Groth. Covalent immobilization of hirudin improves the haemocompatibility of polylactide-polyglycolide in vitro. Biomaterials 18:1495–1502, 1997.

61. CG Gebelein. Methodologies in polymeric medication. In: CG Gebelein, CE Carraher, eds. Polymeric Materials in Medication. New York: Plenum Press, 1985, pp 1–10.

62. VP Torchilin, AV Maksimenko, AV Mazaev. Immobilized enzymes for thrombolytic therapy. Meth Enzymol 137:552–566, 1988.

63. JM Schor, V Steinberger, E Tutko, S Aboulafia, IJ Pachter, R Jacobsen. Fibrolytic enzymes. In: JM Schor, ed. Chemical Control of Fibrinolysis–Thrombolysis. New York: Wiley-Interscience, 1970, pp 114–118.

64. RK Drummond, NA Peppas. Fibrinolytic behaviour of streptokinase-immobilized poly(methacrylic acid-g-ethylene oxide). Biomaterials 12:356–360, 1991.

65. Y Park, E Ryu, H Kim, J Jeong, J Kim, J Shim, S Jeon, Y Jo, W Kim, B Min. Characterization of antithrombotic activity of lumbrokinase-immobilized polyurethane valves in the total artificial heart. Artif Organs 23:210–214, 1999.

66. GH Ryu, S Park, DK Han, YH Kim, B Min. Antithrombotic activity of a lumbrokinase immobilized polyurethane surface. ASAIO J 39:M314–M318, 1993.

67. GH Ryu, S Park, M Kim, DK Han, YH Kim, B Min. Antithrombogenicity of lumbrokinase-immobilized polyurethane. J Biomed Mater Res 28:1069–1077, 1994.

68. GH Ryu, DK Han, S Park, M Kim, YH Kim, B Min. Surface characteristics and properties of lumbrokinase-immobilized polyurethane. J Biomed Mater Res 29:403–409, 1995.

69. SR Torr-Brown, BE Sobel. Antiplatelet effects of urokinase and their clinical implications. Coron Artery Dis 7:63–68, 1996.

70. Y Kitamoto, M Tomita, S Kiyama, T Inoue, Y Yabushita, T Sato, H Ryoda, T Sato. Antithrombotic mechanisms of urokinase immobilized polyurethane. Thrombosis 65:73–76, 1991.

71. RI Forster, F Bernath. Analysis of urokinase immobilization on the polytetrafluoroethylene vascular prosthesis. Am J Surg 156:130–132, 1988.

72. A Sugitachi, M Tanaka, T Kawahara, N Kitamura, K Takagi. A new type of drain tube. Artif Organs 5:69, 1981.

73. LS Liu, Y Ito, Y Imanishi. Biological activity of urokinase immobilized to cross linked poly(2-hydroxyethyl methacrylate). Biomaterials 12:545–549, 1991.

74. T Ohshiro, MC Liu, J Kambayashi, T Mori. Clinical applications of urokinase-treated material. Meth Enzymol 137:529–545, 1988.

75. S Watanabe, Y Shimizu, T Teramatsu, T Murachi, T Hino. The in vitro and in vivo behavior of urokinase immobilized onto collagen-synthetic polymer composite material. J Biomed Mater Res 15:553–563, 1981.

76. J Jean-François, G Fortier. Immobilization of L-asparaginase into a biocompatible poly(ethylene glycol)-albumin hydrogel: I: Preparation and in vitro characterization. Biotechnol Appl Biochem 23:221–226, 1996.

77. J Jean-François, EM D'Urso, G Fortier. Immobilization of L-asparaginase into a biocompatible poly(ethylene glycol)-albumin hydrogel: evaluation of performance in vivo. Biotechnol Appl Biochem 26:203–212, 1997.

78. E Pimentel. Handbook of Growth Factors. Volume 2. Peptide Growth Factors. Boca Raton: CRC Press, 1994.

79. NE Nimni. Polypeptide growth factors: targeted delivery systems. Biomaterials 18:1201–1225, 1997.

80. GL Brown, LB Nanney, J Griffen, AB Cramer, JM Yancey, LJ Curtsinger 3d, L Holtzin, GS Schultz, MJ Jurkiewicz, JB Lynch. Enhancement of wound healing by topical treatment with epidermal growth factor. N Engl J Med 321:76–79, 1989.

81. N Celebi, N Erden, B Gonul, M Koz. Effects of epidermal growth factor dosage forms on dermal wound strength in mice. J Pharm Pharmacol 46:386–387, 1994.

82. PR Kuhl, LG Griffith-Cima. Tethered epidermal growth factor as a paradigm for growth factor-induced stimulation from the solid phase. Nat Med 2:1022–1027, 1996.

83. Y Ito, JS Li, T Takahashi, Y Imanishi, Y Okabayashi, Y Kido, M Kasuga. Enhancement of the mitogenic effect by artificial juxtacrine stimulation using immobilized EGF. J Biochem 121:514–520, 1997.

84. Y Ito, G Chen, Y Imanishi. Micropatterned immobilization of epidermal growth factor to regulate cell function. Bioconjug Chem 9:277–282, 1998.

85. K Doi, T Matsuda. Enhanced vascularization in a microporous polyurethane graft impregnated with basic fibroblast growth factor and heparin. J Biomed Mater Res 34:361–370, 1997.

86. C Gosselin, D Ren, J Ellinger, HP Greisler. In vivo platelet deposition on polytetrafluoroethylene coated with fibrin glue containing fibroblast growth factor 1 and heparin in a canine model. Am J Surg 170:126–130, 1995.

87. A Baird. Potential mechanisms regulating the extracellular activities of basic fibroblast growth factor (FGF-2). Mol Reprod Dev 39:43–48, 1994.

88. BK Mann, AT Tsai, T Scott-Burden, JL West. Modification of surfaces with cell adhesion peptides alters extracellular matrix deposition. Biomaterials 20:2281–2286, 1999.

89. BK Mann, RH Schmedlen, JL West. Tethered-TGF-beta increases extracellular matrix production of vascular smooth muscle cells. Biomaterials 22:439–444, 2001.

90. Y Ito, J Zheng, Y Imanishi, K Yonezawa, M Kasuga. Protein-free cell culture on an artificial substrate with covalently immobilized insulin. Proc Natl Acad Sci USA 93:3598–3601, 1996.

91. JS Li, Y Ito, J Zheng, T Takahashi, Y Imanishi. Enhancement of artificial juxtacrine stimulation of insulin by co-immobilization with adhesion factors. J Biomed Mater Res 37:190–197, 1997.

92. Y Ito, M Inoue, SQ Liu, Y Imanishi. Cell growth on immobilized cell growth factor. 6. Enhancement of fibroblast cell growth by immobilized insulin and/or fibronectin. J Biomed Mater Res 27:901–907, 1993.

93. SQ Liu, Y Ito, Y Imanishi. Cell growth on immobilized cell growth factor. 4: Interaction of fibroblast cells with insulin immobilized on poly(methyl methacrylate) membrane. J Biochem Biophys Meth 25:139–148, 1992.

94. SQ Liu, Y Ito, Y Imanishi. Cell growth on immobilized cell growth factor. 7. Protein-free cell culture by using growth-factor-immobilized polymer membrane. Enzyme Microb Technol 15:167–172, 1993.

95. Y Ito, SQ Liu, Y Imanishi. Enhancement of cell growth on growth factor–immobilized polymer film. Biomaterials 12:449–453, 1991.

96. SQ Liu, Y Ito, Y Imanishi. Cell growth on immobilized cell growth factor. 9. Covalent immobilization of insulin, transferrin, and collagen to enhance growth of bovine endothelial cells. J Biomed Mater Res 27:909–915, 1993.

97. EJ Kim, IK Kang, MK Jang, YB Park. Preparation of insulin-immobilized polyurethanes and their interaction with human fibroblasts. Biomaterials 19:239–249, 1998.

98. Y Ito, J Zheng, Y Imanishi. Enhancement of cell growth on a porous membrane co-immobilized with cell-growth and cell adhesion factors. Biomaterials 18:197–202, 1997.

99. S Moncada, JR Vane. The role of prostacyclin in vascular tissue. Fed Proc 38:66–71, 1979.

100. G Joseph, CP Sharma. Prostacyclin immobilized albuminated surfaces. J Biomed Mater Res 21:937–945, 1987.

101. G Llanos, MV Sefton. Immobilization of prostaglandin $PGF_{2\alpha}$ on poly(vinyl alcohol). Biomaterials 9:429–434, 1988.

102. CD Ebert, ES Lee, SW Kim. The antiplatelet activity of immobilized prostacyclin. J Biomed Mater Res 16:629–638, 1982.

103. T Chandy, CP Sharma. The antithrombotic effect of prostaglandin E1 immobilized on albuminated polymer matrix. J Biomed Mater Res 18:1115–1124, 1984.

104. PL Feldman, OW Griffith, DJ Stuehr. The surprising life of nitric oxide. Chem Eng News 71:26–38, 1993.

105. J Loscalzo. Nitric oxide and restenosis. Clin Appl Thromb Hemostas 2:7–10, 1996.

106. R Sarkar, EG Meinberg, JC Stanley, D Gordon, RC Webb. Nitric oxide reversibly inhibits the migration of cultured vascular smooth muscle cells. Circ Res 78:225–230, 1996.

107. J Loscalzo, G Welch. Nitric oxide and its role in the cardiovascular system. Prog Cardiovasc Dis 38:87–104, 1995.

108. CM Maragos, D Morley, DA Wink, TM Dunams, JE Saavedra, A Hoffman, AA Bove, L Isaac, JA Hrabie, LK Keefer. Complexes of NO with nucleophiles as agents for the controlled biological release of nitric oxide—vasorelaxant effects. J Med Chem 34:3242–3247, 1991.

109. JG Diodati, AA Quyyumi, LK Keefer. Complexes of nitric oxide with nucleophiles as agents for the controlled biological release of nitric oxide: hemodynamic effect in the rabbit. J Cardiovasc Pharmacol 22:287–292, 1993.

110. DS Marks, JA Vita, JD Folts, JF Keaney Jr, GN Welch, J Loscalzo. Inhibition of neointimal proliferation in rabbits after vascular injury by a single treatment with a protein adduct of nitric oxide. J Clin Invest 96:2630–2638, 1995.

111. JG Diodati, AA Quyyumi, N Hussain, LK Keefer. Complexes of nitric oxide with nucleophiles as agents for the controlled biological release of nitric oxide: antiplatelet effect. Thromb Haem 70:654–658, 1993.

112. ZL Yin, GJ Dusting. A nitric oxide donor (spermine-NONOate) prevents the formation of neointima in rabbit carotid artery. Clin Exp Pharmacol Physiol 24:436–438, 1997.

113. A Chaux, XM Ruan, MC Fishbein, Y Ouyang, S Kaul, JA Pass, JM Matloff. Perivascular delivery of a nitric oxide donor inhibits neointimal hyperplasia in vein grafts implanted in the arterial circulation. J Thorac Cardiovasc Surg 115:604–612, 1998.

114. DJ Smith, D Chakravarthy, S Pulfer, ML Simmons, JA Hrabie, ML Citro, JE Saavedra, KM Davies, TC Hutsell, DL Mooradian, SR Hanson, LK Keefer. Nitric oxide-releasing polymers containing the [N(O)NO]-group. J Med Chem 39:1148–1156, 1996.

115. SK Pulfer, D Ott, DJ Smith. Incorporation of nitric oxide-releasing crosslinked polyethyleneimine microspheres into vascular grafts. J Biomed Mater Res 37:182–189, 1997.
116. KA Mowery, MH Schoenfisch, JE Saavedra, LK Keefer, ME Meyerhoff. Preparation and characterization of hydrophobic polymeric films that are thromboresistant via nitric oxide release. Biomaterials 21:9–21, 2000.
117. YB Aldenhoff, LH Koole. Studies on a new strategy for surface modification of polymeric biomaterials. J Biomed Mater Res 29:917–928, 1995.
118. YB Aldenhoff, AP Pijpers, LH Koole. Synthesis of a new photoreactive derivative of dipyridamole and its use in the manufacture of artificial surfaces with low thrombogenicity. Bioconjug Chem 8:296–303, 1997.
119. YB Aldenhoff, FH van der Veen, J ter Woorst, J Habets, LA Poole-Warren, LH Koole. Performance of a polyurethane vascular prosthesis carrying a dipyridamole (Persantin) coating on its lumenal surface. J Biomed Mater Res 54:224–233, 2001.
120. YB Aldenhoff, R Blezer, T Lindhout, LH Koole. Photo-immobilization of dipyridamole (Persantin) at the surface of polyurethane biomaterials: reduction of in-vitro thrombogenicity. Biomaterials 18:167–172, 1997.
121. WD Glanze, KN Anderson, LE Anderson, eds. The Signet Mosby Medical Encyclopedia. New York: Signet, 1996.
122. KH Bouhadir, GM Kruger, KY Lee, DJ Mooney. Sustained and controlled release of daunomycin from cross-linked poly(aldehyde gul5uronate) hydrogels. J Pharm Sci 89:910–919, 2000.
123. MP Hacker, JS Lazo, CA Pritsos, TR Tritton. Immobilized adriamycin: toxic potential in vivo and in vitro. Sel Cancer Ther 5:67–72, 1989.
124. LB Wingard, K Narasimhan. Immobilization of a primary amine-containing drug, adriamycin. Coupling to crosslinked polyvinyl alcohol and mechanistic comparison of hydrolytic stability. Appl Biochem Biotechnol 19:117–127, 1988.
125. LB Wingard, TR Tritton, KA Egler. Cell surface effects of adriamycin and carminomycin immobilized on cross-linked polyvinyl alcohol. Cancer Res 45:3529–3536, 1985.
126. L Erdmann, C Campo, C Bedell, K Uhrich. Polymeric prodrugs: novel polymers with bioactive components. ACS Symp Ser 709:83–91, 1998.
127. E Krogh-Jespersen, T Anastasiou, K Uhrich. Synthesis of a novel aromatic polyanhydride containing aminosalicylic acid. Polym Prepr 41:1048–1049, 2000.
128. L Erdmann, C Campo, D Palms, K Uhrich. Polymer prodrugs with pharmaceutically active degradation products. Polym Prepr 38:570–571, 1997.

18

Biomimetic Lung Surfactant Replacements

Cindy W. Wu and Annelise E. Barron
Northwestern University, Evanston, Illinois

I. INTRODUCTION

Pulmonary surfactant, or lung surfactant (LS), is a natural biomaterial that coats the internal surfaces of mammalian lungs and enables normal breathing. It is a complex mixture composed of about 90% lipids and about 10% surfactant proteins (SPs). Both fractions are critical for its physiological function, which is to decrease the work of breathing by regulating surface tension at the air–liquid interface of the alveoli (the network of air sacs that perform gas exchange within the lung) as a function of alveolar surface area (1,2). A deficiency of functional LS in premature infants results in the development of neonatal respiratory distress syndrome (RDS) (3), a leading cause of infant mortality. Two-thirds of infants born preterm are affected by RDS, with 60% of the incidence in infants born before 28 weeks of gestation (4). Left untreated, an infant with RDS will die. This has led to the development of exogenous lung surfactant replacements that can, if delivered within minutes of birth, either prevent RDS or mitigate its effects.

Exogenous surfactant replacement therapy (SRT) is now a standard form of care in the clinical management of premature infants with RDS. The impact of SRT on neonatal health was demonstrated by a dramatic reduction of 31% in the RDS mortality rate in the United States between 1989 and 1990 (5). In terms of the number of infants involved, another study showed that the incidence of deaths from RDS in the United States dropped from 5498 in 1979 to 1460 in 1995 (6). Each year, about 40,000 infants in the United States are afflicted with neonatal RDS (7), whereas worldwide the number exceeds 2 million (8).

Currently, there are eight different surfactant replacement formulations commercially available for the treatment of RDS (4,9–14). These formulations can be divided into two different classes: "natural" and "synthetic" LS replacements. So-called natural LS replacements are prepared from animal lungs by lavage or by mincing, followed by extraction of surfactant materials with organic solvents and purification. Synthetic surfactant replacements, on the other hand, are always protein free and are made from a blend of synthetic phospholipids with added chemical agents (generally, either lipid or detergent molecules) that facilitate adsorption and spreading of the material at the surface of the lungs.

Motivated by concerns that natural LS replacements are animal derived and hence carry risks of pathogen transmission, whereas the presently available synthetic formulations are less efficacious, extensive research has been conducted on the development of a third, not-yet-commercial class of formulations: biomimetic LS replacements. Formulations of this class are designed to closely mimic the biophysical characteristics and physiological performance of natural LS while not sharing its precise molecular composition. To date, most biomimetic LS formulations contain synthetic phospholipid mixtures in combination with either recombinantly derived or chemically synthesized polypeptide analogues of the hydrophobic surfactant proteins (8,15–33). The successful creation of a good biomimetic LS replacement will facilitate better, and safer, treatment of a medical syndrome that afflicts premature infants throughout the world. A formulation that offers the efficacy of animal surfactant, as well as the safety and relatively low cost of synthetic products, would not only improve current treatment protocols but would offer a feasible product for treating infants in nonindustrialized countries where the cost of currently available replacements remains prohibitive. In addition, there is evidence that a nonimmunogenic biomimetic LS would have applications in the treatment of other lung diseases that have surfactant dysfunction as an element of their pathogenesis, including meconium aspiration syndrome, congenital pneumonia, and acute RDS (34–36).

II. RESPIRATORY DISTRESS SYNDROME

Typically, the premature lungs of infants born after less than 32 weeks' gestation will either have insufficient amounts of, or be completely devoid of, pulmonary surfactant. This deficiency results in higher than normal alveolar surface tension and alveolar instability, factors that lead to the rapid development of respiratory distress syndrome, which is manifested as an inability to breathe and an inability to be respired without secondary lung trauma. RDS is a leading cause of infant mortality in the industrialized world. Since the pioneering efforts of Fujiwara et al. (9), numerous clinical trials have shown the efficacy of the administration of exogenous LS replacements for the rescue of these infants. Surfactant replacement therapy (SRT) improves lung compliance and oxygenation, and hence decreases the requirements for inspired oxygen, reduces the incidence of pulmonary complications, and, most importantly, increases the survival rate (9,37–43). Clearly, exogenous SRT is a successful means of treating premature infants at risk of developing RDS. However, there is a percentage of neonates who do not respond well to LS replacements, for reasons that we will briefly discuss and that remain poorly understood (44,45). Hence, improvements in the current therapeutic biomaterial and its method of administration are still required. Toward this end, researchers have worked on the development of a completely biomimetic LS replacement formulation that will be functional, safe, and cost effective.

III. HISTORICAL PERSPECTIVE ON THE PHYSIOLOGICAL ROLE OF LS AND THE CAUSES OF RDS

The history of LS research dates back to the late 1920s, when von Neergaard illustrated the significance of surface tension in pulmonary physiology. In his demonstration, von Neergaard showed that a greater pressure is required to expand an atelectatic (i.e., collapsed) lung with air, rather than a saline solution, and surmised that this was a result of differences in the relative magnitudes of surface tension forces on the alveoli (46). However, it was not until the mid-1950s that Pattle (2) and Clement (1,47) showed the existence of a surface-active material in the lungs that naturally reduces surface tension.

Shortly after the initial discovery of surface-active agents in the lung in 1959, Avery and Mead demonstrated that a lack of surfactant was central to the pathophysiology of RDS in neonates (3). Specifically, they showed that the deficiency or dysfunction of surfactant reduces lung compliance by increasing surface tension forces at the air–water interface of the alveoli. This knowledge led to the isolation of pulmonary surfactant from calf lung in 1961 (48). After it was recognized that dipalmitoylphosphatidylcholine (DPPC) is a major constituent of the LS mixture (48), clinical trials were conducted to test the efficacy of the first synthetic LS formulation, which was composed of DPPC and delivered as an aerosol (49,50). However, trials were unsuccessful; DPPC alone does not adequately mimic natural LS because of the rigidity of the monolayer that it forms at the air–water interface (51–53).

It was not until 1980 that surfactant replacement therapy became a reality in the treatment of neonatal RDS. That year, Fujiwara et al. successfully rescued 10 preterm infants who were suffering from severe RDS by intratracheal bolus instillation of a bovine-derived LS (9). Although these authors called their bovine surfactant replacement "semiartificial," by today's convention it would be known as natural because it was extracted from animal lungs. Since then, LS replacement treatment has become standard care for preterm infants with RDS. If infants with RDS survive surfactant replacement therapy (requiring up to 4 doses, every 6–8 h after birth), they generally begin to secrete their own pulmonary surfactant within 96 h (54,55).

Although animal-derived LS replacements have been used with success for neonate rescue, improvements to further increase survival rate and to decrease the cost per patient are still needed. Toward this end, researchers are working to develop a new class of biomimetic LS replacements that capture the advantages of both natural and synthetic formulations. In order to design a functional replacement for a complex biomaterial such as pulmonary surfactant, it is necessary to understand the properties of the natural substance and to recognize aspects of the current therapy that require improvement. Therefore, we begin with an introduction to the molecular composition and the biophysical functioning of LS, before discussing strategies for and reviewing recent progress in the development of a useful biomimetic LS replacement.

IV. BIOSYNTHESIS OF LS

Lung surfactant is synthesized in alveolar type II epithelial cells and is stored intracellularly in dense, multilayered membrane structures, referred to as *lamellar bodies* (56). The contents of the lamellar bodies are excreted into the alveoli (57), where they undergo a transformation to lattice-like, tubular double layers, referred to as *tubular myelin* (58,59), the main reservoir of surfactant (60), from which an LS monolayer at the air–liquid interface is formed (61,62) (Fig. 1). The efficient and rapid adsorption of the surfactant to the air–liquid interface imparts a dramatic reduction in alveolar surface tension, which is requisite for breathing.

V. PHYSIOLOGICAL ROLE OF LS

Pulmonary surfactant is a complex mixture of proteins and lipids that coats the internal surfaces of healthy mammalian lungs to enable normal

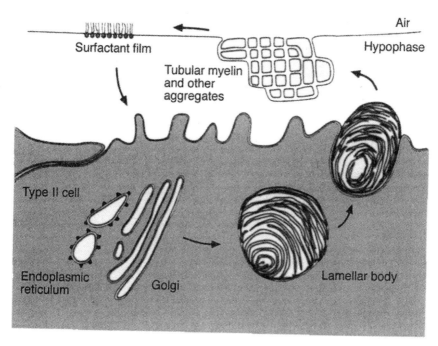

Air

Surfactant film   Hypophase

Tubular myelin
and other
aggregates

Type II cell

Endoplasmic
reticulum   Golgi   Lamellar body

Figure 1   A schematic diagram of natural pulmonary surfactant synthesis and transport to the alveolar surface. Pulmonary surfactant is synthesized in type II alveolar cells as a complex mixture of lipids and surfactant proteins, and assembled into lamellar bodies. These organelles are secreted and transformed into tubular myelin, which then adsorbs to the air–liquid interface where it functions to control the surface tension throughout the breathing cycle. Surfactant materials are eventually taken back into the type II cells for degradation and recycling. (From Ref. 276, with permission.)

respiration (2). By virtue of its unique surface-active properties, which we will soon describe, lung surfactant reduces the pressure required for alveolar expansion and decreases the work of breathing (1,63). Lung surfactant also stabilizes the alveolar network, preventing its collapse upon exhalation (53,64–66).

VI.   MOLECULAR COMPOSITION OF LS AND COMPONENT ROLES IN SURFACTANT ACTIVITY

Lung surfactant is composed of approximately 85–90% phospholipids, 5% neutral lipids, and 8–10% proteins (see Table 1) (66–70). The most abundant

Table 1 Molecular Composition of Lung Surfactant (66–70)

Components	Percentage (%)
Phospholipids	85–90
Phosphatidylcholine (PC)	68–72
Phosphatidylglycerol (PG)	8
Phosphatidylethanolamine (PE)	5
Phosphatidylinositol (PI)	3
Phosphatidylserine (PS)	Trace
Lysophophatidylcholine	Trace
Sphingomyelin	Trace
Neutral lipids	5
Cholesterol	
Cholesterol esters	
Surfactant proteins (SP)	8–10
Hydrophilic Proteins	
SP-A	5
SP-D	2
Hydrophobic Proteins	1.5
SP-B	
SP-C	

component is phosphatidylcholine (PC), which is generally dipalmitoylated and in the saturated form (DPPC). Phosphatidylglycerol (PG), an anionic lipid, accounts for another 8%. Also present are phosphatidylethanolamine (PE, about 5%), phosphatidylinositol (PI, about 3%), and trace amounts of phosphatidylserine (PS), lysophosphatidylcholine, and sphingomyelin. Some neutral lipids are also present, and include both cholesterol and cholesterol esters.

In vitro and in vivo biophysical experiments have shown that the most critical lipid molecules for reduction of alveolar surface tension are DPPC and PG. Although DPPC films are capable of reducing surface tension to near zero upon compression (i.e., DPPC monolayers can sustain high surface pressures before collapse), these phospholipids are slow to adsorb to an interface (51–53). The presence in LS of other, minor lipid components, in particular PG, has been shown to assist in the spreading of DPPC molecules at the air–water interface (52). However, such lipid mixtures alone are also ineffective as lung surfactant replacements because, under physiological conditions and in the absence of other spreading agents, DPPC and PG will not adsorb to the air–liquid interface with sufficient quickness or respread as rapidly as needed for breathing as alveolar surface area changes cyclically (71). Instead, a unique combination of protein-based surfactants function as the necessary spreading agents.

Actually, a total of four different surfactant-specific proteins (SP) are known to be present with phospholipids on the alveolar hypophase (i.e., the aqueous lining of the lung): SP-A, SP-B, SP-C, and SP-D (72). These proteins fall into two major subgroups: the hydrophilic surfactant proteins (SP-A and SP-D), and the hydrophobic, amphipathic surfactant proteins (SP-B and SP-C). SP-A and SP-D aid in the control of surfactant metabolism and also have important immunological roles for defense against inhaled pathogens (73,74). But for therapeutic LS replacements, it is the biophysical properties of surfactant as they affect the mechanical properties of the lung that are important for the treatment of RDS. Even though SP-A is involved in the ordering of LS phospholipids in the presence of calcium, it is typically omitted from LS replacements because it does not have a significant role in reducing surface tension and is also immunogenic (75). For the same reasons, SP-D is also omitted from surfactant replacements (76).

SP-B and SP-C are required for proper biophysical functioning of LS (77), enabling attainment of low surface tensions on the alveolar hypophase and endowing proper dynamic behavior to the mixed lipid monolayers and multilayers that are found there (78–80). It has been suggested by one study that SP-B and SP-C function in a nonsynergistic manner (81); yet, considering the strict conservation of both proteins in mammals and the significant differences in their structures, which we will discuss, it seems likely that each plays a role that is important and distinct in facilitating easy breathing. However, it has been difficult to deconvolute the individual roles of SP-B and SP-C (82). Both proteins have been found to facilitate the rapid adsorption of phospholipids to an air–water interface and to allow rapid respreading of phospholipids as the alveoli expand and contract. Both have a dramatic influence on monolayer phase behavior and reduce the surface tension on alveoli upon compression of surface area (81,83). A variety of studies indicate that SP-B is more effective in enhancing the adsorption rate and dynamic surface activity of phospholipids (81,84–87), particularly in refining the films of surfactant to have enriched DPPC content (88,89). It has been suggested that SP-C is more effective at promoting respreading and film formation from the collapsed phase (88–90).

Below we briefly describe the molecular structures and biophysical properties of the SP-B and SP-C proteins. The reader is referred to recent reviews (91–94) for more comprehensive and detailed discussions of their structure–function relationships.

VII. STRUCTURAL DESCRIPTION AND APPARENT PHYSIOLOGICAL ROLE OF SP-B

SP-B is a small, hydrophobic protein, composed of 79 amino acids, that has an unusually high cysteine content (Fig. 2A) (95–97). In the native SP-B protein, seven cysteine residues form a unique disulfide pattern that includes three intramolecular bonds and one intermolecular bond, the latter of which results in the formation of SP-B dimers (98–100). The numerous positively charged side chains scattered throughout the SP-B sequence are essential for its activity (33). Electrostatic interaction of these groups with negatively charged PG molecules is known to enhance respreading of the phospholipid film, as well as to cause refinement of the monolayer by the enrichment of the DPPC content of the film through the "squeeze-out" of other lipids at the air–liquid interface (52,101–106). The hydrophobic amino acids in the SP-B sequence are known to interact with lipid acyl chains (33). Spectroscopic studies have shown that the secondary structure of SP-B is dominated by α helices, which are likely to be amphipathic given their sequence distribution. The detailed tertiary structure of the protein has yet to be determined by nuclear magnetic resonance (NMR) or crystallographic studies (20,21,107–111).

In a structural model for SP-B that was proposed by Andersson et al., four amphipathic helices are aligned in an antiparallel, left-handed hairpin motif, where one helical face is hydrophobic and the other relatively hydrophilic, as illustrated in Figure 2B (110). With this tertiary structure,

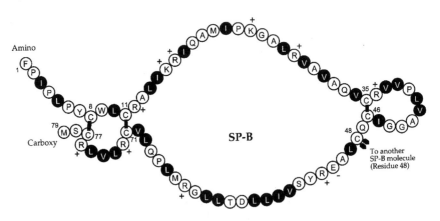

Figure 2A Primary structure of SP-B (human sequence). The identity of each amino acid is given by the one-letter code. Hydrophobic residues are shown in black, and charged residues are identified. (Adapted from Ref. 277, with permission.)

SP-B

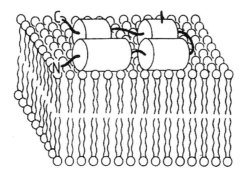

Figure 2B Hypothetical model of SP-B folded structure and its proposed mode of interaction with a phospholipid bilayer. SP-B is suggested to be a dimer of two identical 79-residue four-helix protein chains (cross-linked at Cys48, in the third helix), with the polar face of the amphipathic helix interacting with the lipid headgroups. (From Ref. 278, with permission.)

SP-B would be well suited to interact with a phospholipid monolayer or bilayer (80,112–114), with its polar (mostly cationic) faces interacting with lipid headgroups, particularly those of the anionic phospholipids (115), and the apolar faces interacting with acyl chains in the regions of the headgroup (91). Recently, another hypothetical structural model of SP-B, which reflects the homodimeric structure of native SP-B, was proposed by Zaltash et al. (116). In this model, the two SP-B monomers are linked by disulfide bond at Cys48, with the charged residues lying on one surface of the disk-like structure. The dimer is thought to be stabilized by hydrogen bonds or by ion pairs between Glu51 and Arg52 residues from each of the two monomers (116). This hinged, dimerized structure would provide correlated motion of SP-B monomers that interact with two different monolayers/bilayers, creating "cross-talk" between these organized lipid films (116).

Apparently the main physiological function of SP-B protein is to facilitate phospholipid adsorption to the air–liquid interface, thereby allowing rapid spreading and respreading of the surface tension–lowering phospholipids as alveoli expand and contract. In this way, SP-B has the effect of stabilizing the surface film. It has been shown that the ability of SP-B to induce rapid insertion of phospholipids into the monolayer is essential for the maintenance of alveolar integrity (33,84,85,96,117,118). Hence, SP-B may have a predominant role in facilitating the reduction of surface tension in the lungs. Besides these roles, SP-B may also serve the critical functions of aiding the formation of tubular myelin structures (119–121) and inducing the calcium-dependent fusion of membranes (119,122).

In vivo rescue experiments with premature rabbits (123), in vivo blocking of SP-B with monoclonal antibodies (124), and studies with genetically engineered SP-B-deficient mice (125,126) have all confirmed the critical role of SP-B in functional LS. Furthermore, recent studies of SP-B knockout mice revealed that the presence of covalently linked homodimers of SP-B appears to be important for the optimal functioning of natural LS (127,128). These studies, in addition to the fact that an inherited SP-B deficiency in infants is lethal (129,130), provide strong evidence for the predominant importance of SP-B in LS.

VIII. STRUCTURAL DESCRIPTION AND APPARENT PHYSIOLOGICAL ROLE OF SP-C

The smaller of the two hydrophobic surfactant proteins, SP-C, is composed of 35 amino acids and has an unusual dipalmitoyl modification near the carboxy terminus (Fig. 3A) (131,132). Two-thirds of the protein consists of a long, continuous, valyl-rich hydrophobic stretch, which adopts an α-helical secondary structure as evidenced by both circular dichroism (CD) and NMR structure determination (Fig. 3B) (133–135). The length of this helix, 37 Å, is perfect for the spanning of a fluid DPPC bilayer (136). Consistent with this observation, it has been shown in other studies that the

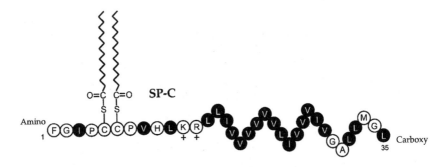

Figure 3A Primary structure of hydrophobic surfactant protein SP-C (human sequence). The identity of each amino acid is given by the one-letter code. Hydrophobic residues are shown in black, and charged residues are identified. The two cysteine residues are palmitoylated. (Adapted from Ref. 277, with permission.)

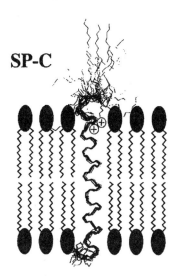

Figure 3B Schematic presentation of SP-C secondary structure and its proposed mode of interaction with a phospholipid bilayer. This SP-C structure was deduced by 2D-NMR, and in this picture is artificially superimposed on a lipid bilayer. In this transbilayer orientation, the hydrophobic part of the protein (residues 13–28) interacts with the lipid acyl chains, while the basic residues at position 11 and 12 (indicated by positive charges) interact with the polar (anionic) lipid headgroup. The two cysteine residues at positions 5 and 6 are palmitoylated; the role of these palmitoyl chains is still disputed in the literature. (From Ref. 278, with permission.)

SP-C α-helix is a transbilayer protein, with the α-helix oriented roughly parallel to the lipid acyl chains at the air–water interface (134,137). Other evidence suggests that in interactions with a DPPC *monolayer*, SP-C is situated to make a 70° tilt relative to the normal of the monolayer plane (138). The issue of whether SP-C preferentially interacts with an LS monolayer or with bilayer or multilayer structures is still under active investigation (82,114,139,140).

Palmitoylation of the two SP-C cysteines at positions 5 and 6 in the sequence has been proposed to promote protein interactions with lipid acyl chains in neighboring, stacked lipid bilayers (141), thereby facilitating SP-C binding to the bilayer (142) and/or orienting the peptide (143). However, the physiological function of the two palymitoyl chains, as well as their necessity for in vivo efficacy of LS replacements, remains to be fully understood (142,144,145). The two adjacent, positively charged lysine and arginine residues at positions 11 and 12 of SP-C most likely interact with the phospholipid headgroups and promote binding to the monolayer or bilayer by ionic interactions (146).

Similarly to SP-B, SP-C seems to promote phospholipid insertion into the air–liquid interface (108), and thereby to enhance the rate of lipid adsorption (145,147) and the respreading of the alveolar films upon inhalation (83). SP-C also stabilizes the surfactant film during the expansion and compression phases of breathing, apparently by regulating phospholipid ordering in such a fashion as to increase the lateral pressure within the bilayer (note that increased surface pressure, Π, correlates with decreased surface tension, γ) (121,148,149). Interestingly, the results of one study have suggested that a single SP-C molecule is capable of influencing the phase behavior of 20–35 lipid molecules (135). In addition, SP-C has been found to stimulate liposomal fusion in vitro (119) and to enhance the binding of lipid vesicles to a cell membrane for endocytosis of lipids (150,151).

In vivo studies of genetically engineered SP-C knockout mice have revealed that SP-C plays an important role in endowing function to LS but is seemingly less critical for breathing than SP-B. SP-C knockout mice are viable at birth and grow normally without altered lung development or function (152,153), but lung mechanics studies reveal abnormalities in lung hysteresivity at low lung volume (153). Furthermore, studies have shown that mutations in the human SP-C gene can result in the expression of an altered proprotein, the precursor that undergoes proteolytic cleavage to yield mature SP-C, which is believed to be involved in the development of interstitial lung disease (152). The deficiency of SP-C in some Belgian blue calves has been shown to increase the likelihood of RDS (154).

IX. INTERFACIAL PROPERTIES OF LS

The physiological roles of LS require it to adsorb and respread quickly upon inhalation and to reduce surface tension upon exhalation. These requirements can be satisfied by envisioning the surface film as being composed of monolayers highly enriched in DPPC, as well as bilayers/multilayers of lipid/protein structures that remain closely attached to the film (80,88). Both selective squeeze-out and insertion of lipids has been proposed to enrich the monolayer with DPPC to enable the attainment of low surface tension observed for LS during exhalation. However, upon reexpansion, DPPC is a poor spreading material. Instead, it is the unsaturated lipids and surfactant proteins that are responsible for the rapid adsorption and respreading of LS upon inhalation (114,140,157,163). These squeezed-out components are stored in multilayers that remain closely associated with the film at the interface (80,155) and respread into the surface film upon alveolar expansion

(156). Replenishment of the surface film occurs by adsorption from the subphase, and by respreading of collapsed phases and excluded material (114,140). The transferring of the lipids to the interface and the formation of surfactant film at the air–liquid interface is enhanced by the presence of the surfactant proteins SP-B and SP-C (157), which perturb the packing of the phospholipids (85,149,158,159).

X. RECONCILIATION OF LS'S DICHOTOMY OF ROLES AS A SURFACE-ACTIVE MATERIAL

For lung surfactant to work effectively, the films that are formed must be *fluid*, so that the material adsorbs and respreads quickly and reversibly to the alveolar interface, to form a monolayer upon expansion; yet it also needs to be *rigid* as a surface film, so that it reaches near-zero surface tension during the alveolar compression accompanying exhalation (82). Hence, there is a dichotomy of the roles of LS. To reconcile the dual actions of LS, the "squeeze-out" theory was postulated (52,53). This theory states that adsorption is facilitated by the presence of the fluidizing agents, which are subsequently removed upon compression, resulting in the formation of a DPPC-enriched monolayer to promote low surface tension (52,101–104). However, this theory does not account for the presence of the surfactant proteins or for their complex roles (80,83,105,160–162).

Recent investigations of LS phase behavior and surface film morphology and 2D phase behavior of different LS components have led to the development of the "monolayer-associated" theory (82). Contrary to the squeeze-out theory, this theory states that the surfactant proteins help to retain the unsaturated fluidizing components of LS within or near monolayers at all surface pressures, even at film collapse (i.e., at high surface pressures and low surface tensions) (82,163–166). Consistent with this, experiments conducted have shown that SP-B and SP-C *prevent* the squeeze-out of unsaturated lipids by altering the film collapse mechanism from a fracturing event to a more reversible buckling or folding of the monolayer (163,164). Particularly for SP-B, it appears that these folds remain in close association with the surface film, thereby allowing facile reincorporation of the material upon expansion (164). To a greater extent for SP-C, it has been observed that the lipid components that are removed from squeeze-out upon compression (83) are stored in a multilayered phase that remains closely attached to the interface (80,155), which upon expansion respreads into the surface film (156,157).

XI. LS REPLACEMENTS FOR TREATMENT OF RDS

Clearly, a good understanding of the surfactant proteins, and their structural links to the underlying mechanisms that endow lung surfactant with its extraordinary surface-active properties, will be critical for successful bioengineering design of a functional, biomimetic LS replacement. Elucidation of the interactions between the various components of this complex protein–lipid mixture entails deconvolution of the phase behavior of both the lipid and protein components. Intense study of whole LS and various fractions thereof in recent years has afforded a number of invaluable insights into the structure–function relationships between proteins and lipids (28,33,80,82,90,112,114,139,140,157,162,166–173), and is beginning to provide enough information to guide well-informed design of novel biomimetic LS replacements.

Delivery of an exogenous LS replacement to a preterm infant is a temporary intervention, intended to maintain respiratory function and to minimize lung injury until maturation of type II cells occurs, generally within 96 hours of birth, permitting an adequate amount of endogenous LS to be produced and transported to the alveolar surface (54,55). A good replacement must capture the physiological characteristics described earlier. In vivo, the surfactant needs to be capable of improving the stability of immature fetal lungs and of providing healthy pressure–volume characteristics to the alveolar network. In terms of in vitro biophysical properties and therapeutic characteristics, this translates to (a) rapid surface adsorption of LS, to generate an equilibrium surface tension of about 25 mN/m within 1 min (60); (b) reduction of the minimal alveolar surface tension to nearly zero upon cyclic compression, to prevent alveolar collapse and to maintain the patency of terminal bronchioles at expiration (174,175); and (c) effective respreading of surfactant after compression beyond the collapse pressure, to replenish surfactant materials during alveolar expansion and to ensure that the maximum surface tension does not rise above an equilibrium level of 25 mN/m during the breathing cycle (53,65,176). LS replacements must provide these benefits and should also be pure, safe, and bioavailable (i.e., they should have no viral, protein, or chemical contamination, and should not elicit an immune response). From a production standpoint and to facilitate wide availability, the ease of surfactant manufacturing, purification, quality control, and cost must also be considered. Therefore, an ideal LS replacement would be highly similar in its properties to the natural material and also cost effective.

From a design perspective, it is not only important to understand the physiological and biophysical activities of lung surfactant but also the factors that can inhibit its performance. LS can be inactivated by the presence of (a) plasma and blood proteins (albumin, fibrinogen, hemoglobin, etc.) (177–180); (b) unsaturated cell membrane phospholipids (178); (c) hysophospholipids (181); (d) cholesterol (182); (e) free fatty acids (183); (f) lytic enzymes (proteases and phospholipases) (184); (g) reactive radicals; and (h) meconium (first feces of a fetus) (185). Investigations of these endogenous molecules have shown that inactivation by these contaminants can, in general, be mitigated by increasing the LS concentration (177,186). This means that, potentially, a patient suffering from RDS or ARDS could be helped by the delivery of additional LS or of a functional replacement.

The design, testing, and benchmarking of any novel LS replacement necessitates in vitro characterization of the material by a number of different approaches, each of which evaluates surface activity in complementary ways. Those formulations that show promise in in vitro studies then undergo in vivo animal studies, including both pharmacological studies to determine the effectiveness of the formulation for treatment of RDS and toxicological studies to identify the proper dose regime. Only those therapeutic agents that are found to be both efficacious and safe in animals will progress to the next stage, in which human clinical trials are carried out in neonates (187).

XII. IN VITRO CHARACTERIZATION OF LS REPLACEMENTS

Three different experimental tools are used extensively to evaluate the surface-active properties of various natural and synthetic LS formulations, including (a) the Langmuir-Wilhelmy surface balance (LWSB), often used in conjunction with fluorescence microscopy (FM) to observe surface phase morphology; (b) the pulsating bubble surfactometer (PBS); and/or, (c) the captive bubble surfactometer (CBS). The Wilhelmy surface balance, first used by Clements for LS studies in 1957 (1), is designed to carry out cyclic film compression on a Langmuir trough and to allow accurate measurement of the very low surface tensions that are characteristic of LS at high levels of monolayer compression. The major utility of the LWSB in the study of LS replacements has been to allow the observation of surface pressure effects that occur within films that are spread directly onto the air–water interface (i.e., not adsorbed from the subphase), although adsorbed films are also sometimes studied. LWSB experiments allow the generation of pressure–area (Π-A) isotherms, as seen in Fig. 4, which are obtained during slow cycling of film surface area at dynamic but nonphysiological rates (188). In conjunction with the LWSB, FM can provide sensitive imaging of the phase

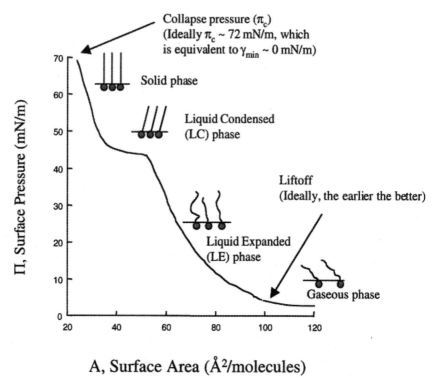

A, Surface Area (Å²/molecules)

Figure 4 Surface pressure–area (Π-A) isotherm of the compression of a hypothetical surfactant film that exhibits gaseous, liquid-expanded, liquid-condensed, and solid phases. As area decreases, the surface pressure increases until the film collapses. Typical lift-off and collapse pressure values of lung surfactant are depicted. (Adapted from Ref. 279, with permission.)

morphology of LS monolayers or multilayers as they undergo compression and expansion on the trough. Interactions between different lipid components and/or between lipids and surfactant proteins, as they influence the film behavior and phase morphology, can be imaged and then correlated with other measures of performance and surface activity, especially the Π-A isotherms (155,171,189).

The PBS was developed in 1977 by Enhorning (190) and applied to the study of LS behavior with the goal of obtaining more physiologically relevant data on the surface tension-lowering ability of dispersed pulmonary surfactants. Experiments carried out on a PBS can provide information on both equilibrium adsorption and dynamic film compression and expansion characteristics of a surfactant. Continuous measurements of surface tension are made on a cyclically expanding and contracting bubble surface covered with surfactant, and can be acquired at a physiological temperature (37°C), cycling rate (20 cycles/min), and film compression ratio (up to 50% area compression). This access to conditions mimicking those of the human lung is a major advantage of the technique. The resultant data are generally plotted as shown in Fig. 5, which shows a curve of surface tension as a function of bubble surface area (168). Particularly important are the low values of the minimal and maximal surface tensions observed during bubble compression and expansion, respectively, as well as the dramatic hysteresis

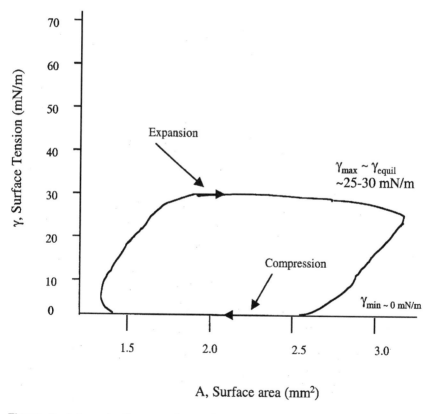

Figure 5 Schematic diagram of a typical surface tension (γ) versus interfacial bubble area (A) loop observed for calf lung surfactant (CLS) in 5 mM $CaCl_2$ and 0.15 M NaCl at 37°C, as measured during dynamic oscillations by a pulsating bubble surfactometer (PBS) at a frequency of 20 cycles/min and a bulk surfactant concentration of 1 mg/mL. (Adapted from Ref. 168, with permission.)

seen in the data curve. Here, of course, the bubble (typically ranging from about 0.8 to 1.0 mm in diameter) mimics a single alveolus. In addition to generating these curves that depict dynamic surface tension, one can also use the PBS to map out adsorption isotherms for LS (i.e., to create plots of surface tension γ versus time t), if the instrument is run in static mode (190–192).

Because of some initial concerns about a possible leakage of surfactant from the bubble surface to the capillary tube from which the bubble is suspended in a PBS, the CBS was developed in 1989 by Schürch et al. (193) to provide similar data with a lower likelihood of surfactant leakage (192,194,195). Therefore, many consider CBS data to be more reliable than PBS data (194). However, disadvantages of the CBS include its unavailability as a commercial instrument, and the time-consuming and complex nature of data analysis (192). In vitro characterization using the LWSB, PBS, and CBS can provide complimentary information. Standards for good in vitro performance have been established for these instruments and can now be used as evaluative parameters for biomimetic surfactant formulations under development.

XIII. IN VIVO CHARACTERIZATION OF LS REPLACEMENTS

Animal studies provide a necessary link between in vitro biophysical studies and clinical therapy. Multiple animal models of RDS have been established and have proven invaluable in the testing and evaluation of surfactant performance. Important evaluation parameters include (a) pressure–volume (P-V) lung mechanics (see Fig. 6); (b) lung functional parameters [i.e, arterial partial pressure of oxygen (PaO_2), arterial partial pressure of carbon dioxide ($PaCO_2$), and arterial/alveolar partial pressure of oxygen (a/AO_2)]; and (c) ventilator-associated parameters [i.e., ventilator rate, fraction of inspired oxygen (FiO_2), mean airway pressure (MAP), peak inspiratory pressure (PIP), and positive end-expiratory pressure (PEEP)]. Some common animal models used to evaluate the efficacy and safety of LS formulations include rats (196) and prematurely born rabbits (197), as well as premature lambs (198–200), baboons (201), and monkeys (202). Typically, in vivo studies evaluate lung function for either short or extended periods of time; clinically relevant procedures and manipulations are also tested.

Building on successful in vitro experiments and animal studies, the efficacy of exogenous LS replacements is evaluated in clinical trials with human infants to determine the onset and duration of the therapeutic action of the LS replacement. Incidence of mortality from RDS, typical severity of

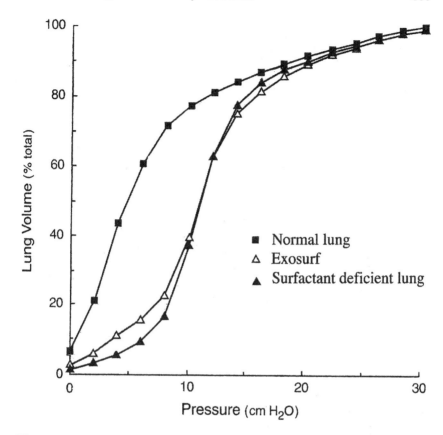

Figure 6 Pressure–volume (P–V) deflation mechanics of rat lung at 37°C: normal lungs, surfactant-deficient excised lungs, and after natural (CLSE) or synthetic (Exosurf) surfactant instillation into depleted excised lungs. Normal curve is obtained postexcision, and surfactant-deficient curve is after multiple lavages to deplete the endogenous surfactant. Exogenous surfactant is instilled at a concentration of 20 mg phospholipid/2.5 mL saline for CLSE, and 37.5 mg lipid/2.5 mL saline for Exosurf. (Adapted from Ref. 276, with permission.)

RDS, rate of recovery, and incidence and severity of bronchopulmonary dysplasias (BPD) and other chronic lung disorders, as well as any safety-related outcomes, are determined (11,203–207). The criteria assessed in human trials of LS replacements are the same as those listed above for the animal studies.

Utilizing these benchmarks for evaluation, surfactant replacement therapies have been developed and are used to effectively minimize alveolar collapse at end-expiration and to increase lung compliance, allowing safe respiration of prematurely born infants. Current LS treatments fall into two main categories: *natural* and *synthetic*. A third, promising but not yet available class of formulations is the *biomimetic lung surfactant replacements*, which will be covered later in this chapter.

XIV. NATURAL LS REPLACEMENTS

A. Animal-Derived Replacements

Natural surfactant replacements are prepared from animal lungs, either by lavaging or mincing followed by organic phase extraction of the phosphopholipids and hydrophobic surfactant proteins. A number of different natural surfactant replacements have been commercialized (Table 2). From bovine lungs, there are surfactant TA (Surfacten, Tokyo Tanabe, Japan) (9), beractant (Survanta, Abbott Laboratories, Columbus, Ohio) (10), Alveofact (Thomae, Biberach/Riss, FRG) (11), and BLES (BLES Biochemicals, Ontario, Canada) (208,209). Both surfactant TA and beractant are obtained from minced cow lung and are spiked with added synthetic lipids [DPPC, palmitic acid (PA), and tripalmitin] to standardize the composition and to improve the physical and physiological properties of the material. From calf lungs, there is calf lung surfactant extract, CLSE (Infasurf, Forest Laboratories) (4), whereas from porcine lungs there is Curosurf (Chiesi Farmaceutici, Parma) (12). CLSE, Alveofact, and BLES are obtained by lung washing and subsequent extraction of the lavage fluid with organic solvents. Curosurf is obtained by mincing of the lung, followed by washing, chloroform-methanol extraction, and liquid–gel chromatography. As a result of this sample preparation, Curosurf is devoid of triglycerides, cholesterol, and cholesteryl esters; it is not really known to what extent this lack may change the manner in which it functions.

In vitro biophysical characterization experiments have shown that natural surfactants generally provide virtually instant surfactant adsorption, efficient surface spreading and respreading, good film compressibility, and the achievement of low surface tension during cyclic film compression and expansion (78,180,210). For example, preparations of surfactant TA and Curosurf rapidly spread to an equilibrium surface tension of 24–27 mN/m, yielding a minimal surface tension upon compression that is below 5 mN/m. (For comparison, the surface tension of a clean water surface at 37°C is about 70 mN/m.) Films of CLSE require only 20% compression to achieve a similarly low surface tension (180). Furthermore, evaluations of material performance based on animal models of RDS have shown that natural surfactants typically provide good oxygenation, pulmonary pressure–

Table 2 Commercially Available LS Replacements (Natural and Synthetic)

Product name	Company	Composition	Formulation	Performance	References
CLSE (Infasurf®)	ONY, Inc. Amherst, NY	Heat-sterilized suspension in 0.15 M NaCl at 35 mg/ml	Calf Extract (93% phospholipid, 5% cholesterol and neutral lipids, 1.5% SP-B/SP-C)	PBS at 0.2 min at 2 mg/ml: $\gamma_{ads} \sim 24$ mN/m; $\gamma_{min} \sim 0$ mN/m (reaches these values at 1 mg/ml) (180) and at 0.063 mg/ml, reduced γ_{ads} to 22 mN/m in 2.5 min (78). P-V mechanics in lavaged rat lungs: Similar to normal lung (78). Two randomized placebo-controlled clinical trials showed positive results of use of CLSE (280-282).	(4,78,180,280-282)
Surfactant-TA (Surfacten®)	Tokyo Tanabe, Tokyo, Japan	Sterile suspension in 0.15 M NaCl at 30 mg/ml	Bovine Minced Supplemented with DPPC, PA, and tripalmitin (84% phospholipid, 7% PA, tripalmitin, 8% PA, and 1% protein) (283)	Three randomized placebo-controlled clinical trials showed positive results with the use of Surfactant-TA (284-286).	(9,283,284-286)
(SF-RI 1) Alveofact®	Thomae GmbH, Biberach, Germany	Sterile suspension in 0.15 M NaCl at 45 mg/ml	Calf Extract (99% phospholipids and neutral lipids, including 4% cholesterol; 1% SP-B/SP-C) (288)	PBS at 0.2 min at 2 mg/ml: $\gamma_{ads} \sim 24$ mN/m; $\gamma_{min} \sim 0$ mN/m (180).	(11,180,288,289)

Table 2 Continued

Product name	Company	Composition	Formulation	Performance	References
BLES®	BLES Biochemicals Inc., Ontario, Canada	Sterile suspension in 0.15 NaCl and 1.5 mM $CaCl_2$ at 25 mg/ml	Bovine Extract (98–99% phospholipids and neutral lipids and 1% SP-B/SP-C)	One randomized placebo-controlled clinical trials showed positive results with the use of Alveofact (11). Two randomized placebo-controlled clinical trials showed positive results with the use of BLES (208, 290).	(208,209,290)
Beractant (Survanta®)	Ross/Abbott Laboratories, Columbus, OH Licensed from Tokyo Tanabe	Auto-claved, sterilized suspension in 0.15 M NaCl at 25 mg/ml	Bovine Minced Supplemented with DPPC, PA, tripalmitin	PBS at 0.2 min at 2 mg/ml: $\gamma_{ads} \sim 24$ mN/m; $\gamma_{min} \sim 4$ mN/m (180) and γ_{ads} reduced to 30 mN/m at 2.5 min at 0.063 mg/ml (78) P-V mechanics in lavaged rat lungs showed improved lung function (78) Seven randomized placebo-controlled clinical trials showed positive results with the use of Survanta (10,214,291–293).	(10,78,214,291–293)
Curosurf®	Chiesi Farmaceutici Parma, Italy and Dey Labs Napa, CA	Suspension in saline at 80 mg/ml	Porcine Minced (99% polar lipids and 1% SP-B/SP-C) (294)	PBS at 0.2 min at 2 mg/ml: $\gamma_{ads} \sim 24$ mN/m (180).	(12,180,294)

Colfosceril palmitate (Exosurf®)	Glaxo Wellcome NC	DPPC: hexadecanol :tyloxapol (13.5:1.5:1)	One randomized placebo-controlled clinical trial showed positive results with the use of Curosurf (12). PBS at 0.063 mg/ml at 20 min: $\gamma_{ads} \sim$ 38 mN/m (78) P-V mechanics in lavaged rat lungs: Slightly improved lung function (78) Nine randomized placebo-controlled clinical trials showed positive results with the use of Exosurf (14,204,295).	(14,78,200,204,295,296)
Pumactant (ALEC®)	Britannia Pharmaceuticals Redhill, Surrey, UK	DPPC:PG (7:3)	Three randomized placebo-controlled clinical trials, with 1 showing positive results (224,297).	(13,224,297)

volume characteristics, and survival rates upon treatment (211). Finally, and more importantly, clinical trials have demonstrated the efficacy of natural surfactants to treat or prevent RDS in premature infants (12,212–215).

Although natural LS formulations are both functional and relatively safe, there are definitely a few potentially grave risks associated with sourcing a human medicine directly from animals. Because natural surfactants are extracted from animal lungs, it is impossible to eliminate the possibility of cross-species transfer of antigenic or infectious agents, such as scrapie prion (216), or other unforeseeable biological contamination (187,217). In addition, because the bovine and porcine sequences of SP-B and SP-C are only about 80% homologous to the human sequences, these animal proteins have the potential to be recognized as foreign by the human immune system (124,218,219). Antibodies developed to these homologous protein sequences could potentially inactivate the natural human proteins and lead to respiratory failure (124). This has not yet been found to occur in newborns, but for adults with ARDS, production of such antibodies could be a serious problem (216). Furthermore, the isolation of LS from animals is an expensive process that can produce variability in LS composition as a result of animal-to-animal inconsistencies. Animal-derived preparations (e.g., porcine Curosurf) are generally two to three times as expensive as some currently available synthetic surfactants (e.g., ALEC) (187,216). Finally, because of limited supply, the clinical use of natural surfactant may be restricted (34).

B. Human-Derived Replacements

As an alternative to animal-derived replacements, human lung surfactant can be harvested from the amniotic fluid of full-term pregnancies. Lung surfactant is secreted by a maturing fetus into the amniotic fluid in utero, and is present along with contaminating lipids and proteins. Whole human surfactant, obtained under sterile conditions from term amniotic fluid, has been used successfully in several studies with premature infants (212,220). However, human LS collected by this method has been shown to have reduced activity in comparison with extracts of animal lung surfactant, for reasons that are not completely understood (221). While the immunogenic risks are reduced as compared to animal-derived substances, they are nevertheless still present in human-derived LS. Furthermore, there is a possibility of disease transmission. Finally, a low supply of good-quality amniotic fluid–derived LS drastically limits its clinical use and makes it commercially unfeasible as a therapeutic replacement.

XV. SYNTHETIC REPLACEMENTS

To obviate the risks associated with natural surfactant replacements, synthetic formulations have been developed. Currently there are two synthetic products commercially available: ALEC (Pumactant, Britannia Pharmaceuticals, Redhill, UK) (13) and Exosurf (Glaxo Wellcome, Research Triangle Park, NC, USA) (14) (Table 2). The "artificial lung expanding compound," ALEC, is composed of DPPC and PG in a ratio of 7:3 and is suspended in saline at 100 mg/mL. In this formulation, PG serves the purpose of promoting the spreading of DPPC at the air–liquid interface (52). In Exosurf, hexadecanol and tyloxapol are added to DPPC to serve as spreading agents, creating a suspension consisting of 13.5:1.5:1 (DPPC:hexadecanol:tyloxapol) by weight in a saline solution, with a DPPC concentration of 13.5 mg/mL. Britannia Pharmaceutical has voluntarily suspended the marketing and distribution of Pumactant (222) pending further investigations of clinical trial results that indicated the inadequacy of this synthetic formulation in comparison with natural surfactant (223).

The advantages of synthetic surfactant replacements include their lower cost as well as a reduced potential for antigenicity, viral and protein contamination, and product variability. Clinically, some synthetic surfactants have been shown to be reasonably effective in the rescue of premature infants. For example, in a 10-center trial of ALEC, mortality was reduced from 30% in control infants to 19% in treated infants (224). However, ALEC has been shown to be less effective in the treatment of babies with established RDS, often taking several hours to produce the desired response, whereas natural surfactants take effect much more rapidly. Similarly, Exosurf also improves lung function in babies with RDS, but the therapeutic response appears to be irregular and may lag material administration by several hours (225). Hence, in comparison with natural surfactant replacements, synthetic surfactant replacements lacking surfactant proteins give inferior performance, with the reported loss of one additional infant per 42 treated (213,216). This increased mortality rate has been attributed to the absence of the surfactant proteins SP-B and SP-C, which are known to potently improve surfactant activity (211).

A meta-analysis of seven clinical trials involving more than 3000 infants was carried out to allow a comparison of the efficacy of natural surfactant replacements (mainly Survanta) with that of the synthetic surfactant replacement Exosurf. The meta-analysis revealed that natural surfactant replacements typically show a slightly superior performance, as observed in the generally lower posttreatment oxygen requirements of treated infants, and a lower risk of neonatal mortality when the natural biomaterial is administered (226,227).

XVI. BIOMIMETIC SURFACTANT REPLACEMENTS UNDER DEVELOPMENT

In light of the disadvantages present in both natural and synthetic surfactant replacements, researchers are working to develop biomimetic surfactant replacements as an improved treatment not only for neonatal RDS but for a broader class of patients and respiratory disorders. From a molecular design aspect this is a tractable bioengineering problem, as a reasonably good understanding of the composition and function of LS, as well as the deficiencies of current LS replacements, has been established. It seems clear that biomimetic LS replacements should be designed to capture the advantages of synthetic products (i.e., to be nonimmunogenic, to exclude all infectious agents and biological risks, and to be chemically pure, consistently formulated, and cost effective) while truly mimicking the performance and efficacy of natural surfactants. Up until this point, the most promising design avenues have focused on utilization of a combination of lipids with spreading agents that somehow mimic the hydrophobic surfactant proteins. Typically, the lipid fraction will include DPPC, PG, and PA. However, the selection of the lipid composition will depend on which SP-B and/or SP-C analogues are used as spreading agents in formulating the LS replacement (160).

Since the inferior performance of synthetic LS has been attributed to the absence of the surfactant proteins, various groups are working to design biomimetic versions of SP-B and SP-C. Approaches being taken range from the use of recombinant molecular biology to direct chemical synthesis of these proteins or fragments thereof, with sequences that are either similar to or completely different from the native human sequence. In all cases, present knowledge of the structure–function relationships of the proteins is taken into account in order to design SP-B and/or SP-C analogues that can serve as effective spreading agents in an LS replacement formulation.

A. Recombinant Surfactant Proteins

One approach to biomimetic LS replacement design is the development of recombinant proteins, with the goal of creating SP analogues that are highly similar to the natural proteins. However, the isolation of recombinant human SP-B and SP-C proteins from a cell culture broth is a nontrivial task. Recombinant SP-C proteins (rSP-C) with the natural human sequence have been expressed in *E. coli* (15,16,228,229,298), but recovery of the protein can be difficult, probably at least in part because of the extreme hydrophobicity and its resultant strong tendency to aggregate with itself (16). This rSP-C is currently being manufactured and researched by Scios-Nova (Sunnyvale,

CA). To increase the chances of good protein recovery, the human SP-C sequence also has been redesigned by some researchers, incorporating amino acid substitutions via standard oliogonucleotide-directed mutagenesis. In the mutant rSP-C (Cys→Ser), the cysteines at positions 4 and 5 (Fig. 3a) are replaced with serines to reduce the likelihood of protein oligomerization via the formation of disulfide bonds (15). Similarly, in the mutant rSP-C (Cys→Phe and Met→Ile), phenylalanines replace the cysteines at positions 4 and 5, whereas isoleucine replaces methionine at position 32 (16,228) to reduce the tendency to aggregate (16). This rSP-C is manufactured by Byk Gulden Pharmaceuticals (Konstanz, Germany) and is currently being investigated (16).

Biomimetic LS replacement formulations that include recombinant SP-C have shown good biophysical activity in vitro and in vivo. However, in animal studies, comparison of these biomimetic formulations, including SP-C only with natural surfactants that include both hydrophobic proteins, revealed that the recombinant surfactant formulations show poorer performance, as indicated by a lower mean PO_2 value and a higher mean FIO_2 value (15,16). It is unclear whether this drop in performance results from a lack of SP-B in the biomimetic formulation, from differences in the SP-C mimic sequence, or from a higher incidence of SP-C protein aggregation and misfolding than in the natural material.

In an alternative approach, the expression of rSP-C has been performed in eukaryotic systems such as baculovirus to enable posttranslational modification of the cysteine residues with the palmitoyl chains that are naturally present in human SP-C. Palmitoylated SP-C was expressed and purified by this method; however, the yield of the desired material was only 15% of the total product isolate (17). In addition, because of the hydrophobicity of the protein and other problems inherent to eukaryotic systems, protein expression levels were low. The activity of this palmitoylated rSP-C in comparison to nonacylated SP-C has not yet been investigated (17). Significant improvements are required to make protein production in insect cells a cost-effective means of producing SP-C for a commercial surfactant replacement. Moreover, although rSP-C-based LS is much safer than animal-derived LS replacements, there still exists the possibility of an unfavorable immune response from foreign proteins present in the vector (e.g., *E. coli* or baculovirus) used for the expression of rSP-C.

Regarding the larger and more complicated hydrophobic surfactant protein, SP-B, attempts have been made to express its mature form in *E. coli* using a truncated human SP-B cDNA (18). This recombinant protein, which ended up to be approximately eight residues larger than natural SP-B, was produced in *E. coli*, but expression levels were extremely low and it was not known to what extent the correct disulfide bonds had formed (Fig. 2a). The limited recovery of this longer length SP-B version most likely relates to the hydrophobicity and surface activity of the protein (18,230). Future efforts to produce the correct sequence in high yield will involve the use of fusion proteins (e.g., fusion of SP-B with β-galactosidase) (18). To date, there has been no publication describing the expression of a functional, active, recombinant SP-B protein. Without a method that yields the correct sequence (with the correct fold and disulfide bonds) in sufficient quantity, the production of recombinant SP-B for therapeutic purposes will not be feasible. Therefore, the development of biomimetic SP mimics by other means is a worthwhile and important bioengineering goal.

B. Synthetic Polypeptides as Surfactant Protein Mimics

A more feasible solution for the development of biomimetic spreading agents is the use of organic chemical methods to synthesize polypeptide versions of SP-B and SP-C. Results from structural and physical experiments that provide structure–function correlations have been invaluable in the efforts to create successful SP mimics by this route (90,107,118,133–135,148,156,162,171,231). Designs for synthetic SP-B analogues have focused on mimicking the important structural features of the protein, including its amphipathic helices with opposing polar (i.e., positively charged) and hydrophobic faces (19,20,32). In the case of SP-C, designs have been created to mimic its hydrophobic helix, with attention also being paid to the two adjacent positive charges near the C terminus (146), palmitoylation of the cysteines (28,145,180), and the length of the valyl-rich helix (37 Å), which supposedly spans a lipid bilayer (27–29,232).

Synthetically engineered peptides circumvent many of the problems associated with current purification procedures for animal-derived surfactants, and should facilitate the production of sufficient quantities of material for its use as a therapeutic agent for treatment of other respiratory diseases, most particularly in children and adults. Moreover, a significant number of these synthetic, biomimetic polypeptide variants (some quite dissimilar in sequence from the natural SP-B and SP-C, as we will discuss) have been found to be biophysically functional in vitro and in vivo. A variety of synthetic polypeptide-based SP mimics have been successful to some degree in promoting the achievement of low surface tensions upon film compression, rapid respreading of surfactant lipids at an interface, and the rescue of prematurely born animals with RDS.

C. Polypeptide Analogues of SP-B

Because the SP-B protein is relatively large (with regard to what can be made on a peptide synthesizer) and structurally complex with its numerous disulfide bonds, both recombinant and chemical synthesis of the full-length human SP-B sequence are challenging endeavors. Based on a strong conservation of the SP-B sequence in various mammalian systems, peptide analogues have been templated on the human SP-B sequence, based on a desire to retain the correct structural configuration of the molecule (see Table 3 for SP-B designs). Researchers have designed, synthesized, and characterized synthetic peptide mimics of the full-length human SP-B protein, as well as truncated peptide sequences that represent different regions or domains of the protein (19–21,163,233,234). Because synthetic versions of full-length SP-B produced so far do not reproduce the three physiological disulfide bridges, heterogeneity and oligomerization of these peptides is highly likely. Nevertheless, this as well as other SP-B analogues based on synthetic peptides have been shown to have respectable biophysical activity both in vitro and in vivo. LS preparations that contain these synthetic peptides provide improved oxygenation and lung compliance in surfactant-deficient animal models (19,235).

Interestingly, the amino-terminal, amphipathic domain of human SP-B (amino acids 1–25) has been shown to adopt a helical conformation (236) and to possess many of the important surface-active properties of full-length SP-B protein, when added to biomimetic lipid mixtures such as the so-called Tanaka lipids [i.e., DPPC:PG:PA in a ratio of 68:22:9 by weight (160)]. Specifically, upon compression, an SP-B (1–25)/Tanaka lipid formulation reached low surface tension and was shown to improve oxygenation in rats in vivo (19,20,233). Interactions of this amino-terminal fragment of SP-B with anionic lipids is believed to induce the coexistence in the film of flat and buckled monolayers upon collapse, thereby reducing surface tension and improving respreading during film compression and expansion (163,164). However, the synthetic system including SP-B (1–25) in place of real SP-B protein has been shown to have a significantly slower rate of adsorption than natural surfactant, a disadvantage that reduces its therapeutic value (19,25,29).

Modification of the natural SP-B amino terminus (1–25), with substitutions of hydrophobic, charged, and/or oligomerizable residues targeted to potentially improve its surface activity, was not found to improve the adsorption rate of the molecule (20). To address this issue, peptides matching sequential, overlapping regions of SP-B were synthesized systematically, and each prepared with a lipid mixture of DPPC:PG (3:1 by weight). In vivo studies in fetal rabbit lung revealed that some of these

Table 3 Designs of SP-B Peptides

Design sequence	In vitro surface activity (mN/m)	In vivo performance	References
Full-length human SP-B (1–78) FPIPLPYCWLCRALIKRIQAMIPKGALAVA VAQVCRVVPLVAGGICQCLAERYSVILLDT LLGRMLPQLVCRLVLRCSM (note, does not have correct disulfide fold) Truncated SP-B SP-B (1–60)	Both SP-B (1–78) and SP-B (1–60) confer biophysical activity to Tanaka lipids, with SP-B (1–78) having better dynamic behavior. However, both SP-B peptides show poor adsorption kinetics in comparison to Surfactant TA. LWSB at 1% (40–100% Area) SP-B (1–78): $\gamma_{min} \sim 0.2$ mN/m, $\gamma_{max} \sim 43.5$ mN/m SP-B (1–60): $\gamma_{min} \sim 2.1$ mN/m; $\gamma_{max} \sim 48$ mN/m Surfactant TA: $\gamma_{min} \sim 4.2$ mN/m; $\gamma_{max} \sim 40$ mN/m PBS at 1% SP-B (1–78): $\gamma_{min} \sim 3.3$ mN/m, $\gamma_{max} \sim 43.5$ mN/m SP-B (1–60): $\gamma_{min} \sim 22$ mN/m; $\gamma_{max} \sim 40.9$ mN/m Surfactant TA: $\gamma_{min} \sim 2.8$ mN/m; $\gamma_{max} \sim 40$ mN/m Adsorption kinetics (Note large standard deviation for SP) SP-B (1–78): $\gamma_{ads} \sim 43$ mN/m (1 min); 36 mN/m (5 min) SP-B (1–60): $\gamma_{ads} \sim 47$ mN/m; (1 min); 42 mN/m (5 min) Surfactant TA: $\gamma_{ads} \sim 30$ mN/m; (1 min); 24.6 mN/m (5 min) (22)	In vivo studies with excised rat lungs showed that SP-B (1–78) and SP-B (1–60) have similar % Total Lung Capacity values at 5 cm H_2O and 10-cm H_2O as Surfactant TA (% TLC $\sim$95) (22) In vivo studies of lavaged rats showed that SP-B (1–78)-DPPC:POPG:PA improves a/A PO_2, and P-V mechanics to a slighter extent increases a/A PO_2 from 0.1 to 0.32 (235)	(22,235,238)

N-terminus of human SP-B (1–25)
FPIPLPYCWLCRALIKRIQAMIPKG
and
SP-B (49–66)
LAERYSVILLDTLLGRnLL-CONH2

Studies with DPPC:POPG:PA
(69:22:9) on LWSB
SP-B (1–78) increases the
hysteresis of compression-
expansion curves when compared
to lipids alone (235)

The combination of SP-B (1–25) and
SP-B(49–66) improves spreading
of lipid mixture of DPPC:PG:PA
(68:21:8). However, the SP-B
peptides have slow adsorption
kinetics in comparison to bovine
LS.

LWSB and PBS at 3 wt%
B1, B2: γ_{min} ~2–9 mN/m;
γ_{max} ~59–44 mN/m;
γ_{ads} ~51 mN/m
Bovine: γ_{min} ~8–7 mN/m;
γ_{max} ~43–37 mN/m;
γ_{ads} ~40 mN/m

In vivo studies with lavaged
adult rats showed
improvement in PaO_2 with
the combo SP-B (1–25) and
SP-B (49–66) after 75 min.
Lipids: ~60 torr
B1, B2: ~150 torr
Bovine: ~250 torr

(19)

Table 3 Continued

Design sequence	In vitro surface activity (mN/m)	In vivo performance	References
Variants of N-terminal human SP-B (1–25)	Adsorption and spreading of Tanaka lipids at 2 minutes were improved (slightly) with the presence of various SP-B mimics. The addition of SP-B (1–25) significantly reduces the minimum surface tension, to values that are acceptable, but the maximum surface tension is still high.	Not available	(20)
SP-B	SP-B: $\gamma_{min} \sim 55\,mN/m$;		
SP-B (C→A)	$\gamma_{max} \sim 56\,mN/m$		
SP-B (L, I→A)	SP-B (C→A): $\gamma_{min} \sim 54\,mN/m$;		
SP-B (R→K)	$\gamma_{max} \sim 7\,mN/m$		
SP-B (R, K→S)	SP-B (L, I→A);		
SP-B (R, K→E)	$\gamma_{min} \sim 51\,mN/m$;		
	$\gamma_{max} \sim 57\,mN/m$		
	SP-B (R→K): $\gamma_{min} \sim 57\,mN/m$;		
	$\gamma_{max} \sim 57\,mN/m$		
	LWSB of SP-B: $\gamma_{max} \sim 60\,mN/m$;		
	$\gamma_{min} \sim 5\,mN/m$		
	LWSB of lipids:		
	$\gamma_{max} \sim 70\,mN/m$;		
	$\gamma_{min} \sim 55\,mN/m$		

N-terminus of human SP-B (1–25)
FPIPLPYCWLCRALIKRIQAMIPKG

Investigation with various lipid mixtures shows that SP-B (1–25) improves surface activity by increasing the collapse pressure (i.e, reducing minimum surface tension) and altering it to be more reversible to enable respreading. Increases collapse pressure and alters the type of collapse as observed on LWSB and FM (164) 3 wt% SP-B (1–25) increases the hysteresis of P-A curve and retains this upon cycling of DPPC:PG:PA (68:21:9), liftoff ~ 90% trough area and π_c of 65 mN/m ~ 50% trough area (lipids alone, liftoff ~45% and π_c of 50 mN/m ~ 15% trough area) (165)

3 wt% SP-B (1–25) increases the π_c (alters it to a more reversible fold) of PA at 25°C (163, 165) 10 wt% SP-B (1–25) has activity comparable to SP-B (1–78) in confering surface activity to DPPG:POPG (3:1): SP-B (1–25) or SP-B (1–78)–π_c ~ 60 mN/m and lipids–π_c ~ 52 mN/m (82)

Monomeric SP-B (1–25) in DPPC:POPG:PA (69:22:9) improves lung function in either premature rabbits or lavaged rats

(25,82,163,165)

Table 3 Continued

Design sequence	In vitro surface activity (mN/m)	In vivo performance	References
	However, dynamic adsorption surface tension is too high in comparison to native SP-B when added to DPPC:POPG (8:2) vesicles, as measured on CBS 1% SP-B 1–25: $\gamma_{ads} \sim 40.6$ mN/m 1% hSP-B: $\gamma_{ads} \sim 22.6$ mN/m (25)		
Fragments of human SP-B (1–81) FPIPLPYCWLCRALIKRIQAMIPKGALAVA VAQVCRVVPL_VAGGICQCLAERYSVILLD TLLGRMLPQLVCRLVLRCSMDD e.g., SP-B (59–80) SP-B (64–80) SP-B (52–81) SP-B (66–81)	Accelerated spreading of lipids: PBS; DPPG:PG (3:1) 10 mg/ml, with 10 wt% SP-B (64–80): $\gamma_{min} \sim 0$ mN/m in 5 min SP-B (59–80): $\gamma_{min} \sim 2.7$ mN/m in 5 min Native SP-B: $\gamma_{min} \sim 3$ mN/m in 15 sec	Improvement in static lung compliance in fetal lungs of rabbit with SP-B (52–81) and SP-B (66–81) Slower adsorption but shows improvement in lung compliance compared to native human surfactant for SP-B (64–80)	(21,233)
Bovine variants SP-1: LLGRLPNLVCGLRLRCSG SP-2: RLPNLVCGLRLRCSG Human variants SP-3: RMLPQLVCRLVLRCSMD SP-4: RMLPQLVCRLVLRCSM	Wilhelmy plate; DPPC:PG (3:1) SP-1: $\gamma_{ads} \sim 45$ mN/m in 5 min; $\gamma_{spread} \sim 60$ mN/m in 60 sec SP-3: $\gamma_{ads} \sim 65$ mN/m in 5 min; $\gamma_{spread} \sim 55$ mN/m in 1 min Bovine SP-B: $\gamma_{ads} \sim 30$ mN/m; $\gamma_{spread} \sim 20$ mN/m in 20 sec Crude bovine LS: $\gamma_{ads} \sim 20$ mN/m; $\gamma_{spread} \sim 15$ mN/m in 20 sec	Not available	(23)

Human SP-B bend (35–46) and variant NB: Cys_{35}RVVPLVAGGICys_{46}-$CONH_2$ MB: Ac-Cys_{35}RVVPDSerHisGGIC$ys_{46}$$CONH_2$	Not available	Not available	(115)
Dimeric N-terminal human SP-B (1–25) FPIPLPYCWLARALIKRIQAMIPKG FPIPLPYCWLARALIKRIQAMIPKG	CBS; DPPC:POPG:PA (7:2:1) vesicle $\gamma_{ads} \sim 40$ mN/m (compare to 23 mN/m for hSP-B); $\gamma_{min} \sim 0$ mN/m; $\gamma_{max} \sim 42$ mN/m Requires larger compression to reach zero surface tension when compared to hSP-B	Not available	(25)

synthetic peptide surfactants did provide an increase in lung compliance but that their adsorption rates were still substantially slower than that of native human surfactant (233). Other studies of the activity of different regions of SP-B peptide have revealed that peptide fragments including the carboxyl-terminal residues and composed of at least 17 amino acids accelerate surfactant spreading and improve static lung compliance in premature rabbits (21,22,233). Other modified, truncated SP-B fragments derived from both bovine and human sequences have been synthesized and characterized; the surface activities of these peptides have been studied on an LWSB. Interestingly, higher activity was observed in analogues that also showed greater overall helicity by circular dichroism (CD) spectroscopy (23).

Since the natural, dimeric form of SP-B protein is considered to be of importance for optimal function of LS replacements, a dimeric version of the *N*-terminal segment of SP-B has been synthesized. In particular, a dimeric form of SP-B (1–25) was engineered by the replacement of the cysteine at position 11 with an alanine, whereas the remaining cysteine at position 8 was used for dimerization via disulfide bonding. Comparison of monomeric and dimeric SP-B (1–25) in premature rabbit and lavaged rat models show that the dimeric form is more efficient than the monomer in improving lung function (25). However, natural SP-B is dimerized through residue 48 in its sequence, distal from the 1–25 sequence used in this mimic.

D. Polypeptide Analogues of SP-C

In contrast to SP-B, the SP-C protein is monomeric and quite small; therefore, it is feasible to chemically synthesize a full-length version of it. SP-C analogues have been designed to mimic both the sequence and the folded conformation of the human protein (see Table 4). A challenging aspect in the synthesis of human SP-C is engineering the attachment of the two adjacent palmitoyl groups at positions 5 and 6, the absence of which can lead to the formation of irreversible β-sheet aggregates of SP-C (237) and to an accompanying reduction in surface activity (142). Two different approaches that have been taken for synthetic SP-C palmitoylation are (a) use of succinylamidyl palmitate derivatives (238) and (b) formation of a thioester linkage via a palmitoyl chloride reaction (239).

Full-length and truncated *non*palmitoylated versions of human SP-C protein have already been evaluated as components of an artificial surfactant (26). These SP-C mimics, in conjunction with a DPPC:PG:PA lipid mixture (75:25:10 by weight), display promising activity in vitro on an LWSB, as well as in vivo in lung pressure–volume curves obtained for premature rabbits treated with the material. Moreover, it was shown that a nonpalmitoylated core sequence containing residues 5–31 or 6–32 of the

Table 4 Designs of SP-C

Sequence	In vitro activity	In vivo activity	References
rSP-C (Cys)2 Scios-Nova Inc, Sunnyvale, CA, USA	Not available	Good surface activity but reduced inhibition of protein plasma disruption as compared to native SP-B (298) Acylation influences physical properties (142), but does not increase physiological activity of rSP-C(Cys)2 in premature rabbits (15)	(15,298,299)
rSP-C(Cys→Phe; Met→Ile) Byk Gulden Pharmaceuticals, Konstanz, Germany	Wilhelmy surface balance with DPPC:POPG (70:30): 5% PA:2% rSP-C showed good surface activity as compared to natural surfactant (16).	Improved lung function, but to lesser extent than natural surfactant in ventilated preterm lambs and rabbits (16)	(16,229,300,301)
Fragment of modified canine SP-C (nonpalmitoylated) IPCFPSSLKRLLAVAVAVALAVAVIAGLLMGL	PBS with DPPC:PG:PA (68:22:9) with 1wt%SP-C (canine, 1–31): $\gamma_{ads} \sim 26\,mN/m$ (compared to bovine $\sim 26\,mN/m$) $\gamma_{min} \sim 20\,mN/m$	Not available	(238)

Table 4 Continued

Sequence	In vitro activity	In vivo activity	References
Fragments of human SP-C (nonpalmitoylated) SP-C (6–32) SP-C (5–31)	LWSB with DPPC:PG:PA (75:25:1) With SP-C: $\gamma_{spread} \sim 31$ mN/m within 30 sec; $\gamma_{ads} \sim 41$ mN/m within 60 sec Alone: $\gamma_{spread} \sim 48$ mN/m within 30 sec; $\gamma_{ads} \sim 55$ mN/m Bovine SP-C: $\gamma_{ads} \sim 37$ mN/m	Tracheal instillation in immature rabbits improved P-V characteristics to level similar to mature neonates	(26)
Variant of human SP-C Dipalmitolyated SP-C(A) FGIPC*C*PVHLKRLLAVAVAVALAVAVAVGALLMGL:	Wilhelmy balance with DPPC:POPG:PA shows that dipalmitolyated SP-C (A) confers surface activity	Improves lung function in ventilated, lavaged rats and premature rabbits (235, 240)	(24,235,240)
Variants of porcine SP-C LRIPCCPVNLKRLLVVVVVVVLVVVVVIVGALLMGL SP-C (CC): C nonpalmitoylated SP-C (FF): C→F SP-C (SS): C→S SP-C (AAA): R1, L10, K11→A SP-C/BR: LRIPCCPVNLKRFYAITTLVAAIAFTLYLSLLLGY	Wihelmy balance with DPPC:PG:PA (68:22:9) Native porcine SP-C: $\gamma_{spread} \sim 37$ mN/m at 20 sec SP-C (CC): $\gamma_{spread} \sim 37$ mN/m at 30 sec	Not available	(28)

Variants of porcine SP-C (nonpalmitoylated) SP-C (1–12) SP-C (1–17) SP-C (1–21)	SP-C (FF); SP-C (SS); SP-C (AAA): SP-C/ BR: $\gamma_{spread} \sim 42\,mN/m$ at 30 sec Platinum Plate with DPPC:PG (7:3) Adsorption kinetics (π_{ads}): only SP-C (CC) reproduce native with $\pi_{ads} \sim 48\,mN/m$	Not available	(232)
Variant of human SP-C SP-C (Leu) FGIPSSPVLKRLLILLLLLLLLLILGALLMGL: Dipalmitoylated SP-C (Leu)	SP-C (Leu) has similar activity to native SP-C. However, both SP-C mimics give relatively high maximum surface tension when compared to Curosurf, which contains both SP-B and SP-C. PBS with DPPC:PG:PA (68:22:9) at 10 mg/ml SP-C (Leu): $\gamma_{min} \sim 0\,mN/m$ and $\gamma_{max} \sim 35\text{–}43\,mN/m$ Native SP-C: $\gamma_{min} \sim 0\,mN/m$ and $\gamma_{max} \sim 42\,mN/m$	Airway instillation in preterm rabbits improved dynamic lung compliance by 30% compared with untreated controls with SP-C (Leu)	(29,239,302)

Table 4 Continued

Sequence	In vitro activity	In vivo activity	References
	Curosurf: $\gamma_{min} \sim 0\,mN/m$ and $\gamma_{max} \sim 30\,mN/m$ Wilhelmy balance (10 mg/ml) SP-C (Leu): $\gamma_{spread} \sim 25$–$30\,mN/m$ native SP-C: $\gamma_{spread} \sim 25$–$30\,mN/m$		
Variant of human SP-C SP-C (LKS) FGIPSSPVHLKRLLIKLLLKILLKILLKLGALLMGL	SP-C (LKS) improves surface activity of the lipids PBS with DPPC:PG:PA(68:22:9) or DPPC:PG (7:3) SP-C (LKS): $\gamma_{min} < 1$; mN/m; $\gamma_{max} \sim 42\,mN/m$ Wilhelmy balance with DPPC:PG (7:3): SP-C (LKS): $\gamma_{spread} \sim 28\,mN/m$ after 3 sec	Not available	(30)

total 35 amino acids seems to be sufficient to mimic virtually full biophysical activity both in vitro and in vivo (26). However, other researchers have synthesized the full-length SP-C peptide and palmitoylated it with succinylamidyl palmitate, and have reported that the hexadecyl modification of cysteine residues 5 and 6 is critical for the protein's surface activity and biophysical function (145,147). Furthermore, modified, dipalmitoylated SP-C peptide in combination with the Tanaka lipid formulation was also shown to improve lung function in lavaged rats (235) and in premature rabbits (240).

In the canine SP-C protein, a phenylalanine residue is substituted for one of the palmitoylated cysteines (28,98). Hence, another approach to the synthesis of SP-C mimics has been the replacement of palmitoylated cysteine residues with phenylalanine residues, a mimic that has been called SP-Cff (28). Other analogues have introduced serine substitutions for the two cysteine residues (28); however, in vitro results that differ substantially from natural SP-C performance have been reported. Specifically, both Ser- and Phe-substituted SP-C analogues, in combination with the Tanaka lipid mixture, were found to have inferior spreading properties in comparison to a formulation that contains natural or native SP-C (28).

Studies have shown that the α-helical conformation of SP-C protein is important for the rapid spreading and low surface tension that are exhibited by lung surfactant (28,232). Thus, the poor performance generally observed for LS replacements that contain synthetic SP-C has been attributed to a low α-helical content of the polypeptide (28) due to incorrect folding of chemically synthesized SP-C (241). In its physiological environment, SP-C protein exists in complexation with a high concentration of lipids, which enable the proper folding and subsequent structural stability of the natural chain configuration. In the absence of lipids, the native polyvaline stretch, which is extraordinarily hydrophobic, has a strong tendency to misfold into β sheets and aggregate in nonphysiological environments (241).

To overcome these challenges in synthetic SP-C production, several SP-C analogues have been designed with modified sequences in the hydrophobic stretch to maximize helicity and minimize β-sheet formation and aggregation. In one design, the polyvaline stretch was replaced with the transmembrane helical region (42–64) of bacteriorhodopsin (BR), reportedly resulting in an SP-C/BR analogue with secondary structure and spreading kinetics similar to native SP-C (28). In other SP-C analogues, replacement of the valine residues with either polyleucine or polynorleucine residues was shown to enable the rapid surface spreading activity of the natural protein in vitro, and to improve static lung compliance in preterm rabbits to levels comparable with that of natural lung surfactant (e.g., Beractant) (27). Another design approach prescribed the replacement of all the valine residues with leucine residues, the substitution of both palmitoylcysteines with serines, and the deletion of histidine from the sequence. This SP-C (Val→Leu; Cys→Ser) analogue was determined to have a helical, transbilayer orientation by Fourier transform infrared spectroscopy (29) and reportedly to exhibit in vitro surface activity resembling that of native SP-C (29,30). In vivo studies of this SP-C mimic, in combination with the Tanaka lipid cocktail in rabbits, showed 30% improvement in dynamic lung compliance when compared with untreated premature rabbits (29). However, unlike modified natural surfactant (242), this SP-C analogue did not succeed in restoring dynamic compliance to healthy levels (29). Then again, the material that was tested lacked SP-B, having only a mimic of SP-C, so this may not have been a fair comparison to natural LS, which contains both SPs.

Part of the problem with the modified SP-C (Val→Leu; Cys→Ser) peptide may arise from its ability to aggregate via hydrophobic association of the polyleucine stretch (29). To circumvent this difficulty, one group introduced lysine residues at positions 17, 22, and 27 of this region to locate positive charges around the helical circumference and thus prevent hydrophobic aggregation by ionic repulsion. This SP-C (LKS) analogue showed good surface activity but was inferior to native surfactant, and showed a particularly high dynamic maximum surface tension ($\gamma \sim 42\,\text{mN/m}$) (30).

What is striking about these studies is that many groups have designed peptide mimics of surfactant proteins B and C, and all have achieved some degree of success in creating useful LS replacements using these diverse SP mimics (Tables 4 and 5). This provides strong evidence that this biomaterial system is tolerant to modification, at least for its use in acute replacement therapy. This is perhaps to be expected, since it seems that surfactant proteins interact primarily with lipids, which is likely to be an interaction with much less specificity than many types of biomolecular associations. Researchers are also making progress in the development and characterization of simplified peptide mimics of SP-B and SP-C for use as biomimetic spreading agents in exogenous LS replacements.

E. Simplified Peptide Mimics of SP-B and SP-C

Strict sequence conservation may not be necessary to retain the proper, helical secondary structure and surface activity of the native surfactant proteins. Some groups have created simplified, amphipathic peptides and tested them as mimics of SP-B and SP-C (Table 5). Small peptides offer the advantages of being less immunogenic (243), easier to produce, and less costly than long-chain peptides.

Biomimetic Lung Surfactant Replacements

Table 5 Simplified SP-Mimics Based on Synthetic Polypeptides

Sequence	In vitro activity	In vivo activity	References
KL4: KLLLLKLLLLKLLLLKLLLL K	PBS with DPPC:POPG (3:1):15 wt% PA: 3 WT% KL4	Increases dynamic lung compliance and oxygenation in premature rabbits and monkeys	(29,33,244,245,247,302)
	Wilhelmy with DPPC:PG:PA (68:22:9) with 2 wt% $\gamma_{spread} \sim 37$ mN/m at 60 sec (29, 244)	Improves lung expansion and gas exchange in infants: a/A $PO_2 \sim$ 0.4 by 12 h (normal is 0.4)	
KL2,3: LLLLKLLLLKLLKLLLLKLL L	Wilhelmy with DPPC:PG:PA (68:22:9) with 2 wt% $\gamma_{spread} \sim 50$ mN/m at 60 sec	Not available	(29,244)
WMAP10: Suc-LLEKLLLEWLK-CONH$_2$	PBS with DPPC $\gamma_{max} > 45$ mN/m (canine LS $\sim$ 30 mN/m) and $\gamma_{min} < 4$ mN/m (canine LS $\sim$ 8)	Almost complete restoration (92%) of static pulmonary compliance in lung-lavaged rats	(29,32)
	Wilhelmy with DPPC:PG:PA Slow spreading kinetics: $\gamma_{spread} \sim 45$ mN/m at 60 s	Restore a/A PO_2 in lung-lavaged guinea pigs (> 85%)	

Taking the advantages of small peptides into account, water-soluble synthetic peptides have been designed with sequences unrelated to native protein SP-B, but also coding for helical amphipathic structures, in the hope that these molecules will have suitable physical properties for an LS replacement. An amphipathic α-helical peptide called 18As (a 24-residue peptide from the lipid binding region of plasma apolipoprotein) was designed and was shown, in combination with DPPC, to be reasonably effective as an LS replacement both in vitro and in vivo (31). The success of this DPPC/18As formulation led McClean et al. (32) to develop a series of model amphipathic α-helical peptides (MAP) to be tested as potential spreading agents for DPPC. Of these, WMAP10 (succinyl-LLEKLLEWLK amide) has shown the greatest promise as a spreading agent, purportedly because it was designed to be optimally helical, by (a) facilitating the formation of salt bridges between side chains; (b) neutralizing the negative charge on the C terminus; and (c) introducing a negative charge at the N terminus. In vivo testing of WMAP10 function demonstrated the restoration of acceptable pulmonary compliance (32), but in vitro experiments showed slow spreading of the material at the air–liquid interface (reaching $\gamma_{\text{spread}} \sim 45\,\text{mN/m}$, which is also a relatively high surface tension for an LS replacement) (29,32).

In work along the same lines, Cochrane et al. (33) developed the 21-residue peptide KL4, with a repeat sequence of lysine followed by four leucine residues. The design of KL4 was patterned after the amphipathic characteristics of the SP-B helical domain (SP-B 59–80), which had been shown in prior experiments to be biophysically active as a peptide fragment (233). KL4 is also reasonably active as an LS spreading agent. It has been proposed that the KL4 peptide associates with the peripheral regions of the lipid bilayer in such a way that positively charged residues interact with the polar lipid headgroup while the hydrophobic stretch interacts with lipid acyl side chains (33). Contrary results, which seem more likely to be correct, suggest that the KL4 peptide is in a transbilayer orientation in a lipid environment (244). Regardless of the orientation of KL4, in combination with a lipid mixture of DPPC:POPG (3:1), the peptide has been shown to create an active exogenous surfactant for the treatment of immature newborn rabbits (33) and rhesus monkeys (245,246). However, concerns about the poor spreading kinetics of the KL4/lipid mixture (to $\gamma_{\text{spread}} \sim 37\,\text{mN/m}$) have been raised, and are evidenced by a reduced efficiency of this novel formulation in comparison with native SP-C and SP-C/BR in combination with a Tanaka lipid mixture (244). This may explain why, when KL4 was added to a bovine-derived LS with low SP-B content (Survanta), oxygenation was not improved in lavaged adult rats as compared to the use of Survanta alone (24). Nevertheless, and more importantly, premature infants treated with a mixed KL4-Surfacten formulation (DPPC:POPG with a ratio of 3:1 with 15% PA and 3% KL4, by weight) do show restoration of arterial-to-alveolar oxygen tension ratios to a normal range within 12 h, suggesting a reasonably good efficacy of this surfactant replacement (247). Though promising, the clinical efficacy and safety of this formulation has yet to be fully established because of the limited number of patients in which it has been studied. Furthermore, comparisons with other commercially available surfactants are so far unavailable. Currently, this formulation is referred to as Surfaxin (U.S.-adopted name Sinapultide) and is produced by Discovery Laboratory (Doylestown, PA). Pivotal phase 3 trials are now being established to evaluate the efficacy and safety of Surfaxin for treatment of premature infants with idiopathic RDS (8). This trial will study approximately 1500 premature infants in Latin America and is designed to compare Surfaxin with currently available surfactant replacements (248).

F. Polypeptoid-Based SP Mimics

A more unusual approach to biomimicry of the SP proteins is to develop analogues based on nonnatural peptide mimics that offer greater in vivo stability and easier production while still mimicking the helical, amphipathic structure of the natural molecules. Along these lines, an alternative and novel biomimetic surfactant replacement currently under development in our laboratory is based on the use of poly-*N*-substituted glycine, or *polypeptoid*, SP mimics as additives to lipid mixtures. Polypeptoids are nonnatural, sequence-specific polymers that are based on a peptide backbone but differ from peptides in that their side chains are appended to the tertiary amide nitrogen rather than to the α carbon (Fig. 7) (249). This difference in structure has been shown to result in virtually complete protease resistance for peptoid analogues (250). Peptoids also offer the advantages of low immunogenicity (251), facile production on a peptide synthesizer (252), and a low cost relative to synthetic peptides. Peptoids with α-chiral side chains have been designed and shown to form stable, helical, secondary structures by CD (252,253), 2D-NMR (254), and molecular modeling (255). Because peptoids are N-substituted and hence lack amide hydrogen bonds, they cannot form β-sheets. Previous studies have established that polypeptoid helices are extremely stable and monomeric, with no tendency to misfold and aggregate (252,253,256). Therefore, peptoids seem to be quite promising for the development of effective spreading agents for LS formulations.

Exploiting similar strategies as have been used in the design of peptide-based SP-B and SP-C analogues, sequence-specific peptoid-based SP mimics

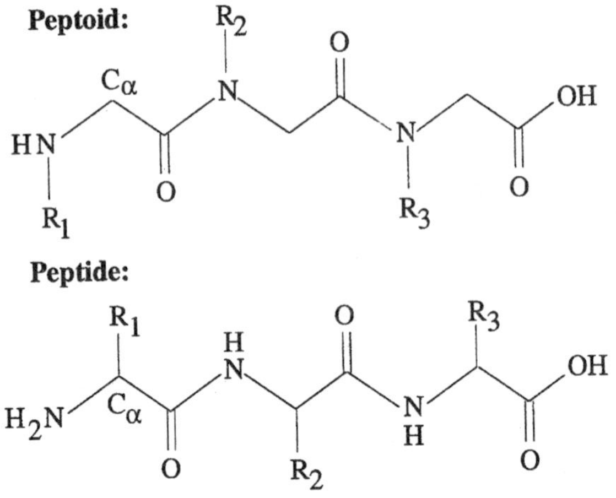

Figure 7 Comparison of the structures of peptide and peptoid trimers with arbitrary side chains R_1, R_2, and R_3. Peptoid structure differs from peptides in that the side chains are appended to the backbone nitrogen instead of the α carbon. (Adapted from Ref. 249, with permission.)

have been designed to capture both the amphipathic and three-dimensional structural characteristics of these proteins that are critical for their proper biophysical functioning. Studies so far have focused on SP-C analogues, which have been designed with a hydrophobic, helical stretch that spans a DPPC bilayer and that conserves the patterning of charged and hydrophilic residues found in natural protein. These peptoid-based SP mimics have been shown to be stably helical by CD and highly surface active by LWSB. In conjunction with various lipid mixtures (e.g., DPPC:POPG, 7:3, or Tanaka lipids), peptoid-based SP mimics have shown promise in vitro on the Langmuir-Wilhelmy surface balance and pulsating bubble surfactometer (257). Further investigations are necessary for evaluation of the efficacy and safety of these nonnatural materials, but these biostable analogues hold promise for treatment not only of RDS but of other respiratory diseases caused by the deficiency and dysfunction of LS.

XVII. FUTURE DIRECTIONS IN THE DEVELOPMENT OF BIOMIMETIC LS REPLACEMENTS

The development of a functional, reliable, safe, less immunogenic, and lower cost biomimetic lung surfactant replacement will be beneficial for the effective prevention and improved treatment of preterm infant RDS (258). The eventual impact of such a formulation on neonatal and perinatal health could be great (34–36), as it is likely that the indications for surfactant replacement therapy in infants will expand in the future to include other lung diseases that have surfactant dysfunction as an element of their pathogenesis (259,260), including meconium aspiration syndrome (261), congenital pneumonia (262), pulmonary hypoplasia, and pulmonary hemorrhage. To make the use of surfactant replacement therapy feasible for an expanded list of infant respiratory disorders and a greater number of patients worldwide, both the immunogenicity and the cost of exogenous surfactant replacements must be minimized (259).

Adults and children will also benefit from the development of a less immunogenic and less expensive synthetic formulation (34–36). The dysfunction of lung surfactant is a major contributor to the lethal "acute RDS (ARDS)," which can occur in adults and children after shock, bacterial sepsis, hyperoxia, near-drowning, or apiration (263–265). RDS is the leading cause of death in intensive care units, and there is no generally effective and economically viable treatment for it (266–268). The dysfunction of lung surfactant in adults and children most typically results from the encroachment of blood serum or other foreign fluids into the lungs. Serum proteins can disrupt and inhibit the spreading of the natural surfactant monolayer by a number of mechanisms (71,269). There has been indication in a few studies that LS replacement therapy may be effective for treatment of adult and child ARDS (270–273). However, adult therapy requires much larger dosage, making this treatment prohibitively expensive and unfeasible (274). In addition, there are important issues of LS inactivation and immunogenicity using LS replacements in adults because of their highly developed adaptive immune systems. Recent clinical work also suggests that surfactant dysfunction may play a role in the pathogenesis of cystic fibrosis and that specially designed surfactant replacements could prove beneficial to cystic fibrosis patients (275).

XVIII. CONCLUSIONS

The design of biomaterials that effectively mimic the structure and function of natural materials but that have the advantages of low immunogenicity and good bioavailability is a challenging area of bioengineering. An important and tractable problem in biomaterials research is the need for more effective and bioavailable LS replacements for the treatment of respiratory disease.

Before venturing into the development of complex material such as a biomimetic LS replacement, we must begin by recognizing both the need for this material and the specific areas for improvement in the present therapy. An integral step in the development process is to exploit knowledge of the structure–function relationships of the natural system to provide the design criteria. In vitro and in vivo studies are providing a better understanding of the role of LS components. The saturated lipids, particularly DPPC, are involved in reducing surface tension to near zero, whereas the unsaturated lipids and proteins have a role in facilitating adsorption and respreading of the LS films. In particular, the surfactant proteins B and C are responsible for enhancing lipid adsorption, respreading, and for stabilizing the surface film.

We are beginning to understand the composition and functions of LS, allowing improved designs of novel LS replacements. Researchers are currently developing biomimetic LS replacements based on recombinant and chemical production of SP-B and SP-C analogues. Successful expression and isolation of recombinant SP offers the advantage of producing a large quantity of material, potentially at a relatively low cost. However, production of recombinant SP mimics is challenging because of the difficulty in expressing these proteins with the correct conformation and in purifying them in high yield due to their highly hydrophobic nature. An alternative approach has been to chemically synthesize full-length, truncated, and modified versions of the SP. The chemical synthesis route offers ease of production and has enabled the investigation of numerous peptide analogues. Additionally, this synthetic route offers the reduction/ elimination of viral contamination and immunogenicity risks. It is chemically challenging to synthesize peptide analogues of SP-B and/or SP-C with the correct fold, but this may not necessarily be requisite for a functional LS replacement. It is interesting to note that a number of different amphipathic peptide designs have been successful in mimicking the biophysical and physiological roles of LS, to some extent. Most of the LS formulations have been based on the use of either SP-B or SP-C mimics (not both). Since both SP-B and SP-C are present in natural LS, biomimetic LS formulations most likely would be improved by the presence of both SP analogues. In addition, a better understanding of the individual roles of SP-B and SP-C would facilitate the design of improved biomimetic LS replacements.

An exciting aspect of developing these biomimetic LS replacements is the capacity to tailor their formulation to treat respiratory diseases with varying degrees of surfactant deficiency, insufficiency, and inactivation. There is an indication that LS therapy may also be effective for treating adult RDS, meconium aspiration syndrome, and pneumonia. However, the use of current commercially available LS replacements (natural and synthetic) is not yet viable for the treatment of adults; treatment of adult respiratory dysfunction will be one major application of a biomimetic LS replacement.

ACKNOWLEDGMENTS

We are grateful to Ka Yee C. Lee, Edward Ingenito, Michael Caplan, and Mark Johnson for helpful discussions. We acknowledge funding for this work provided by the National Science Foundation (Grant No. BES-0093806). C.W.W. was supported by an NIH Biophysics Training Grant (Grant No. 5T32 GM08382-10).

REFERENCES

1. JA Clements. Surface tension of lung extracts. Proc Soc Exp Bio Med 95:170–172, 1957.
2. RE Pattle. Properties, function and origin of the alveolar lining layer. Nature 175:1125–1126, 1955.
3. ME Avery, J Mead. Surface properties in relation to atelectasis and hyaline membrane disease. Am J Dis Child 97:517–523, 1959.
4. JW Kendig, RH Notter, C Cox, LJ Reubens, JM Davis, WM Maniscalco, RA Sinkin, A Bartoletti, HS Dweck, MJ Horgan, H Risemberg, DL Phelps, DL Shapiro. A Comparison of surfactant as immediate prophylaxis and as rescue therapy in newborns of less than 30 weeks gestation. N Engl J Med 324:865–871, 1991.
5. AI Eidelman. Economical consequences of surfactant therapy. J Perinatol 13:137–139, 1993.
6. B Guyer, DM Strobino, SJ Ventura, M MacDorman, JA Martin. Annual summary of vital statistics—1995. Pediatrics 98:1007–1019, 1995.
7. RM Schwartz, AM Luby, JW Scanlon, RJ Kellogg. Effect of surfactant on morbidity, mortality, and resource use in newborn infants weighing 500 to 1500 g. N Engl J Med 330:1476–1480, 1994.
8. Discovery Laboratories, Inc. addresses plans to conduct a Surfaxin trial in Latin America. February 23, 2001.
9. T Fujiwara, H Maeta, S Chida, T Morita, Y Watabe, T Abe. Artificial surfactant therapy in hyaline-membrane disease. Lancet 1:55–59, 1980.
10. RE Hoekstra, JC Jackson, TF Meyers, ID Frantz, ME Stern, WF Powers, M Maurer, JR Raye, ST Carrier, JH Gunkel, AJ Gold. Improved neonatal survival following multiple doses of bovine surfactant in very premature neonates at risk of respiratory distress syndrome. Pediatrics 88:19–28, 1991.

11. LA Gortner, U Bernsau, HH Hellwege, G Heironimi, G Jorch, HL Reiter. A multicenter randomized controlled trial of bovine surfactant for prevention of respiratory distress syndrome. Lung 168 (Suppl):864–869, 1990.

12. Collaborative European Multicenter Study Group. Surfactant replacement therapy in severe neonatal respiratory distress syndrome: An international randomized clinical trial. Pediatrics 82:683–691, 1988.

13. CJ Morley, AD Bangham, N Miller, JA Davis. Dry artificial lung surfactant and its effect on very premature babies. Lancet 1:64–68, 1981.

14. RH Phibbs, RA Ballard, JA Clements, DC Heilbron, CS Phibbs, MA Schlueter, SH Sniderman, WH Tooley, A Wakely. Initial clinical trial of Exosurf, a protein-free synthetic surfactant, for the prophylaxis and early treatment of hyaline membrane disease. Pediatrics 88:1–9, 1991.

15. S Hawgood, A Ogawa, K Yukitake, M Schlueter, C Brown, T White, D Buckley, D Lesikar, B Benson. Lung function in premature rabbits treated with recombinant human surfactant protein-C. Am J Respir Crit Care Med 154:484–490, 1996.

16. AJ Davis, AH Jobe, D Häfner, M Ikegami. Lung function in premature lambs and rabbits with a recombinant SP-C surfactant. Am J Respir Crit Care Med 157:553–559, 1998.

17. EJA Veldhuizen, JJ Batenburg, G Vandenbussche, G Putz, LMG van Golde, HP Haagsman. Production of surfactant protein C in the baculovirus expression: the information required for correct folding and palmitoylation. Biochim Biophys Acta 1416:295–308, 1999.

18. L-J Yao, C Richardson, C Ford, N Mathialagan, G Mackie, GL Hammond, PGR Harding, F Possmayer. Expression of mature pulmonary surfactant-associated protein B (SP-B) in Escherichia coli using truncated human SP-B cDNAs. Biochem Cell Biol 68:559–566, 1990.

19. A Waring, W Taeusch, R Bruni, J Amirkhanian, B Fan, R Stevens, J Young. Synthetic amphipathic sequences of surfactant protein-B mimic several physiochemical and in vivo properties of native pulmonary surfactant proteins. Peptide Res 2:308–313, 1989.

20. R Bruni, HW Taeusch, AJ Waring. Surfactant protein B: lipid interactions of synthetic peptides representing the amino-terminal amphipathic domain. Proc Natl Acad Sci USA 88:7451–7455, 1991.

21. JE Baatz, V Sarin, DR Absolom, C Baxter, JA Whitsett. Effects of surfactant-associated protein SP-B synthetic analogs on the structure and surface activity of model membrane bilayers. Chem Phys Lipids 60:163–178, 1991.

22. VK Sarin, S Gupta, TK Leung, VE Taylor, BL Ohning, JA Whitsett, JL Fox. Biophysical and biological activity of a synthetic 8.7-kDa hydrophobic pulmonary surfactant protein SP-B. Proc Natl Acad Sci USA 87:2633–2637, 1990.

23. JH Kang, MK Lee, KL Kim, K-S Hahm. The relationships between biophysical activity and the secondary structure of synthetic peptides from the pulmonary surfactant protein SP-B. Biochem Mol Biol Int 40:617–627, 1996.

24. FJ Walther, J Hernández-Juviel, R Bruni, AJ Waring. Spiking Survanta® with synthetic surfactant peptides improves oxygenation in surfactant-deficient rats. Am J Respir Crit Care Med 156:855–861, 1997.

25. EJA Veldhuizen, AJ Waring, FJ Walther, JJ Batenburg, LMG Van Golde, HP Haagsman. Dimeric N-terminal segment of human surfactant protein B (dSP-B1-25) has enhanced surface properties compared to monomeric SP-B1-25. Biophys J 79:377–384, 2000.

26. T Takei, Y Hashimoto, T Aiba, K Sakai, T Fujiwara. The surface properties of chemically synthesized peptides analogous to human pulmonary surfactant protein SP-C. Biol Pharm Bull 19:1247–1253, 1996.

27. T Takei, Y Hashimoto, E Ohtsubo, H Ohkawa. Characterization of polyleucine substituted analogues of human surfactant protein SP-C. Biol Pharm Bull 19:1550–1555, 1996.

28. J Johansson, G Nilsson, R Stromberg, B Robertson, H Jornvall, T Curstedt. Secondary structure and biophysical activity of synthetic analogs of the pulmonary surfactant polypeptide SP-C. Biochem J 307:535–541, 1995.

29. G Nilsson, M Gustafsson, G Vandenbusshe, E Veldhuizen, WJ Griffiths, J Sjovall, HP Haagsman, JM Ruysschaert, B Robertson, T Curstedt, J Johansson. Synthetic peptide-containing surfactants: evaluation of transmembrane versus amphipathic helices and SP-C poly-valyl to polyleucyl substitution. Eur J Biochem 225:116–124, 1998.

30. M Palmblad, J Johansson, B Robertson, T Curstedt. Biophysical activity of an artificial surfactant containing an analogue of surfactant protein (SP)-C and native SP-B. Biochem J 339:381–386, 1999.

31. LR McLean, RL Jackson, JL Krstenansky, KA Hagaman, KF Olsen, JE Lewis. Mixtures of synthetic peptides and dipalmitoylphosphatidylcholine as lung surfactants. Am J Physiol 262:L292–L300, 1992.

32. L McLean, J Lewis, J Krstenansky, K Hagaman, A Cope, K Olsen, E Matthews, D Uhrhammer, T Owen, M Payne. An amphipathic alpha-helical decapeptide in phosphatidylcholine is an effective synthetic lung surfactant. Am Rev Respir Dis 147:462–465, 1993.

33. CG Cochrane, SD Revak. Pulmonary surfactant protein (SP-B): structure–function relationships. Science 254:566–568, 1991.

34. B Robertson, J Johansson, T Curstedt. Synthetic surfactants to treat neonatal lung disease. Mol Med Today 6:119–124, 2000.

35. FJ Walther, LM Gordon, JA Zasadzinski, MA Sherman, AJ Waring. Surfactant protein B and C analogues. Mol Genet Metab 71:342–351, 2000.

36. J Johansson, M Gustafsson, M Palmblad, S Zaltash, B Robertson, T Curstedt. Pulmonary surfactant emerging protein analogues. BioDrugs 2:71–77, 1999.

37. AH Jobe. Respiratory distress syndrome: new therapeutic approaches to a complex pathophysiology. Adv Pediatr Chicago 30:93–130, 1984.

38. H O'Brodovich, V Hannam. Exogenous surfactant rapidly increases PaO2 in mature rabbits with lungs that contain large amounts of saline. Am Rev Respir Dis 147:1087–1090, 1993.

39. B Robertson. Surfactant substitution: experimental models and clinical applications. Lung 158:57–68, 1980.

40. C Vilstrup, D Gommers, JAH Bos, B Lachmann, O Werner, A Larson. Natural surfactant instilled in premature lambs increases lung volume and improves ventilation homogeneity within five minutes. Pediatr Res 32:595–599, 1992.

41. W Long, A Corbet, R Cotton, S Courtney, G McGuiness, D Walter, J Watts, J Smyth, H Bard, V Chernick. A controlled trial of synthetic surfactant in infants weighing 1250 g or more with respiratory distress syndrome. N Engl J Med 325:1696–1703, 1991.

42. JA Mauskopf, ME Backhouse, D Jones, DE Wold, MC Mammel, M Mullet, R Guthrie, WA Long. Synthetic surfactant for rescue treatment of respiratory distress syndrome in premature infants weighing from 700 to 1350 grams: impact on hospital resource use and charges. J Pediatr 126:94–101, 1995.

43. CE Mercier, RF Soll. Clinical trials of natural surfactant extract in respiratory distress syndrome. In: WA Long, ed. Clinics in Perinatology. Philadelphia: WB Saunders, 1993, pp 711–735.

44. A Charon, HW Taeusch, C Fitzgibon, GB Smith, ST Treves, DS Phelps. Pediatrics 83:348–354, 1989.

45. JD Amirkhanian, HW Taeusch. Reversible and irreversible inactivation of preformed pulmonary surfactant surface films by changes in subphase constituents. Biochim Biophys Acta 1165:321–326, 1993.

46. K von Neergaard. Neue Aufassungen uber einen Grundbegriff der Atemmechanik. Die Retraktionskraft der Lunge, abhangig von der Oberflachenspannung in den Alveolen. Gesamete Exp Med 66:373–394, 1929.

47. JA Clements. Dependence of pressure-volume characteristics of lungs on intrinsic surface active material. Am J Physiol 187:592, 1956.

48. MH Klaus, JA Clements, RJ Havel. Composition of surface-active material isolated from beef lung. Proc Natl Acad Sci USA 47:1858–1859, 1961.

49. E Robillard, Y Alarie, P Dagenais-Perusse, E Baril, A Guilbeault. Microaerosol administration of synthetic beta-gamma-dipalmitoyl-L-alpha-lecithin in the respiratory distress syndrome: a preliminary report. Can Med Assoc J 90:55–57, 1964.

50. J Chu, JA Clements, EK Cotton, MH Klaus, AY Sweet, WH Tooley. Neonatal pulmonary ischemia. Pediatrics 40:709–782, 1967.

51. MC Phillips, BD Ladbrooke, D Chapman. Molecular interactions in mixed lecithin systems. Biochim Biophys Acta 196:35–44, 1970.

52. A Bangham, C Morley, M Phillips. The physical properties of an effective lung surfactant. Biochim Biophys Acta 573:552–556, 1979.

53. J Goerke, JA Clements. Alveolar surface tension and lung surfactant. ed. Handbook of Physiology: The Respiratory System—Control of Breathing. Bethesda: American Physiology Society, 1986, pp 247–261.

54. RH Notter. Surface chemistry of pulmonary surfactant: the role of individual components. In: B Robertson, LMG van Golde, and JJ Batenburg, ed. Pulmonary Surfactant. Amsterdam: Elsevier, 1984, pp 17–53.

55. RH Notter. The physical chemistry and physiological activity of pulmonary surfactant. In: DL Shapiro, RH Notter, eds. Surfactant Replacement Therapy. New York: Alan R. Liss, 1989, pp 19–70.

56. FB Askin, C Kuhn. The cellular origin of pulmonary surfactant. Lab Invest 25:260–268, 1971.

57. US Ryan, JW Ryan, DS Smith. Alveolar type II cells: studies on the mode of release of lamellar bodies. Tissue Cell 3:587–599, 1975.

58. ER Weiber, GS Kistler, G Töndury. A stereological electron microscope study of "tubular myelin figures" in alveolar fluids of rat lungs. Z Zellforsch 69:418–427, 1966.

59. MC Williams. Conversion of lamellar body membranes into tubular myelin in alveoli of fetal rat lungs. J Cell Biol 72:260–277, 1977.

60. J Goerke. Lung surfactant. Biochim Biophys Acta 344:241–261, 1974.

61. RH Notter, DP Penney, JN Finkelstein, DL Shapiro. Adsorption of natural lung surfactant and phospholipid extracts related to tubular myelin formations. Pediatr Res 20:97–101, 1986.

62. E Putman, LAJM Creuwels, LMG van Golde, HP Haagsman. Surface properties, morphology, and protein composition of pulmonary surfactant subtypes. Biochem J 320:599–605, 1996.

63. JA Clements, ES Brown, RP Johnson. Pulmonary surface tension and the mucus lining of the lungs: some theoretical considerations. J Appl Physiol 12:262–268, 1958.

64. JA Clements. Functions of the alveolar lining. Am Rev Respir Dis 115:67–71, 1977.

65. RH Notter. The physical and physiological activity of pulmonary surfactant. In: DL Shapiro, RH Notter, eds. Surfactant Replacement Therapy. New York: Alan R. Liss, 1989, pp 19–70.

66. LMG van Golde, JJ Batenburg, B Robertson. The pulmonary surfactant system: biochemical aspects and functional significance. Physiol Rev 68:374–455, 1988.

67. AM Cockshutt, F Possmayer. Metabolism of surfactant lipids and proteins in developing lung. In: B Robertson, LMG van Golde, JJ Batenbur, eds. Pulmonary Surfactant: From Molecular Biology to Clinical Practice. Amsterdam: Elsevier, 1992, pp 339–378.

68. RL Sanders. The composition of pulmonary surfactant. In: PM Farrell, ed. Lung development: biological and clinical perspectives. New York: Academic Press, 1982, pp 193–219.

69. RJ King. Isolation and chemical composition of pulmonary surfactant. In: B Robertson, LMG van Golde, JJ Batenburg, eds. Pulmonary Surfactant. Amsterdam: Elsevier, 1984, pp 1–15.

70. S Hawgood, JA Clements. Pulmonary surfactant and its aproproteins. J Clin Invest 86:1–6, 1990.

71. A Cockshutt, D Absolom, F Possmayer. The role of palmitic acid in pulmonary surfactant: enhancement of surface activity and prevention of inhibition by blook proteins. Biochim Biophys Acta 1085:248–256, 1991.

72. J Johansson, T Curstedt, B Robertson. The proteins of the surfactant system. Eur Respir J 7:372–391, 1994.

73. A Khoor, ME Gray, WM Hull, JA Whitsett, MT Stahlman. Developmental expression of SP-A and SP-A mRNA in the proximal and distal epithelium in the human fetus and newborn. J Histochem Cytochem 41:1311–1319, 1993.

74. K Miyamura, EA Leigh, J Lu, J Hopkins, A Lopez-Bernal, KBM Reid. Surfactant protein D to alveolar macrophages. Biochem J 300:237–242, 1994.

75. S Hawgood. The hydrophilic surfactant protein SP-A: Molecular biology, structure and function. In: B Robertson, L van Golde, JE Batenburg, eds. Pulmonary Surfactant: From Molecular Biology to Clinical Practice. Amsterdam: Elsevier, 1992, pp 33–45.

76. HP Haagsman. Surfactant protein A and D. Biochem Soc Trans 22:100–106, 1994.

77. RJ King, JA Clements. Surface active materials from dog lung. II. Composition and physiological correlations. Am J Physiol 223:715–726, 1972.

78. SB Hall, AR Venkitaraman, J Whitsett, BA Holm, RH Notter. Importance of hydrophobic apoproteins as constituents of clinical exogenous surfactants. Am Rev Respir Dis 145:24–30, 1992.

79. Z Wang, SB Hall, RH Notter. Roles of different hydrophobic constituents in the adsorption of pulmonary surfactant. J Lipid Res 37:790–798, 1996.

80. S Schürch, R Qanbar, H Bachofen, F Possmayer. The surface-associated surfactant reservoir in the alveolar lining. Biol Neonate 67:61–76, 1995.

81. Z Wang, O Gurel, JE Baatz, RH Notter. Differential activity and lack of synergy of lung surfactant proteins SP-B and SP-C interactions. J Lipid Res 37:1749-1760, 1996.

82. DY Takamoto, MM Lipp, A von Nahmen, KYC Lee, AJ Waring, JA Zasadzinski. Interaction of lung surfactant proteins with anionic phospholipids. Biophys J 81:153–169, 2001.

83. S Taneva, KMW Keogh. Pulmonary surfactant proteins SP-B and SP-C in spread monolayers at the air–water interface. III. Proteins SP-B plus SP-C with phospholipids in spread monolayers. Biophys J 66:1158–1166, 1994.

84. T Curstedt, H Jornvall, B Robertson, T Bergman, P Berggren. Two hydrophobic low-molecular mass protein fractions of pulmonary surfactant: characterization and biophysical activity. Eur J Biochem 168:255–262, 1987.

85. MA Oosterlaken-Dijksterhuis, HP Haagsman, LMG van Golde, RA Demel. Characterization of lipid insertion into monomolecular layers mediated by lung surfactant proteins SP-B and SP-C. Biochemistry 30:10965–10971, 1991.

86. SD Revak, TA Merritt, E Degryse, L Stefani, M Courtney, M Hallman, CG Cochrane. The use of human low molecular weight (LMW) apoproteins in the reconstitution of surfactant biological activity. J Clin Invest 81:826–833, 1988.

87. SH Yu, F Possmayer. Comparative studies of the biophysical activities of the low molecular weight proteins purified from bovine pulmonary surfactant. Biochim Biophys Acta 961:337–350, 1988.

88. S Schürch, FY Green, H Bachofen. Formation and structure of surface films: captive bubble surfactometry. Biochim Biophys Acta 1408:180–202, 1998.

89. K Nag, JG Munro, K Inchley, S Schürch, NO Petersen, F Possmayer. SP-B refining of pulmonary surfactant phospholipid films. Am J Physiol 277:L1179–L1189, 1999.

90. S Krol, A Janshoff, M Ross, H-J Galla. Structure and function of surfactant protein B and C in lipid monolayers: a scanning force microscopy study. Phys Chem Chem Phys 2:4586–4593, 2000.

91. J Johansson, T Curstedt. Molecular structures and interactions of pulmonary components. Eur J Biochem 244:675–693, 1997.

92. S Hawgood, M Derrick, F Poulain. Structure and properties of surfactant protein B. Biochim Biophys Acta 1408:150–160, 1998.

93. J Johansson. Structure and properties of surfactant protein C. Biochim Biophys Acta 1408:161–172, 1998.

94. TE Weaver, JJ Conkright. Functions of surfactant proteins B and C. Annu Rev Physiol 63:555–578, 2001.

95. SW Glasser, TR Korfhagen, TE Weaver, T Pilot-Matias, JL Fox, JA Whitsett. cDNA and deduced amino acid sequence of human pulmonary surfactant-associated proteolipid SPL (phe). Proc Natl Acad Sci USA 84:4007–4011, 1987.

96. S Hawgood, BJ Benson, J Schilling, D Damm, JA Clements, RT White. Nucleotide and amino acid sequences of pulmonary surfactant protein SP 18 and evidence for cooperation between SP 18 and SP 28-36 in surfactant lipid adsorption. Proc Natl Acad Sci 84:66–70, 1987.

97. T Curstedt, J Johansson, J Barros-Soderling, B Robertson, G Nilsson, M Westberg, H Jornvall. Low molecular-mass surfactant protein type 1: the primary structure of a hydrophobic 8 kDa polypeptide with eight half-cystine residues. Eur J Biochem 172:521–525, 1988.

98. J Johansson, T Curstedt, H Jörnvall. Surfactant protein B: disulfide bridges, structural properties, and kringle similarities. Biochemistry 30:6917–6921, 1991.

99. J Johansson, H Jörnvall, T Curstedt. Human surfactant polypeptide SP-B disulfide bridges, C-terminal end, and peptide analysis of the airway form. FEBS Lett 301:165–167, 1992.

100. A Takahashi, AJ Waring, J Amirkhanian, B Fan, HW Taeusch. Structure–function relationships of bovine surfactant proteins: SP-B and SP-C. Biochem Biophys Acta 1044:43–49, 1990.

101. J Watkins. The surface properties of pure phospholipids in relation to those of lung extracts. Biochim Biophys Acta 152:293–306, 1968.

102. JN Hildebran, J Goerke, JA Clements. Pulmonary surface film stability and composition. J App Physiol 47:604–611, 1979.

103. MS Hawco, PJ Davis, KMW Keough. Lipid fluidity in lung surfactant monolayers of saturated and unsaturated lechitins. J Appl Physiol 51:509–515, 1981.

104. J Egbert, H Sloot, A Mazure. Minimal surface tension, squeeze-out and transition temperatures of binary mixtures of dipalmitoylphosphatidylcholine and unsaturated phospholipids. Biochim Biophys Acta 1002:109–113, 1989.

105. SH Yu, F Possmayer. Effect of pulmonary surfactant protein (SP-B) and calcium on phospholipid adsorption and squeeze-out of phosphatidylglycerol from binary phospholipid monolayers containing dipalmitoylphosphatidylcholine. Biochim Biophys Acta 1126:26–34, 1992.

106. L Camacho, A Cruz, R Castro, C Casals, J Perez-Gil. Effect of pH on the interfacial adsorption activity of pulmonary surfactant. Colloids Surf B Biointerf 5:271–277, 1996.

107. G Vandenbussche, A Clercx, M Clercx, T Curstedt, J Johansson, H Jornvall, JM Ruysschaert. Secondary structure and orientation of hydrophobicthe surfactant protein B in a lipid environment: a Fourier transform infrared spectroscopy study. Biochemistry 31:9169–9176, 1992.

108. MA Oosterlaken-Dijksterhuis, HP Haagsman, LMG van Golde, RA Demel. Interaction of lipid vesicles with monomolecular layers containing lung surfactant proteins SP-B or SP-C. Biochemistry 30:8276–8281, 1991.

109. J Perez-Gil, A Cruz, C Casals. Solubility of hydrophobic surfactant proteins in organic solvent/water mixtures: structural studies on SP-B and SP-C in aqueous organic solvents and lipids. Biochim Biophys Acta 1168:261–270, 1993.

110. M Andersson, T Curstedt, H Jornvall, J Johansson. An amphipathic helical motif common to tumourolytic polypeptide NK-lysin and pulmonary surfactant polypeptide SP-B. FEBS Lett 362:328–332, 1995.

111. G Vandenbussche, J Johansson, T Clercx, T Curstedt, JM Ruysschaert. Structure and orientation of hydrophobic surfactant-associated proteins in a lipid environment. In: H Jornhall, P Jolles, eds. Interfaces Between Chemistry and Biochemistry. Basel: Birkhauser, 1995, pp 27–47.

112. JA Whitsett, JE Baatz. Hydrophobic surfactant proteins SP-B and SP-C: molecular biology, structure, and function. In: B Robertson, LMG van Golde, JJ Batenburg, eds. Pulmonary Surfactant: From Molecular Biology to Clinical Practice. Amsterdam: Elsevier, 1992, pp 55–75.

113. KMW Keough. Physical chemistry of pulmonary surfactant in the terminal air spaces. In: B Robertson, LMG van Golde, JJ Batenburg, eds. Pulmonary Surfactant: From Molecular Biology to Clinical Practice. Amsterdam: Elsevier, 1992, pp 109–164.

114. J Pérez-Gil, MW Keough. Interfacial properties of surfactant proteins. Biochim Biophys Acta 1408:203–217, 1998.

115. AJ Waring, KF Faull, C Leung, A Chang-Chien, P Mercado, HW Taeusch, LM Gordon. Synthesis, secondary structure and folding of the bend region of lung surfactant protein B. Pept Res 9:28–39, 1996.

116. S Zaltash, M Palmblad, T Curstedt, J Johansson, B Persson. Pulmonary surfactant protein B: A structural model and a functional analogue. Biochim Biophys Acta 1466:179–186, 2000.

117. J Perez-Gil, T Tucker, G Simatos, KMW Keough. Cell Biol 70:332–338, 1991.

118. JS Vincent, SD Revak, CG Cochrane, IW Levin. Raman spectroscopic studies of model human pulmonary surfactant systems: phospholipid interactions with peptide paradigms for the surfactant protein SP-B. Biochemistry 30:8395–8401, 1991.

119. FR Poulain, L Allen, MC Williams, RL Hamilton, S Hawgood. Effects of surfactant apolipoproteins on liposome structure: implications for tubular myelin formation. Am J Physiol 262:L730–L739, 1992.

120. Y Suzuki, Y Fujita, K Kogishi. Reconstitution of tubular myelin from synthetic lipids and proteins associated with pig pulmonary surfactant. Am Rev Respir Dis 140:75–81, 1989.

121. MC Williams, S Hawgood, SC Hamilton. Changes in lipid structure produced by surfactant proteins SP-A, SP-B, and SP-C. Am J Respir Cell Mol Biol 5:41–50, 1991.

122. MA Oosterlaken-Dijksterhuis, LMG van Golde, HP Haagsman. Lipid mixing is mediated by the hydrophobic surfactant protein SP-B but not by SP-C. Biochim Biophys Acta 1110:45–50, 1992.

123. ED Rider, M Ikegami, JA Whitsett, W Hull, D Absolom, AH Jobe. Treatment responses to surfactants containing natural surfactant proteins in preterm rabbits. Am Rev Respir Dis 147:669–676, 1993.

124. B Robertson, T Kobayashi, M Ganzuka, G Grossman, W-Z Li, Y Suzuki. Experimental neonatal respiratory failure induced by a monoclonal antibody to the hydrophobic surfactant-associated protein SP-B. Pediatr Res 30:239–243, 1991.

125. JC Clark, SE Wert, CJ Bachurski, MT Stahlman, BR Stripp, TE Weaver, JA Whitsett. Targeted disruption of the surfactant protein B gene disrupts surfactant homeostasis, causing respiratory failure in newborn mice. Proc Natl Acad Sci USA 92:7794–7798, 1995.

126. K Tokeida, JA Whitsett, JC Clark, TE Weaver, K Ikeda, KB McConnell, AH Jobe, M Ikegami, HS Iwamoto. Pulmonary dysfunction in neonatal SP-B-deficient mice. Am J Physiol 273:L875–L882, 1997.

127. DC Beck, M Ikegami, C-L Na, S Zaltash, J Johansson, JA Whitsett, TE Weaver. The role of homodimers in surfactant protein B function in vivo. J Biol Chem 275:3365–3370, 2000.

128. DC Beck, CL Na, JA Whitsett, TE Weaver. Ablation of a critical surfactant protein B intramolecular disulfide bonds in transgenic mice. J Biol Chem 275:3371–3376, 2000.

129. LM Nogee, G Garnier, HC Dietz, L Singer, AM Murphy, DE Demello, HR Colten. A mutation in the surfactant protein B gene responsible for fatal neonatal respiratory disease in multiple kindreds. J Clin Invest 93:1860–1863, 1994.

130. LM Nogee, DE deMello, LP Dehner, HR Colten. Pulmonary surfactant B deficiency in congenital pulmonary alveolar proteinosis. N Engl J Med 328:406–410, 1993.

131. J Johansson, T Curstedt, B Robertson, H Jörnvall. Size and structure of the hydrophobic low molecular weight surfactant-associated polypeptide. Biochemistry 27:3544–3547, 1988.

132. J Johansson, H Jörnvall, A Eklund, N Christensen, B Robertson, T Curstedt. Hydrophobic 3.7 kDa surfactant polypeptide: structural characterization of the human and bovine forms. FEBS Lett 232:61–64, 1988.

133. J Johansson, T Szyperki, T Curstedt, K Wüthrich. The NMR structure of the pulmonary surfactant-associated polypeptide SP-C in an apolar solvent contains a valyl-rich α-helix. Biochemistry 33:6015–6023, 1994.

134. B Pastrana, AJ Mautone, R Mendelsohn. FTIR studies of secondary structure and orientation of pulmonary surfactant SP-C and its effect on the dynamic surface properties of phospholipids. Biochemistry 30:10058–10064, 1991.

135. K Shiffer, S Hawgood, HP Haagsman, B Benson, JA Clements, J Goerke. Lung surfactant proteins SP-B and SP-C alter the thermodynamic properties of the phospholipid membrane: a differential calorimetry study. Biochemistry 32:590–597, 1993.

136. MR Morrow, S Taneva, GA Simatos, LA Allwood, KMW Keough. ^{2}H-NMR studies of the effect of pulmonary surfactant SP-C on the 1,2-dipalmitoyl-sn-glycerol-3-phosphocholine headgroup: a model for transbilayer peptides in surfactant and biological membranes. Biochemistry 32:11338–11344, 1993.

137. G Vandenbussche, A Clercx, T Curstedt, J Johansson, H Jörnvall, JM Ruysschaert. Structure and orientation of the surfactant-associated protein C in a lipid bilayer. Eur J Biochem 203:201–209, 1992.

138. A Gericke, CR Flach, R Mendelsohn. Structure and orientation of lung surfactant SP-C and L-α-dipalmitoylphophatidylcholine in aqueous monolayers. Biophys J 73:492–499, 1997.

139. H-J Galla, N Buordos, A von Nahmen, M Amrein, M Sieber. The role of pulmonary surfactant C during the breathing cycle. Thin Solid Films 327–329:632–635, 1998.

140. EJA Veldhuizen, HP Haagsman. Role of pulmonary surfactant components in surface film formation and dynamics. Biochim Biophys Acta 1467:255–270, 2000.

141. T Curstedt, J Johansson, P Persson, A Eklund, B Robertson, B Lowenadler, H Jornvall. Hydrophobic surfactant-associated polypeptides: SP-C is a lipopeptide with two palmitoylated cysteine residues, whereas SP-B lacks covalently linked fatty acyl groups. Proc Natl Acad Sci USA 87:2985–2989, 1990.

142. LAJM Creuwels, RA Demel, LMG van Golde, BJ Benson, HP Haagsman. Effect of acylation on structure and function of surfactant protein C at the air–liquid interface. J Biol Chem 268:26752–26758, 1993.

143. T Kato, S Lee, S Ono, Y Agawa, H Aoyagi, M Ohno, N Nishino. Conformational studies of amphipathic α-helical peptides containing an amino acid with a long alkyl chain and their anchoring to lipid bilayer liposomes. Biochim Biophys Acta 1063:191–196, 1991.

144. R Qanbar, F Possmayer. On the surface activity of surfactant-associated protein C (SP-C): effects of palmitoylation and pH. Biochim Biophys Acta 1255:251–259, 1995.

145. Z Wang, O Gurel, GE Baatz, RH Notter. Acylation of pulmonary surfactant protein-C is required for its optimal surface active interactions with phospholipids. J Biol Chem 271:19104–19109, 1996.

146. LAJM Creuwels, EH Boer, RA Demel, LMG van Golde, HP Haagsman. Neutralization of the positive charges of surfactant protein C: effects on structure and function. J Biol Chem 270:16225–16229, 1995.

147. R Qanbar, S Cheng, F Possmayer, S Schurch. Role of palmitoylation of surfactant-associated protein C in surfactant film formation and stability. Am J Physiol 271:L572–L580, 1996.

148. AD Horowitz, B Elledge, JA Whitsett, JE Baatz. Effects of lung sufactant proteolipid SP-C on the organization of model membrane lipids: a fluorescence study. Biochim Biophys Acta 1107:44–54, 1992.

149. J Perez-Gil, K Nag, S Taneva, KMW Keough. Pulmonary surfactant protein SP-C causes packing rearrangements of dipalmitoyl phosphatidylcholine in spread monolayers. Biophys J 63:197–204, 1992.

150. AD Horowitz, B Moussavian, JA Whitsett. Roles of SP-A, SP-B, and SP-C in modulation of lipid uptake by pulmonary epithelial cells in vitro. Am J Physiol 270:L69–L79, 1996.

151. WR Rice, VK Sarin, JL Fox, J Baatz, J Wert, JA Whitsett. Surfactant peptides stimulate uptake of phosphatidylcholine by isolated cells. Biochim Biophys Acta 1006:237–242, 1989.

152. LM Nogee, AE Dunbar, SE Wert, F Askin, A Hamvas, JA Whitsett. A mutation in the surfactant protein C gene associated with familial interstitial lung disease. N Engl J Med 344:573–579, 2001.

153. SW Glasser, MS Burhans, TR Korfhagen, C-L Na, PD Sly, GF Ross, M Ikegami, JA Whitsett. Altered stability of pulmonary surfactant in SP-C deficient mice. Proc Natl Acad Sci USA, in press.

154. F Danlois, S Zaltash, J Johansson, B Robertson, HP Haagsman, M van Eijk, MF Beers, F Rollin, J-M Ruysschaert, G Vandenbussche. Very low surfactant protein C, contents in newborn Belgian white and blue calves with respiratory distress syndrome. Biochem J 351:779–787, 2000.

155. A von Nahmen, A Post, HJ Galla, M Sieber. The phase behavior of lipid monolayers containing pulmonary surfactant protein C studied by fluorescence light microscopy. Eur Biophys J:359–369, 1997.

156. M Amrein, A von Nahmen, M Sieber. Scanning force and fluorescence light microscopy study of structure and function of a model pulmonary surfactant. Eur Biophys J 26:349–357, 1997.

157. G Putz, M Walch, M Van Eijk, HP Haagsman. Hydrophobic lung surfactant proteins B and C remain associated during dynamic cyclic area changes. Biochim Biophys Acta 1453:126–134, 1999.

158. S-H Yu, F Possmayer. Role of bovine pulmonary surfactant-associated proteins in the surface-active property of phospholipid mixtures. Biochim Biophys Acta 1046:233–241, 1990.

159. K Nag, J Perez-Gil, A Cruz, KMW Keough. Fluorescently labeled pulmonary surfactant protein C in spread phospholipid monolayers. Biophys J 71:246–256, 1996.

160. Y Tanaka, T Takei, T Aiba, K Masuda, A Kiuchi, T Fujiwara. Development of synthetic lung surfactant. J Lipid Res 27:475–485, 1986.

161. A Post, A von Nahmen, M Schmitt, J Ruths, H Riegler, M Sieber, H-J Galla. Pulmonary surfactant protein C containing lipid films at the air–water interface as a model for the surface of lung alveoli. Mol Membrane Biol 12:93–99, 1995.

162. A von Nahmen, M Schenk, M Sieber, M Amrein. The structure of a model pulmonary surfactant as revealed by scanning force microscopy. Biophys J 72:463–469, 1997.

163. MM Lipp, KYC Lee, JA Zasadzinski, AJ Waring. Phase and morphology changes in lipid monolayers induced by SP-B protein and its amino-terminal peptide. Science 273:1196–1199, 1996.

164. MM Lipp, KY Lee, DY Takamoto, JA Zasadzinski, AJ Waring. Coexistence of buckled and flat monolayers. Phys Rev Lett 81:1650–1653, 1998.

165. M Longo, A Bisagno, J Zasadzinski, R Bruni, A Waring. A function of lung surfactant protein SP-B. Science 261:453–456, 1993.

166. J Ding, DY Takamoto, A von Nahmen, MM Lipp, KYC Lee, A Waring, J Zasadzinski. Effects of lung surfactant proteins SP-B and SP-C and palmitic acid and monolayer stability. Biophys J 80:2262–2272, 2001.

167. R Bruni, JM Hernandez-Juviel, R Tanoviceanu, FJ Walther. Synthetic mimics of surfactant proteins B and C: in vitro surface activity and effects on lung compliance in two animal models of surfactant deficiency. Mol Gene Metab 63:116–125, 1998.

168. EP Ingenito, L Mark, J Morris, FF Espinosa, RD Kamm, M Johnson. Biophysical characterization and modeling of lung surfactant components. J Appl Physiol 86:1702–1714, 1999.

169. EP Ingenito, R Mora, L Mark. Pivotal role of anionic phospholipids in determining dynamic behavior of lung surfactant. Am J Respir Crit Care Med 161:831–838, 2000.

170. P Krüger, M Schalke, Z Wang, RH Notter, RA Dluhy, M Lösche. Effect of hydrophobic surfactant peptides SP-B and SP-C on binary phospholipid monolayers I. Fluorescence and dark-field microscopy. Biophys J 77:903–914, 1999.

171. MM Lipp, KYC Lee, A Waring, JA Zasadzinski. Fluorescence, polarized fluorescence, and Brewster angle microscopy of palmitic acid and lung surfactant protein B monolayers. Biophys J 72:2783–2804, 1997.

172. K Nag, J Perez-Gil, MLF Ruano, LAD Worthman, J Stewart, C Casals, KMW Keough. Phase transitions in films of lung surfactant at the air–water interface. Biophys J 74:2983–2995, 1998.

173. K Rodriguez-Capote, K Nag, S Schürch, F Possmayer. Surfactant protein interactions with neutral and acidic phospholipid films. Am J Physiol Lung Cell Mol Physiol 281:L231–L242, 2001.

174. J Goerke, J Gonzales. Temperature dependence of dipalmitoyl phosphatidylcholine monolayer stability. J Appl Physiol 51:1108–1114, 1981.

175. S Schürch. Surface tension at low lung volumes: dependence on time and alveolar size. Respir Physiol 48:339–355, 1982.

176. RJ King. The surfactant system of the lung. Fed Proc 33:2238–2247, 1974.

177. BA Holm, G Enhorning, RH Notter. A biophysical mechanism by which plasma protein inhibit lung surfactant activity. Chem Phys Lipids 49:49–55, 1988.

178. BA Holm, RH Notter. Effects of hemoglobin and cell membrane lipids on pulmonary surfactant activity. J Appl Physiol 63:1434–1442, 1987.

179. M Ikegami, A Jobe, H Jacobs, R Lam. A protein from airways of premature lambs that inhibits surfactant function. J Appl Physiol 57:1134–1142, 1984.

180. W Seeger, C Grube, A Gunther, R Schmidt. Surfactants inhibition by plasma proteins: differential sensitivity of various surfactant preparations. Eur Respir J 6:971–977, 1993.

181. A Cockshutt, F Possmayer. Lysophosphatidylcholine sensitizes lipid extracts of pulmonary surfactant to inhibition by plasma proteins. Biochim Biophys Acta 1086:63–71, 1991.

182. RH Notter, SA Tabak, RD Mavis. Surface properties of binary mixtures of some pulmonary surfactant components. J Lipid Res 21:10–22, 1980.

183. SB Hall, ZR Lu, AR Venkitaraman, RW Hyde, RH Notter. Inhibition of pulmonary surfactant by oleic acid: mechanisms and characteristics. J Appl Physiol 72:1708–1716, 1992.

184. U Pison. Proteolytic inactivation of dog lung surfactant associated proteins by neutrophil elastase. Biochim Biophys Acta 992:251–257, 1989.

185. DA Clark, GF Nieman, AM Thompson, JE Paskanik, CE Bredenburg. Surfactant displacement by meconium free fatty acids: an alternative explanation for atelectasis in meconium aspiration syndrome. J Pediatr 110:765–770, 1987.

186. BA Holm, RH Notter, JH Finkelstein. Surface property changes from interactions of albumin with natural lung surfactant and extracted lung lipids. Chem Phys Lipids 38:287–298, 1985.

187. W Long. Synthetic surfactant. Semin Perinatol 17:275–284, 1993.

188. SA Tabak, RH Notter. A modified technique for dynamic surface pressure and relaxation measurements at the air–water interface. Rev Sci Instrum 48:1196–1201, 1977.

189. K Nag, C Boland, NH Rich, KMW Keough. Epifluorescence microscopic observation of monolayers of dipalmitoyl phosphatidylcholine: dependence of domain size on compression rates. Biochim Biophys Acta 1068:157–160, 1991.

190. G Enhorning. Pulsating bubble technique for evaluating pulmonary surfactant. J Appl Physiol Respir Environ Exercise Physiol 43:198–203, 1977.

191. SB Hall, MS Bermel, YT Ko, HJ Palmer, G Enhorning, RH Notter. Approximations in the measurement of surface tension on the oscillating bubble surfactometer. J Appl Physiol 75:468–477, 1993.

192. G Putz, J Goerke, HW Taeusch, JA Clements. Comparison of captive and pulsating bubble surfactometers with use of lung surfactants. J Appl Physiol 76:1425–1431, 1994.

193. S Schürch, H Bachofen, J Goerke, F Possmayer. A captive bubble method reproduces the in situ behavior of lung surfactant monolayers. J Appl Physiol 67:2389–2396, 1989.

194. S Schürch, H Bachofen, J Goerke, F Green. Surface properties of rat pulmonary surfactant studied with the captive bubble method: adsorption, hysteresis, stability. Biochim Biophys Acta 1103:127–136, 1992.

195. G Putz, J Goerke, S Schürch, JA Clements. Evaluation of pressure-driven captive bubble surfactometer. J Appl Physiol 76:1417–1424, 1994.

196. MS Bermel, JT McBride, RH Notter. Lavaged excised rat lungs as model of surfactant deficiency. Lung 162:99–113, 1984.

197. G Enhorning, B Robertson. Lung expansion in the premature rabbit fetus after tracheal deposition of surfactant. Pediatrics 50:59–66, 1972.

198. FH Adams, B Tower, AB Osher, M Ikegam, T Fujiwara. Effect of tracheal instillation of natural surfactant in premature lambs. I. Clinical and autospy findings. Pediatr Res 12:841–848, 1978.

199. EA Egan, RH Noter, MS Kwong, DL Shapiro. Natural and artificial lung surfactant replacement therapy in premature lambs. J Appl Physiol 55:875–883, 1983.

200. DJ Durand, RI Clyman, MA Heymann, JA Clements, F Mauray, J Kitterman, P Ballard. Effects of protein-free, synthetic surfactant on survival and pulmonary function in preterm lambs. J Pediatr 107:775–780, 1985.

201. H Maeta, D Vidyasagar, T Raju, R Bhat, H Matsuda. Responses to bovine surfactant (Surfactant TA) in two different HMD models (lambs and baboons). Eur J Pediatr 147:162–167, 1988.

202. G Enhorning, D Hill, G Sherwood, E Cutz, et al. Improved ventilation in prematurely derived primates following tracheal deposition of surfactant. Am J Obstet Gynecol 132:529–536, 1978.

203. C Bose, A Corbet, G Bose, J Garciaprats, L Lombardy, D Wold, D Donlon, W Long. Improved outcome at 28 days of very low birth weight infants treated with a single dose of synthetic surfactant. J Pediatr 117:947–953, 1990.

204. AJ Corbet, R Bucciarelli, SA Goldman, M Mammel, D Wold, W Long. Decreased mortality in small premature infants treated at birth a single dose of synthetic surfactant: a multicenter trial. J Pediatr 118:277–284, 1991.

205. MS Dunn, AT Shennan, F Possmayer. Single- versus multiple-dose surfactant replacement therapy in neonates at 30–36 weeks gestation with respiratory distress syndrome. Pediatrics 86:564–571, 1990.

206. H Halliday. Overview of clinical trials comparing natural and synthetic surfactants. Biol Neonate 67 Suppl 1:32–37, 1995.

207. ML Hudak, DJ Martin, EA Egan, EJ Matteson, J Cummings, AL Jung, LV Kimberlin, RL Auten, AA Rosenberg, JM Asselin, MR Belcastro, PK Donohue, CR Hamm, RD Jansen, AS Brody. A multicenter randomized masked comparison trial of synthetic surfactant versus calf lung surfactant extract in the prevention of neonatal respiratory distress syndrome. Pediatrics 100:39–50, 1997.

208. G Enhorning, A Shennan, F Possmayer, M Dunn, CP Chen, J Milligan. Prevention of neonatal respiratory distress syndrome by tracheal instillation of surfactant: a randomized clinical trial. Pediatrics 76:145–153, 1985.

209. J Smyth, I Metcalfe, P Duffy, F Possmayer, M Bryan, G Enhorning. Hyaline membrane disease treated with bovine surfactants. Pediatrics 71:913–917, 1983.

210. M Ikegami, Y Agata, T Elkady, M Hallman, D Berry, A Jobe. Comparison of four surfactants: in vitro surface properties and responses of preterm lambs to treatment at birth. Pediatrics 79:38–46, 1987.

211. JJ Cummings, BA Holm, ML Hudak, WH Ferguson, EA Egan. A controlled clinical comparison of four different surfactant preparations in surfactant-deficient preterm lambs. Am Rev Respir Dis 145:999–1004, 1992.

212. M Hallman, TA Merritt, AL Jarvenpaa, B Boynton, F Mannino, L Gluck, DK Edwards. Exogenous human surfactant for treatment of severe respiratory distress syndrome: a randomized prospective clinical trial. J Pediatr 106:963–969, 1985.

213. JD Horbar, LL Wright, RF Soll, EC Wright, A Fanaroff, SB Korones, S Shankaran, W Oh, BD Fletcher, CR Bauer, JE Tyson, JA Lemons. A multicentre randomised trial comparing two surfactants for the treatment of neonatal respiratory distress syndrome. J Pediatr 123:757–766, 1993.

214. RF Soll, RE Hoekstra, JJ Fangham, AJ Corbet, JM Adams, K Schulze, W Oh, JD Roberts, JP Dorst, SS Kramer, AJ Gold, EM Zola, JD Horbar, TL McAuliffe, JF Lucey. Multicenter trial of single-dosed modified surfactant extract (Survanta) for preventon of respiratory distress syndrome. Pediatrics 85:1092–1102, 1990.

215. CP Speer, O Gefeller, P Groneck, E Laufkotter, C Roll, L Hanssler, K Harms, E Herting, H Boenisch, J Windeler, B Robertson. Randomized clinical trial of 2 treatment regimens of natural surfactant preparations in neonatal respiratory distress syndrome. Arch Dis Child 72:F8–F13, 1995.

216. A Whitelaw. Controversies: synthetic or natural surfactant treatment for respiratory distress syndrome? The case for synthetic surfactant. J Perinat Med 24:427–435, 1996.

217. FR Moya, DR Hoffman, B Zhao, JM Johnston. Platelet-activating factor in surfactant preparations. Lancet 341:858–860, 1993.

218. DS Strayer, TA Merritt, J Lwebuga-Mukasa, M Hallman. Surfactant anti-surfactant immune complexes in infants with respiratory distress syndrome. Am J Pathol 122:353–362, 1986.

219. S Chida, DS Phelps, RF Soll, HW Taeusch. Surfactant proteins and anti-surfactant antibodies in sera from infants with respiratory distress syndrome. Pediatrics 88:84–89, 1991.

220. TA Merritt, M Hallman, BT Bloom, C Berry, K Benirschke, D Sahn, T Key, D Edwards, AL Jarvenpaa, M Pohjavriori, K Kanakaanpaa, M Kunnas, M Paatero, J Rapola, J Jaaskelainen. Prophylactic treatment of very premature infants with human surfactant. N Engl J Med 315:785–790, 1986.

221. BT Bloom, P Delmore, T Rose, T Rawlins. Human and calf lung surfactant: a comparison. Neonat Intens Care, March/April:31–35, 1993.

222. Use of pumactant suspended. April 29, 2000.

223. SB Ainsworth, MW Beresford, DWA Milligan, NJ Shaw, JNS Matthews, AC Fenton, MPW Platt. Pumactant and poractant alfa for treatment of respiratory distress syndrome in neonates born at 25–29 weeks' gestation: a randomised trial. Lancet 355:1387–1392, 2000.

224. TCS Group. Ten centre trial of artificial surfactant (artificial lung expanding compound) in very premature babies. Br Med J 294:991, 1987.

225. ML Choukroun, B Llanas, H Apere, M Fayon, RI Galperine, H Guenard, JC Demarquez. Pulmonary mechanics in ventilated preterm infants with respiratory distress syndrome after exogenous surfactant administration: a comparison between two surfactant preparations. Pediatr Pulmonol 18:272–278, 1994.

226. H Halliday. Natural vs synthetic surfactants in neonatal respiratory distress syndrome. Drugs 51:226–237, 1996.

227. RF Soll. Surfactant therapy in the USA: trials and current routines. Biol Neonate 71:1–7, 1997.

228. JW Schilling, RT White, B Cordell. Recombinant alveolar surfactant protein. U.S. Patent No. 4,659,805, 1987.

229. D Hafner, P-G Germann, D Hauschke. Effects of rSP-C surfactant on oxygenation and histology in a rat-lung-lavage model of acute lung injury. Am J Respir Crit Care Med 158:270–278, 1998.

230. JH Weiner, BD Lemire, ML Elmes, RD Bradley, DG Scraba. Overproduction of fumarate reductase in Escherichia coli induces a novel intracellular lipid-protein organelle. J Bacteriol 158:590–596, 1984.

231. J Pérez-Gil, C Casals, D March. Interactions of hydrophobic lung surfactant proteins SP-B and SP-C with dipalmitoylphosphatidylcholine and dipalmitoylphosphatidylglycerol bilayers studies by electron spin resonance spectroscopy. Biochemistry 34:3964–3791, 1995.

232. A Clercx, G Vandenbussche, T Curstedt, J Johansson, H Jornvall, J-M Ruysschaert. Structural and functional importance of the C-terminal part of the pulmonary surfactant polypeptide SP-C. Eur J Biochem 228:465–472, 1995.

233. SD Revak, TA Merritt, M Hallman, G Heldth, RG La Polla, K Hoey, RA Houghton, CG Cochrane. The use of synthetic peptides in the formation of biophysically and biologically active pulmonary surfactant. Pediat Res 29:460–465, 1991.

234. LM Gordon, S Horvath, ML Longo, JAN Zasadzinski, HW Taeusch, K Faull, C Leung, AJ Waring. Conformation and molecular topography of the N-terminal segment of surfactant protein B in structure-promoting environments. Protein Sci 5:1662–1675, 1996.

235. FJ Walther, J Hernandez-Juviel, R Bruni, AJ Waring. Protein composition of synthetic surfactant affects gas exchange in surfactant-deficient rats. Pediatr Res 43:666–673, 1998.

236. LM Gordon, KYC Lee, MM Lipp, JA Zasadzinski, FJ Walther, MA Sherman, AJ Waring. Conformational mapping of the N-terminal segment of surfactant protein B in lipid using ^{13}C-enhanced Fourier transform infrared spectroscopy. J Pept Res 55:330–347, 2000.

237. M Gustafsson, J Thyberg, J Naslund, E Eliasson, J Johansson. Amyloid fibril formation by pulmonary surfactant protein C. FEBS Lett 464:138–142, 1999.

238. JD Amirkhanian, R Bruni, AJ Waring, C Navar, HW Taeusch. Full-length synthetic surfactant proteins, SP-C and SP-C, reduce surfactant inactivation by serum. Biochim Biophys Acta 1168:315–320, 1993.

239. E Yousefi-Salakdeh, J Johansson, R Stromberg. A method for S- and O-palmitoylation of peptides: synthesis of pulmonary surfactant-C models. Biochim J 343:557–562, 1999.

240. N Mbagwu, R Bruni, JM Hernandez-Juviel, AJ Waring, FJ Walther. Sensitivity of synthetic surfactant to albumin inhibition in preterm rabbits. Mol Genet Metab 66:40–48, 1999.

241. T Szyperski, G Vandenbussche, T Curstedt, J-M Ruysschaert, K Wüthrich, J Johansson. Pulmonary surfactant–associated polypeptide in a mixed organic solvent transforms from a monomeric α-helical state into insoluble β-sheet aggregates. Protein Sci 7:2533–2540, 1998.

242. B Sun, T Kobayashi, T Curstedt, G Grossman, B Robertson. Eur Respir J 4:364–370, 1991.

243. B Frisch, S Muller, JP Briand, MHV van Regenmortel, F Schuber. Parameters affecting the immunogenicity of a liposome-associated synthetic hexapeptide antigen. Eur J Immunol 21:185–193, 1991.

244. M Gustafsson, G Vandenbussche, T Curstedt, J-M Ruysschaert, J Johansson. The 21-residue surfactant peptide (LysLeu4)4Lys(KL4) is a transmembrane alpha-helix with a mixed nonpolar/polar surface. FEBS Lett 384:185–188, 1996.

245. CG Cochrane, SD Revak. Protein and phospholipid interaction in pulmonary surfactant. Chest 105:57S–62S, 1994.

246. SD Revak, TA Merritt, CG Cochrane, GP Heldt, MS Alberts, DW Anderson, A Kheiter. Efficacy of synthetic peptide-containing surfactant in treatment of respiratory distress syndrome in preterm infant Rhesus monkeys. Pediatr Res 39:715–724, 1996.

247. CG Cochrane, SD Revak, TA Merritt, GP Heldt, M Hallman, MD Cunningham, D Easa, A Pramanik, DK Edwards, MS Alberts. The efficacy and safety of KL4 surfactant in preterm infants with respiratory distress syndrome. Am J Respir Crit Care Med 153:404–410, 1996.

248. U. S. drug firm revamps Latin American baby trial. CNN, April 5, 2001.

249. RN Zuckermann, JM Kerr, SBH Kent, WH Moos. Efficient method for the preparation of peptoids [oligo (N-substituted) glycines] by submonomer solid-phase synthesis. J Am Chem Soc 114:10646–10647, 1992.

250. SM Miller, RJ Simon, S Ng, RN Zuckermann, JM Kerr, WH Moos. Comparison of the proteolytic susceptibilities of homologous L-amino acid, D-amino acid, and N-substituted glycine peptide and peptoid oligomers. Drug Dev Res 35:20–32, 1995.

251. JA Gibbons, AA Hancock, CR Vitt, S Knepper, SA Buckner, ME Brune, I Milicic, JF Kerwin, LS Richter, EW Taylor, KL Spear, RN Zuckermann, DC Spellmeyer, RA Braeckman, WH Moos. Pharmacologic characterization of

CHIR 2279, an N-substituted glycine peptoid with high-affinity binding for α_1-adrenocepters. J Pharm Exp Ther 277:885–899, 1996.

252. CW Wu, TJ Sanborn, RN Zuckermann, AE Barron. Peptoid oligomers with α-chiral, aromatic sidechains: effects of chain length on secondary structure. J Am Chem Soc 123:2958–2963, 2001.

253. K Kirshenbaum, AE Barron, P Armand, R Goldsmith, E Bradley, FE Cohen, KA Dill, RN Zuckermann. Sequence-specific polypeptoids: a diverse family of heteropolymers with stable secondary structure. Proc Natl Acad Sci USA 95:4303–4308, 1998.

254. P Armand, K Kirshenbaum, RA Goldsmith, S Farr-Jones, AE Barron, KTV Truong, KA Dill, DF Mierke, FE Cohen, RN Zuckermann, EK Bradley. NMR determination of the major solution conformation of a peptoid pentamer with chiral side chains. Proc Natl Acad Sci USA 95:4309–4314, 1998.

255. P Armand, K Kirshenbaum, A Falicov, RL Dunbrack Jr., KA Dill, RN Zuckermann, FE Cohen. Chiral N-alkylated glycines can form stable helical conformations. Fold Design 2:369–375, 1997.

256. CW Wu, TJ Sanborn, AE Barron. Peptoid oligomers with α-chiral, aromatic sidechains: Sequence requirements for the formation of stable peptoid helices. J Am Chem Soc 123:6778–6784, 2001.

257. CW Wu, KYC Lee, AE Barron. Polypeptoids for biological mimicry of surfactant proteins: a novel exogenous lung surfactant replacement. Biophys J 80:2553, 2001.

258. HL Halliday. Synthetic or natural surfactants. Acta Paediatr 86:233–237, 1997.

259. AK Pramanik, RB Holtzman, TA Merritt. Surfactant replacement therapy for pulmonary diseases. Update Neonatol 40:913–936, 1993.

260. B Robertson. New targets for surfactant replacement therapy: experimental and clinical aspects. Arch Dis Child 75:F1–F3, 1996.

261. B Sun, E Herting, T Curstedt, B Robertson. Exogenous surfactant improves lung compliance and oxygenation in adult rats with meconium aspiration. J Appl Physiol 77:1961–1971, 1994.

262. E Herting, C Jarstrand, O Rasool, T Curstedt, B Sun, B Robertson. Experimental neonatal group-B streptococcal pneumonia: effects of a modified porcine surfactant on bacterial proliferation in ventilated near-term rabbits. Pediatr Res 36:784–791, 1994.

263. JF Lewis, AH Jobe. Surfactant and adult respiratory distress syndrome. Am Rev Respir Dis 147:218–233, 1993.

264. RG Spragg, et al. The adult respiratory distress syndrome: clinical aspects relevant to surfactant supplementation. In: B Robertson, ed. Pulmonary Surfactant from Molecular Biology to Clinical Practice. Amsterdam: Elsevier, 1992, pp 685–703.

265. FX McCormack. Molecular biology of the surfactant apoprotein. SEM Respir Crit Care Med 16:29–38, 1995.

266. GR Bernard, A Artigas, KL Brigham, J Carlet, K Falke, L Hudson, M Lamy, JR Legall, A Morris, R Spragg. The American–European consensus

conference on ARDS: definitions, mechanisms, relevant outcomes, and clinical trial coordination. Am J Respir Crit Care Med 149:818–824, 1994.

267. JE Heffner, LK Brown, CA Barbieri, KS Harpel, J Deleo. Prospective validation of an acute respiratory distress syndrome predictive score. Am J Respir Care Med 152:1518–1526, 1995.

268. P Krafft, P Fridrich, T Pernerstorfer, RD Fitzgerald, D Koc, B Schneider, AF Hammerle, H Steltzer. The acute respiratory distress syndrom; definitions, severity, and clinical outcome. An analysis of 101 clinical investigations. Intens Care Med 22:519–529, 1996.

269. A Jobe, M Ikegami, H Jacobs, S Jones, D Conaway. Permeability of premature lamb lungs to protein and the effect of surfactant on that permeability. J Appl Physiol 55:169–176, 1983.

270. TJ Gregory, JE Gadek, JE Weiland, et al. Survanta supplementation in patients with acute respiratory distress syndrome (ARDS). Am J Resp Cell Mol Biol 149:A567, 1994.

271. RG Spragg, N Gilliard, P Richman, RM Smith, D Hite, D Pappert, B Robertson, T Curstedt, D Strayer. Acute effects of a single dose of porcine surfactant on patients with adult respiratory distress syndrome. Chest 105:195–202, 1994.

272. D Häfner, R Beume, U Kilian, G Kraznai, B Lachmann. Dose response comparisons of five lung surfactant factor (LSF) preparations in an animal model of adult respiratory distress syndrome (ARDS). Br J Pharmacol 116:451–458, 1995.

273. DF Willson, JH Jiao, LA Bauman, A Zaritsky, H Craft, K Dockery, D Conrad, H Dalton. Calf's lung surfactant extract in acute hypoxemic respiratory failure in children. Crit Care Med 24:1316–1322, 1996.

274. J Kattwinkel. Surfactant: evolving issues. Clin Perinatol 25:17–32, 1998.

275. M Griese, P Birrer, A Demirsoy. Pulmonary surfactant in cystic fibrosis. Eur Respir J 10:1983–1988, 1997.

276. RH Notter. Lung Surfactants: Basic Science and Clinical Applications. New York: Marcel Dekker, 2000.

277. LAJM Creuwels, MG van Golde, HP Haagsman. The pulmonary surfactant system: biochemical and clinical aspects. Lung 175:1–39, 1997.

278. J Johansson, T Curstedt, B Robertson. Synthetic protein analogues in artificial surfactants. Acta Paediatr 85:642–646, 1996.

279. G Gaines. Insoluble Monolayers at Liquid–Gas Interfaces. New York: Interscience, 1966.

280. JW Kendig, RH Notter, C Cox, JL Aschner, S Benn, RM Bernstein, K Hendricks-Munoz, WM Maniscalco, LA Metlay, DL Phelps, DL Shapiro. Surfactant replacement therapy at birth: final analysis of a clinical trial and comparisons with similar trials. Pediatrics 82:756–762, 1988.

281. MS Kwong, EA Egan, RH Notter, DL Shapiro. A double blind clinical trial of calf lung surfactant extract for the prevention of hyaline membrane disease in extremely premature infants. Pediatrics 76:585–592, 1985.

282. DL Shapiro, RH Notter, F Morin, KS Deluga, LM Golub, RA Sinkin, KI Weiss, C Cox. A double blind randomized trial of calf lung surfactant extract administered at birth to very premature infants for prevention of respiratory distress syndrome. Pediatrics 76:593–599, 1985.

283. T Fujiwara, B Robertson. Pharmacology of exogenous surfactant. In: B Robertson, LMG van Golde, JJ Batenburg, eds. Pulmonary Surfactant. Amsterdam: Elsevier, 1992, pp 561–592.

284. T Fujiwara, M Konishi, S Chida, Y Okuyama, Y Takeuchi, H Nishida, H Kito, M Fujiwar, H Nakamura. Surfactant replacement therapy with a single post-ventilatory dose of a reconstituted bovine surfactant in preterm neonates with respiratory distress syndrome: final analysis of a multicenter, double-blind, randomized trial and comparison with similar trials. Pediatrics 86:753–764, 1990.

285. M Konishi, T Fujiwara, T Naito, Y Takeuchi, Y Ogawa, K Inukai, M Fujiwara, H Nakamura, T Hashimoto. Surfactant replacement therapy in neonatal respiratory distress syndrome—a multicenter, randomized clinical trial: comparison of high versus low dose of surfactant-TA. Eur J Pediatr 147:20–25, 1988.

286. JD Gitlin, RF Soll, RB Parad, JD Horbar, HA Feldman, JF Lucey, HW Tauesch. Randomized controlled trial of exogenous surfactant for treatment of hyaline membrane disease. Pediatrics 79:31–37, 1987.

287. HW Taeusch, KMW Keough, W Williams, R Slavin, E Steele, AS Lee, D Phelps, N Kariel, J Floros, ME Avery. Characterization of bovine surfactant for infants with respiratory distress syndrome. Pediatrics 77:572–581, 1986.

288. L Gortner, F Pohlandt, B Disse, E Weller. Effects of bovine surfactant in premature lambs after intratracheal application. Eur J Pediatr 149:280–283, 1990.

289. P Bartmann, U Bamberger, F Pohlandt, L Gortner. Immunogenicity and immunomodulatory activity of bovine surfactant (SF-RI 1). Acta Paediatr 81:383–388, 1992.

290. MS Dunn, AT Shennan, D Zayack, F Possmayer. Bovine surfactant replacement in neonates of less than 30 weeks gestation: a randomized controlled trial of prophylaxis vs. treatment. Pediatrics 87:377–386, 1991.

291. JD Horbar, R Soll, JM Sutherland, U Kotagal, AG Philip, DL Kessler, GA Little, WH Edwards, D Vidyasagar, TN Raju. A multicenter randomized, placebo-controlled trial of surfactant therapy for respiratory distress syndrome. N Engl J Med 320:959–965, 1989.

292. JD Horbar, RF Soll, H Schachinder, G Kewitz, HT Versmold, W Linder, G Duc, D Mieth, O Linkerkamp, EP Zilow. A European multicenter randomized trial of single dose surfactant therapy for idiopathic respiratory distress syndrome. Eur J Pediatr 320:959–965, 1990.

293. EA Liechty, E Donovan, D Purohit, J Gilhooly, B Feldman, A Noguchi, SE Denson, SS Sehgal, I Gross, D Stevens, M Ikegami, RD Zachman, ST Carrier, JH Gunkel, AJ Gold. Reduction of neonatal mortality after multiple

doses of bovine surfactant in low birth weight neonates with respiratory distress syndrome. Pediatrics 88:19–28, 1991.

294. E Redenti, T Peveri, P Ventura, M Zanol, A Selva. Characterization of phospholipidic components of the natural pulmonary surfactant Curosurf. Il Farmaco 49:285–289, 1994.

295. W Long, R Cotton, A Corbet, S Courtney, G McGuiness, D Walter, J Watts, J Smyth, H Bard, V Chernick. A controlled trial of synthetic surfactant in infants weighing 1250 G or more with respiratory distress syndrome. N Engl J Med 325:1696–1703, 1991.

296. W Long, T Thompson, H Sundell, R Schumacher, F Volberg, R Guthrie. Effects of two rescue doses of a synthetic surfactant on mortality in 700–1300 gram infants with RDS. J Pediatr 118:595–605, 1991.

297. A Wilkinson, PA Jenkins, JA Jeffrey. Two controlled trials of dry artificial surfactant: early effects and later outcome in babies with surfactant deficiency. Lancet 2:287–291, 1985.

298. W Seeger, C Thede, A Günther, C Grube. Surface properties and sensitivity to protein-inhibition of a recombinant aproprotein C-based phospholipid mixture in vitro: comparison to natural surfactant. Biochim Biophys Acta 1081:45–52, 1991.

299. BJ Benson. Genetically engineered human pulmonary surfactant. Clin Perinatol 20:791–811, 1993.

300. M Ikegami, AH Jobe. Surfactant protein-C in ventilated premature lamb lung. Pediatr Res 44:860–864, 1998.

301. J Lewis, L McCraig, D Hafner, R Spragg, R Veldhuizen, C Kerr. Dosing and delivery of recombinant surfactant in lung-injured sheep. Am J Respir Crit Care Med 159:741–747, 1999.

302. M Gustafsson, M Palmblad, T Curstedt, J Johansson, S Schurch. Palmitoylation of a pulmonary surfactant protein C analogue affects the surface-associated lipid reservoir and film stability. Biochim Biophys Acta 1466:169–178, 2000.

303. TA Merritt, A Kheiter, CG Cochrane. Positive end-expiratory pressure during KL4 surfactant instillation enhances intrapulmonary distribution in a simian model of respiratory distress syndrome. Pediatr Res 38:211–217, 1995.

19

Peptide Nucleic Acid (PNA) Conjugates in Biotechnology

James W. Schneider
Carnegie Mellon University, Pittsburgh, Pennsylvania

Peptide nucleic acid (PNA) exemplifies the power of biomimetic strategies in molecular design. PNA was developed in the early 1990s by a Danish group led by Peter Nielsen and coworkers as a mimic of triple-helix-forming DNA nucleotides (1–3). PNA is remarkably resistant to degradation by nucleases and proteases, and antisense therapeutic applications for PNA were soon envisioned. PNA makes more stable, more sequence-specific hybridizations with complementary DNA and RNA oligonucleotides. Recently, Boc- and Fmoc-protected PNA monomers have become commercially available so that PNA oligomers can be readily conjugated to natural peptides, biotin, proteins, and lipophilic materials using standard peptide chemistry methods. PNA conjugation strategies enable biochemists to modify DNA with cellular signals, separate DNA oligomers in a sequence-specific way, identify point mutations in genes, and sense femtomolar concentrations of nucleic acid analytes. The observation that PNA can perform the same recognition function as DNA has even prompted some speculation that PNA may have been the first genetic material, and a recent study concluded that PNA-like monomers can be formed from electrical discharge reactions simulating primordial conditions (4).

There have been several excellent reviews of PNA technology in recent years (5–8) focusing on therapeutic applications, synthesis, and binding properties. Recently, the potential to use PNA sequences as a handle for the attachment of various ligands to DNA has led to the development of a wider range of applications of PNA in biotechnology. In this chapter, we will begin with an overview of PNA synthesis and physical properties, and then discuss some of the emerging applications for PNA conjugates in biotechnology.

I. PNA STRUCTURE AND PROPERTIES

A. PNA Interactions with ssDNA and ssRNA

While several isoforms exist, the classic PNA structure has the sugar-phosphate backbone of DNA replaced by an N-(2-aminoethyl)glycine polyamide (Fig. 1). To accommodate the bulky nucleotides, two glycine backbone units are incorporated for each base. The structure of PNA monomers is such that the C terminus of the PNA peptide corresponds to the 3' end of a DNA strand. Despite the fact that the polyamide backbone is considerably more flexible than the phosphodiester backbone, nuclear

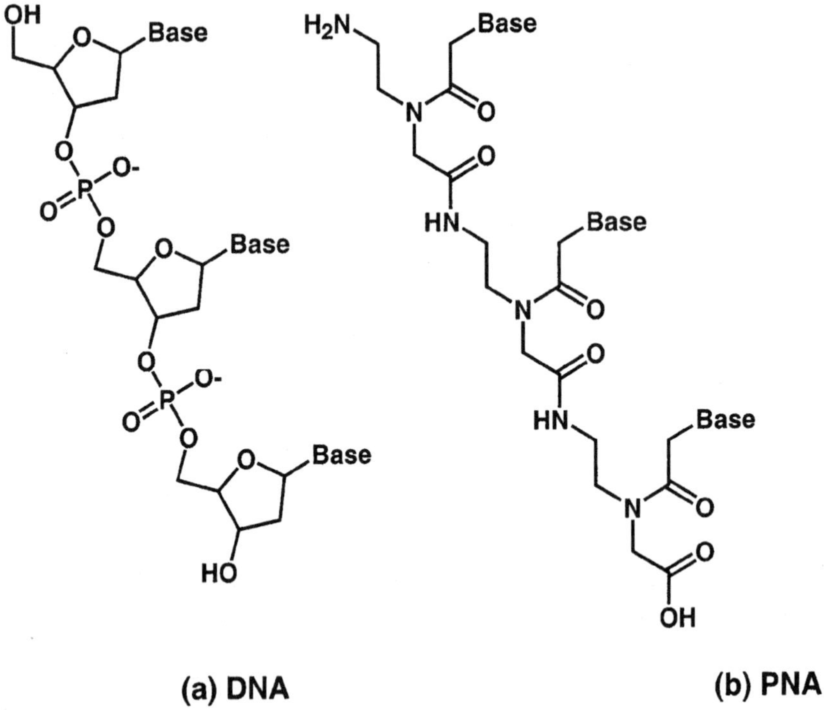

(a) DNA   **(b) PNA**

Figure 1   Chemical structures of (a) DNA and (b) PNA.

magnetic resonance (NMR) and x-ray crystallography have confirmed that single-stranded (ss) PNA oligomers bind complementary ssDNA, RNA, and ssPNA oligomers in a sequence-specific way, forming an antiparallel double-helical duplex (9–12). PNA-DNA and PNA-RNA duplexes are very similar to B and A forms, respectively, but the PNA-PNA helix ("P" form) is wider and has a longer pitch (13).

The replacement of the phosphodiester backbone with a polyamide backbone confers a number of unique DNA binding properties on PNA. By greatly reducing interstrand electrostatic repulsion, particularly at low ionic strength, PNA-containing duplexes have a greater thermal stability than their phosphodiester counterparts. By tracking hypochromic decreases in UV absorbance on strand hybridization (14), Egholm and coworkers (15) found that the melting temperature (T_m) of PNA-DNA duplexes is approximately 1°C higher per monomer unit compared to sequence-similar DNA-DNA duplexes in pure water. As the ionic strength is increased, differences in T_m are diminished due to Debye screening of the DNA-DNA repulsion, and at an ionic strength equivalent to 1 M NaCl the T_m values are identical (Table 1). PNA binding to RNA is especially strong, leading to a nearly 2°C enhancement in stability per base pair. Precise measurements of thermodynamics of PNA–nucleic acid hybridization using UV absorbance (16) and isothermal titration calorimetry (17) have been made, and an empirical model predicting T_m based on a nearest-neighbor model for DNA-DNA hybridization has been developed. (18)

Table 1 Comparison of UV-Melting Data for PNA-PNA and DNA-DNA Duplexes

Duplex	T_m
15-mer PNA/DNA	69°C
15-mer DNA/DNA	54°C
15-mer PNA/RNA	72°C
15-mer DNA/RNA	50°C

[NaCl] (mM)	PNA-DNA T_m	DPNA-DNA T_m
0	72°C	38°C
140	69°C	56°C
1000	65°C	65°C

PNA-DNA duplex binding can also be regarded as more sequence specific than for DNA duplexes. UV melting studies of these duplexes demonstrate that a single-base mismatch in a PNA-DNA duplex gives rise to an 8–10°C decrease in T_m, making PNA much less tolerant to base pair mismatches than other DNA binders. This property makes PNA an attractive candidate for the detection of single-nucleotide polymorphisms (SNPs) in genomic DNA.

B. PNA Interactions with Double-Stranded DNA

The increased stability of PNA-DNA duplexes in comparison with DNA-DNA duplexes can actually bring about the displacement of a single DNA strand from a DNA-DNA duplex by PNA in some instances (1,19). The potential of PNA to achieve this "strand invasion" has great promise in biotechnology, since it allows for the functionalization of plasmid and even genomic DNA without fully separating each strand. Since the invasion triplex is the energetically favorable configuration, maximizing invasion efficiency amounts to lowering the kinetic barriers to invasion. A detailed kinetic analysis of homopyrimidine (C and T bases) PNA invasion of homopurine DNA (A and G) revealed that the complex formed is a triplex, with the homopyrimidine DNA strand displaced by two PNA oligomers binding to one of the DNA strands (Fig. 2) (20). One PNA oligomer binds in the antiparallel orientation to ssDNA and one binds in the parallel orientation to the same strand. The unbound ssDNA section remains in a loop configuration, susceptible to degradation by ssDNA nucleases.

The efficient strand invasion of homopurine dsDNA target sequences is a result of a greater availability of hydrogen bonds in the purine nucleobases compared to pyrimidines (Fig. 3). Since two PNA strands bind

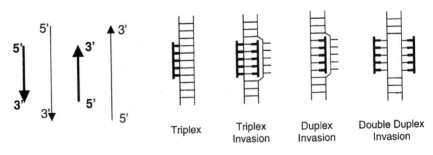

Figure 2 Binding configurations for strand invasion of dsDNA by PNA.

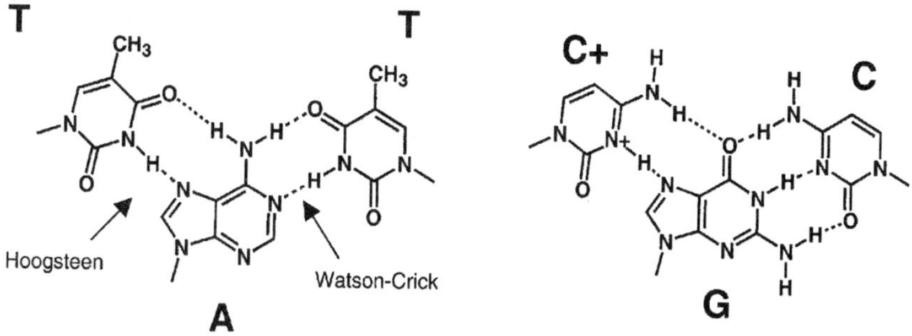

Figure 3 Purine (A/G) DNA targets accommodate hydrogen bonding to parallel and antiparallel PNA strands in the triplex invasion process. For cytosine, triplex invasion is greatly facilitated at pH <5.5, where the cytosines are protonated for Hoogsteen hydrogen bonding. As an alternative, the unnatural nucleobase pseudoisocytosine (J) can be incorporated to provide for Hoogsteen hydrogen bonding at physiological pH.

a single strand of DNA, the DNA target must bind one PNA strand in the antiparallel (Watson-Crick) orientation and another must bind in the parallel (Hoogsteen) orientation, and only the purines can accommodate both simultaneously. Guanine targets show a pronounced pH dependence on (PNA)$_2$-DNA triplex formation since the PNA cytosines must be protonated (pH <5.5) to effect Hoogsteen base pairing. The pH dependence is removed by replacing the PNA cytosines with pseudoisocytosine (J base, see Fig. 7a), and protected PNA J bases are now commercially available specifically for this purpose.

Since the DNA duplex must be separated for strand invasion to occur, conditions that destabilize the DNA duplex act to attenuate the kinetic barriers to strand invasion. Strand invasion is encouraged at low ionic strength (<50 mM NaCl) so that the electrostatic repulsion between the DNA strands is unscreened, destabilizing the DNA duplex. However, once formed the (PNA)$_2$-DNA triplex is very stable even in high ionic strength (up to 500 mM NaCl) buffers (19). Target sequences of DNA with a low GC content are also more suitable for strand invasion due to the lower stability of the DNA duplex. Highly efficient strand invasion has been observed using homothymine PNA at low ionic strength, so that the target dsDNA (homoadenine) has a low stability and a propensity for Hoogsteen base pairing with PNA. Strand invasion is also encouraged by the presence of the DNA intercalators ethidium bromide and 9-aminoacridine, whereas it is slowed by the major and minor groove binders (21). Strand invasion of supercoiled plasmid DNA is 2–3 times more efficient than with linear DNA, likely due to a higher rate of transient base pair unbinding or "breathing" (22). The attachment of the cationic peptide (AAKK)$_4$, which increases DNA-PNA hybridization rates 48,000-fold, has been shown to increase the rate of strand invasion by a factor of 2–4 (23).

The efficiency of strand invasion can be increased further by linking symmetrical PNA oligomers by a flexible spacer to form a bis-PNA clamp (Fig. 4) (24,25). This improves the rate of strand invasion by effectively replacing a trimolecular reaction with a bimolecular one. Again, the thymines in the Hoogsteen PNA branch are often replaced by J bases to improve the hydrogen bonding (26). The flexible spacer has been made of a series of natural amino acids that promote β-turn structures (24), 8-amino-3,6-dioxaoctanoic acid units (26), polyethylene glycol spacers, and lysinated linkers (25). The lysinated linkers show improved binding to DNA owing to their positive charge. Bis-PNAs have the greatest potential for binding plasmid and genomic DNA at physiological conditions and therefore are of great interest in biotechnology.

Recent work has expanded the dsDNA recognition repertoire of PNA oligomers. Witting et al. (27) have observed the formation of a PNA-(DNA)$_2$ triplex without separation of dsDNA (Fig. 2) for a cytosine-rich homopyrimide PNA probe of dsDNA. In addition, they found that homopurine or alternating TG sequences invade complementary dsDNA to form PNA-DNA duplexes rather than triplexes. A double-duplex invasion complex has also been reported (28) for PNAs containing the sterically compromised unnatural nucleobases 2,6-diaminopurine and thiouracil (Fig. 7b, d). A thorough study of a series of about 20 base pair targets within pUC19 plasmid DNA by Corey and coworkers (29) found that PNA complementary to inverted repeats within AT-rich regions of

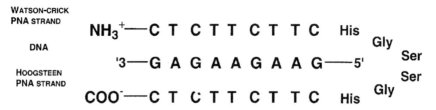

Figure 4 Bis-PNA clamp for highly efficient dsDNA binding, even under high ionic strength conditions. The cytosines on the Hoogsteen strand are often replaced by pseudoisocytosine (J) for improved hydrogen bonding.

dsDNA hybridize with very high efficiency, whereas those adjacent to those regions hybridize with moderate efficiency. Other targets did not detectably hybridize without the addition of positive charge. Inverted repeats typically form cruciform structures, which are more accessible to PNA for strand invasion. These observations argue for a wide range of possible dsDNA targets, expanding the utility of PNA conjugates for biotechnology applications.

C. Chemical and Biological Stability of PNA

PNA has demonstrated a greater chemical stability and resistance to nuclease and protease degradation than DNA or RNA. PNA does not suffer from depurination in strong acid as DNA does, although some slow rearrangements may occur under alkaline conditions (30). PNA has also proven highly resistant to degradation in human serum and cellular extracts (31). The stability of PNA makes it more amenable to synthetic modification, conjugation, cellular delivery, and high-throughput diagnostics than DNA.

D. PNA Solubility in Aqueous Solutions

A major difficulty in working with PNA is its poor solubility and tendency to self-aggregate in aqueous solution. Generally, PNA solubility decreases with increasing length and increasing purine content. Pure PNA oligomers are sparingly soluble in water; however, the addition of a single C-terminal lysine amide can greatly improve water solubility. For example, a homothymine PNA decamer is water-soluble at concentrations above 5 mg/mL (2). Solubility of PNA oligomers can be improved by constructing PNA monomers with an N-(2-aminoethyl)-D-lysine polyamide backbone. Substitution of only two N-(2-aminoethyl)-D-lysine monomers into a PNA dodecamer has yielded a fivefold increase in its solubility (32). Because only the N-(2-aminoethyl)glycine-protected monomers are commercially available, the addition of natural amino acids is often the most expeditious approach. Interestingly, the addition of positively charged groups to PNA oligomers does not appear to diminish the sequence specificity of PNA–DNA duplex binding.

E. Kinetics of PNA–Nucleic Acid Hybridization

Several studies have focused on the experimental measurement of association and dissociation kinetics of PNA–nucleic acid duplexes and triplexes by tracking the time course using UV absorbance, shifts in gel mobility, and optical biosensors. PNA–nucleic acid duplexes have association rate constants $(k_a) \sim 1.17\,\mathrm{mM}^{-1}\,\mathrm{s}^{-1}$ for a fully complementary PNA-DNA 15-mer, and $k_a = 22\,\mathrm{mM}^{-1}\,\mathrm{s}^{-1}$ for an identical PNA-RNA duplex (PBS buffer) (33). A single mismatch dropped the rate constants by about one order of magnitude. Demidov (20) measured kinetics for the association of decamer $(PNA)_2$-DNA triplexes and measured pseudo-first-order k_a of $4.2 \times 10^{-4}\,\mathrm{min}^{-1}$ for a fully complementary triplex and $3.2 \times 10^{-2}\,\mathrm{min}^{-1}$ for a 50% mismatched triplex (10 mM Tris buffer). The pseudo-first-order rate constant had a power-law exponent of approximately 2–3 with PNA concentration, consistent with the triplex invasion model described above. Kinetics of decamer bis-PNA-DNA triplex formation are fast (34), with $k_a = 1$–$0.1\,\mathrm{min}^{-1}$ when incorporating J bases in the Hoogsteen branch of the clamp. Association kinetics are about four to five orders of magnitude slower at moderate to high pH without the C for J substitution, highlighting the necessity of this approach. Dissociation kinetics of decamer bis-PNA-DNA triplexes (35) are slow $(k_d = 10^{-4}\,\mathrm{min}^{-1})$, and do not exhibit a strong dependence on temperature or salt concentration below 0.1 M NaCl, with much faster dissociation kinetics at high ionic strength.

II. SYNTHETIC VARIANTS OF PNA

Several PNA backbone modifications have been investigated with the goal of improving PNA solubility and establishing structure–property relationships for general nucleic acid binding. It should be emphasized that the original PNA backbone structure is perfectly acceptable for most applications; in fact, most modifications decreased the thermal stability of the resulting duplexes. Still, they shed light on the mechanism of PNA–DNA interactions and will be discussed briefly here.

A. PNA Monomer Modifications

The success of the classical PNA structure has encouraged many to optimize the monomeric structure to improve binding efficiency (Fig. 5). Many of these efforts focused on constraining the comparably flexible polyamide backbone to provide a smaller entropic penalty for hybridization. Replacement of the ethylene part of the PNA monomer (Fig. 5a) with a cyclohexyl structure (Fig. 5b) was a partial success (36). While the PNA-DNA duplex stability was not improved by this modification, the entropic penalty was reduced, but with a concomitant decrease in binding enthalpy.

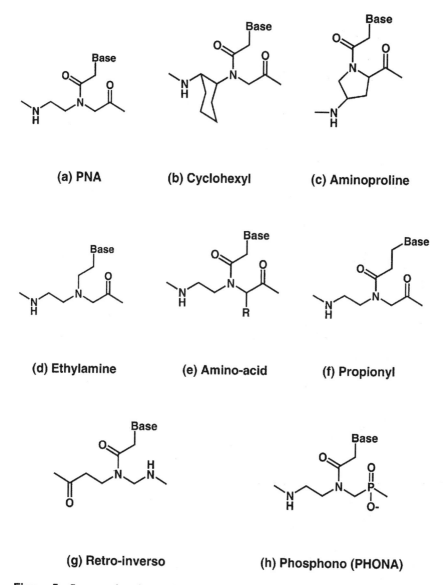

Figure 5 Structural variants of PNA monomers. (Adapted from Ref. 6.)

Aminoproline substitution was more successful (Fig. 5c), yielding a 6–7°C increase in PNA-DNA duplex stability (octa- and dodecamers) (37). These materials were also capable of strand invasion and showed excellent stability against enzymatic degradation. The synthesis of related proline-containing PNA monomers and their effect on resulting duplex conformation have also been reported (38–40).

In contrast, Hyrup and coworkers (41) synthesized a PNA monomer with an ethylamine linker (Fig. 5d), which is more flexible than the classical PNA structure owing to the relief of the conformational constraint imposed by the amide side group. This modification also introduced a positive charge at the backbone amide group. This modification greatly destabilized both PNA-DNA duplexes and (PNA)$_2$-DNA triplexes, highlighting the importance of the PNA backbone as a director for nucleobase hydrogen bonding.

With the goal of further functionalizing the PNA backbone, and to introduce chirality, Haaima et al. (32) modified the N-2(aminoethyl)glycine backbone to accommodate amino acids other than glycine (Fig. 5e). PNA monomers of L-lysine, D- and L-serine, D-glutamic acid, L-aspartic acid, and L-isoleucine were synthesized, but only the D-lysine modification showed a stabilizing effect (about 3°C per introduced monomer.) The added stability was attributed to the favorable electrostatic interaction with the DNA phosphodiester backbone, yet the sequence specificity of binding was not adversely impacted by the modification. As mentioned above, the incorporation of D-lysine in the PNA backbone also increases PNA water solubility, and this represents one of the more promising improvements to the classical PNA structure. Hyrup et al. (42) replaced the N-2(aminoethyl)-glycine backbone with a N-(3-aminopropyl)glycine (Fig. 5f), also with a reduction in thermal stability for PNA-DNA hybrids, but with no reduction in sequence specificity.

A common strategy in the design of peptide mimics is to reverse the peptide bond to form an isomer having the side chain shifted along the backbone. Such "retro-inverso" PNAs have been synthesized (43) (Fig. 5g), with an N-(aminomethyl) β-alanine backbone. This substitution also destabilized PNA-DNA and PNA-RNA duplexes, in this case by about 7°C per substitution for DNA and 3°C for RNA. Molecular dynamics simulations identified sequestering of the backbone amide group from the aqueous medium and new repulsive electrostatic "clashes" between carbonyls on the backbone and linker (44).

The lack of negative charge on the classical PNA backbone has been implicated in its poor water solubility and its poor cellular uptake. Negative charge can be incorporated into the PNA backbone with only small changes in DNA binding properties by replacing the peptide bond with a phosphonic acid bridge. These "PHONAs" (Fig. 5h) have been synthesized as pure oligomers and as co-oligomers with PNA, and have demonstrated PHONA-DNA duplex stability comparable with PNA-DNA duplexes.

(PHONA)$_2$-DNA triplex melting transitions are somewhat lower than those of (PNA)-DNA due to electrostatic interactions (45).

B. PNA Backbone Modifications

An alternative to monomer modification is to intersperse PNA monomers together with monomers having a modified backbone architecture. This methodology is less time consuming from a synthetic standpoint because monomers of each nucleotide do not have to be created.

PNA/DNA chimeras (Fig. 6a), which are co-oligomers of each material, have been investigated largely in the hope that the negative charge of the DNA part would improve the solubility and cellular uptake of the PNA. PNA/DNA chimeras are produced either by the linking of presynthesized PNA and DNA oligomers in solution, or by their on-line

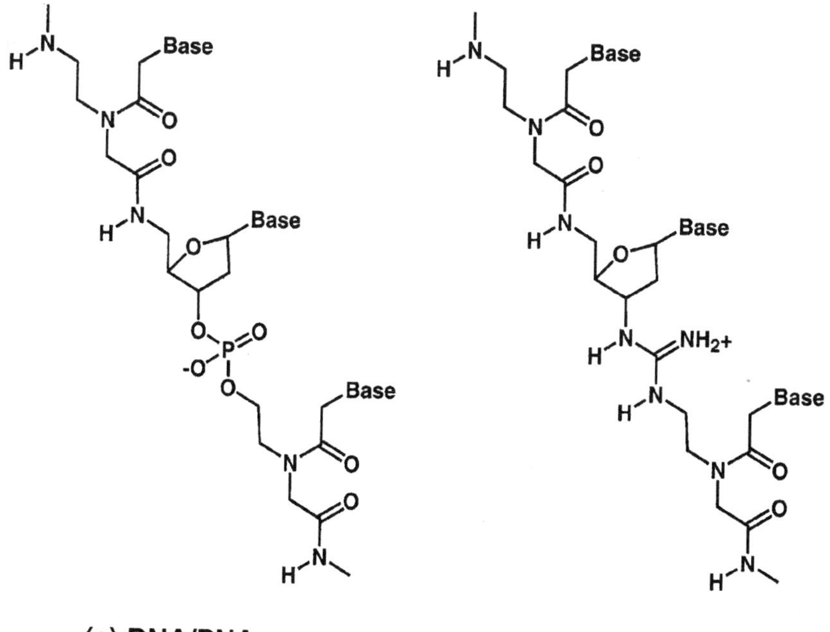

(a) DNA/PNA   **(b) DNG/PNA**

Figure 6   PNA and its chimeras. The negative charges of DNA (a) promote water solubility and cellular uptake, while the guanidinium groups of the DNG (b) promote DNA binding kinetics.

solid phase synthesis with suitably protected DNA and PNA monomers and special linker molecules. The second approach has been more successful and also makes interspersing DNA and PNA possible [reviewed in (8)]. Bergmann reported the first synthesis of PNA/DNA chimeras, but only using acid-stable pyrimidine nucleotides (46). Later, Uhlmann developed a new series of protected monomers that expanded the repertoire to all PNA nucleotides using the acid-labile protecting group monomethoxytrityl (Mmt), which is compatible with DNA solid phase methods (47). PNA/DNA chimeras hybridze with complementary DNA with a stability intermediate between DNA-DNA and PNA-DNA duplexes. Cellular uptake of a homothymine PNA/hexamer/DNA/hexamer chimera was found to be as high as uptake of a DNA homothymine dodecamer (47). PHONA/PNA chimeras have been explored for their improved water solubility and cellular uptake, again with intermediate duplex stability (48). The implementation of PNA/DNA chimeras in cellular delivery remains an area of active research.

Other backbone modifications involve interspersing positive charge in the backbone, by conjoining DNA binding molecules to PNA oligomers. Gangamani appended a C-terminal cationic spermine molecule, which gave rise to a 10°C enhancement in PNA-DNA duplex stability for a complementary 13-mer (49). A kinetic study also showed a twofold acceleration in the bimolecular association process. Conjugation of spermine to PNA oligomers is readily performed during the solid phase synthesis of the oligomer. Also using an on-line solid phase synthesis method, Bruice and coworkers (50) incorporated positively charged guanidine groups into PNA oligomers to form deoxynucleic guanidine (DNG)/PNA chimeras (Fig. 6b) DNG/PNA-DNA duplexes, while not more thermally stable than PNA-DNA duplexes, show a significant increase in association rates. The kinetics of (DNG/PNA)$_2$-DNA triplex formation were also faster and sequence specific. It was surmised that the introduction of guanidinium linkages resulted in unfavorable structural changes in the backbone that compensated for the electrostatic stabilization of the triplex.

Lately, attempts to incorporate secondary structure into unbound PNA have led to some exciting results. Howarth and Wakelin (51) built an α-helical peptide with pendant nucleobases by solid phase synthesis of novel, Boc-protected L-α-amino acids with nucleobase side chains. An improved α-PNA was conceived by Garner et al. (52) who created a series of protected L-serine molecules with nucleobase side chains (Ser^B). The α-PNA had the sequence Ac-Lys$_2$-(Ser^B-Ala$_2$-Lys)$_4$-Ser^B-Gly-Cys'-NH$_2$, where "Ac" is an acyl group and "Cys" is S-acetamidomethyl-L-cysteine. An α-PNA pentamer formed a duplex with DNA having a 35°C higher melting

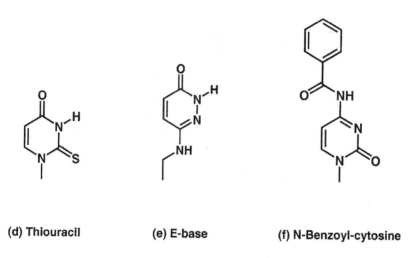

(a) Pseudoisocytosine   (b) 2,6-Diaminopurine   (c) 2-Aminopurine

(d) Thiouracil   (e) E-base   (f) N-Benzoyl-cytosine

Figure 7 Unnatural nucleotides incorporated in PNA oligomers. (Adapted from Ref. 6.)

transition temperature than the corresponding DNA-DNA duplex. Additionally, the water solubility was higher than that of PNA. The α-helical character of the α-PNA both before and after DNA hybridization was confirmed by CD spectroscopy. This approach is very promising, since amino acid side groups required for water solubility or other purposes can be directed away from the nucleobases involved in base pairing, in principle.

C. PNAs with Unnatural Nucleobases

PNAs with unnatural nucleobases have the potential to overcome some of the binding limitations of the natural nucleobases. Earlier, we described the use of pseudoisocytosine (J, Fig. 7a) as a replacement for cytosine for the pH-independent Hoogsteen bonding with guanine groups in (PNA)$_2$-DNA triplexes and bis-PNA clamps (26). We also described a double-duplex invasion complex using unnatural amino acids thiouracil (Fig. 7d) and 2,6-diaminopurine (Fig. 7b) (28). 2,6-Diaminopurine (D) is a naturally occurring nucleobase in some organisms, where it replaces adenine to form three hydrogen bonds with thymine. Incorporation of D monomers into PNA oligomers in place of A led to increases in T_m of about 2.5–6.5°C per substitution, along with a substantial increase in sequence specificity (53). 2-Aminopurine (Fig. 7c) is intrinsically fluorescent and is a less efficient but capable binder of thymine in comparison with adenine (A). In addition, the fluorescence intensity of 2-aminopurine decreases in the presence of other nucleases, making possible the fluorescent detection of PNA-DNA hybridization. Replacement of a single A with 2-aminopurine leads to a T_m decrease of only 2–3°C, while providing this useful fluorescent probe (54).

The inability to form stable, hydrogen-bonded triplexes with pyrimidine DNA targets limits the potential of PNA as a DNA probe. As an alternative, Eldrup et al. (55) synthesized PNA monomers hosting the unnatural nucleobase 3-oxo-2,3-dihydropyridazine (E). The "E base" can form a triplex with bonded A-T pairs in dsDNA to form a triplex without strand displacement (Fig. 2). Eldrup et al. incorporated the E base at two positions in the Hoogsteen strand of bis-PNA and found triplex T_m increases of about 5–7°C over bis-PNAs with a guanine (G) or no base at the same positions. This important achievement should expand the binding repertoire of PNA for dsDNA.

Finally, Christensen et al. (56) incorporated the unnatural nucleobase N-benzoylcytosine (C^{Bz}) in an attempt to prevent the formation of triplexes under controlled conditions. A computer model of C^{Bz+}-G-C^{Bz} triplexes indicated a strong steric interference between benzoyl groups of C^{Bz} in the triplex. UV melting data identified duplex rather than triplex formation when one C residue was replaced by a C^{Bz}, with a 30°C decrease in T_m. These researchers showed that duplex or triplex formation can be controlled by judicious choice of PNA nucleotides. Computer modeling should reveal additional candidate unnatural nucleotides for other important uses in DNA or RNA recognition.

III. APPLICATIONS FOR PNA CONJUGATES

In the previous decade, numerous biotechnology applications for PNA and its conjugates have been envisioned and explored. Virtually all biosystems that involve nucleic acids and their recognition, analysis, and separation have been candidates for implementation of PNAs and their unique DNA binding properties. Originally, the primary application of PNA technology was to treat genetic disease, but lately efforts have focused on single-nucleotide polymorphism (SNP) detection for genomic analysis as well.

A. Cellular Delivery of PNA for Therapeutic Applications

While the unique binding properties and biostability of PNA encouraged its early development as a therapeutic, it was soon realized that the uptake of PNA in cell lines is much less efficient than that of naked DNA. Wittung (57) studied the passive diffusion of unmodified PNA through model liposome membranes and measured very low efflux rates (half-times of 5.5–11 days). In addition, the lack of negative charge on the PNA backbone obviates its use in standard DNA delivery vehicles like cationic liposomes or polyethylene imine. As a result, most of the early development of PNA drugs focused on PNA delivery using targeting methods. Simmons and coworkers (58) achieved a high-efficiency uptake of PNA to mammalian cells when conjoined to a delivery peptide from Antennapedia. Basu and Wickstrom (59) conjoined a PNA to a peptide analogue of insulin-like growth factor type I (IGF-I) for PNA delivery to murine and human cells, and observed much higher PNA uptake for those cell lines that expressed the IGF-I receptor. Observing that the blood–brain barrier has a high concentration of transferrin receptor, the Pardridge group (60) effected PNA delivery across the blood–brain barrier by attaching an antitransferrin receptor antibody to a PNA peptide by a biotin/streptavidin linkage. Chinnery (61) used a peptidyl targeting presequence to deliver PNA to human mitochondria. A more general approach was described by the Nielsen group (62) who studied the cellular uptake of hydrophobically modified PNAs incorporated into cationic liposomes. The effectiveness of the method was strongly dependent on cell type, but a substantial improvement in uptake was reported in some cases.

Solution-based studies of PNA–nucleic acid interactions provide ample evidence that PNA can bring about significant changes in gene expression when properly delivered to living cells. The capacity of PNA to inhibit RNA translation ("antisense therapy") in solution has been ascribed to either a steric blockage of the translation machinery or an RNase-mediated cleavage of the PNA-RNA duplex (63). Nielsen et al. demonstrated that transcription elongation by RNA polymerase is arrested when complementary PNA is bound to the template strand. Later, the Nielsen group made the interesting observation that the act of transcription itself increases the rate of PNA binding to the template strand, resulting in a "suicide transcription" (64) process in which RNA polymerase is down-regulated by its own action. PNA can also be used as a transcription promoter by forming a strand invasion complex from dsDNA that allows for the binding of RNA polymerase to the displaced strand (65). Such PNA-induced promotion can be as efficient as that of natural promoters in some cases. Mologni et al. (66) observed an additive effect when targeting three different regions of a human oncogene in solution, in which all three PNAs were necessary to effectively inhibit expression.

Despite the challenges of PNA delivery to cells to alter gene expression there are many success stories. Praseuth reported an inhibition of interleukin-2 receptor (IL-2Rα) synthesis by delivery of naked PNA complementary to IL-2Rα regulatory sequences (67). Good and Nielsen delivered PNA designed to target the start codon regions of β-galactosidase and β-lactamase genes in *E. coli*. Dose-dependent and specific gene inhibition was identified by a decrease in the velocity of reactions catalyzed by these enzymes (68). The inhibition was more efficient for a mutant strain of "permeable" *E. coli*, indicating that PNA delivery is a limiting step. In a separate study (69), they implemented PNA as an artificial antibiotic by targeting ribosomal RNA to shut down protein synthesis, leading to a significant inhibition of *E. coli* growth. Using a particular retro-inverso delivery peptide, PNA was rapidly internalized by neuronal cells, leading to a decreased production of the hormone oxytocin, active in controlling certain types of behavior (70).

In addition to its use as an antisense inhibitor, PNA can perform many other functions in cells. PNA has been used to block the reverse transcription activity of an HIV strain by complexing with the primer binding site of the HIV-1 genome (71,72). Faruqi et al. (73) employed PNA for the in vitro site-directed mutation of a reporter gene delivered to mouse cells. Specific binding of PNA led to triplex formation and mutagenesis by a repair-dependent pathway. A radiolabeled PNA probe was used to simultaneously regulate and image the expression of a luciferase reporter gene in a rat model (74). Telomerase is a DNA-binding enzyme responsible for the lengthening of telomeres, whose progressive shortening with cell division leads to the apoptosis (programmed death) of cells. The immortality of most tumor cell lines has been connected to high levels of telomerase in the cells, and its inhibition is an important potential cancer therapy. The DNA binding properties of PNA have also been exploited to bind the active site of telomerase, inhibiting its activity in human cell culture (75).

Despite the enormous potential of PNA antisense therapies, the delivery of PNA is a major difficulty, even in in vitro situations. The successes described above should motivate the increased exploration of PNA delivery strategies.

B. PNA Conjugates as DNA Shuttles

Apart from the difficulties in delivering PNA to cells, DNA delivery to cells is challenging in its own right. DNA is much more susceptible to degradation by nucleases in the cytoplasm and therefore must be quickly shuttled from the exterior of the cell to the nucleus. Several "delivery barriers" stand in the way, including the transport of DNA across the cell membrane (by either a targeted or passive mechanism), escape from the harsh environment of the endocytotic endosome, and, finally, import into the nucleus through nanoscopic pores (76). While cationic liposomes have received the most attention from biomedical researchers as a nonviral delivery vehicle, naked DNA shows a reasonable transfection efficiency in many cases. Recently, researchers have been exploring the use of PNA as a means of attaching various cellular signals and surface-active peptides to plasmid DNA for improved delivery efficiency of naked DNA. Liang et al. (77) conjugated a bis-PNA to transferrin via a reversible disulfide bond and then studied its uptake in myoblasts and myotubes. Significant transfection was observed when the naked DNA was incubated with polyethylene imine. The efficiency was inhibited by excess transferrin, indicating that targeting function of PNA-conjugated transferrin was achieved. A more general approach was described by Zelphati et al. (78) who outlined chemistries to append biotin and maleimide to bis-PNA for the attachment of a wide range of peptides and oligonucleotides to plasmid DNA, including peptidyl nuclear localization signals. This PNA-dependent gene chemistry promises to be a very powerful technique for achieving a better understanding and development of nonviral delivery vectors.

C. Genomic Analysis via PNA

Polymerase chain reaction (PCR) is a ubiquitous method in biotechnology used to amplify nucleic acids for analysis. A more specific application is in the amplification of "variable number of tandem repeat (VNTR)" loci for genetic typing purposes. Due to the inter- and intrastrand associations of longer strands, small products are amplified to a greater extent than large ones. In the case of VNTR typing this amplification can lead to improper typing, particularly in heterozygous samples. Small PNA oligomers can be used to block the PCR template strand to prevent these associations without impeding primer extension (79). Interestingly, recent studies of PNA and PNA/DNA chimeras demonstrate that these molecules can function as PCR primers, but only for a few polymerases. This indicates that the shape of the duplex region rather than specific interaction with the backbone phosphate group is a critical factor in polymerase recognition (80–82).

PNA technology can be used to assist in or prevent the cleavage of nucleic acids at particular sequences. The Nielsen group (83) showed that PNA oligomers targeted to restriction enzyme sites on plasmid DNA completely inhibited the enzymatic cleavage. (PNA)$_2$-DNA triplexes leave one DNA strand displaced and subject to digestion by S1 nuclease, and as such, PNA and S1 nuclease together form an "artificial restriction enzyme" system in which a targeted sequence can be cleaved (84). The specificity of cleavage can be greatly enhanced by a PNA-assisted rare cleavage method (85) that uses bis-PNA to shield rare sequences from enzymatic methylation. Subsequent digestion by restriction enzymes effects cleavage at the protected sites alone with very high selectivity. The double-duplex invasion complex formed by unnatural nucleobases in PNA has also shown resistance to restriction and methylation enzymes (86), expanding these methods to encompass a wider range of target sequences.

PNA-mediated PCR clamping is a highly sensitive method for detecting point mutations. The key concept is that PNAs targeted against primer binding sites on the template strand will block the formation of PCR product (87). Detection of mutations occurs by selective amplification/ suppression of various target sequences or, alternatively, by suppressing the amplification of the wild-type sequence and analyzing amplified products as potential mutants (88). By taking advantage of the high sequence specificity of PNA binding, this technique can identify point mutations over a 4- to 6-8 base-pair region by a single test. Recently, PNA-mediated PCR clamping methods have been extended to include integration with on-line fluorescence detection (89) detection of mitochondrial DNA (90), and formalin-fixed, paraffin-embedded samples (91).

D. Nucleic Acid Biosensors Using PNA

The highly sequence-sensitive binding of PNA to nucleic acids has motivated the use in biosensors for the analysis of SNPs. These small changes in DNA sequence can have remarkable impact on gene function and expression, and the detection of SNPs in biosensors will someday be used for the identification of genetic diseases. An early report by Ross (92) used PNA hybridization as a method to discriminate SNPs in the human mitochondrial genome using MALDI-TOF (matrix-assisted laser desorption ionization–time of flight) mass spectroscopy. A 268-base-pair target from a human blood extract was PCR amplified and biotinylated for attachment to magnetic particles. PNA oligomer probes were hybridized to immobilized DNA. After a washing step, the molecular weights of the PNA-DNA complexes were measured by MALDI-TOF to assay PNA hybridization. Since different probes have different molecular weights, it is possible to identify the probe, and therefore the allele, unambiguously. The Nielsen group (93) has developed a quartz crystal microbalance (QCM) platform for SNP detection using PNA immobilized to the QCM crystal by gold-thiol chemistry, and reported very fast (3–5 min) detection for a complementary DNA oligomer. No effect on the frequency response was observed when a large excess of single-base mismatched DNA was analyzed, again indicating the highly selective nature of PNA binding. In a later study, they studied both the mass and shear dissipation in a similar system (94). Burgener et al. (95) have described a surface-plasmon resonance detection system for PNA-DNA hybridization, exhibiting detection of an ssDNA target at 1% concentrations combined with ssDNA having a single point mutation. Efimov outlined a strategy to attach PNA probes to surface-grafted polyamide polymers in an attempt to improve the potency of PNA hybridization in biosensors, with promising results (96).

Of course, PNA can be used to detect DNA by linking radioactive or fluorescent moieties to the complementary DNA as well. Svanik et al. (97) took this approach one step further and combined the excellent binding properties of PNA with the fluorescence enhancement properties of cyanine dyes to yield a "light-up probe" hybridization detection system. Binding of a complementary PNA to target ssDNA causes the cyanine dye (thiazole orange) to become fluorescent ("light up"), providing a fast, readily identifiable, and sequence-selective detection method.

E. Bioseparations Using PNA

There is a growing need to develop sequence-specific means of purifying nucleic acids, both for genomic analysis and for the larger scale purification of plasmid DNA for gene therapy. The sequence-specific binding properties of PNA can be used in affinity separations of DNA as an alternative to standard DNA purification methods such as anion exchange chromatography and density gradient techniques. With genomic analysis as a goal, Perry-O'Keefe et al. (98) developed a prehybridization technique using PNA in gel electrophoresis as a fast, efficient alternative to Southern blotting. At plasmid or PCR sample was incubated with PNA probe at low ionic strength conditions, which are amenable to PNA-DNA duplex formation but not DNA-DNA. Ensuing electrophoresis simultaneously separated and detected the target in a single step. The separation was found to be highly specific using both slab and capillary electrophoresis formats. Rose (99) measured (PNA)$_2$-DNA binding kinetics and stoichiometry using capillary electrophoresis by evaluating the relative amounts of bound and unbound DNA after a given hybridization time. Igloi (100) prepared an affinity gel hosting PNA oligomers and measured shifts in migration for complementary but mismatched DNA oligomers via fluorescence. Shifts in migration relative to a fully noncomplementary standard gave a real-time visualization of the hybridization and yielded dissociation constants in good agreement with gel mobility shift and CD data cited above.

Larger scale purification of nucleic acids using PNA probes have also been explored. The Nielsen group synthesized a PNA-peptide chimera with six histidine groups to separate DNA oligonucleotides and larger RNAs using metal ion affinity chromatography (101). The strong interaction between the Ni^{2+} column and the histidine groups bound the target nucleic acid to the column, which could then be washed and the target eluted by heating to 95°C. The operation was found to be highly sequence specific to facilitate discrimination of single-base mismatches. Boffa et al. (102) used streptavidin-agarose magnetic beads to separate target nucleic acids with biotinylated PNA probes. The targets were tandem CAG repeats, which have been implicated in hereditary neurodegenerative diseases. Cellular extracts of chromatin were digested by restriction endonuclease and incubated with the biotinylated PNA for hybridization followed by the functionalized beads. Some decrease in the (PNA)$_2$-DNA binding efficiency was reported when using these cellular extracts, likely due to interference by nucleosomal proteins. Recently, Chandler et al. (103) compared the recovery efficiency of biotinylated DNA and PNA probes in a streptavidin-magnetic bead system and found no significant difference between PNA and DNA probes at moderately high (0.4 M phosphate) buffer concentration, but significant advantage for PNA probes at low ionic strength. As these separation schemes move to the less pristine conditions of cellular extracts, it may become necessary to predialyze or prefilter extracts for the comparative advantage of PNA to be realized.

IV. SYNTHESIS AND PROPERTIES OF PNA AMPHIPHILES

Recent work in our group has focused on the development of PNA conjugates with various synthetic lipophilic groups attached. These "PNA amphiphiles" hold great promise for the separation of nucleic acids using hydrophobically driven operations such as reversed-phase high-performance liquid chromatography (HPLC) and aqueous two-phase extraction. Additionally, PNA amphiphiles can be incorporated into liposomes to serve as molecular switches for their controlled aggregation and dispersion in drug delivery systems and colloidal processing. Because PNA has limited solubility and a tendency to self-aggregate, our initial efforts have been on improving the water solubility of the PNA amphiphiles while incorporating a large enough nonpolar "tag" to provide separation resolution. In this section, we will describe the synthesis and characterization of these molecules, along with some preliminary data concerning their interfacial, solubility, and DNA binding properties. For the most part, these methods are similar to those used to characterize PNA oligomers and will be instructive for those interested in working with other PNA oligomers and conjugates as well.

A. Chemical Structure of PNA Amphiphiles

The structure of a typical PNA amphiphile is shown in Fig. 8. By a flexible synthetic technique (104) we can alter the tail architecture, tail length, and peptide–tail spacer length, along with the sequence of the PNA-peptide headgroup. PNA amphiphiles are synthesized using a manual solid phase synthesis in which the PNA peptide is built on a resin support one residue at a time. A synthetic "base amphiphile" or fatty acid is added to the peptide chain as a final step. At least one lysine residue is incorporated to ensure water solubility. The base amphiphile notation describes the tail architecture, where "$(C_{16})_2$" refers to the 16 carbon dialkyl tails, "glu" refers to the glumatic acid linker, and "C_2" refers to the two methylene groups of the succinic anhydric spacer. Conventional names were used for the fatty acid–modified PNA oligomers.

B. Synthesis of Base Amphiphile

The base amphiphiles were synthesized by a two-step solution procedure. Additional synthesis and characterization details are available from Berndt et al. (104). For the tail linking step, 100 mmol hexadecanol (Aldrich), 50 mmol L-aspartic acid (Aldrich), and 75 mmol p-toluenesulfonate

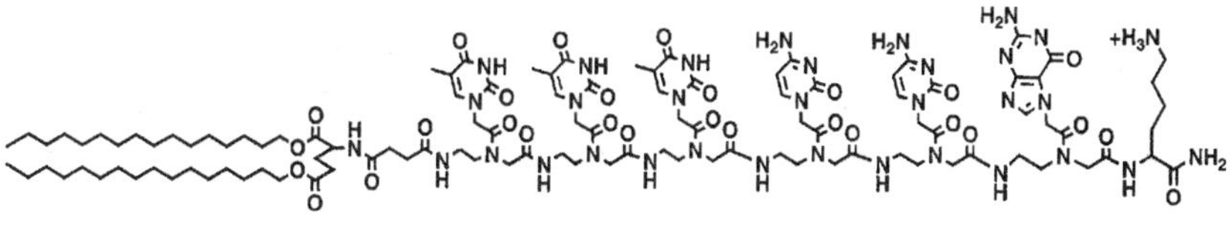

Figure 8 Chemical structure of PNA-amphiphile "$(C_{16})_2$-glu-C_2-TTTCCGK."

monohydrate (Aldrich) were dissolved in about 500 mL toluene. The mixture was heated until a stoichiometric amount of water was recovered in a Dean–Stark trap. Toluene was removed by rotary evaporation and the product was recrystallized several times in acetone. The yield of the linking reaction was 80%. Purity was high as judged by electrospray mass spectroscopy, ^{1}H NMR, and FTIR spectroscopy. The second step is a succinylation step, for which 20 mmol of linking reaction product and 25 mmol of N,N-diisopropylethylamine (DIPEA) were dissolved in about 50 mL of a 1:1 tetrahydrofuran (THF)/chloroform solution. After stirrings 23 mmol succinic anhydride (Aldrich) was added. The mixture was heated to 40°C for 2 h of reaction. The solvent was removed by rotary evaporation and the product was recrystallized several times in acetone. The yield of the succinylation reaction was 90%. Purity of the base amphiphile product was high as judged by electrospray mass spectroscopy, ^{1}H NMR, and FTIR.

C. Synthesis of PNA Amphiphiles

PNA amphiphiles were synthesized via a manual solid phase peptide synthesis method (105). Synthesis was performed using an Fmoc-PEG-PAL-PS resin (Peptides International). The resin was swelled for 1 h in dichloromethane (DCM) to increase the accessibility of reagents to the functional groups on the support. Deprotection was performed by agitating the resin in 20% piperidine in N,N-dimethylformamide (DMF) for 4 min three separate times. DCM and DMF were used to wash the resin after deprotection. A ninhydrin test (Applied Biosystems) was used to test for active amines on the resin prior to coupling of the first lysine residue. Once deprotection was verified, coupling was performed using an HATU activator (O-(7-azabenzotriazol-1-yl)-1,1,3,3-tetramethyluronium hexafluor-ophosphate, Applied Biosystems) in a base solution (DMF, DIPEA, and 2,6-lutidine; Applied Biosystems) with the monomer solution. The protected monomer was added in fivefold excess to ensure efficient coupling. After a 2-min incubation with the activator, the coupling solution was added to the resin and allowed to react for 1 h in the case of the initial lysine, and 20 min for subsequent residues. After coupling, the resin was washed with DCM and DMF and a ninhydrin test was performed to verify coupling. A capping solution made up of acetic anhydride, 1-methyl-2-pyrrolidinone, and pyridine was then added to block unreacted amino groups, preventing elongation of failure sequences. A final wash with DCM was done to complete the cycle. This procedure was followed for subsequent monomer additions until the peptide sequence was complete. The terminal base amphiphile or carboxylic acid was added following the same procedures as the protected monomers.

Following synthesis, the PNA amphiphile was cleaved from the solid resin support by reaction with trifluoroacetic acid (TFA) and m-cresol in a 4:1 ratio (2 mL total, for 2 h). The TFA cleaves the peptide from the resin and removes the Bhoc protecting groups while the m-cresol acts as a proton scavenger for the cleaved protecting groups. The solution was separated from the beads using a glass frit and transferred to a glass centrifuge tube. A fivefold excess of dry ether was added to precipitate the PNA amphiphile. The mixture was placed in a $-80°C$ freezer for 10 min to fully precipitate the peptide, then centrifuged for 5 min to separate the ether from the solid PNA amphiphile. The supernatant was decanted and fresh ether added once again, following which mixing was done to resuspend the pellet. This procedure was repeated three times. Once complete the PNA amphiphile was dried with a gentle stream of nitrogen and then dissolved in water.

D. Purification and Characterization of PNA Amphiphiles

PNA amphiphile was purified by reversed-phase HPLC (Waters Delta 600) using a C_4 HPLC column (Waters Symmetry 300, 300-Å pore size, 5-μm particle size). A linear acetonitrile/water gradient (0–60% acetonitrile) was eluted over 30 min. The product peak eluted at different times depending on the base amphiphile and peptide sequence. The yield of the reaction was about 25% based on the available reactive sites on the resin. Purity of the product was high as judged by FTIR, ^1H NMR, and MALDI mass spectroscopy (Voyager, PerSeptive Biosystems.)

Pressure–area isotherms and LB depositions were carried out using a computer-controlled, liquid-cooled KSV 5000 Langmuir trough (KSV Instruments) in a dust-free laminar flow hood. Surface pressure measurements were made using a platinum Wilhelmy plate. The pure water subphase was equilibrated to $25 \pm 0.5°C$. About 100-μL of a 1 mg/mL amphiphile solution (in 9:1 chloroform/methanol) was spread on the water surface using a 100-μL syringe. The solvent was allowed to dry for 5 min prior to monolayer compression. The movement of the barrier was controlled by a computer algorithm that continually decreased the speed of the barrier movement in response to the increase in surface pressure.

Purified, desalted DNA oligomers (5'-CGGAAA-3' and 5'-ATAGCC-3') were obtained in 10-nmol amounts from a commercial supplier (Integrated DNA Technologies). Five hundred microliters of 10 mM phosphate buffer (pH = 7.0) was added to the oligomer sample and vortexed to ensure complete mixing. DNA concentration was determined by measuring the absorbance at 260 nm and 70°C using tabulated extinction coefficients. The sample was then transferred to a quartz cuvette (Starna) and placed in a thermostated block in the UV spectrometer (CARY-300).

Absorbance at 260 nm was monitored as the temperature was ramped from 60°C to 10°C and back to 60°C. At least two full cycles were performed for each sample. Melting transition temperature (T_m) and other thermodynamic data were obtained using software provided with the UV instrument.

E. Solubility of PNA Amphiphiles

To investigate the water solubility and self-aggregating properties of PNA amphiphiles, we synthesized a number of synthetic variants. Table 2 summarizes the PNA amphiphiles we have synthesized, along with their HPLC retention times for elution via a acetonitrile/water gradient (0–60% acetonitrile). The double-tailed surfactants have a much higher retention time than the single-tailed surfactants, indicating the poorer water solubility of the double-tailed surfactants. This observation was confirmed by pressure–area isotherms measured on both the single- and double-tailed PNA amphiphiles (Fig. 9). The double-tailed surfactants exhibited stable pressure–area isotherms with high collapse pressures, attesting to both the interfacial stability and purity of the samples.

Table 2 Summary of PNA-Amphiphiles Synthesized

PNA-amphiphile	MW, expected (g/mol)	MW, MALDI (g/mol)	C_4 retention time (min)
$(C_{12})_2$-glu-C_2- TTTCCGK	2305.71	2306.19	14.1 ± 0.3
$(C_{14})_2$-glu-C_2- TTTCCGK	2361.71	—	16.2 ± 0.2
$(C_{16})_2$-glu-C_2- TTTCCGK	2417.71	2418.16	18.3 ± 0.3
Lauric- TTTCCGK	1922.03	1921.95	4.4 ± 0.7
Lauric- TTTCCGKK	2051.21	2072.31 (M + Na)	—
Stearic- TTTCCGK	2006.19	2028.01 (M + Na)	11.3 ± 0.2
Stearic- TTTCCGKK	2135.37	2156.67 (M + Na)	11.9 ± 0.3
Stearic- KTTCCGK	2135.37	2134.58	10.1 ± 0.3

Retention times are for a C_4 analytical column with a linear acetonitrile/water gradient (0–60% acetonitrile) eluted over 30 min. MALDI molecular weights are for the primary ion or a sodium complex of the primary ion (M + Na).

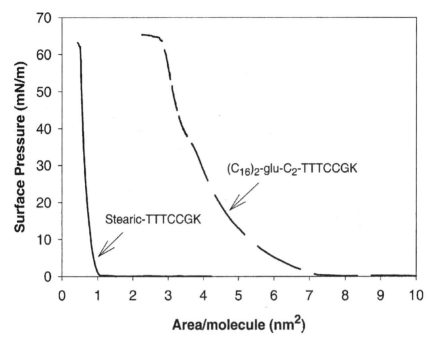

Figure 9 Pressure–area isotherms for insoluble PNA amphiphiles.

The $(C_{16})_2$-glu-C_2-TTTCCGK isotherm begins at an area per molecule of about $8\,nm^2$ and has an ultimate area per molecule of about $3\,nm^2$—much larger than the dialkyl tail cross section ($0.4\,nm^2$). For comparison, the PNA-DNA duplex has a cross-sectional area of $6.2\,nm^2$, and a single-stranded nucleic acid has a cross-sectional area closer to $1.0\,nm^2$. The inability of the PNA headgroups to closely pack prior to collapse is likely due to a combination of electrostatic and excluded volume interactions between the PNA amphiphiles. For the single-tailed surfactants, observed collapse pressures were very low ($<20\,mN/m$) and the ultimate area per molecule was much less than $1.0\,nm^2$, indicating desorption of these soluble PNA amphiphiles from the air–water interface.

A notable exception is the "stearic-TTTCCGK" sample, which yielded a stable isotherm with an ultimate area per molecule of $0.6\,nm^2$, and we have observed some heat-induced precipitation with this molecule. Generally, single-tailed PNA amphiphiles require two lysine groups to be appended to the C terminus for moderate water solubility (about $5\,mM$). The water solubility appears to be lower when using a $0.15\,M$ sodium phosphate buffer (pH 7.0). Some precipitation of PNA amphiphile has been observed at temperatures above 60°C, an effect we are studying in more detail using light scattering techniques.

F. DNA Hybridization Properties of PNA Amphiphiles

We have also performed some preliminary studies to assess the DNA binding properties of PNA amphiphiles using UV spectroscopy (Fig. 10). To avoid complications with precipitation on heating and micellization, we used the lauric-TTTCCGKK molecule at concentrations below the CMC (about 0.4 mg/mL) for these studies. In both pure water and pH 7.0 buffer, the temperature profiles gave the sigmoidal increase in absorbance typical for nucleic acid hybridization, along with a small hysteresis. The hysteresis was minimized at slower ramps (0.5°C/min), indicating the hysteresis is due to slow association kinetics. Temperature profiles for the PNA amphiphile alone or with a scrambled-sequence DNA oligomer control showed no sigmoidal transition and an overall change in absorbance of less than 0.1 absorbance unit. This demonstrates that the binding of DNA oligomers to PNA amphiphiles is sequence specific and not caused by self-aggregation.

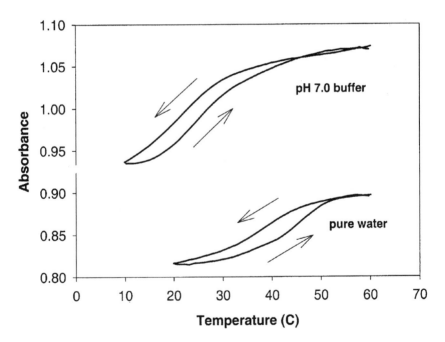

Figure 10 UV absorbance vs. temperature profiles for lauric-TTTCCGKK with a complementary DNA oligomer.

Table 3 Summary of Thermal Stability Data for PNA Oligomer TTTCCGKK and Its Lauric Conjugate with a Complementary DNA Oligomer

Sample	T_m (°C)	Hysteresis (C)
Lauric-TTTCCGKK Pure water	42.3 ± 1.0	4.4
Lauric-TTTCCGKK pH 7.0 buffer	26.8 ± 1.0	2.8
TTTCCGKK Pure water	39.2 ± 1.0	11.2
TTTCCGKK pH 7.0 buffer	22.0 ± 1.0	3.0

Comparing the UV melting data for the lauric-modified and unmodified peptide (Table 3), we find that the presence of the lauric tail has a significant impact on both the thermal stability and binding kinetics of PNA-DNA duplexes. The thermal stability of the lauric-modified PNA was significantly higher in both pure water (2°C higher) and pH 7.0 buffer (5°C higher). In addition, the hysteresis in the curves was lower for the lauric-modified PNA in pure water (4.4°C compared to 11.2°C), but not significantly different in buffer. These effects are likely due to attractive hydrophobic interactions between the nucleotides and the fatty acid tail.

V. CONCLUSIONS

The stable binding and ready modification of PNA can be exploited in rapid, specific bioseparations, and in biosensors that can readily identify SNPs and other genomic information. Its high nuclease and protease stability makes it a very attractive candidate for antisense therapies. Strand invasion of dsDNA by PNA is a very useful tool in genomic analysis by PCR and as a rare-cutter. While the unique binding properties of PNAs hold great promise, for PNA technology to move from the laboratory to the marketplace issues regarding water solubility and cellular delivery remain to be tackled. Still, good progress has been made using unnatural nucleobases in PNA to target a wider variety of nucleic acid sequences. The continued development of PNA technology will require researchers to refine this biomimetic material using a combination of molecular insight and modern biotechniques.

REFERENCES

1. PE Nielsen, et al. Sequence-selective recognition of DNA by strand displacement with a thymine-substitutede polyamide. Science 254:1497–1500, 1991.
2. M Egholm, et al. Peptide nucleic acids (PNA). Oligonucleotide analogues with an achiral peptide backbone. J Am Chem Soc 114:1895–1897, 1992.
3. M Egholm, et al. Recognition of guanine and adenine in DNA by cytosine and thymine containing peptide nucleic acids (PNA). J Am Chem Soc 114:9677–9678, 1992.
4. KE Nelson, M Levy, SL Miller. Peptide nucleic acids rather than RNA may have been the first genetic molecule. Proc Natl Acad Sci USA 97:3868–3871, 2000.
5. A Ray, B Nordén. Peptide nucleic acid (PNA): its medical and biotechnical applications and promise for the future. FASEB J 14:1041–1060, 2000.
6. PE Nielsen. Peptide nucleic acid. A molecule with two identities. Acc Chem Res 32:624–630, 1999.
7. PE Nielsen. Peptide nucleic acids as therapeutic agents. Curr Opin Struct Biol 9:353–357, 1999.
8. E Uhlmann, et al. PNA: synthetic polyamide nucleic acids with unusual binding properties. Angew Chem Int Ed 37:2796–2823, 1998.
9. SC Brown, et al. NMR solution structure of a peptide nucleic acid complexed with RNA. Science 265:777–780, 1994.
10. M Eriksson, PE Nielsen. Solution structure of a peptide nucleic acid–DNA duplex. Nat Struct Biol 3:410–413, 1996.
11. H Rasmussen, et al. Crystal structure of a peptide nucleic acid (PNA) duplex at 1.7 Å resolution. Nat Struct Biol 4:98–101, 1997.
12. M Leijon, et al. Structural characterization of PNA-DNA duplexes by NMR. Evidence for DNA in a B-like conformation. Biochemistry 33:9820–9825, 1994.
13. M Eriksson, PE Nielsen. PNA–nucleic acid complexes. Structure, stability, and dynamics. Q Rev Biophys 29:369–394, 1996.
14. CR Cantor, PR Schimmel. Biophysical chemistry. Part II: Techniques for the study of Biological Structure and Function. New York: WH Freeman, 1980.
15. M Egholm, et al. PNA Hybridizes to complementary oligonucleotides obeying the Watson-Crick hydrogen-bonding rules. Nature 365:566–568, 1993.
16. T Ratilainen, et al. Thermodynamics of sequence-specific binding of PNA to DNA. Biochemistry 39:7781–7791, 2000.
17. FP Schwarz, S Robinson, JM Butler. Thermodynamic comparison of PNA/DNA and DNA/DNA hybridization reactions at ambient temperature. Nucl Acids Res 27:4792–4800, 1999.
18. U Giesen, et al. A formula for the thermal stability (T_m) prediction of PNA/DNA duplexes. Nucl Acids Res 26:5004–5006, 1998.
19. DY Cherny, et al. DNA unwinding upon strand-displacement binding of a thymine-substituted polyamide to double-stranded DNA. Proc Natl Acad Sci USA 90:1667–1670, 1993.

20. VV Demidov, et al. Kinetics and mechanism of polyamide ("peptide") nucleic acid binding to duplex DNA. Proc Natl Acad Sci USA 92:2637–2641, 1995.

21. P Wittung, P Nielsen, B Nordén. Direct observation of strand invasion by peptide nucleic acid (PNA) into double-stranded DNA. J Am Chem Soc 118:7049–7054, 1996.

22. T Bentin, PE Nielsen. Enhanced peptide nucleic acid binding to supercoiled DNA: possible implications for DNA "breathing" dynamics. Biochemistry 35:8863–8869, 1996.

23. X Zhang, T Ishihara, DR Corey. Strand invasion by mixed base PNAs and a PNA-peptide chimera. Nucl Acids Res 28:3332–3338, 2000.

24. L Betts, et al. A nucleic acid triple helix formed by a peptide nucleic acid–DNA complex. Science 270:1838–1841, 1995.

25. MC Griffith, et al. Single and bis peptide nucleic acids as triplexing agents: binding and stoichiometry. J Am Chem Soc 117:831–832, 1995.

26. M Egholm, et al. Efficient pH-independent sequence-specific DNA binding by pseudoisocytosine-containing bis-PNA. Nucl Acids Res 23:217–222, 1995.

27. P Wittung, P Nielsen, B Nordén. Extended DNA-recognition repertoire of peptide nucleic acid (PNA): PNA-dsDNA triplex formed with cytosine-rich homopyrimidine PNA. Biochemistry 36:7973–7979, 1997.

28. J Lohse, O Dahl, PE Nielsen. Double duplex invasion by peptide nucleic acid: a general principle for sequence-specific targeting of double-stranded DNA. Proc Natl Acad Sci USA 96:11804–11808, 1999.

29. T Ishihara, DR Corey. Rules for strand invasion by chemically modified oligonucleotides. J Am Chem Soc 121:2012–2020, 1999.

30. M Eriksson, et al. Sequence dependent N-terminal rearrangement and degradation of peptide nucleic acid (PNA) in aqueous solution. New J Chem 1055–1059, 1998.

31. V Demidov, et al. Stability of peptide nucleic acids in human serum and cellular extracts. Biochem Pharmacol 48:1309–1313, 1994.

32. G Haaima, et al. Peptide nucleic acids (PNAs) containing thymine monomers derived from chiral amino acids: hybridization and solubility properties of D-lysine PNA. Angew Chem Int Ed Engl 35:1939–1942, 1996.

33. KK Jensen, et al. Kinetics for hybridization of peptide nucleic acid (PNA) with DNA and RNA studied with the BIAcore technique. Biochemistry 36:5072–5077, 1997.

34. H Kuhn, et al. An experimental study of mechanism and specificity of peptide nucleic acid (PNA) binding to duplex DNA. J Mol Biol 286:1337–1345, 1999.

35. YN Kosaganov, et al. Effect of temperature and ionic strength on the dissociation kinetics and lifetime of PNA-DNA triplexes. Biochemistry 39:11742–11747, 2000.

36. P Lagriffoule, et al. Peptide nucleic acids (PNAs) with a conformationally constrained, chiral cyclohexyl derived backbone. Chem Eur J 3:912–919, 1997.

37. S Jordan, et al. New hetero-oligomeric peptide nucleic acids with improved binding properties to complementary DNA. Bioorg Med Chem Lett 7:687–690, 1997.

38. G Lowe, T Vilaivan. Dipeptides bearing nucleobases for the synthesis of novel peptide nucleic acids. J Chem Soc Perkin Trans I:547–554, 1997.

39. G Lowe, T Vilavan. Amino acids bearing nucleobases for the synthesis of novel peptide nucleic acids. J Chem Soc Perkin Trans I:539–545, 1997.

40. BP Gangamani, VA Kumar, KN Ganesh. Chiral analogues of peptide nucleic acids: synthesis of 4-aminoprolyl nucleic acids and DNA complementation studies using UV/CD spectroscopy. Tetrahedron 55:177–192, 1999.

41. B Hyrup, et al. A flexible and positively charged PNA analogue with an ethylene-linker to the nucleobase: synthesis and hybridization properties. Bioorg Med Chem Lett 6:1083–1088, 1996.

42. B Hyrup, et al. Structure–activity studies of the binding of modified peptide nucleic acids (PNAs) to DNA. J Am Chem Soc 116:7964–7970, 1994.

43. AH Krotz, O Buchardt, PE Nielsen. Synthesis of "Retro-Inverso" peptide nucleic acids: 1. Characterization of the monomers. Tetrahedron Lett 36:6937–6940, 1995.

44. AH Krotz, et al. A "Retro-Inverso" PNA: structural implications for DNA and RNA binding. Bioorg Med Chem 6:1983–1992, 1998.

45. A Peyman, et al. PHONO-PNA co-oligomers: nucleic acid mimetics with interesting properties. Angew Chem Int Ed Engl 36:2809–2812, 1997.

46. F Bergmann, W Bannwarth, S Tam. Solid phase synthesis of directly linked PNA-DNA-hybrids. Tetrahedron Lett 36:6823–6826, 1995.

47. E Uhlmann, et al. Synthesis and properties of PNA/DNA chimeras. Angew Chem Int Ed Engl 35:2632–2635, 1996.

48. VA Efimov, et al. Synthesis and evaluation of some properties of chimeric oligomers containing PNA and phosphono-PNA residues. Nucl Acid Res 26:566–575, 1998.

49. BP Gangamani, VA Kumar, KN Ganesh. Spermine conjugated peptide nucleic acids (sppNA): UV and fluoresence studies of PNA-DNA hybrids with improved stability. Biochem Biophys Res Commun 240:778–782, 1997.

50. DA Barawkar, et al. Deoxynucleic guanidine/peptide nucleic acid chimeras: synthesis, binding and invasion studies with DNA. J Am Chem Soc 122:5244–5250, 2000.

51. NM Howarth, LPG Wakelin. α-PNA: a novel peptide nucleic acid analogue of DNA. J Org Chem 62:5441–5450, 1997.

52. P Garner, S Dey, Y Huang. α-Helical peptide nucleic acids (αPNAs): a new paradigm for DNA-binding molecules. J Am Chem Soc 122:2405–2406, 2000.

53. G Haaima, et al. Increased DNA binding and sequence discrimination of PNA oligomers containing 2,6-diaminopurine. Nucl Acids Res 25:4639–4643, 1997.

54. BP Gangamani, VA Kumar, KN Ganesh. 2-Aminopurine peptide nucleic acids (2-apPNA): intrinsic fluorescent PNA analogues for probing PNA-DNA interaction dynamics. Chem Commun 1913–1914, 1997.

55. AB Eldrup, O Dahl, PE Nielsen. A novel peptide nucleic acid monomer for recognition of thymine in triple-helix structures. J Am Chem Soc 119:11116–11117, 1997.

56. L Christensen, et al. Inhibition of PNA triplex formation by N_4-benzoylated cytosine. Nucl Acids Res 26:2735–2739, 1998.

57. P Wittung, et al. Phospholipid membrane permeability of peptide nucleic acid. FEBS Lett 375:27–29, 1995.

58. CG Simmons, et al. Synthesis and membrane permeability of PNA-peptide conjugates. Bioorg Med Chem Lett 7:3001–3006, 1997.

59. S Basu, E Wickstrom. Synthesis and characterization of a peptide nucleic acid conjugated to a D-peptide analog of insulin-like growth factor 1 for increased cellular uptake. Bioconj Chem 8:481–488, 1997.

60. WM Pardridge, RJ Boado, Y-S Kang. Vector-mediated delivery of a polyamide ("peptide") nucleic acid analogue through the blood–brain barrier in vivo. Proc Natl Acad Sci USA 92:5592–5596, 1995.

61. PF Chinnery, et al. Peptide nucleic acid delivery to human mitochondria. Gene Ther 6:1919–1928, 1999.

62. T Ljungstrøm, H Knudsen, PE Nielsen. Cellular uptake of adamantyl conjugated peptide nucleic acids. Bioconj Chem 10:955–972, 1999.

63. H Knudsen, PE Nielsen. Antisense properties of duplex- and triplex-forming PNAs. Nucl Acids Res 24:494–500, 1996.

64. HJ Larsen, PE Nielsen. Transcription-mediated binding of peptide nucleic acid (PNA) to double-stranded DNA: sequence-specific suicide transcription. Nucl Acids Res 24:458–463, 1996.

65. NE Mollegaard, et al. Peptide nucleic acid. DNA strand displacement loops as artificial transcription promoters. Proc Natl Acad Sci 91:3892–3895, 1994.

66. L Mologni, et al. Additive antisense effects of different PNAs on the in vivo translation of the PML/RARα gene. Nucl Acids Res 26:1934–1938, 1998.

67. D Praseuth, et al. Peptide nucleic acids directed to the promoter of the α-chain of the interleukin-2 receptor. Biochim Biophys Acta 1309:226–238, 1996.

68. L Good, PE Nielsen. Antisense inhibition of gene expression in bacteria by PNA targeted to mRNA. Nat Biotechnol 16:355–358, 1998.

69. L Good, PE Nielsen. Inhibition of translation and bacterial growth by peptide nucleic acid targeted to ribosomal RNA. Proc Natl Acad Sci USA 95:2073–2076, 1998.

70. G Aldrian-Herrada, et al. A peptide nucleic acid (PNA) is more rapidly internalized in cultured neurons when coupled to a Retro-Inverso delivery peptide. The antisense activity depresses the target mRNA and protein in magnocellular oxytocin neurons. Nucl Acids Res 26:4910–4916, 1998.

71. U Koppelhus, et al. Efficient in vitro inhibition of HIV-1 gag reverse by peptide nucleic acid (PNA) at minimal ratios of PNA/RNA. Nucl Acids Res 25:2167–2173, 1997.

72. R Lee, et al. Polyamide nucleic acid targeted to the primer binding site of the HIV-1 reverse transcription. Biochemistry 37:900–910, 1998.

73. AF Farqui, M Egholm, PM Glazer. Peptide nucleic acid–targeted mutagenesis of a chromosomal gene in mouse cells. Proc Natl Acad Sci USA 95:1398–1403, 1998.

74. N Shi, RJ Boado, WM Pardridge. Antisense imaging of gene expression in the brain in vivo. Proc Natl Acad Sci 97:14709–14714, 2000.

75. B-S Herbert, et al. Inhibition of human telomerase in immortal human cells leads to progressive telomere shortening and cell death. Proc Natl Acad Sci USA 96:14276–14281, 1999.

76. L Huang, MC Hung, E Wagner, eds. Nonviral Vectors for Gene Therapy. San Diego: Academic Press, 1999.

77. KW Liang, EP Hoffman, L Huang. Targeted delivery of plasmid DNA to myogenic cells via transferrin-conjugated peptide nucleic acid. Mol Ther 1:236–243, 2000.

78. O Zelphati, et al. PNA-dependent gene chemistry: stable coupling of peptides and oligonucleotides to plasmid DNA. Biotechniques 28:304–316, 2000.

79. DB Demers, et al. Enhanced PCR amplification of VTNR locus D1S80 using peptide nucleic acid. Nucl Acids Res 23:3050–3055, 1995.

80. MJ Lutz, et al. Recognition of uncharged polyamide-linked nucleic acid analogs by DNA polymerases and reverse transcriptases. J Am Chem Soc 119:3177–3178, 1997.

81. HS Misra, et al. Polyamide nucleic acid–DNA chimera lacking the phosphate backbone are novel primers for polymerase chain reaction catalyzed by DNA polymerases. Biochemistry 37:1917–1925, 1998.

82. M Koppitz, PE Nielsen, LE Orgel. Formation of oligonucleotide-PNA-chimeras by template-directed ligation. J Am Chem Soc 120:4563–4569, 1998.

83. PE Nielsen, et al. Sequence specific inhibition of DNA restriction enzyme cleavage by PNA. Nucl Acids Res 21:197–200, 1993.

84. V Demidov, et al. Sequence-selective double strand DNA cleavage by peptide nucleic acid (PNA) targeting using nuclease S1. Nucl Acids Res 21:2103–2107, 1993.

85. AG Veselkov, et al. A new class of genome rare cutters. Nucl Acids Res 24:2483–2487, 1996.

86. KI Izvolsky, et al. Sequence-specific protection of duplex DNA against restriction and methylation enzymes by pseudocomplementary PNAs. Biochemistry 39:10908–10913, 2000.

87. H Ørum, et al. Single base pair mutation analysis by PNA directed PCR clamping. Nucl Acids Res 21:5332–5336, 1993.

88. C Theide, et al. Simple and sensitive detection of mutations in the ras proto-oncogenes using PNA-mediated PCR clamping. Nucl Acids Res 24:983–984, 1996.

89. EM Kyger, MD Krevolin, MJ Powell. Detection of the hereditary hemochromatosis gene mutation by real-time fluorescence polymerase chain reaction and peptide nucleic acid clamping. Anal Biochem 260:142–148, 1998.

90. DG Murdock, NC Christacos, DC Wallace. The age-related accumulation of a mitochondrial DNA control region mutation in muscle, but not brain,

detected by a sensitive PNA-directed PCR clamping based method. Nucl Acids Res 28:4350–4355, 2000.

91. Y Myal, et al. Detection of genetic point mutations by peptide nucleic acid–mediated polymerase chain reaction clamping using paraffin-embedded specimens. Anal Biochem 285:169–172, 2000.

92. PL Ross, K Lee, P Belgrader. Discrimination of single-nucleotide polymorphisms in human DNA using peptide nucleic acid probes detected by MALDI-TOF mass spectrometry. Anal Chem 69:4197–4202, 1997.

93. J Wang, et al. Mismatch-sensitive hybridization detection by peptide nucleic acids immobilized on a quartz crystal microbalance. Anal Chem 69:5200–5202, 1997.

94. P Wittung-Stafshede, et al. Detection of point mutations in DNA by PNA-based quartz-crystal biosensor. Coll Surf 174:269–273, 2000.

95. M Burgener, M Sänger, U Candrian. Synthesis of a stable and specific surface plasmon resonance biosensor surface employing covalently immobilized peptide nucleic acids. Bioconj Chem 11:749–754, 2000.

96. VA Efimov, AA Buryakova, OG Chakhmakhcheva. Synthesis of polyacrylamides N-substituted with PNA-like oligonucleotide mimics for molecular diagnostic applications. Nucl Acids Res 27:4416–4426, 1999.

97. N Svanvik, et al. Light-up probes: thiazole orange–conjugated peptide nucleic acid for detection of target nucleic acid in homogeneous solution. Anal Biochem 281:26–35, 1999.

98. H Perry-O'Keefe, et al. Peptide nucleic acid pre-gel hybridization: an alternative to southern hybridization. Proc Natl Acad Sci USA 93:14670–14675, 1996.

99. DJ Rose. Characterization of antisense binding properties of peptide nucleic acids by capillary gel electrophoresis. Anal Chem 65:3545–3549, 1993.

100. GL Igloi. Variability in the stability of DNA-peptide nucleic acid (PNA) single-base mismatched duplexes: real-time hybridization during affinity electrophoresis in PNA-containing gels. Proc Natl Acad Sci USA 95:8562–8567, 1998.

101. H Ørum. et al. Sequence-specific purification of nucleic acids by PNA-controlled hybrid selection. Biotechniques 19:472–480, 1995.

102. LC Boffa, EM Carpaneto, VG Allfrey. Isolation of active genes containing CAG repeats by DNA strand invasion by a peptide nucleic acid. Proc Natl Acad Sci USA 92:1901–1905, 1995.

103. DP Chandler, et al. Affinity capture and recovery of DNA at femtomolar concentrations with peptide nucleic acid probes. Anal Biochem 283:241–249, 2000.

104. P Berndt, GB Fields, M Tirrell. Synthetic lipidation of peptides and amino acids: monolayer structure and properties. J Am Chem Soc 117:9515–9522, 1995.

105. M Bodansky, A Bodansky. The practice of peptide synthesis. Heidelberg; Springer-Verlag, 1984.

Index

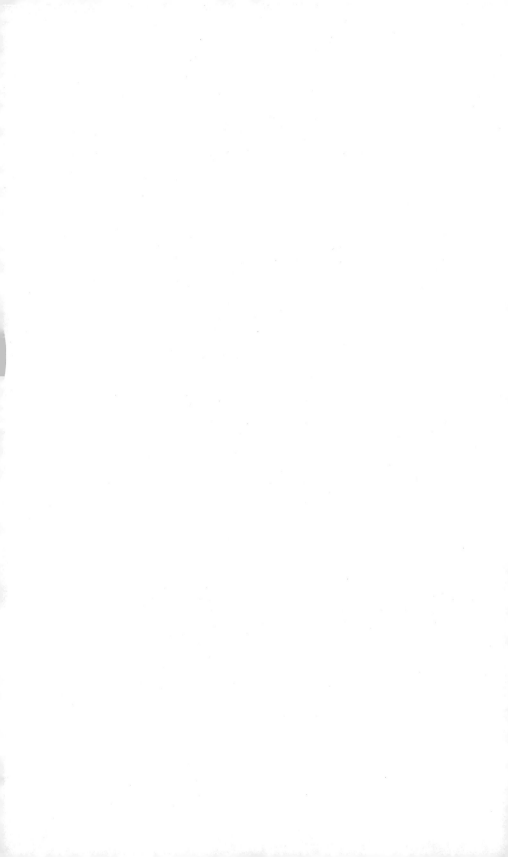

Ollscoil na hÉireann, Gaillimh

3 1111 40104 5537